Healthy Aging and Immune System

Healthy Aging and Immune System

Editor: Holden Miller

AMERICAN
MEDICAL PUBLISHERS
www.americanmedicalpublishers.com

AMERICAN
MEDICAL PUBLISHERS
www.americanmedicalpublishers.com

Cataloging-in-Publication Data

Healthy aging and immune system / edited by Holden Miller.
p. cm.
Includes bibliographical references and index.
ISBN 979-8-88740-170-6
1. Older people--Diseases--Immunological aspects. 2. Geriatrics--Immunological aspects.
3. Aging. 4. Immunologic diseases--Age factors. 5. Aging. I. Miller, Holden.
RC952.5 .H43 2023
618.97--dc23

American Medical Publishers,
41 Flatbush Avenue,
1st Floor, New York,
NY 11217, USA

ISBN 979-8-88740-170-6 (Hardback)

Contents

Preface

The process of growing older is known as aging. Among humans, it refers to the gradual accumulation of changes in a person's physical, psychological, and social characteristics over time. At the molecular and cellular level, ageing is caused by the accumulation of a range of molecular and cellular damage throughout time. This results in a gradual loss of physical and mental capacity, and an increased risk of disease and, eventually, death. These changes are not linear or continuous, and they are only tangentially related to a person's chronological age. Aging has an impact on both innate and adaptive immunity. Proinflammatory cytokines, such as IL-6 and TNF-and acute-phase reactants, such as C-reactive protein and blood clotting factors, all rise paradoxically as humans' innate immune system ages. The readers would gain knowledge that would broaden their perspective about healthy aging and the immune system through this book. Those in search of information to further their knowledge will be greatly assisted by it.

After months of intensive research and writing, this book is the end result of all who devoted their time and efforts in the initiation and progress of this book. It will surely be a source of reference in enhancing the required knowledge of the new developments in the area. During the course of developing this book, certain measures such as accuracy, authenticity and research focused analytical studies were given preference in order to produce a comprehensive book in the area of study.

This book would not have been possible without the efforts of the authors and the publisher. I extend my sincere thanks to them. Secondly, I express my gratitude to my family and well-wishers. And most importantly, I thank my students for constantly expressing their willingness and curiosity in enhancing their knowledge in the field, which encourages me to take up further research projects for the advancement of the area.

Editor

1

Abnormal Epigenetic Regulation of Immune System during Aging

*Miriam G. Jasiulionis**

Laboratory of Ontogeny and Epigenetics, Pharmacology Department, Universidade Federal de São Paulo, São Paulo, Brazil

Correspondence:
Miriam G. Jasiulionis
mjasiulionis@gmail.com

Epigenetics refers to the study of mechanisms controlling the chromatin structure, which has fundamental role in the regulation of gene expression and genome stability. Epigenetic marks, such as DNA methylation and histone modifications, are established during embryonic development and epigenetic profiles are stably inherited during mitosis, ensuring cell differentiation and fate. Under the effect of intrinsic and extrinsic factors, such as metabolic profile, hormones, nutrition, drugs, smoke, and stress, epigenetic marks are actively modulated. In this sense, the lifestyle may affect significantly the epigenome, and as a result, the gene expression profile and cell function. Epigenetic alterations are a hallmark of aging and diseases, such as cancer. Among biological systems compromised with aging is the decline of immune response. Different regulators of immune response have their promoters and enhancers susceptible to the modulation by epigenetic marks, which is fundamental to the differentiation and function of immune cells. Consistent evidence has showed the regulation of innate immune cells, and T and B lymphocytes by epigenetic mechanisms. Therefore, age-dependent alterations in epigenetic marks may result in the decline of immune function and this might contribute to the increased incidence of diseases in old people. In order to maintain health, we need to better understand how to avoid epigenetic alterations related to immune aging. In this review, the contribution of epigenetic mechanisms to the loss of immune function during aging will be discussed, and the promise of new means of disease prevention and management will be pointed.

Keywords: immune aging, epigenetics, DNA methylation, histones, environment, age-related diseases

EPIGENETICS: HOW THE GENOME TALKS WITH THE ENVIRONMENT

Epigenetics (epi = beyond) refers to the study of the heritable information on the chromatin beyond that given by the DNA sequence. Epigenetic marks, represented by different chemical groups added on both the DNA molecule and histone proteins, play key roles in the control of chromatin structure and function (1, 2). Among the most studied epigenetic mechanisms are DNA methylation

---

Abbreviations: ncRNA, noncoding RNA; 5mC, 5-methylcytosine; DNMT, DNA methyltransferase; SAM, *S*-adenosylmethionine; TET, ten-eleven translocation; 5hmC, 5-hydroxymethylcytosine; 5fC, 5-methylformylcytosine; 5caC, 5-caboxylcytosine; PTM, posttranslational modification; 8-OHdG, 8-hydroxy-2′-deoxy-guanosine; DC, dendritic cell; NK, natural killer; APC, antigen-presenting cell; IFN-γ, interferon-gamma; IL, interleukin; MIP-1α, macrophage inflammatory protein 1-alpha; LPS, lipopolysaccharide; PRR, pattern recognition receptor; DAMP, damage-associated molecular pattern; PAMP, pathogen-associated molecular pattern; TCR, T cell receptor; NFAT, nuclear factor of activated T cells; MHC, major histocompatibility complex; CIITA, class II transactivator; Treg cell, regulatory T cell; TGFβ, transforming growth factor β; RORC, RAR-related orphan receptor C; FOXP3, forkhead box P3; Pax5, paired box 5; AID, activation-induced cytidine deaminase; Ezh2, enhancer of zeste homolog 2; MOZ, monocytic leukemia zinc finger protein; HPC, hematopoietic progenitor cell; TNF-α, tumor necrosis factor-alpha; TLR-2, toll-like receptor 2; CRAT, carnitine *O*-acetyltransferase; F3, coagulation factor III; CRP, C-reactive protein; EWAS, epigenome wide association studies; HSC, hematopoietic stem cell.

and posttranslational histone modifications. The chromatin remodeling, the presence of structural and functional variants of histones, and the regulation by noncoding RNAs are additional epigenetic mechanisms working together with DNA methylation and histone modifications to maintain genome stability and control gene expression.

DNA Methylation

In mammals, each cytosine in the context of a CpG dinucleotide is a potential site for the covalent addition of a methyl group, yielding 5-methylcytosine (5mC) (3). This reaction is catalyzed by DNA methyltransferases (DNMTs)—DNMT1, 3A, and 3B, which transfer the methyl group from *S*-adenosylmethionine (SAM) to the 5-carbon of the cytosine (5mC) (4). SAM, a component of methionine cycle, is considered the universal donor of methyl groups to various biomolecules, including DNA and histones (5). Different components coming from the diet, such as B6 and B12 vitamin, choline, and betaine act as cofactors in reactions taking part in methionine cycle, and the folate cycle is coupled to the methionine cycle, bringing up how cellular nutrient status may modulate epigenetic marks (6). In normal cells, most CpG-rich (CpG islands) gene promoters are unmethylated, making these genes permissive to transcription. Hypermethylated CpG-rich promoters are typically associated with gene silencing, since methylated CpGs can both impair the binding of transcriptional factors and recruit repressive complexes (7, 8). Regions, such as repetitive DNA sequences and transposons, present in high number in our genome, have CpGs heavily methylated in normal cells. The loss of methylation in these regions favors homologous recombination and the expression of undesirable elements, contributing to chromosomal instability (9). The technological advances in genome-wide chromatin profiling have revealed that in fact the role of DNA methylation in gene regulation depends on its position and context. While in promoters it is associated with transcriptional silencing, in other regions it can modulate enhancer activity and splicing (10). The methylation at gene bodies is frequent in ubiquitously expressed genes and correlated with transcriptional activation (11). The tissue-specific DNA methylation seems to occur not at CpG islands, but at regions of lower CpG density about 2 kb distant from CpG islands, named CpG island shores (12). In addition, other non-CpG sites were more recently described as sites for DNA methylation in humans, such as CHG and CHH sites (where H is A, C, or T) (13), but the mechanisms involved in this process are still unknown. The complexity of the covalent modification of DNA has additionally increased with the recent identification of a new family of enzymes known as ten-eleven translocation 1-3 (TET1-3), which are able to oxidize 5mC to 5-hydroxymethylcytosine (5hmC) in a reaction that generates other intermediates (5-methylformylcytosine and 5-carboxylcytosine) (14, 15). These modified bases may be excised by thymine DNA glycosylases (TDG) and, through the base excision repair (BER) process, yield demethylated cytosines (16), which makes this process a mechanism of active DNA demethylation. The DNA can be also actively demethylated by the deamination of 5mC and 5hmC by the activation-induced deaminase/apolipoprotein B editing complex enzymes, followed by BER/TDG activity (17). Alternatively, 5hmC can be passively demethylated during DNA replication, since it is not recognized by DNMT1, yielding in this position non-methylated cytosine in the newly synthesized DNA strand.

Histone Modifications

In the nucleosomes, not only the DNA molecule but also histone proteins carry chemical modifications, which are fundamental for chromatin-dependent gene regulation (18). Several post-translational histone modifications (PTMs) regulate the chromatin structure, by affecting inter-nucleosomal interactions, and recruit proteins and complexes that influence not only the gene transcription but also mediate processes, such as DNA replication, DNA repair, alternative splicing, and recombination (19). A large number of proteins acting as writers, erasers, and readers have been described as components of histone modifier machinery, targeting all core histones H2A, H2B, H3, and H4, and the linker H1 histone, which have their amino acids subjected to covalent modifications mainly in the *N*-terminal tails. Among these modifications are acetylation, phosphorylation, methylation, ubiquitylation, sumoylation, and ADP ribosylation (19). By decreasing the positive charge of histones, acetylation and phosphorylation weaken interactions between histones and DNA, facilitating transcription machinery to access the DNA. Histone methylation occurs mainly on lysines and arginines, which can be, respectively, mono-, di- or trimethylated, and mono- and dimethylated, resulting in a high level of complexity regarding their effects. For example, high levels of trimethylated H3K4, H3K36, and H3K79 are associated with actively transcribed chromatin, while methylated H3K9, H3K27, and H4K20 are associated with transcriptionally inactive chromatin (20). The covalent attachment of the large ubiquitin molecule changes the nucleosome conformation, affecting both intra-nucleosomal interactions and interactions with effector proteins. Sumoylation involves the addition of small ubitiquin-like molecules to histones, and has been associated with repressive functions. Histone mono- and poly-ADP ribosylation has been correlated with a relaxed chromatin state. The number of possible histone modifications has increased with the continuous identification of novel histone PTMs, such as lysine propionylation (21, 22), butyrylation (21), crotonylation (23), succinylation, and malonylation (24), coupling cell metabolism with chromatin structure and function. It is important to keep in mind that a single histone mark is not responsible for the final effect on chromatin, but rather the combination of all marks in a chromatin region defines the biological outcome (25, 26). Besides that, there is interplay of DNA methylation, histone modifications, and nucleosome positioning, and the outcome is a result of the sum of these interactions.

The Plasticity of the Epigenetic Marks

Although presenting the same genome, each cell type in the same individual has a specific group of epigenetic marks, named epigenome. Epigenetic marks are established during embryonic development and transmitted through mitosis, stabilizing gene expression programs, and defining cell-type identities and function (27). In addition to their role in cell differentiation, these marks are fundamental to X chromosome inactivation in females and genomic imprinting during development (28, 29). Although being relatively stable over time, epigenetic marks can change dynamically in response to cellular conditions and environmental cues (2, 30, 31). Recent studies have shown that the methylation patterns determined by the binding of factors on DNA motifs are less responsive to environment within the lifetime of an individual, and that these patterns would persist across generations (32, 33). However, other DNA regions would have their epigenetic marks more susceptible to internal and external environment, such as stress, smoke, drugs, hormones, circadian rhythms, and metabolic variations caused by diet. In this way, the environment can modulate the epigenotype, and consequently the phenotype, being decisive to direct to health or disease states. In fact, many studies have shown the relation between epigenetic alterations and a wide variety of diseases, including aging-related diseases (34–36).

CHANGES IN EPIGENETIC MARKS DURING AGING

During the aging of an organism, there is a gradual decline of normal physiological functions. In humans, these include decreased immune function, chronic inflammation, sarcopenia, and most importantly increased susceptibility to diseases, such as cancer, cardiovascular disorders, and metabolic and neurodegenerative diseases. Although systemic, these phenotypes are a result of alterations in different cellular processes, such as DNA damage response, mitochondrial and proteasome function, and cell death regulation (37–40). At the molecular level, transcriptional dysregulation is observed with aging, resulting in gene expression changes (41, 42). Epigenetic alterations are important contributors to these changes in the aged transcriptome, and are known as "epigenetic drift" (43–45).

DNA Methylation

Regarding DNA methylation, a progressive global hypomethylation occurs invariably with advanced age (46). Repetitive DNA sequences normally silenced by epigenetic marks become expressed, being at least partly responsible for the well-characterized loss of heterochromatin observed during aging (47, 48). An age-dependent hypomethylation of specific gene promoters, such as *IL17RC*, occurs and induces their transcription (49). At the same time, some gene promoters become hypermethylated and abnormally silenced (50–52). Regarding 5hmC, it was shown that although the global level of 5hmC in the brain increases with aging both in mice (53) and humans (54), it decreases in other tissues, such as blood (55).

Besides the epigenetic drift, which is stochastic non-site-specific changes in DNA methylation that contributes to variability during aging, DNA methylation signatures in specific CpGs, both tissue-specific and present in several tissue types, were identified as associated with chronological age (56). Although age-related DNA methylation alterations are more frequent in CpG islands, tissue-specific changes occur in other genomic regions (57). In a comprehensive study of DNA methylation, Yuan and colleagues (58) showed that besides hypermethylated CpG islands, a great number of age-related differentially methylated regions fell into open sea (regions of megabase extension characterized by low CG content) or shore/shelf regions, which were found hypomethylated with age. These authors have also identified large age-associated hypomethylated blocks, similar to those described associated with cancer (59). Based on the genome-wide methylation profile of whole blood from 656 individuals spanning a wide age range, a quantitative model was built to determine the rate at which an individual's methylome ages, and was shown to represent a strong and reproducible mean to discriminate relevant factors in aging (60).

Histone Modifications

The global DNA hypomethylation observed during aging was shown to be associated with changes in histone modification patterns (61, 62). Changes in the activity, function, and abundance of enzymes of the epigenetic machinery are present with aging (63, 64). Genes identified as hypermethylated in blood cells during aging were associated with the presence of bivalent chromatin domains in embryonic stem cells and with the repressive histone marks H3K27me3 and H3K9me3 in differentiated cells (65–67). A global loss of histones, as well as an imbalance of activating and repressive histone marks, occurs with age (68, 69). For example, a diminished content of acetylated H3K9 (70) and trimethylated H3K27 (71) was described in aged cells. Reduced levels of H3K9me3, which can be a result of the downregulation of SUV39H1/2 (72), were found with age in human and murine tissues and cells and seem to contribute to the loss of heterochromatin (72, 73). An age-decrease in the expression of HP1 (74) and DNMTs (75) could favor DNA demethylation in the heterochromatin. Another alteration that could contribute to a more opened chromatin state is the increased level of H4K16Ac with replicative age, as described in human fibroblasts in culture (76). H4K16 is among the targets of the NAD^+-dependent histone deacetylase SIRT1, which is associated with aging extent and genome maintenance in different organisms (77).

While the levels of the canonical histones decrease during aging, alterations in the replication-independent incorporation of histone variants occur during aging. The replication-independent histone variant H3.3 becomes more abundant with age in general, not just in non-replicating cells, such as neurons (78). Again, this could favor a chromatin state more accessible to the transcription machinery. Another replication-independent histone variant that seems to be linked to aging is the H2A.Z, since H2A.Z knockdown fibroblasts were shown to develop premature senescence (79). The H2A variant macroH2A is characteristic of senescence-associated heterochromatin foci, heterochromatin regions over proliferation-promoting genes in senescent cells (80). An age-dependent increase in the macroH2A level was described both during replicative senescence in cultured human fibroblasts and in many tissues of aged mammals (81).

Effects of the Environmental and Lifestyle Factors on Epigenetic Changes and Aging

A classical study by Esteller's group (82) showed significant differences in epigenetic marks in old monozygotic twin pairs compared to very young twin pairs, which presented these marks indistinguishable. More interestingly, those old twin pairs that had spent less of their lifetime together and/or had a more different natural health-medical history were those presenting the greatest differences in epigenetic marks. Studies with human population have shown that genetic factors cause no more than 20–30% of the differences observed in the lifespan of identical twins, the epigenetic drift being the main responsible for variation during the lifetime (83, 84). These and other studies (85–88) illustrate how epigenetic marks change with aging and are under the effect of environment. As a whole, these alterations change the chromatin accessibility, resulting in abnormal gene transcription and genomic instability, and have been proposed to be key regulators of the aging process, contributors to the development of age-related diseases and even predictors of the chronological age (52, 89–93). Age-related changes in multiple CpG sites across the genome were shown to accurately predict the biological age of an individual. This epigenetic clock has been shown a potential biomarker of aging in humans and associated with several aging-related disease phenotypes (60, 90, 94, 95). Epigenetic age assessed in blood was able to predict, independently of chronological age, all-cause mortality in different cohorts, including different racial/ethnic groups (93, 95–97).

It is important to emphasize that the epigenome acts as a molecular interface between the genome and the environment. In this way, the lifestyle, including diet habits, exercises, life stressors, smoke, substance abuse, chemical exposition, among others, could alter the epigenetic landscape, affecting the chromatin structure and function, and, consequently, favoring the development of aging-related disease phenotypes. Exercise and nutritional habits remodel epigenetic marks in human skeletal muscle and adipose tissue (98–100). The effect of exercise on the improved cardiorespiratory fitness and running performance, as well as on the decreased low-density lipoprotein levels, was accompanied by a widespread demethylation of CpG islands, opposed of the methylation changes observed during aging (101, 102). Several studies have demonstrated the adverse effect of smoke associated with changes in epigenetic marks. Prenatal smoke exposure affects DNA methylation of blood cells from children of smoking mothers (103). Epigenetic alterations caused by chronic cigarette smoke sensitize bronchial epithelial cells to malignant transformation (104). Tobacco smoking may induce DNA methylation alterations in cell types of both the innate and adaptive immune system (105). Offspring DNA methylation alterations were associated with maternal alcohol consumption (106). The turnover of histones and histone variants was shown to be affected by the alcohol exposure in rats (107). Many of these effects of the environment on aging involve oxidative stress, both in humans and animal models. Although severe acute or chronic stress exposure accelerates aging by favoring error accumulation due to exhausting defense mechanisms, moderate stress has shown to delay aging process by activating defense mechanisms to prevent and/or eliminate errors (108). In the last years, several studies have demonstrated the relation between cellular stress and epigenetic alterations (104, 109–114). Reactive oxygen species (ROS) lead to oxidized DNA lesions that can contribute to DNA methylation alterations. One of the major DNA oxidative damage products is 8-hydroxy-2′-deoxy-guanosine that impairs binding of DNMTs and methyl-CpG binding proteins to DNA (115). In addition, ROS may interfere with TET-mediated DNA demethylation (116). SAM availability can also be decreased by the depletion of glutathione (GSH) because of redox status, inhibiting all methylation reactions (117). Sirtuins play important role in response to a variety of stresses, such as oxidative or genotoxic stress and are crucial for cell metabolism. ROS can both induce DNA damage and SIRT1 relocation to these damage sites, for where SIRT1 recruits other epigenetic machinery components, such as DNMTs and polycomb proteins in order to silence these regions. O'Hagan and coworkers (110, 112) showed that this process could result in stable aberrant epigenetic and gene transcription changes, similarly to alterations observed in cancer. In murine embryonic mesenchymal fibroblasts, increased levels of hydrogen peroxide induce SIRT1 to relocate from repressed DNA sequences to DNA breaks to promote repair, resulting in transcriptional changes that parallel those in the aging mouse brain (118). By responding to environmental stress, sirtuins promote cell survival and, as a result, increase replicative and chronological lifespan. Although not clearly established in mammals, the association of sirtuins with aging and lifespan is suggested by the overexpression of SIRT1 in murine tissues during caloric restriction (CR) (119), the requirement of Sirt1 to the increased physical activity and extended lifespan during caloric restriction (120), and the improved health and survival of mice submitted to a high-calorie diet after resveratrol treatment, which activates Sirt1 (121). Several studies in different model organisms show the role of sirtuins in lifespan extension by CR (122–125), and evidences indicate that epigenetic mechanisms have crucial roles in this process (126, 127). In this context, new and known compounds have been tested as "CR mimetics," including sirtuin-activating compounds, such as resveratrol (128). Compounds inhibiting histone acetylation, such as spermidine, also extend lifespan (129).

As mentioned before, ROS may modify the TET-mediated DNA demethylation (116). Both the increase in endogenous antioxidants and caloric restriction were shown to impair the increase in 5hmC levels in murine aged brains (130). The demethylase activity of TET enzymes can be stimulated by nutrients, such as ascorbic acid (131, 132). Since the activity of many epigenetic enzymes depend on intracellular levels of essential metabolites (methionine, iron, ketoglutarate, NAD^+, acetyl-CoA, SAM), the cellular metabolism controls epigenetic modifications and may regulate longevity (133, 134).

In another aspect, studies in human cohorts have shown that life stressors, in special during early development, can induce lasting epigenome alterations (135–139). Stress and glucocorticoids may induce long-lasting changes in DNA methylation both at the genome-wide level and within selective gene loci, as observed both in humans and rodent models (140–142).

EPIGENETIC REGULATION OF THE IMMUNE SYSTEM

An important characteristic of the immune system is its adaptive capacity to recognize self from non-self to protect the organism in response to environmental signals of different types and duration, such as potentially pathogenic agents and substances. Several immune cell populations act against potentially hazard environment by both innate and adaptive mechanisms, and their functions depend on highly controlled regulation of hematopoietic cell differentiation. Increasing number of studies have demonstrated the crucial role of epigenetic mechanisms in the development and differentiation of immune system, as well as in related pathologies (143–145). With age, the immunocompetence becomes compromised and this has been linked to the repression of immune cell differentiation genes along with the activation of autoimmunity genes because of DNA methylation alterations (49, 146–148).

Innate Immune Cells

The innate immune system, consisting of macrophages, neutrophils, dendritic cells (DCs), and natural killer (NK) cells, is the first response to pathogenic agents. Macrophages and DCs are professional antigen-presenting cells (APCs) able to capture antigens for processing and presentation to lymphocytes. When activated, resident macrophages can act directly by destroying their targets or indirectly *via* initiating an acute inflammatory response by producing cytokines, chemoattractants, and inflammatory mediators, and recruiting neutrophils, monocytes, and DCs (149). Activated macrophages release different factors in response to the extracellular environment, being able to acquire functionally distinct phenotypes, classic M1 and alternative M2. Activated M1 macrophages are induced by the cytokine interferon-gamma (IFN-γ) and bacterial products and have a pro-inflammatory profile, playing an important role in host defense. Differently, M2 macrophages are induced by interleukin-4 and -10 (IL-4 and IL-10) and helminthic products and have an anti-inflammatory profile, promoting tissue repair. Since mature cells of the immune system have to rapidly respond to pathogens, the contribution of epigenetic mechanisms to the regulation of genes involved in these responses has been substantially described. In this context, epigenetic mechanisms were shown to be involved in the modulation of macrophage polarization, mainly by histone marks present in enhancers of specific genes (150). The first study showing the epigenetic regulation of inflammation was that by Saccani and Natoli (151). They demonstrated the induction of inflammatory cytokines, such as IL-8 and macrophage inflammatory protein 1-alpha (MIP-1α), by the loss of H3K9 methylation at the promoter regions after exposing cultured human monocyte-derived DCs to bacterial endotoxin lipopolysaccharide (LPS). Innate immune cells have a degree of specificity by presenting pattern recognition receptors (PRRs) to recognize damage- or pathogen-associated molecular patterns in non-infectious substances or microbes, respectively (152). Recent evidences indicate that, different from previously believed, cells of innate immune system may keep a memory of past stimulations, named "trained immunity," changing the response upon new stimuli and becoming able to respond to a larger number of microbes than the initial agent (153, 154). This immunological memory involves changes in transcriptional programs by reprogramming epigenetic marks. For example, metabolic changes in monocytes activated by β-glucan from *Candida* are associated with increased levels of the active histone marks, H3K4 trimethylation, and H3K27 acetylation, leading to increased production of IL-6 and TNF cytokines, inflammation, and "trained immunity" (155). Macrophages restimulated with LPS induce an attenuated inflammatory response, although maintaining an intact antimicrobial response. Foster and colleagues (156) showed that genes involved in LPS-tolerance lose the active histone marks H3K4me3 and H4Ac in their promoters during restimulation with LPS, while non-tolerizeable genes maintain these active marks after a secondary challenge with LPS, correlated with a permissive gene transcription. Epigenetic mechanisms also regulate the differentiation of human monocytes into DCs under specific stimuli. For example, the observed increased expression of CD209 during differentiation was shown to be a result of the acquisition of H3K9Ac and loss of H3K9me3, H4K20me3, and DNA methylation in its promoter (157).

T Lymphocytes

The age-dependent deterioration of the immune system, named immunesenescence, is accompanied by alterations in epigenetic marks. Kuwahara and colleagues (158) showed that CD4 T-cell senescence and cytokine homeostasis is controlled by the maintenance of histone acetylation on the *Bach2* locus promoted by the binding of menin. In addition, the increased genomic instability in the thymus with age is associated with a loss of heterochromatin marks, including H3K9me3 with corresponding reduction in SUV39H1 expression (159). The senescence seems to be also activated by DNA hypomethylation since the hypomethylation is observed in senescing but not in immortalized cells (160), and the DNA methylation inhibition leads immortal cells to cell arrest (161).

Cells from the innate immune system present antigens to both B and T lymphocytes, activating them to proliferate and differentiate into effector cells. APCs activate T cell receptor and costimulatory molecules of naïve T cells, initiating T cell differentiation by the activation of the nuclear factor of activated T cells and production of interleukin-2 (IL-2). IL-2 orchestrates the molecular switch of transcriptional programs of immune-responsive genes in response to T cell activation. Naïve and resting CD4$^+$ T cells do not express IL-2, but this cytokine is expressed in T cells under antigen stimulation. Murayama and colleagues (162) showed that demethylation of a single specific CpG site in an enhancer region is a prerequisite for IL-2 transcription and, more interestingly, that this epigenetic change constitutes a memory that CD4$^+$ T cells encountered the antigen.

Peptide antigens are presented by APCs to T cells in the context of the major histocompatibility complex (MHC) molecules. Cytotoxic T cells, expressing CD8, recognize antigens presented by normal cells in the context of MHC class I molecules, being able to directly destroy the infected cells. Activated CD8$^+$ T cells have increased levels of H3Ac at the *IFN-γ* promoter and enhancer, modification that is maintained through memory CD8$^+$ T cells, and permits a quicker and stronger cytotoxic response to additional antigen stimulation (163). MHC class II are the MHC molecules involved in the antigen presentation to CD4$^+$ helper T cells. The class II transactivator (CIITA) is a key factor controlling the expression of MHC-II, and both CIITA expression and CIITA-dependent MHC-II expression are epigenetically regulated (164). Analysis of chromatin accessibility in PBMCs identified memory CD8+ T cells as the subpopulation with the most profound chromatin remodeling with aging (165, 166).

After antigen recognition, depending on cytokine environment, naïve T lymphocytes differentiate into effector T "helper" (Th1, Th2, and Th17) or regulatory (Treg) CD4+ T cells, and coordinate specific immune responses by producing distinct sets of cytokines (167). The differentiation toward a Th1 profile is induced by IFN-γ, IL-12, or IL-15, whereas differentiation toward the Th2 profile—by IL-4, IL-10, or IL-13; both pathways involve the regulated expression of multiple effector genes. Transforming growth factor beta and IL-6 are responsible for inducing naïve T cell differentiation into Th17 cells. The CD4+ T cells differentiation into these different profiles is tightly regulated to assure specific cytokine signatures and changes in the epigenetic marks are fundamental to complete this process. The *IFNG* promoter, hypermethylated in human naïve T cells, becomes demethylated during the differentiation into Th1 profile (168). Specific histone marks were identified across the *IFNG* locus, where H4Ac and H3K4me3 are present in Th1 cells and H3K27me2 and H3K27me3 in Th2 cells (169). Naïve and Th1 cells present *IL-4* promoter highly methylated, while Th2 cells have the intron 2 of *IL-4* partly demethylated (170). Th17 cells are characterized by the expression of IL-17 cytokine and RAR-related orphan receptor C (RORC) transcription factor. The demethylation of both *IL-17A* and *RORC* loci correlates with gene expression in human Th17 cells (171), and the active histone marks H3Ac and H3K4me3 were found in the *IL-17* locus (172). The demethylation of *Foxp3* locus, as well the hyperacetylation of histones, was shown to be important to maintain the stable expression of forkhead box P3 (FOXP3) and stabilize the regulatory phenotype in Treg cells (173, 174).

B Lymphocytes

After binding to an antigen and be induced by T helper cells, B cells differentiate into antibody-secreting plasma cells. Antibodies bind to the specific antigen, leading to a better recognition and destruction of the pathogen (such as bacteria, virus, and tumor cells) by activating complement and/or interacting with lytic cells. During B cell differentiation, lineage-specific genes are expressed, whereas genes related to multipotent progenitors and alternative lineages are repressed. Complex epigenetic regulatory mechanisms coordinate B cell differentiation and function, including monoallelic V(D)J rearrangement and antibody diversity (175–178). A key transcriptional factor involved in B cell commitment is paired box 5 (Pax5) that, besides having its expression regulated by epigenetic mechanisms (179, 180), recruits chromatin-modifying proteins to regulate the expression of its targets. For example, *CD79a* gene promoter, hypermethylated in the progenitor stage, becomes demethylated during early stages of B cell differentiation, followed by the action of histone acetyltransferases recruited by Pax5, allowing gene expression (181). Pax5 can also interact with chromatin-modifying enzymes to repress genes specific for other lineages (182). V(D)J rearrangement and antibody diversity are necessary for the production of effective antibodies and require the activation-induced cytidine deaminase (AID), expressed by B cells at specific stages of differentiation. In naïve B cells, *AID* gene promoter is hypermethylated and the gene is not expressed. Upon B cells activation, *AID* gene becomes demethylated and acquires increased levels of the active histone mark H3Ac (183). The acquisition of this histone mark in active promoters and distal enhancers is also crucial for gene expression changes occurring during the differentiation of B cells to plasma cells (184). Blimp-1, a transcriptional repressor that maintains plasma cell identity, has its expression epigenetically induced and epigenetically suppresses the expression of mature B cell genes by recruiting histone modifiers (185, 186). After V(D)J rearrangement and antibody diversity processes, B cells can differentiate into memory B cells, which acquire additional epigenetic marks beyond those acquired during B cell activation (187). Different epigenetic modifications, as well as epigenetic enzymes, such as enhancer of zeste homolog 2 (188), histone acetyltransferase monocytic leukemia zinc finger protein (189), and DNMT3a (190), are observed in resting and activated B cells, and indicate that the memory B cell epigenome could favor a faster and more efficient activation than that of naïve cells.

CONTRIBUTION OF EPIGENETIC ALTERATIONS TO IMMUNE AGING

Age-associated defects are observed in all cells from the immune system, affecting their activation and cytokines production.

Innate Immune Cells

Regarding the innate immune system, many immune responses decrease during aging, but at the same time hyperreactivity of some responses are also observed (191). Epigenetic alterations seem to affect the monocyte differentiation with age, since older hematopoietic progenitor cells (HPCs) present hypomethylation of differentiation-related genes compared to progenitor cells from umbilical cord blood (192). It could be related to the reduced pluripotency and decreased potential of differentiation of HPCs from older donors (193). At the same time, older HPCs presented *de novo* methylation of a subset of genes associated with the Polycomb repressive complex that could contribute to the reduced phenotypic plasticity of aged stem cells (192). Indeed, epigenetic dysfunction could be a precursor to hematologic disease in elderly individuals (194). In macrophages, epigenetic mechanisms contribute to the decreased expression of MHC-II observed with age (195). Although the number of NK cells increases in older individuals, their cytotoxic activity decrease, and DNA methylation regulation of IFN-γ and IL-2 seems to contribute to this defected function of NK cells (196). Aging is well characterized by an imbalance between inflammatory and anti-inflammatory responses, where increased levels of inflammatory mediators, such as IL-6 and tumor necrosis factor-alpha (TNF-α), are observed even in the absence of acute infection or other physiologic stress (process known as "inflammaging") (197). TNF-α has its expression increased during aging linked to its promoter demethylation (198). This epigenetic alteration contributes to the increased levels of TNF-α and also IL-1α (199, 200), which initiate the low-grade inflammation associated with resting neutrophils from aged donors. A major cause of worldwide morbidity in the elderly is the age-associated inflammatory lung disease (201). In this context, promoter hypomethylation of inflammatory genes, such as toll-like receptor 2, carnitine *O*-acetyltransferase, and coagulation factor III, were associated with decreased lung function (202). Zinc is a micronutrient crucial for the development and function of immune system, and its deficiency, frequently observed during aging, contributes to a wide range of immune defects (203), including an enhanced inflammatory response by inducing *IL-6* promoter demethylation (204). Using the C-reactive protein (CRP) as an inflammatory biomarker, Ligthart and coworkers (205) performed a meta-analysis of epigenome wide association studies of DNA methylation on chronic low-grade inflammation. In this study, the authors demonstrated that several inflammation-related CpG sites were associated with the expression of nearby genes, and that many of these CpGs presented association with cardiometabolic phenotypes and incident coronary heart disease. Among these genes is *AIM2*, important in innate immune response since it takes part of host defense mechanisms against bacterial and viral pathogens, and that was found hypermethylated and expressed at low levels in samples with low levels of CRP.

T Lymphocytes

The involution of thymic structure and function, characterized by a reduced number and functional defects of thymic naïve T cells, is other process contributing to the immune aging (206). By analyzing the methylome of $CD4^+$ T cells from newborn and centenarian individuals, Heyn and coworkers (207) showed these immune cells present the same DNA methylation changes that are observed in other tissues during aging, a global DNA hypomethylation and a higher variability of DNA methylation. Later, by an integrated analysis of transcriptome, methylome, and miRNAome in the same $CD4^+$ T cells, Zhao and colleagues (148) found a potential relationship between gene transcription and DNA methylation for age- or immune-related genes, indicating the involvement of DNA methylation in the transcription regulation related to the development and functions of T cells in aging. Mice with a heterozygous *Dnmt1* null mutation have hypomethylated DNA and showed to be phenotypically normal, but presented immune senescence and developed early autoimmunity compared with normal mice of the same age (208). By analyzing naïve $CD4^+$ T cells from 74 healthy 19- to 66-year-old individuals, Dozmorov and colleagues (209) identified sites hypomethylated with age presenting T cell-specific enrichment in active enhancers marked with H3K27Ac and H3K4me1, suggesting a progressive age-associated shift in T-cell epigenomes toward pro-inflammatory and T cell activating phenotype that could contribute to increased autoimmunity with age. It was also shown that aged individuals, who have higher levels of autoantibodies, have T cells presenting demethylation and overexpression in the same genes demethylated and overexpressed in T cells from lupus patients (146). The progressive loss of the costimulatory molecule CD28 in $CD4^+$ T lymphocytes during aging is associated with impaired immune response. Recently, a unique DNA methylation landscape was described in $CD28^{null}$ T cells, leading to the expression of inflammasome-related genes (210). Other recent study found two CpG sites present in the promoter region of *KLF14*, involved in $CD4^+$ T cell differentiation *via* suppression of FOXP3, that exhibit stable methylation early in life and a rapid increase late in life in peripheral whole blood, monocytes, and isolated $CD4^+$ T cells (211). Dysfunctional Treg cells have been considered to be contributors to immune senescence and increased susceptibility to age-associated diseases by suppressing T cell responses. Garg and colleagues (212) showed that the high number of Treg cells observed in aged mice is associated with hypomethylation of the upstream *FoxP3* enhancer, resulting in its increased expression. They also demonstrated that Treg cells from aged mice release more IL-10, are more efficient in downregulating the costimulatory molecule CD86 on DCs, and modulate the extracellular redox environment, suppressing T cells proliferation.

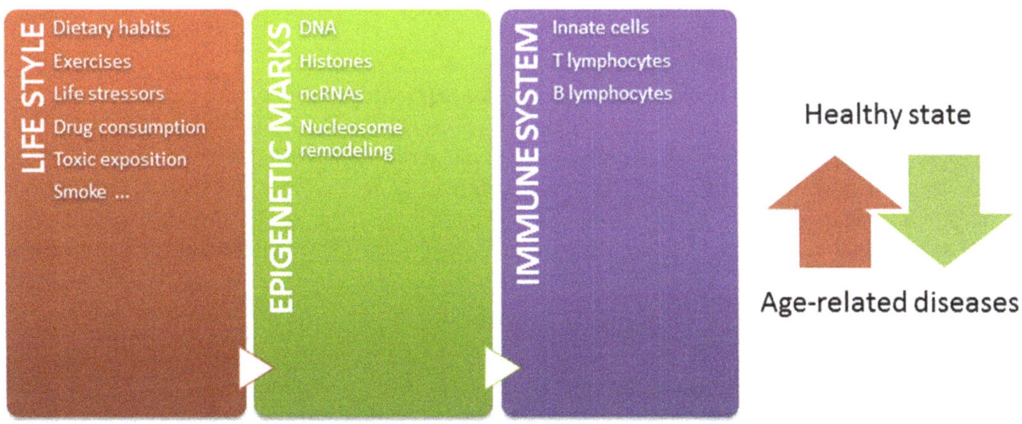

FIGURE 1 | The epigenetic landscape, modulated by intrinsic and extrinsic factors, regulates immune system and contributes to define a healthy or pathological state. Our life style, including nutritional habit, exercises, life stressor, drugs, toxics exposition, and smoke, dynamically sculpts our epigenome along lifetime. The immune system is one of the systems in which functions are importantly regulated by epigenetic mechanisms. In this way, the accumulation of abnormal epigenetic marks in immune cells might contribute to the development of age-related diseases.

Immune senescence is also characterized by a loss of naïve and central memory cells and an expansion of effector memory cells within the $CD8^+$ T cell compartment. A shift toward more differentiated state of chromatin openness was observed in naïve and central memory cells from older individuals, as well a loss of chromatin accessibility at gene promoters mediated in part by the loss of nuclear respiratory factor 1 (NRF1) binding in aged naïve cells (213). By analyzing PBMCs methylation data set in an Italian population, Horvath and colleagues (214) showed that the centenarians are younger than expected based on their chronological age. McEwen and colleagues (215), by examining one of the highest old-age life expectancies populations from Costa Rica (Nicoyans), found this population to possess a significant higher abundance of predicted $CD8^+$ T naïve cells and a lower abundance of estimated $CD8^+$ T memory cells compared with non-Nicoyans, suggesting a younger immune cell profile. In addition, they showed a lower variability in the DNA methylation in Nicoyans compared with non-Nicoyans as an epigenetic characteristic of the longevity in this population.

B Lymphocytes

Considering the role of epigenetic mechanisms in B cell differentiation and function, age-associated epigenetic changes could be the responsible for the decline of humoral immunity in elderly individuals. Loss of function of B cells and their progenitors, reduction in the immunoglobulin diversity and affinity, and shifts in the proportion of naïve and antigen-experienced peripheral B cells subpopulation are characteristics of immune aging (216, 217). Hematopoietic stem cells (HSCs) lose their capacity to differentiate with age, and epigenetic alterations are important contributors to this change. Aged mice present HSCs with an aberrant gene expression profile because of epigenetic deregulation (218). Defects on both B-lineage commitment and transit through early development stage are observed during aging (219).

CONCLUSION AND PERSPECTIVES

Considerable progress has been made in understanding epigenetic alterations involved in aging over the recent years. Most of recent knowledge about epigenetics and aging is almost lack regarding immune aging. Many gaps and questions are still open and should be deeply investigated in this area. However, there are also important challenges and limitations in this study. For example, several analyses in this field use samples contained mixed cell types, instead isolated cells, which may bring confusion in the data interpretation. The dynamic nature of the immune system *per se* becomes challenging to study plastic molecular alterations involved in immune responses. It remains to be determined which epigenetic changes are causally related to aging process, and how they cause immune aging. Future studies are needed to determine the overlapping epigenetic signatures between immune aging and age-related immune diseases.

Independently of these challenges, and taking into account that: (1) epigenetic mechanisms modulate chromatin states, defining gene expression profiles, (2) epigenetic mechanisms play crucial roles in the development and function of immune system, (3) a tightly regulated functioning of immune system is necessary to maintain a healthy state, (4) the environment modifies epigenetic marks throughout lifetime, and (5) epigenetic marks are potentially reversible, the knowledge about how the environment modulates the immune system by epigenetic mechanisms contributing to age-related diseases may lead to the design of novel strategies for prevention and therapeutics. Since some age-related epigenetic alterations are similar across a range of tissues (52, 220), these alterations could be also potentially used as biomarkers for aging-related disease phenotypes in biological samples, such as blood or saliva. But most importantly, considering that both intrinsic and external factors modify epigenetic marks throughout life, it is important to have in mind that healthier lifestyle may be still the most effective way to prevent diseases later in life (**Figure 1**) (221). In conclusion, huge efforts should be undertaken to better understand the relation among epigenetics, immune aging and age-related diseases, in order to define interventions in the lifestyle able to modulate our epigenome for a healthy aging.

AUTHOR CONTRIBUTIONS

The author confirms being the sole contributor of this work and approved it for publication.

FUNDING

This work was supported by the Fundação de Amparo à Pesquisa do Estado de São Paulo (FAPESP, grant 2014/13663-0) and the Conselho Nacional de Desenvolvimento Científico e Tecnológico (CNPq, grant 400036/2016-9).

REFERENCES

1. Putiri EL, Robertson KD. Epigenetic mechanisms and genome stability. *Clin Epigenetics* (2011) 2(2):299–314. doi:10.1007/s13148-010-0017-z
2. Jaenisch R, Bird A. Epigenetic regulation of gene expression: how the genome integrates intrinsic and environmental signals. *Nat Genet* (2003) 33:245–54. doi:10.1038/ng1089
3. Bestor TH. DNA methylation: evolution of a bacterial immune function into a regulator of gene expression and genome structure in higher eukaryotes. *Philos Trans R Soc Lond B Biol Sci* (1990) 326:179–87. doi:10.1098/rstb.1990.0002
4. Goll MG, Bestor TH. Eukaryotic cytosine methyltransferases. *Annu Rev Biochem* (2005) 74:481–514. doi:10.1146/annurev.biochem.74.010904.153721
5. Struck AW, Thompson ML, Wong LS, Micklefield J. S-adenosyl-methionine-dependent methyltransferases: highly versatile enzymes in biocatalysis, biosynthesis and other biotechnological applications. *Chembiochem* (2012) 13:2642–55. doi:10.1002/cbic.201200556
6. Anderson OS, Sant KE, Dolinoy DC. Nutrition and epigenetics: an interplay of dietary methyl donors, one-carbon metabolism, and DNA methylation. *J Nutr Biochem* (2012) 23(8):853–9. doi:10.1016/j.jnutbio.2012.03.003

7. Bird A, Wolffe AP. Methylation-induced repression – belts, braces, and chromatin. *Cell* (1999) 99:451–4. doi:10.1016/S0092-8674(00)81532-9
8. Jones PA, Takai D. The role of DNA methylation in mammalian epigenetics. *Science* (2001) 293:1068–70. doi:10.1126/science.1063852
9. Jones PA, Gonzalgo ML. Altered DNA methylation and genome instability: a new pathway to cancer? *Proc Natl Acad Sci U S A* (1997) 94(6):2103–5. doi:10.1073/pnas.94.6.2103
10. Jones PA. Functions of DNA methylation: islands, start sites, gene bodies and beyond. *Nat Rev Genet* (2012) 13(7):484–92. doi:10.1038/nrg3230
11. Lee SM, Choi WY, Lee J. The regulatory mechanisms of intragenic DNA methylation. *Epigenomics* (2015) 7(4):527–31. doi:10.2217/epi.15.38
12. Doi A, Park IH, Wen B, Murakami P, Aryee MJ, Irizarry R, et al. Differential methylation of tissue- and cancer-specific CpG island shores distinguishes human induced pluripotent stem cells, embryonic stem cells and fibroblasts. *Nat Genet* (2009) 41:1350–3. doi:10.1038/ng.471
13. Laurent L, Wong E, Li G, Huynh T, Tsirigos A, Ong CT, et al. Dynamic changes in the human methylome during differentiation. *Genome Res* (2010) 20:320–31. doi:10.1101/gr.101907.109
14. Tahiliani M, Koh KP, Shen Y, Pastor WA, Bandukwala H, Brudno Y, et al. Conversion of 5-methylcytosine to 5-hydroxymethylcytosine in mammalian DNA by MLL partner TET1. *Science* (2009) 324(5929):930–5. doi:10.1126/science.1170116
15. Ito S, D'Alessio AC, Taranova OV, Hong K, Sowers LC, Zhang Y. Role of Tet proteins in 5mC to 5hmC conversion, ES-cell self-renewal and inner cell mass specification. *Nature* (2010) 466(7310):1129–33. doi:10.1038/nature09303
16. He YF, Li BZ, Li Z, Liu P, Wang Y, Tang Q, et al. Tet-mediated formation of 5-carboxylcytosine and its excision by TDG in mammalian DNA. *Science* (2011) 333(6047):1303–7. doi:10.1126/science.1210944
17. Delatte B, Deplus R, Fuks F. Playing TETris with DNA modifications. *EMBO J* (2014) 33:1198–211. doi:10.15252/embj.201488290
18. Allis CD, Jenuwein T. The molecular hallmarks of epigenetic control. *Nat Rev Genet* (2016) 17:487–500. doi:10.1038/nrg.2016.59
19. Bannister AJ, Kouzarides T. Regulation of chromatin by histone modifications. *Cell Res* (2011) 21:381–95. doi:10.1038/cr.2011.22
20. Li B, Carey M, Workman JL. The role of chromatin during transcription. *Cell* (2007) 128:707–19. doi:10.1016/j.cell.2007.01.015
21. Chen Y, Sprung R, Tang Y, Ball H, Sangras B, Kim SC, et al. Lysine propionylation and butyrylation are novel post-translational modifications in histones. *Mol Cell Proteomics* (2007) 6:812–9. doi:10.1074/mcp.M700021-MCP200
22. Kebede AF, Nieborak A, Sharidian LZ, Gras SL, Richter F, Gómez DA, et al. Histone propionylation is a mark of active chromatin. *Nat Struct Mol Biol* (2017) 24(12):1048–56. doi:10.1038/nsmb.3490
23. Tan M, Luo H, Lee S, Jin F, Yang JS, Montellier E, et al. Identification of 67 histone marks and histone lysine crotonylation as a new type of histone modification. *Cell* (2011) 146:1016–28. doi:10.1016/j.cell.2011.08.008
24. Xie Z, Dai J, Dai L, Tan M, Cheng Z, Wu Y, et al. Lysine succinylation and lysine malonylation in histones. *Mol Cell Proteomics* (2012) 11:100–7. doi:10.1074/mcp.M111.015875
25. Wang Z, Zang C, Rosenfeld JA, Schones DE, Barski A, Cuddapah S, et al. Combinatorial patterns of histone acetylations and methylations in the human genome. *Nat Genet* (2008) 40(7):897–903. doi:10.1038/ng.154
26. Ernst J, Kellis M. Discovery and characterization of chromatin states for systematic annotation of the human genome. *Nat Biotechnol* (2010) 28:817–25. doi:10.1038/nbt.1662
27. Barrero MJ, Boué S, Izpisúa Belmonte JC. Epigenetic mechanisms that regulate cell identity. *Cell Stem Cell* (2010) 7(5):565–70. doi:10.1016/j.stem.2010.10.009
28. Kacem S, Feil R. Chromatin mechanisms in genomic imprinting. *Mamm Genome* (2009) 20:544–56. doi:10.1007/s00335-009-9223-4
29. Reik W, Lewis A. Co-evolution of X-chromosome inactivation and imprinting in mammals. *Nat Rev Genet* (2005) 6:403–10. doi:10.1038/nrg1602
30. Tobi EW, Lumey LH, Talens RP, Kremer D, Putter H, Stein AD, et al. DNA methylation differences after exposure to prenatal famine are common and timing- and sex-specific. *Hum Mol Genet* (2009) 18(21):4046–53. doi:10.1093/hmg/ddp353
31. Aguilera O, Fernández AF, Muñoz A, Fraga MF. Epigenetics and environment: a complex relationship. *J Appl Physiol* (2010) 10(1):243–51. doi:10.1152/japplphysiol.00068.2010
32. Teh AL, Pan H, Chen L, Ong ML, Dogra S, Wong J, et al. The effect of genotype and in utero environment on interindividual variation in neonate DNA methylomes. *Genome Res* (2014) 24(7):1064–74. doi:10.1101/gr.171439.113
33. Whitaker JW, Chen Z, Wang W. Predicting the human epigenome from DNA motifs. *Nat Methods* (2015) 12(3):265–72. doi:10.1038/nmeth.3065
34. Egger G, Liang G, Aparicio A, Jones PA. Epigenetics in human disease and prospects for epigenetic therapy. *Nature* (2004) 429(6990):457–63. doi:10.1038/nature02625
35. Portela A, Esteller M. Epigenetic modifications and human disease. *Nat Biotechnol* (2010) 28(10):1057–68. doi:10.1038/nbt.1685
36. Brunet A, Berger SL. Epigenetics of aging and aging-related disease. *J Gerontol* (2014) 69(1):S1–20. doi:10.1093/gerona/glu042
37. Rajawat YS, Hilioti Z, Bossis J. Aging: central role for autophagy and the lysosomal degradative system. *Aging Res Rev* (2009) 8:199–213. doi:10.1016/j.arr.2009.05.001
38. Freitas AA, de Magalhães JP. A review and appraisal of the DNA damage theory of aging. *Mutat Res* (2011) 728:12–22. doi:10.1016/j.mrrev.2011.05.001
39. Saez I, Vilchez D. The mechanistic links between proteasome activity, aging and age-related diseases. *Curr Genomics* (2014) 15(1):38–51. doi:10.2174/138920291501140306113344
40. Payne BAI, Chinnery PF. Mitochondrial dysfunction in aging: much progress but many unresolved questions. *Biochim Biophys Acta* (2015) 1847(11):1347–53. doi:10.1016/j.bbabio.2015.05.022
41. Tan Q, Christensen K, Christiansen L, Frederiksen H, Bathum L, Dahlgaard J, et al. Genetic dissection of gene expression observed in whole blood samples of elderly Danish twins. *Hum Genet* (2005) 117(2–3):267–74. doi:10.1007/s00439-005-1308-x
42. Zahn JM, Sonu R, Vogel H, Crane E, Mazan-Mamczarz K, Rabkin R, et al. Transcriptional profiling of aging in human muscle reveals a common aging signature. *PLoS Genet* (2006) 2(7):e115. doi:10.1371/journal.pgen.0020115
43. Feser J, Tyler J. Chromatin structure as a mediator of aging. *FEBS Lett* (2011) 585:2041–8. doi:10.1016/j.febslet.2010.11.016
44. Tsurumi A, Li WX. Global heterochromatin loss: a unifying theory of aging? *Epigenetics* (2012) 7:680–8. doi:10.4161/epi.20540
45. Moskalev AA, Aliper AM, Smit-McBride Z, Buzdin A, Zhavoronkov A. Genetics and epigenetics of aging and longevity. *Cell Cycle* (2014) 13:1063–77. doi:10.4161/cc.28433
46. Wilson VL, Smith RA, Ma S, Cutler RG. Genomic 5-methyldeoxycytidine decreases with age. *J Biol Chem* (1987) 262:9948–51.
47. Bolati V, Schwartz J, Wright R, Litonjua A, Tarantini L, Suh H, et al. Decline in genomic DNA methylation through aging in a cohort of eldery subjects. *Mech Ageing Dev* (2009) 130:234–9. doi:10.1016/j.mad.2008.12.003
48. Barbot W, Dupressoir A, Lazar V, Heidmann T. Epigenetic regulation of an IAP retrotransposon in the aging mouse: progressive demethylation and de-silencing of the element by its repetitive induction. *Nucleic Acids Res* (2012) 30:2365–73. doi:10.1093/nar/30.11.2365
49. Wei L, Liu B, Tuo J, Shen D, Chen P, Li Z, et al. Hypomethylation of the IL17RC promoter associates with age-related macular degeneration. *Cell Rep* (2012) 2(5):1151–8. doi:10.1016/j.celrep.2012.10.013
50. Narita M, Nunez S, Heard E, Narita M, Lin AW, Hearn SA, et al. Rb-mediated heterochromatin formation and silencing of E2F target genes during cellular senescence. *Cell* (2003) 113:703–16. doi:10.1016/S0092-8674(03)00401-X
51. Salpea P, Russanova VR, Hirai TH, Sourlingas TG, Sekeri-Pataryas KE, Romero R, et al. Postnatal development- and age-related changes in DNA-methylation patterns in the human genome. *Nucleic Acids Res* (2012) 40:6477–94. doi:10.1093/nar/gks312
52. Horvath S. DNA methylation age of human tissues and cell types. *Genome Biol* (2013) 14:R115. doi:10.1186/gb-2013-14-10-r115
53. Chen H, Dzitoyeva S, Manev H. Effect of aging on 5-hydroxymethylcytosine in the mouse hippocampus. *Restorat Neurol Neurosci* (2012) 30:237–45. doi:10.3233/RNN-2012-110223
54. Wagner M, Steinbacher J, Kraus TF, Michalakis S, Hackner B, Pfaffeneder T, et al. Age-dependent levels of 5-methyl-, 5-hydroxymethyl-, and 5-formylcytosine in human and mouse brain tissues. *Angew Chem Int Ed Engl* (2015) 54:12511–4. doi:10.1002/anie.201502722

55. Xiong J, Jiang HP, Peng CY, Deng QY, Lan MD, Zeng H, et al. DNA hydroxymethylation age of human blood determined by capillary hydrophilic-interaction liquid chromatography/mass spectrometry. *Clin Epigenetics* (2015) 7:72. doi:10.1186/s13148-015-0109-x
56. Farré P, Jones MJ, Meaney MJ, Emberly E, Turecki G, Kobor MS. Concordant and discordant DNA methylation signatures of aging in human blood and brain. *Epigenetics Chromatin* (2015) 8:19. doi:10.1186/s13072-015-0011-y
57. Weidner CI, Wagner W. The epigenetics tracks of aging. *Biol Chem* (2014) 395:1307–14. doi:10.1515/hsz-2014-0180
58. Yuan T, Jiao Y, Jong S, Ophoff RA, Beck S, Teschendorff AE. An integrative multi-scale analysis of the dynamic DNA methylation landscape in aging. *PLoS Genet* (2015) 11(2):e1004996. doi:10.1371/journal.pgen.1004996
59. Timp W, Bravo HC, McDonald OG, Goggins M, Umbricht C, Zeiger M, et al. Large hypomethylated blocks as a universal defining epigenetic alteration in human solid tumors. *Genome Med* (2014) 6(8):61. doi:10.1186/s13073-014-0061-y
60. Hannum G, Guinney J, Zhao L, Zhang L, Hughes G, Sadda S, et al. Genome-wide methylation profiles reveal quantitative views of human aging rates. *Mol Cell* (2013) 49(2):359–67. doi:10.1016/j.molcel.2012.10.016
61. Xu Z, Taylor JA. Genome-wide age-related DNA methylation changes in blood and other tissues relate to histone modification, expression and cancer. *Carcinogenesis* (2014) 35:356–64. doi:10.1093/carcin/bgt391
62. Sidler C, Kovalchuk O, Kovalchuk I. Epigenetic regulation of cellular senescence and aging. *Front Genet* (2017) 8:138. doi:10.3389/fgene.2017.00138
63. Pogribny IP, Vanyushin BF. Age-related genomic hypomethylation. In: Tollefsbol TO, editor. *Epigenetics of Aging*. New York: Springer (2010). p. 11–26.
64. McCauley BS, Dang W. Histone methylation and aging: lessons learned from model systems. *Biochim Biophys Acta* (2014) 1839(12):1454–62. doi:10.1016/j.bbagrm.2014.05.008
65. Rakyan VK, Down TA, Maslau S, Andrew T, Yang TP, Beyan H, et al. Human aging-associated DNA hypermethylation occurs preferentially at bivalent chromatin domains. *Genome Res* (2010) 20:434–9. doi:10.1101/gr.103101.109
66. Fernández AF, Assenov Y, Martin-Subero JI, Balint B, Siebert R, Taniguchi H, et al. A DNA methylation fingerprint of 1628 human samples. *Genome Res* (2012) 22:407–19. doi:10.1101/gr.119867.110
67. Fernández AF, Bayón GF, Urdinguio RG, Toraño EG, García MG, Carella A, et al. H3K4me1 marks DNA regions hypomethylated during aging in human stem and differentiated cells. *Genome Res* (2015) 25(1):27–40. doi:10.1101/gr.169011.113
68. Dang W, Steffen KK, Perry R, Dorsey JA, Johnson FB, Shilatifard A, et al. Histone H4 lysine 16 acetylation regulates cellular lifespan. *Nature* (2009) 459:802–7. doi:10.1038/nature08085
69. Sen P, Shah PP, Nativio R, Berger SL. Epigenetic mechanisms of longevity and aging. *Cell* (2016) 166(4):822–39. doi:10.1016/j.cell.2016.07.050
70. Kawakami K, Nakamura A, Ishigami A, Goto S, Takahashi R. Age-related difference of site-specific histone modifications in rat liver. *Biogerontology* (2009) 10(4):415–21. doi:10.1007/s10522-008-9176-0
71. Bracken AP, Kleine-Kohlbrecher D, Dietrich N, Pasini D, Gargiulo G, Beekman C, et al. The polycomb group proteins bind throughout the INK4A-ARF locus and are disassociated in senescent cells. *Genes Dev* (2007) 21(5):525–30. doi:10.1101/gad.415507
72. Djeghloul D, Kuranda K, Kuzniak I, Barbieri D, Naguibneva I, Choisy C, et al. Age-associated decrease of the histone methyltransferase SUV39H1 in HSC perturbs heterochromatin and B lymphoid differentiation. *Stem Cell Reports* (2016) 6:970–84. doi:10.1016/j.stemcr.2016.05.007
73. Sidler C, Woycicki R, Li D, Wang B, Kovalchuk I, Kovalchuk O. A role for SUV39H1-mediated H3K9 trimethylation in the control of genome stability and senescence in WI38 human diploid lung fibroblasts. *Aging* (2014) 6:545–63. doi:10.18632/aging.100678
74. Zhang W, Li J, Suzuki K, Qu J, Wang P, Zhou J, et al. A Werner syndrome stem cell model unveils heterochromatin alterations as a driver of human aging. *Science* (2015) 348:1160–3. doi:10.1126/science.aaa1356
75. Casillas MA Jr, Lopatina N, Andrews LG, Tollefsbol TO. Transcriptional control of the DNA methyltransferases is altered in aging and neoplastically-transformed human fibroblasts. *Mol Cell Biochem* (2003) 252:33–43. doi:10.1023/A:1025548623524
76. O'Sullivan RJ, Kubicek S, Schreiber SL, Karlseder J. Reduced histone biosynthesis and chromatin changes arising from a damage signal at telomeres. *Nat Struct Mol Biol* (2010) 17(10):1218–25. doi:10.1038/nsmb.1897
77. Grabowska W, Sikora E, Bielak-Zmijewska A. Sirtuins, a promising target in slowing down the ageing process. *Biogerontology* (2017) 18(4):447–76. doi:10.1007/s10522-017-9685-9
78. Urban MK, Zweidler A. Changes in nucleosomal core histone variants during chicken development and maturation. *Dev Biol* (1983) 95(2):421–8. doi:10.1016/0012-1606(83)90043-X
79. Gevry N, Chan HM, Laflamme L, Livingston DM, Gaudreau L. p21 transcription is regulated by differential localization of histone H2A.Z. *Genes Dev* (2007) 21:1869–81. doi:10.1101/gad.1545707
80. Zhang R, Poustovoitov MV, Ye X, Santos HA, Chen W, Daganzo SM, et al. Formation of MacroH2A-containing senescence-associated heterochromatin foci and senescence driven by ASF1a and HIRA. *Dev Cell* (2005) 8(1):19–30. doi:10.1016/j.devcel.2004.10.019
81. Kreiling JA, Tamamori-Adachi M, Sexton AN, Jeyapalan JC, Munoz-Najar U, Peterson AL, et al. Age-associated increase in heterochromatic marks in murine and primate tissues. *Aging Cell* (2011) 10(2):292–304. doi:10.1111/j.1474-9726.2010.00666.x
82. Fraga MF, Ballestar E, Paz MF, Ropero S, Setien F, Ballestar ML, et al. Epigenetic differences arise during the lifetime of monozygotic twins. *Proc Natl Acad Sci U S A* (2005) 102(30):10604–9. doi:10.1073/pnas.0500398102
83. Herskind AM, McGue M, Holm NV, Sørensen TI, Harvald B, Vaupel JW. The heritability of human longevity: a population-based study of 2872 Danish twin pairs born 1870-1900. *Hum Genet* (1996) 97(3):319–23. doi:10.1007/BF02185763
84. Poulsen P, Esteller M, Vaag A, Fraga MF. The epigenetic basis of twin discordance in age-related diseases. *Pediatr Res* (2007) 61(5 Pt 2):38R–42R. doi:10.1203/pdr.0b013e31803c7b98
85. Kaminsky ZA, Tang T, Wang SC, Ptak C, Oh GH, Wong AH, et al. DNA methylation profiles in monozygotic and dizygotic twins. *Nat Genet* (2009) 41(2):240–5. doi:10.1038/ng.286
86. Javierre BM, Fernandez AF, Richter J, Al-Shahrour F, Martin-Subero JI, Rodriguez-Ubreva J, et al. Changes in the pattern of DNA methylation associate with twin discordance in systemic lupus erythematosus. *Genome Res* (2010) 20(2):170–9. doi:10.1101/gr.100289.109
87. Sargent M. Why twins age differently. *Nature* (2010) 464:1130–1. doi:10.1038/4641130a
88. Bell JT, Tsai PC, Yang TP, Pidsley R, Nisber J, Glass D, et al. Epigenome-wide scans identify differentially methylated regions for age and age-related phenotypes in a healthy ageing population. *PLoS Genet* (2012) 8:e1002629. doi:10.1371/journal.pgen.1002629
89. López-Otín C, Blasco MA, Partridge L, Serrano M, Kroemer G. The hallmarks of aging. *Cell* (2013) 153:1194–217. doi:10.1016/j.cell.2013.05.039
90. Bocklandt S, Lin W, Sehl ME, Sanchez FJ, Sinsheimer JS, Horvath S, et al. Epigenetic predictor of age. *PLoS One* (2011) 6:e14821. doi:10.1371/journal.pone.0014821
91. O'Sullivan RJ, Karlseder J. The great unravelling: chromatin as a modulator of the aging process. *Trends Biochem Sci* (2012) 37(11):466–76. doi:10.1016/j.tibs.2012.08.001
92. Cruickshanks HA, McBryan T, Nelson DM, Vanderkraats ND, Shah PP, van Tuyn J, et al. Senescent cells harbour features of the cancer epigenome. *Nat Cell Biol* (2013) 15:1495–506. doi:10.1038/ncb2879
93. Marioni RE, Shah S, McRae AF, Chen BH, Colicino E, Harris SE, et al. DNA methylation age of blood predicts all-cause mortality in later life. *Genome Biol* (2015) 16:25. doi:10.1186/s13059-015-0584-6
94. Lin Q, Weidner CI, Costa IG, Marioni RE, Ferreira MR, Deary IJ, et al. DNA methylation levels at individual age-associated CpG sites can be indicative for life expectancy. *Aging* (2016) 8:394–401. doi:10.18632/aging.100908
95. Chen BH, Marioni RE, Colicino E, Peters MJ, Ward-Caviness CK, Tsai PC, et al. DNA methylation-based measures of biological age: meta-analysis predicting time to death. *Aging* (2016) 8(9):1844–65. doi:10.18632/aging.101020
96. Christiansen L, Lenart A, Tan Q, Vaupel JW, Aviv A, McGue M, et al. DNA methylation age is associated with mortality in a longitudinal Danish twin study. *Aging Cell* (2016) 15:149–54. doi:10.1111/acel.12421
97. Perna L, Zhang Y, Mons U, Holleczek B, Saum KU, Brenner H. Epigenetic age acceleration predicts cancer, cardiovascular, and all-cause mortality

in a German case cohort. *Clin Epigenetics* (2016) 8:64. doi:10.1186/s13148-016-0228-z
98. Barrès R, Yan J, Egan B, Treebak JT, Rasmussen M, Fritz T, et al. Acute exercise remodels promoter methylation in human skeletal muscle. *Cell Metab* (2012) 15(3):405–11. doi:10.1016/j.cmet.2012.01.001
99. Barrès R, Kirchner H, Rasmussen M, Yan J, Kantor FR, Krook A, et al. Weight loss after gastric bypass surgery in human obesity remodels promoter methylation. *Cell Rep* (2013) 3(4):1020–7. doi:10.1016/j.celrep.2013.03.018
100. Rönn T, Volkov P, Davegårdh C, Dayeh T, Hall E, Olsson AH, et al. A six months exercise intervention influences the genome-wide DNA methylation pattern in human adipose tissue. *PLoS Genet* (2013) 9(6):e1003572. doi:10.1371/journal.pgen.1003572
101. Denham J, O'Brien BJ, Harvey JT, Charchar FJ. Genome-wide sperm DNA methylation changes after 3 months of exercise training in humans. *Epigenomics* (2015) 7(5):717–31. doi:10.2217/epi.15.29
102. Maejima H, Kanemura N, Kokubun T, Murata K, Takayanagi K. Exercise enhances cognitive function and neurotrophin expression in the hippocampus accompanied by changes in epigenetic programming in senescence-accelerated mice. *Neurosci Lett* (2017) 665:67–73. doi:10.1016/j.neulet.2017.11.023
103. Meyer KF, Verkaik-Schakel RN, Timens W, Kobzik L, Plösch T, Hylkema MN. The fetal programming effect of prenatal smoking on Igf1r and Igf1 methylation is organ- and sex-specific. *Epigenetics* (2017) 21:1–49. doi:10.1080/15592294.2017.1403691
104. Vaz M, Hwang SY, Kagiampakis I, Phallen J, Patil A, O'Hagan HM, et al. Chronic cigarette smoke-induced epigenomic changes precede sensitization of bronchial epithelial cells to single-step transformation by KRAS mutations. *Cancer Cell* (2017) 32(3):360–76. doi:10.1016/j.ccell.2017.08.006
105. Bauer M, Fink B, Thürmann L, Eszlinger M, Herberth G, Lehmann I. Tobacco smoking differently influences cell types of the innate and adaptive immune system-indications from CpG site methylation. *Clin Epigenetics* (2016) 7:83. doi:10.1186/s13148-016-0249-7
106. Sharp GC, Arathimos R, Reese SE, Page CM, Felix J, Küpers LK, et al. Maternal alcohol consumption and offspring DNA methylation: findings from six general population-based birth cohorts. *Epigenomics* (2018) 10(1):27–42. doi:10.2217/epi-2017-0095
107. Rachdaoui N, Li L, Willard B, Kasumov T, Previs S, Sarkar D. Turnover of histones and histone variants in postnatal rat brain: effects of alcohol exposure. *Clin Epigenetics* (2017) 9:117. doi:10.1186/s13148-017-0416-5
108. Gems D, Partridge L. Stress-response hormesis and aging: "that which does not kill us makes us stronger". *Cell Metab* (2008) 7:200–3. doi:10.1016/j.cmet.2008.01.001
109. Campos AC, Molognoni F, Melo FH, Galdieri LC, Carneiro CR, D'Almeida V, et al. Oxidative stress modulates DNA methylation during melanocyte anchorage blockade associated with malignant transformation. *Neoplasia* (2007) 9(12):1111–21. doi:10.1593/neo.07712
110. O'Hagan HM, Mohammad HP, Baylin SB. Double strand breaks can initiate gene silencing and SIRT1-dependent onset of DNA methylation in an exogenous promoter CpG island. *PLoS Genet* (2008) 4(8):e1000155. doi:10.1371/journal.pgen.1000155
111. Molognoni F, Cruz AT, Meliso FM, Morais AS, Souza CF, Xander P, et al. Epigenetic reprogramming as a key contributor to melanocyte malignant transformation. *Epigenetics* (2011) 6(4):450–64. doi:10.4161/epi.6.4.14917
112. O'Hagan HM, Wang W, Sen S, Destefano Shields C, Lee SS, Zhang YW, et al. Oxidative damage targets complexes containing DNA methyltransferases, SIRT1, and polycomb members to promoter CpG Islands. *Cancer Cell* (2011) 20(5):606–19. doi:10.1016/j.ccr.2011.09.012
113. Molognoni F, de Melo FH, da Silva CT, Jasiulionis MG. Ras and Rac1, frequently mutated in melanomas, are activated by superoxide anion, modulate Dnmt1 level and are causally related to melanocyte malignant transformation. *PLoS One* (2013) 8(12):e81937. doi:10.1371/journal.pone.0081937
114. Meliso FM, Micali D, Silva CT, Sabedot TS, Jasiulionis MG. SIRT1 regulates Mxd1 during malignant melanoma progression. *Oncotarget* (2017) 8(70):114540–53. doi:10.18632/oncotarget.21457
115. Valinluck V, Sowers LC. Endogenous cytosine damage products alter the site selectivity of human DNA maintenance methyltransferase DNMT1. *Cancer Res* (2007) 67(3):946–50. doi:10.1158/0008-5472.CAN-06-3123
116. Chia N, Wang L, Lu X, Senut MC, Brenner C, Ruden DM. Hypothesis: environmental regulation of 5-hydroxymethylcytosine by oxidative stress. *Epigenetics* (2011) 6(7):853–6. doi:10.4161/epi.6.7.16461
117. Hitchler MU, Domann FE. Redox regulation of the epigenetic landscape in cancer: a role for metabolic reprogramming in remodeling the epigenome. *Free Radic Biol Med* (2012) 53(11):2178–87. doi:10.1016/j.freeradbiomed.2012.09.028
118. Oberdoerffer P, Michan S, McVay M, Mostoslavsky R, Vann J, Park SK, et al. SIRT1 redistribution on chromatin promotes genomic stability but alters gene expression during aging. *Cell* (2008) 135(5):907–18. doi:10.1016/j.cell.2008.10.025
119. Cohen HY, Miller C, Bitterman KJ, Wall NR, Hekking B, Kessler B, et al. Caloric restriction promotes mammalian cell survival by inducing the Sirt1 deacetylase. *Science* (2004) 305(5682):390–2. doi:10.1126/science.1099196
120. Chen D, Steele AD, Lindquist S, Guarente L. Increase in activity during calorie restriction requires Sirt1. *Science* (2005) 310(5754):1641. doi:10.1126/science.1118357
121. Bauer JA, Pearson KJ, Price NL, Jamieson HA, Lerin C, Kalra A, et al. Resveratrol improves health and survival of mice on a high-calorie diet. *Nature* (2006) 444(7117):337–42. doi:10.1038/nature05354
122. Lin SJ, Kaeberlein M, Andalis AA, Sturtz LA, Defossez PA, Culotta VC, et al. Caloric restriction extends *Saccharomyces cerevisiae* lifespan by increasing respiration. *Nature* (2002) 418(6895):344–8. doi:10.1038/nature00829
123. Howitz KT, Bitterman KJ, Cohen HY, Lamming DW, Lavu S, Wood JG, et al. Small molecule activators of sirtuins extend *Saccharomyces cerevisiae* lifespan. *Nature* (2003) 425(6954):191–6. doi:10.1038/nature01960
124. Wood JG, Rogina B, Lavu S, Howitz K, Helfand SL, Tatar M, et al. Sirtuin activators mimic caloric restriction and delay ageing in metazoans. *Nature* (2004) 430(7000):686–9. doi:10.1038/nature02789
125. Lee C, Longo V. Dietary restriction with and without caloric restriction for healthy aging. *F1000Res* (2016) 5:F1000. doi:10.12688/f1000research.7136.1
126. Vaquero A, Reinberg D. Calorie restriction and the exercise of chromatin. *Genes Dev* (2009) 23(16):1849–69. doi:10.1101/gad.1807009
127. Li Y, Daniel M, Tollefsbol TO. Epigenetic regulation of caloric restriction in aging. *BMC Med* (2011) 25(9):98. doi:10.1186/1741-7015-9-98
128. Hubbard BP, Sinclair DA. Small molecule SIRT1 activators for the treatment of aging and age-related diseases. *Trends Pharmacol Sci* (2014) 35(3):146–54. doi:10.1016/j.tips.2013.12.004
129. Eisenberg T, Knauer H, Schauer A, Büttner S, Ruckenstuhl C, Carmona-Gutierrez D, et al. Induction of autophagy by spermidine promotes longevity. *Nat Cell Biol* (2009) 11(11):1305–14. doi:10.1038/ncb1975
130. Chouliaras L, van den Hove DL, Kenis G, Keitel S, Hof PR, van Os J, et al. Age-related increase in levels of 5-hydroxymethylcytosine in mouse hippocampus is prevented by caloric restriction. *Curr Alzheimer Res* (2012) 9(5):536–44. doi:10.2174/156720512800618035
131. Yin R, Mao SQ, Zhao B, Chong Z, Yang Y, Zhao C, et al. Ascorbic acid enhances Tet-mediated 5-methylcytosine oxidation and promotes DNA demethylation in mammals. *J Am Chem Soc* (2013) 135(28):10396–403. doi:10.1021/ja4028346
132. Blaschke K, Ebata KT, Karimi MM, Zepeda-Martínez JA, Goyal P, Mahapatra S, et al. Vitamin C induces Tet-dependent DNA demethylation and a blastocyst-like state in ES cells. *Nature* (2013) 500(7461):222–6. doi:10.1038/nature12362
133. Salminen A, Kauppinen A, Hiltunen M, Kaarniranta K. Krebs cycle intermediates regulate DNA and histone methylation: epigenetic impact on the aging process. *Ageing Res Rev* (2014) 16:45–65. doi:10.1016/j.arr.2014.05.004
134. Sharma U, Rando OJ. Metabolic input into the epigenome. *Cell Metab* (2017) 25:544–58. doi:10.1016/j.cmet.2017.02.003
135. McGowan PO, Sasaki A, D'Alessio AC, Dymov S, Labonte B, Szyf M, et al. Epigenetic regulation of the glucocorticoid receptor in human brain associates with childhood abuse. *Nat Neurosci* (2009) 12:342–8. doi:10.1038/nn.2270
136. Perroud N, Paoloni-Giacobino A, Prada P, Olie E, Salzmann A, Nicastro R, et al. Increased methylation of glucocorticoid receptor gene (NR3C1) in

adults with a history of childhood maltreatment: a link with the severity and type of trauma. *Transl Psychiatry* (2011) 1:e59. doi:10.1038/tp.2011.60
137. Klengel T, Mehta KB, Anacker C, Rex-Haffner M, Pruessner JC, Pariante CM, et al. Allele-specific FKBP5 DNA demethylation mediates gene-childhood trauma interactions. *Nat Neurosci* (2013) 16:33–41. doi:10.1038/nn.3275
138. Non AL, Binder AM, Kubzansky LD, Michels KB. Genome-wide DNA methylation in neonates exposed to maternal depression, anxiety, or SSRI medication during pregnancy. *Epigenetics* (2014) 9:964–72. doi:10.4161/epi.28853
139. Yehuda R, Daskalakis NP, Bierer LM, Bader HN, Klengel T, Holsboer F, et al. Holocaust exposure induced intergenerational effects on FKBP5 methylation. *Biol Psychiatry* (2015) 80(5):372–80. doi:10.1016/j.biopsych.2015.08.005
140. Weaver IC, Meaney MJ, Szyf M. Maternal care effects on the hippocampal transcriptome and anxiety-mediated behaviors in the offspring that are reversible in adulthood. *Proc Natl Acad Sci U S A* (2006) 103:3480–5. doi:10.1073/pnas.0507526103
141. Murgatroyd C, Patchev AV, Wu Y, Micale V, Bockmuhl Y, Fischer D, et al. Dynamic DNA methylation programs persistent adverse effects of early-life stress. *Nat Neurosci* (2009) 12:1559–66. doi:10.1038/nn.2436
142. Schmauss C, Lee-McDermott Z, Medina LR. Trans-generational effects of early life stress: the role of maternal behavior. *Sci Rep* (2014) 4:4873. doi:10.1038/srep04873
143. Fernández-Morera JL, Calvanese V, Rodríguez-Rodero S, Menéndez-Torre E, Fraga MF. Epigenetic regulation of the immune system in health and disease. *Tissue Antigens* (2010) 76:431–9. doi:10.1111/j.1399-0039.2010.01587.x
144. Rodriguez-Cortez VC, Hernando H, de la Rica L, Vento R, Ballestar E. Epigenomic deregulation in the immune system. *Epigenomics* (2011) 3:697–713. doi:10.2217/epi.11.99
145. Busslinger M, Tarakhovsky A. Epigenetic control of immunity. *Cold Spring Harb Perspect Biol* (2014) 6:a019307. doi:10.1101/cshperspect.a019307
146. Zhang Z, Deng C, Lu Q, Richardson B. Age-dependent DNA methylation changes in the ITGAL (CD11a) promoter. *Mech Ageing Dev* (2002) 123(9):1257–68. doi:10.1016/S0047-6374(02)00014-3
147. Marttila S, Kananen L, Hayrynen S, Jylhava J, Nevalainen T, Hervonen A, et al. Ageing-associated changes in the human DNA methylome: genomic locations and effects on gene expression. *BMC Genomics* (2015) 16:179. doi:10.1186/s12864-015-1381-z
148. Zhao M, Qin J, Yin H, Tan Y, Liao W, Liu Q, et al. Distinct epigenomes in CD4+ T cells of newborns, middle-ages and centenarians. *Sci Rep* (2016) 6:38411. doi:10.1038/srep38411
149. Shi C, Pamer EG. Monocyte recruitment during infection and inflammation. *Nat Rev Immunol* (2011) 11:762–74. doi:10.1038/nri3070
150. van den Bossche J, Neele AE, Hoeksema MA, Winther MP. Macropaheg polarization: the epigenetic point of view. *Curr Opin Lipidol* (2014) 25(5):367–73. doi:10.1097/MOL.0000000000000109
151. Saccani S, Natoli G. Dynamic changes in histone H3 Lys9 methylation occurring at tightly regulated inducible inflammatory genes. *Genes Dev* (2002) 16:2219–24. doi:10.1101/gad.232502
152. Akira S, Uematsu S, Takeuchi O. Pathogen recognition and innate immunity. *Cell* (2006) 124(4):783–801. doi:10.1016/j.cell.2006.02.015
153. Netea MG, Quintin J, van der Meer JW. Trained immunity: a memory for innate host defense. *Cell Host Microbe* (2011) 9(5):355–61. doi:10.1016/j.chom.2011.04.006
154. Crisan TO, Netea MG, Joosten LAB. Innate immune memory: implications for host responses to damage-associated molecular patterns. *Eur J Immunol* (2016) 46:817–28. doi:10.1002/eji.201545497
155. Kleinnijenhuis J, Quintin J, Preijers F, Joosten LA, Ifrim DC, Saeed S, et al. Bacille Calmette-Guerin induces NOD2-dependent nonspecific protection from reinfection via epigenetic reprogramming of monocytes. *Proc Natl Acad Sci U S A* (2012) 109:17537–42. doi:10.1073/pnas.1202870109
156. Foster SL, Hargreaves DC, Medzhitov R. Gene-specific control of inflammation by TLR-induced chromatin modifications. *Nature* (2007) 447:972–8. doi:10.1038/nature05836
157. Bullwinkel J, Ludermann A, Debarry J, Singh PB. Epigenotype switching at the CD14 and CD209 genes during differentiation of human monocytes to dendritic cells. *Epigenetics* (2011) 6:45–51. doi:10.4161/epi.6.1.13314
158. Kuwahara M, Suzuki J, Tofukuji S, Yamada T, Kanoh M, Matsumoto A, et al. The Menin-Bach2 axis is critical for regulating CD4 T-cell senescence and cytokine homeostasis. *Nat Commun* (2014) 5:3555. doi:10.1038/ncomms4555
159. Sidler C, Woycicki R, Ilnytskyy Y, Metz G, Kovalchuk I, Kovalchuk O. Immunosenescence is associated with altered gene expression and epigenetic regulation in primary and secondary immune organs. *Front Genet* (2013) 4:211. doi:10.3389/fgene.2013.00211
160. Degerman S, Landfors M, Siwicki JK, Revie J, Borssen M, Evelonn E, et al. Immortalization of T-cells is accompanied by gradual changes in CpG methylation resulting in a profile resembling a subset of T-cell leukemias. *Neoplasia* (2014) 16:606–15. doi:10.1016/j.neo.2014.07.001
161. Vogt M, Haggblom C, Yeargin J, Christiansen-Weber T, Haas M. Independent induction of senescence by p16INK4a and p21CIP1 in spontaneously immortalized human fibroblasts. *Cell Growth Differ* (1998) 9:139–46.
162. Murayama A, Sakura K, Nakama M, Yasuzawa-Tanaka K, Fujita E, Tateishi Y, et al. A specific CpG site demethylation in the human interleukin 2 gene promoter is an epigenetic memory. *EMBO J* (2006) 25:1081–92. doi:10.1038/sj.emboj.7601012
163. Northrop JK, Thomas RM, Wells AD, Shen H. Epigenetic remodeling of the IL-2 and IFN-γ loci in memory CD8 T cells is influenced by CD4 T cells. *J Immunol* (2006) 177:1062–9. doi:10.4049/jimmunol.177.2.1062
164. Wright KL, Ting JP. Epigenetic regulation of MHC-II and CIITA genes. *Trends Immunol* (2006) 27:405–12. doi:10.1016/j.it.2006.07.007
165. Ucar D, Márquez EJ, Chung CH, Marches R, Rossi RJ, Uyar A, et al. The chromatin accessibility signature of human immune aging stems from CD8+ T cells. *J Exp Med* (2017) 214(10):3123–44. doi:10.1084/jem.20170416
166. Tserel L, Kolde R, Limbach M, Tretyakov K, Kasela S, Kisand K, et al. Age-related profiling of DNA methylation in CD8+ T cells reveals changes in immune response and transcriptional regulator genes. *Sci Rep* (2015) 5:13107. doi:10.1038/srep13107
167. Zhu J, Paul WE. CD4 T cells: fates, functions, and faults. *Blood* (2008) 112:1557–69. doi:10.1182/blood-2008-05-078154
168. Schoenborn JR, Dorschner MO, Sekimata M, Santer DM, Shnyreva M, Fitzpatrick DR, et al. Comprehensive epigenetic profiling identifies multiple distal regulatory elements directing transcription of the gene encoding interferon-gamma. *Nat Immunol* (2007) 8:732–42. doi:10.1038/ni0807-893b
169. Aune TM, Collins PL, Chang S. Epigenetics and T helper 1 differentiation. *Immunology* (2009) 126:299–305. doi:10.1111/j.1365-2567.2008.03026.x
170. Santangelo S, Cousins DJ, Winkelmann N, Triantaphyllopoulos K, Staynov DZ. Chromatin structure and DNa methylation of the IL4 gene in human T(H)2 cells. *Chromosome Res* (2009) 17:485–96. doi:10.1007/s10577-009-9040-3
171. Cohen CJ, Crome SQ, MacDonald KG, Dai EL, Mager DL, Levings MK. Human Th1 and Th17 exhibit stability at signature cytokine and transcription factor loci. *J Immunol* (2011) 187:5615–26. doi:10.4049/jimmunol.1101058
172. Akimzhanov AM, Yang XO, Dong C. Chromatin remodeling of interleukin-17 (IL-17)-IL-17F cytokine gene locus during inflammatory helper T cell differentiation. *J Biol Chem* (2007) 282(9):5969–72. doi:10.1074/jbc.C600322200
173. Baron U, Floess S, Wieczorek G, Baumann K, Grützkau A, Dong J, et al. DNA demethylation in the human FOXP3 locus discriminates regulatory T cells from activated FOXP3(+) conventional T cells. *Eur J Immunol* (2007) 37(9):2378–89. doi:10.1002/eji.200737594
174. van Loosdregt J, Vercoulen Y, Guichelaar T, Gent YY, Beekman JM, van Beekum O, et al. Regulation of Treg functionality by acetylation-mediated Foxp3 protein stabilization. *Blood* (2010) 115(5):965–74. doi:10.1182/blood-2009-02-207118
175. Parra M. Epigenetic events during B lymphocyte development. *Epigenetics* (2009) 4(7):462–8. doi:10.4161/epi.4.7.10052
176. Lee ST, Xiao Y, Muench MO, Xiao J, Fomin ME, Wiencke JK, et al. A global DNA methylation and gene expression analysis of early human B-cell development reveals a demethylation signature and transcription factor network. *Nucleic Acids Res* (2012) 40(22):11339–51. doi:10.1093/nar/gks957
177. Zan H, Casali P. Epigenetics of peripheral B-cell differentiation and the antibody response. *Front Immunol* (2015) 6:631. doi:10.3389/fimmu.2015.00631
178. Bao Y, Cao X. Epigenetic control of B cell development and B-cell-related immune disorders. *Clin Rev Allergy Immunol* (2016) 50(3):301–11. doi:10.1007/s12016-015-8494-7
179. Oguro H, Yuan J, Ichikawa H, Ikawa T, Yamazaki S, Kawamoto H, et al. Poised lineage specification in multipotential hematopoietic stem and progenitor

cells by the polycomb protein Bmi1. *Cell Stem Cell* (2010) 6(3):279–86. doi:10.1016/j.stem.2010.01.005
180. McManus S, Ebert A, Salvagiotto G, Medvedovic J, Sun Q, Tamir I, et al. The transcription factor Pax5 regulates its target genes by recruiting chromatin-modifying proteins in committed B cells. *EMBO J* (2011) 30(12):2388–404. doi:10.1038/emboj.2011.140
181. Maier H, Ostraat R, Gao H, Fields S, Shinton SA, Medina KL, et al. Early B cell factor cooperates with Runx1 and mediates epigenetic changes associated with mb-1 transcription. *Nat Immunol* (2004) 5(10):1069–77. doi:10.1038/ni1119
182. Linderson Y, Eberhard D, Malin S, Johansson A, Busslinger M, Pettersson S. Corecruitment of the Grg4 repressor by PU.1 is critical for Pax5-mediated repression of B-cell-specific genes. *EMBO Rep* (2004) 5(3):291–6. doi:10.1038/sj.embor.7400089
183. Crouch EE, Li Z, Takizawa M, Fichtner-Feigl S, Gourzi P, Montano C, et al. Regulation of AID expression in the immune response. *J Exp Med* (2007) 204:1145–56. doi:10.1084/jem.20061952
184. Shi W, Liao Y, Willis SN, Taubenheim N, Inouye M, Tarlinton DM, et al. Transcriptional profiling of mouse B cell terminal differentiation defines a signature for antibody-secreting plasma cells. *Nat Immunol* (2015) 16:663–73. doi:10.1038/ni.3154
185. Yu J, Angelin-Duclos C, Greenwood J, Liao J, Calame K. Transcriptional repression by blimp-1 (PRDI-BF1) involves recruitment of histone deacetylase. *Mol Cell Biol* (2000) 20:2592–603. doi:10.1128/MCB.20.7.2592-2603.2000
186. Su ST, Ying HY, Chiu YK, Lin FR, Chen MY, Lin KI. Involvement of histone demethylase LSD1 in Blimp-1-mediated gene repression during plasma cell differentiation. *Mol Cell Biol* (2009) 29:1421–31. doi:10.1128/MCB.01158-08
187. Kurosaki T, Kometani K, Ise W. Memory B cells. *Nat Rev Immunol* (2015) 15:149–59. doi:10.1038/nri3802
188. Caganova M, Carrisi C, Varano G, Mainoldi F, Zanardi F, Germain PL, et al. Germinal center dysregulation by histone methyltransferase EZH2 promotes lymphomagenesis. *J Clin Invest* (2013) 123:5009–22. doi:10.1172/JCI70626
189. Good-Jacobson KL. Regulation of germinal center, B-cell memory, and plasma cell formation by histone modifiers. *Front Immunol* (2014) 5:596. doi:10.3389/fimmu.2014.00596
190. Luckey CJ, Bhattacharya D, Goldrath AW, Weissman IL, Benoist C, Mathis D. Memory T and memory B cells share a transcriptional program of self-renewal with long-term hematopoietic stem cells. *Proc Natl Acad Sci U S A* (2006) 103:3304–9. doi:10.1073/pnas.0511137103
191. Panda A, Arjona A, Sapey E, Bai F, Fikrig E, Montgomery RR, et al. Human innate immunosenescence: causes and consequences for immunity in old age. *Trends Immunol* (2009) 30:325–33. doi:10.1016/j.it.2009.05.004
192. Bocker MT, Hellwig I, Breiling A, Eckstein V, Ho AD, Lyko F. Genome-wide promoter DNA methylation dynamics of human hematopoietic progenitor cells during differentiation and aging. *Blood* (2011) 117:e182–9. doi:10.1182/blood-2011-01-331926
193. Beerman I, Maloney WJ, Weissmann IL, Rossi DJ. Stem cells and the aging hematopoietic system. *Curr Opin Immunol* (2010) 22(4):500–6. doi:10.1016/j.coi.2010.06.007
194. Kramer A, Challen GA. The epigenetic basis of hematopoietic stem cell aging. *Sem Hematol* (2017) 54:19–24. doi:10.1053/j.seminhematol.2016.10.006
195. Chang YC, Chen TC, Lee CT, Yang CY, Wang HW, Wang CC, et al. Epigenetic control of MHC class II expression in tumor-associated macrophages by decoy receptor 3. *Blood* (2008) 111(10):5054–63. doi:10.1182/blood-2007-12-130609
196. Kutza J, Murasko DM. Effects of aging on natural killer cell activity and activation by interleukin-2 and IFN-alpha. *Cell Immunol* (1994) 155(1):195–204. doi:10.1006/cimm.1994.1112
197. Baylis D, Bartlett DB, Patel HP, Roberts HC. Understanding how we age: insights into inflammaging. *Longev Healthspan* (2013) 2(1):8. doi:10.1186/2046-2395-2-8
198. Gowers IR, Walters K, Kiss-Toth E, Read RC, Duff GW, Wilson AG. Age-related loss of CpG methylation in the tumour necrosis factor promoter. *Cytokine* (2011) 56(3):792–7. doi:10.1016/j.cyto.2011.09.009
199. Sullivan KE, Reddy AB, Dietzmann K, Suriano AR, Kocieda VP, Stewart M, et al. Epigenetic regulation of tumor necrosis factor alpha. *Mol Cell Biol* (2007) 27(14):5147–60. doi:10.1128/MCB.02429-06
200. van Rietschoten JG, Gal-Yam EN, Jeong S, Cortez CC, Verweij CL, Jones PA. Epigenetic regulation and nucleosome positioning in the human TATA-less IL-1 alpha promoter. *Genes Immun* (2008) 9(7):582–90. doi:10.1038/gene.2008.53
201. Budinger GRS, Kohanski RA, Gan W, Kobor MS, Amaral LA, Armanios M, et al. The intersection of aging biology and the pathobiology of lung diseases: a joint NHLBI/NIA workshop. *J Gerontol A Biol Sci Med Sci* (2017) 72(11):1492–500. doi:10.1093/gerona/glx090
202. Lepeule J, Baccarelli A, Motta V, Cantone L, Litonjua AA, Sparrow D, et al. Gene promoter methylation is associated with lung function in the elderly: the Normative Aging study. *Epigenetics* (2012) 7(3):261–9. doi:10.4161/epi.7.3.19216
203. Haase H, Rink L. The immune system and the impact of zinc during aging. *Immun Ageing* (2009) 6:9. doi:10.1186/1742-4933-6-9
204. Wong CP, Rinaldi NA, Ho E. Zinc deficiency enahnced inflammatory response by increasing imune cell activation and inducing IL6 promoter demethylation. *Mol Nutr Food Res* (2015) 59(5):991–9. doi:10.1002/mnfr.201400761
205. Ligthart S, Marzi C, Aslibekyan S, Mendelson MM, Conneely KN, Tanaka T, et al. DNA methylation signatures of chronic low-grade inflammation are associated with complex diseases. *Genome Biol* (2016) 17(1):255. doi:10.1186/s13059-016-1119-5
206. Aspinall R, Andrew D. Thymic involution in aging. *J Clin Immunol* (2000) 20:250–6. doi:10.1023/A:1006611518223
207. Heyn H, Li N, Ferreira HJ, Moran S, Pisano DG, Gomez A, et al. Distinct DNA methylation of newborn and centenarians. *Proc Natl Acad Sci U S A* (2012) 109:10522–7. doi:10.1073/pnas.1120658109
208. Yung R, Ray D, Eisenbraun JK, Deng C, Attwood J, Eisenbraun MD, et al. Unexpected effects of a heterozygous dnmt1 null mutation on age-dependent DNA hypomethylation and autoimmunity. *J Gerontol A Biol Sci Med Sci* (2001) 56(6):B268–76. doi:10.1093/gerona/56.6.B268
209. Dozmorov MG, Coit P, Maksimowicz-McKinnon K, Sawalha AH. Age-associated DNA methylation changes in naive CD4+ T cells suggest an evolving autoimmune epigenotype in aging T cells. *Epigenomics* (2017) 9(4):429–45. doi:10.2217/epi-2016-0143
210. Suarez-Álvarez B, Rodríguez RM, Schlangen K, Raneros AB, Márquez-Kisinousky L, Fernández AF, et al. Phenotypic characteristics of aged CD4+ CD28null T lymphocytes are determined by changes in the whole-genome DNA methylation pattern. *Aging Cell* (2017) 16(2):293–303. doi:10.1111/acel.12552
211. Johnson ND, Wiener HW, Smith AK, Nishitani S, Absher DM, Arnett DK, et al. Non-linear patterns in age-related DNA methylation may reflect CD4+ T cell differentiation. *Epigenetics* (2017) 12(6):492–503. doi:10.1080/15592294.2017.1314419
212. Garg SK, Delaney C, Toubai T, Ghosh A, Reddy P, Banerjee R, et al. Aging is associated with increased regulatory T-cell function. *Aging Cell* (2014) 13(3):441–8. doi:10.1111/acel.12191
213. Moskowitz DM, Zhang DW, Hu B, Le Saux S, Yanes RE, Ye Z, et al. Epigenomics of human CD8 T cell differentiation and aging. *Sci Immunol* (2017) 2(8):eaag0192. doi:10.1126/sciimmunol.aag0192
214. Horvath S, Pirazzini C, Bacalini MG, Gentilini D, Di Blasio AM, Delledonne M, et al. Decreased epigenetic age of PBMCs from Italian semi-supercentenarians and their offspring. *Aging* (2015) 7(12):1159–66. doi:10.18632/aging.100861
215. McEwen LM, Morin AM, Edgar RD, MacIssac JL, Jones MJ, Dow WH, et al. Differential DNA methylation and lymphocyte proportions in a Costa Rican high longevity region. *Epigenetics Chromatin* (2017) 10:21–34. doi:10.1186/s13072-017-0128-2
216. Klinman NR, Riley RL, Stone MR, Wylie D, Zharhary D. The specificity repertoire of prereceptor and mature B cells. *Ann N Y Acad Sci* (1983) 418:130–9. doi:10.1111/j.1749-6632.1983.tb18061.x
217. Nicoletti C, Yang X, Cerny J. Repertoire diversity of antibody response to bacterial antigens in aged mice. III. Phosphorylcholine antibody from young and aged mice differ in structure and protective activity against infection with *Streptococcus pneumoniae*. *J Immunol* (1993) 150:543–9.

218. Chambers SM, Shaw CA, Gatza C, Fisk CJ, Donehower LA, Goodell MA. Aging hematopoietic stem cells decline in function and exhibit epigenetic dysregulation. *PLoS Biol* (2007) 5:e201. doi:10.1371/journal.pbio.0050201
219. Johnson KM, Owen K, Witte PL. Aging and developmental transitions in the B cell lineage. *Int Immunol* (2002) 14:1313–23. doi:10.1093/intimm/dxf092
220. Farré P, Jones MJ, Meaney MJ, Emberly E, Turecki G, Kobor MS. Concordant and discordant DNA methylation signatures of aging in human blood and brain. *Epigenetics Chromatin* (2015) 8:19. doi:10.1186/s13072-015-0011-y
221. Thunders M. Epigenetics: its understanding is crucial to a sustainable healthcare system. *Healthcare (Basel)* (2015) 3:194–204. doi:10.3390/healthcare3020194

2

An Explorative Biomarker Study for Vaccine Responsiveness after a Primary Meningococcal Vaccination in Middle-Aged Adults

*Marieke van der Heiden[1,2], Guy A. M. Berbers[1], Susana Fuentes[1], Menno C. van Zelm[3,4], Annemieke M. H. Boots[2] and Anne-Marie Buisman[1]**

[1] Centre for Infectious Disease Control (Cib), National Institute for Public Health and the Environment (RIVM), Bilthoven, Netherlands, [2] Department of Rheumatology and Clinical Immunology, University of Groningen, University Medical Centre Groningen, Groningen, Netherlands, [3] Department of Immunology, Erasmus MC, Rotterdam, Netherlands, [4] Department of Immunology and Pathology, Monash University and Alfred Hospital, Melbourne, VIC, Australia

***Correspondence:**
Anne-Marie Buisman
annemarie.buisman@rivm.nl

Introduction: Prevention of infectious diseases in the elderly is essential to establish healthy aging. Yet, immunological aging impairs successful vaccination of the elderly. Predictive biomarkers for vaccine responsiveness in middle-aged adults may help to identify responders and non-responders before reaching old age. Therefore, we aimed to determine biomarkers associated with low and high responsiveness toward a primary vaccination in middle-aged adults, for which a tetravalent meningococcal vaccine was used as a model.

Methods: Middle-aged adults (50–65 years of age, N = 100), receiving a tetravalent meningococcal vaccination, were divided into low and high responders using the functional antibody titers at 28 days postvaccination. A total of 48 parameters, including absolute numbers of immune cells and serum levels of cytokines and biochemical markers, were determined prevaccination in all participants. Heat maps and multivariate redundancy analysis (RDA) were used to reveal immune phenotype characteristics and associations of the low and high responders.

Results: Several significant differences in prevaccination immune markers were observed between the low and high vaccine responders. Moreover, RDA analysis revealed a significant association between the prevaccination immune phenotype and vaccine responsiveness. In particular, our analysis pointed at high numbers of CD4 T cells, especially naïve CD4 and regulatory T subsets, to be associated with low vaccine responsiveness. In addition, low responders showed lower prevaccination IL-1Ra levels than high responders.

Conclusion: This explorative biomarker study shows associations between the prevaccination immune phenotype and vaccine responsiveness after a primary meningococcal vaccination in middle-aged adults. Consequently, these results provide a basis for predictive biomarker discovery for vaccine responsiveness that will require validation in larger cohort studies.

Keywords: biomarkers, vaccine responsiveness, middle-aged adults, regulatory T cells, CD4 T cells, primary vaccination

INTRODUCTION

Prevention of infectious diseases in the elderly is essential to establish healthy aging in the rapidly growing aging population. Yet, immunological aging impairs successful vaccination in the elderly (1–3). Timely vaccination of middle-aged adults may be an alternative option to strengthen the memory immunity before reaching old age. Previously, we showed that a primary meningococcal vaccination, containing antigens toward which no or very low prevaccination immunity exists, was highly immunogenic in middle-aged adults (4). Moreover, we described the induction of T cell responses by the tetanus toxoid (TT) carrier protein that are in favor of efficient T cell help (5). Current research focusses on the identification of immune markers in older individuals to be able to predict the vaccine responders and non-responders (6, 7). At present, the discovery of these predictive immune markers at advanced age is challenging and results are not unambiguous.

Potential biomarkers for vaccine responsiveness may relate to shifts in the immune phenotype from naïve to more memory cells during aging. This phenomenon occurs especially in the T cell compartment and is caused by thymus involution (8–13). Accordingly, the responsiveness to a yellow fever vaccine was found positively associated with the numbers of circulating naïve CD4 T cells that had recently left the thymus (14). Infection with persistent viruses, such as cytomegalovirus (CMV), enhances the numbers of late-differentiated T cells and consequently may accelerate immunological aging (15, 16). High numbers of these late-differentiated T cells were negatively associated with influenza and varicella zoster (VZV) vaccine responses (17, 18). In addition, increased numbers of regulatory T (Treg) cells are observed at old age (19, 20) which may underlie the lower responsiveness to the influenza and VZV vaccinations (18, 21).

Age-associated changes in the B cell compartment have also been reported and include a decrease in naïve B cells and a subsequent increase in late-differentiated and exhausted B cells, as well as B cells with inflammatory characteristics (22–24). Several vaccination studies described a positive correlation between the frequencies of prevaccination Ig switched memory B cells and the responsiveness to influenza and hepatitis B vaccines (17, 23, 25–27), whereas late/exhausted (CD27–IgD–) memory B cells were negatively correlated with the response to the influenza vaccine (23). Moreover, B cell expression levels of activation-induced cytidine deaminase (AID) and TFN-α after *in vitro* stimulation were found predictive for humoral responses after influenza vaccination (23, 26, 28–30).

In addition, several innate immune functions, gene signatures, or miRNA expressions were associated with influenza vaccine responsiveness (25, 31, 32). Moreover, the age-associated increase in inflammatory mediators, also known as "inflammageing" (33–36), as well as modified expression of biochemical markers, such as dehydroepiandosterone sulfate (DHEAs) (37) and vitamin D (38), might affect the immune function at advancing age (39). Also, a range of vaccination responses, for example, to diphtheria, tetanus, and influenza, are substantially influenced by vaccine-specific prevaccination immunity (27, 31).

The studies mentioned provide some promising predictive biomarkers that require validation in other cohort studies. In the present study, we aimed to explore differences in the prevaccination immune phenotype between low and high vaccine responders toward a primary immune response upon a meningococcal vaccination in middle-aged adults.

MATERIALS AND METHODS

Study Design

Data from 100 middle-aged (50–65 years of age, 50% males) adults who received the tetravalent meningococcal vaccine conjugated to TT were used in this explorative biomarker study. These participants were included in a larger cohort study, of which exclusion criteria and study procedures are described elsewhere (4). In short, prevaccination blood samples were drawn from all participants as well as 28 days, and 1-year postvaccination blood samples. Serum samples were collected at the different time points using serum clotting tubes (BD Biosciences) and were immediately kept cold and stored within 4 h in aliquots at −20 and −80°C before further use. Blood samples were collected in tubes containing lithium heparin (BD Biosciences) for detailed cellular immune phenotyping prior to vaccination. Subsequently, different immune parameters, i.e., absolute immune cell counts, serum cytokines, CMV-specific antibodies, and biochemical markers were measured in the prevaccination blood samples of these participants. Meningococcal-specific functional antibody titers were measured in the prevaccination, as well as 28 days and 1-year postvaccination samples. A schematic overview of the study outline is depicted in **Figure 1**. In addition, all participants filled in a short health questionnaire.

Participant Selection

Functional antibody titers for the three different meningococcal groups (Meningococci C, W, and Y) were measured with the serum bactericidal antibody assay in 100 middle-aged adults, as previously described (4, 40, 41). Meningococci-A-specific analysis was left out, due to interference of cross-reactive antibodies in the antibody assays. A functional antibody titer of 8 was considered to be protective, whereas a functional antibody titer of 128 was applied as a more conservative long-term correlate of protection (4, 40).

The quartiles of the functional antibody titers 28 days postvaccination were calculated. Participants with a functional antibody titer matching the corresponding titer of the first quartile or below were considered low responders, whereas those matching the titer of the third quartile or above were considered high responders. Since part of the participants showed antibody titers equal to the cutoff value, the lowest and highest quartile do not include 25% of the participants. In total, 25, 46, and 40 low responders and 27, 35, and 34 high responders were defined for MenC, MenW, and MenY, respectively.

Flow Cytometric Analysis

At the prevaccination time point, the absolute numbers of a broad range of immune cell subsets were determined as described previously (42–44). In brief, the absolute numbers of lymphocytes, T cells, B cells, NK cells, monocytes, and granulocytes

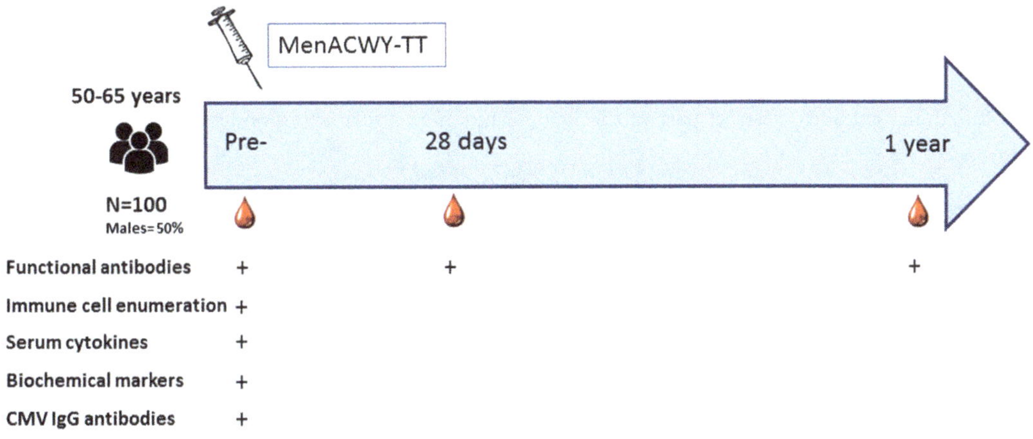

FIGURE 1 | Study outline.

were measured in fresh whole blood samples (within 18 h after collection) using TruCOUNT tubes. Gating strategies as well as a detailed description of the antibodies used were as published previously (42). Example gating strategies are shown in Figure S4 in Supplementary Material. An overview of the phenotype definitions of the different cellular subsets measured is depicted in Table S1 in Supplementary Material. These absolute cell numbers were also used to calculate the ratios between the (memory) Treg cells and the CD4$^+$CD45RO$^+$ effector memory T (TemRO) cells as well as between the CD4 naïve or CD4$^+$CD45RA$^+$CD25^{dim} cells and the CD4 memory cells. The CD4 memory cells were defined as the sum of the CD4 central memory (CM), CD4 TemRO, and CD4$^+$CD45RA$^+$ effector memory T (TemRA) cells.

Serum Cytokines

A set of inflammatory (TNF-α, MCP-1, soluble CD40L, and IL-6) and one anti-inflammatory (IL1 receptor antagonist (IL-1Ra)) serum cytokines were measured in serum samples that were kept cool right after harvest and stored at −80°C within 4 h and prevented from freeze-thaw cycles. Multiplex immunoassays (MIAs) were used to measure the serum cytokine levels as described previously (45, 46). Since serum levels of IL-6 were below detection limit, IL-6 was left out of the analysis.

Serum Biochemical Parameters

Serum levels of C-reactive protein (CRP; mg/L), Rheumatoid factor (RF; IU/mL), reactive oxygen metabolites (ROM; IU/L), and total thiol (TTT; μmol/L) were measured with a clinical auto-analyzer (Dx5, Beckman-Coulter). Dehydroepiandrosterone sulfate (DHEAs; μmol/L) and 25-hydroxyvitamin D (VitD; nmol/L) were measured using the immuno-analyzer Acces-2 from Beckman Counter.

Statistical Analyses

The functional antibody titers were compared between the high and low responders with the Mann–Whitney *U*-test. The geometric means with the 95% confidence intervals (CIs) are indicated in the graphs. The chi-square test was used to determine significant differences in patient characteristics between the high and low vaccine responders.

The different immune markers were compared between the high and low responders using the Mann–Whitney *U*-test. Furthermore, the group-specific geometric mean values of the different immune markers were normalized to *z*-scores using the geometric means and standard deviation of the total group of 100 participants. The normalized *z*-scores were displayed on a color scale in the heat maps, ranging from red (below the geometric mean of the total group) to blue (above the geometric mean of the total group). The color darkness is representative of the deviation from the total group geometric mean. For these analyses, SPSS V22.0 and Graphpad Prism V7 were used.

Multivariate redundancy analysis (RDA) was used to asses associations between vaccine responsiveness and the prevaccination immune phenotype. The absolute numbers of immune cells as well as the levels of serum cytokines and biochemical markers were imported in the analysis as biological variables, whereas vaccine responsiveness, age, sex, and CMV were included as explanatory variables. Significance of the explanatory variables was assessed by Monte Carlo permutation testing (MCPT). The *p*-values as well as the false discovery rates (FDRs) are given. Biological variables with the highest variation explained by the explanatory variables are depicted in the plots (FitE > 15). Canoco5 software for Windows (47) was used to perform this analysis. A value of p of < 0.05 was considered statistically significant.

RESULTS

Participant Characteristics

The functional antibody titers of the low and high vaccine responders 28 days postvaccination are depicted in **Figure 2A**. Although the low responders possess a functional antibody titer below or matching the first quartile of that of the total group, most of these values were above the protection level (functional antibody titer of 8). The fold differences in functional antibody titers between the low and high vaccine responders at 28 days postvaccination is 141.5, 15.2, and 16.7, for MenC, MenW, and MenY, respectively. No difference in prevaccination functional antibody titers was found between the low and high responders (**Figure 2B**). The functional antibody titers of part of the low vaccine responders had declined below the protection level at 1-year postvaccination, whereas all high responders were still highly protected (**Figure 2C**).

Participant characteristics were compared between the low and high vaccine responders (**Table 1**). Only for MenC, the

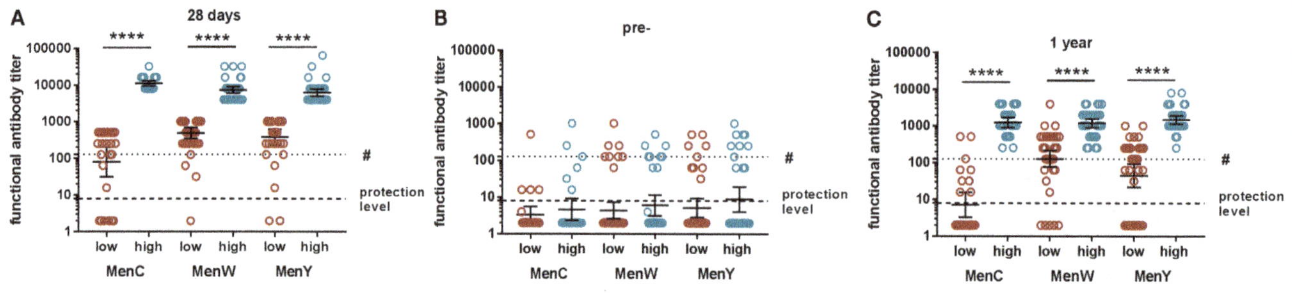

FIGURE 2 | The meningococcal group-specific functional antibody titers of the low (red) and high (blue) vaccine responders. The functional antibody titers 28 days **(A)** postvaccination, prevaccination **(B)** and 1-year postvaccination **(C)** of the low (red) and high (blue) vaccine responders. The protection level is indicated by the lowest dotted line. A more conservative long-term protection level is indicated by the # in the figures. The functional antibody titers were compared between the low and high responders using the Mann–Whitney *U*-test. MenC: low *N* = 25, high *N* = 27; MenW: low *N* = 46, high *N* = 35; and MenY: low *N* = 40, high *N* = 34. ****$p < 0.0001$.

TABLE 1 | Participant characteristics.

	MenC		MenW		MenY	
	Low	High	Low	High	Low	High
	N = 25	*N* = 27	*N* = 46	*N* = 35	*N* = 40	*N* = 34
Age (95% CI)	**59.1* (57.5–60.7)**	**56.1* (54.5–57.7)**	58.3 (57.1–59.6)	56.9 (55.5–58.4)	57.7 (56.4–59.1)	56.6 (55.0–58.1)
Males (%)	13 (52%)	16 (59%)	21 (45.6%)	19 (54.3%)	20 (50%)	17 (50%)
CMV seropositive (%)	10 (40%)	17 (63%)	21 (45.6%)	18 (51.4%)	15 (37.5%)	17 (50%)
BMI (95% CI)	24.9 (23.5–26.3)	24.8 (23.5–26.2)	25.2 (24.2–26.4)	25.8 (24.7–27.0)	24.8 (23.7–26.0)	26.5 (25.2–27.8)
TT-specific prevaccination IgG Geomean (95% CI)	0.72 (0.47–1.11)	1.20 (0.77–1.88)	0.84 (0.5–1.28)	0.87 (0.55–1.37)	1.08 (0.76–1.53)	0.78 (0.51–1.17)
Disease in last year (number, %)						
Diabetes type II	0 (0%)	1 (3.7%)	2 (4.3%)	3 (8.6%)	1 (2.5%)	2 (5.9%)
High blood pressure	5 (20.0%)	3 (11.1%)	8 (17.4%)	5 (14.3%)	6 (15%)	8 (23.5%)
Vascular diseases	0 (0%)	0 (0%)	0 (0%)	0 (0%)	1 (2.5%)	0 (0%)
Lung diseases	1 (4.0%)	1 (3.7%)	0 (0%)	4 (11.4%)	2 (5%)	2 (5.9%)
Rheumatic diseases	1 (4.0%)	1 (3.7%)	2 (4.3%)	0 (0%)	2 (5%)	0 (0%)
Gastro-intestinal diseases	0 (0%)	2 (7.4%)	2 (4.3%)	1 (2.9%)	2 (5%)	2 (5.9%)
Other diseases	1 (4.0%)	1 (3.7%)	1 (2.2%)	3 (8.6%)	1 (2.5%)	3 (8.8%)
No serious disease	18 (72%)	19 (70.4%)	35 (76.1%)	26 (74.3%)	31 (77.5%)	24 (70.6%)
Medication last 6 months (number, %)						
Medication for infection[a]	0 (0%)	4 (14.8%)	3 (6.5%)	4 (11.4%)	2 (5%)	2 (5.9%)
Cholesterol lowering medication	2 (8.0%)	2 (7.4%)	5 (10.9%)	5 (14.3%)	3 (7.5%)	4 (11.8%)
Diabetic medication	0 (0%)	1 (3.7%)	1 (2.2%)	3 (8.6%)	0 (0%)	2 (5.9%)
Blood pressure lowering medication	7 (28.0%)	3 (11.1%)	9 (19.6%)	6 (17.1%)	7 (17.5%)	8 (23.5%)
Immunosuppressive medication	0 (0%)	1 (3.7%)	1 (2.2%)	2 (5.7%)	1 (2.5%)	1 (2.9%)
No medication	18 (72%)	19 (70.4%)	32 (69.6%)	23 (65.7%)	30 (75%)	23 (67.6%)
Infections (number, %)						
Influenza < 4 weeks	0 (0%)	1 (3.7%)	1 (2.2%)	0 (0%)	1 (2.5%)	0 (0%)
Cold < 4 weeks	6 (24.0%)	3 (11.1%)	7 (15.2%)	10 (28.6%)	7 (17.5%)	6 (17.6%)
No infection < 4 weeks	19 (76.0%)	25 (92.6%)	39 (85.8%)	26 (74.3%)	33 (82.5%)	29 (85.3%)
Smoking (number, %)						
Cigarette smoking	6 (24.0%)	3 (11.1%)	6 (13%)	3 (8.6%)	6 (15%)	4 (11.8%)
Cigars, pipe smoking	1 (4.0%)	0 (0%)	3 (6.5%)	1 (2.9%)	3 (7.5%)	1 (2.9%)
No smoking	18 (72%)	25 (92.6%)	38 (82.6%)	32 (91.4%)	32 (80%)	30 (88.2%)
Physical activity (number, %)						
Weekly or more	17 (68.0%)	19 (70.4%)	31 (67.4%)	24 (68.6%)	27 (67.5%)	25 (73.5%)
Less than weekly	4 (16.0%)	2 (7.4%)	8 (17.4%)	4 (11.4%)	6 (15%)	4 (11.8%)
No activity	4 (16.0%)	7 (25.9%)	7 (15.2%)	8 (22.9%)	7 (17.5%)	6 (17.6%)

[a]*Medication used more than 3 months ago and mainly consisting of corticosteroids and antibiotics.*

**$p < 0.05$, significant differences are depicted in bold and underlined. The chi-square test was used to determine statistical significances.*

low responders were significantly older as compared with the high responders. All participants possessed prevaccination TT-specific antibodies. Sex distribution, the number of CMV seropositive participants, and BMI were comparable between the low and high responders. Moreover, no significant differences in disease incidence (within the last year), medication use (within the last 6 months), the incidence of recent infections (within the last 4 weeks), smoking, or physical activity were observed. Not all participants were identified as low or high responder consistently for all meningococcal groups.

Differences in Prevaccination Immune Markers between High and Low Vaccine Responders

At first, the absolute numbers of immune cells were compared between the high and low responders for the different meningococcal groups separately (**Figure 3A**). Low responders to MenC possessed significantly higher absolute numbers of naïve Treg ($p = 0.033$), CD45RA⁺CD25^{dim} ($p = 0.005$), CD4 naïve ($p = 0.021$), CD4 TemRA early ($p = 0.024$), and CD8 CM ($p = 0.038$) cells as compared with the high responders (**Figure 3A**; Figures S1A,C,D,F,G in Supplementary Material). Moreover, trends toward higher absolute numbers of memory Treg ($p = 0.084$) and CD4 TemRA ($p = 0.057$) cells were found in the low responders (**Figure 3A**; Figures S1B,E in Supplementary Material). In addition, the low responders to MenC showed lower serum levels of IL-1Ra ($p = 0.035$) as compared with the high responders (**Figure 3B**; Figures S1H,I in Supplementary Material), as well as a trend toward lower VitD levels ($p = 0.075$) (**Figure 3B**; Figure S1J in Supplementary Material).

Low responders for MenW possessed significantly higher absolute numbers of memory Treg cells ($p = 0.039$) (**Figure 3A**; Figure S2A in Supplementary Material) as well as a trend toward lower levels of IL-1Ra ($p = 0.057$) (**Figure 3B**; Figure S2B in Supplementary Material) as compared with the high responders.

Finally, the low responders for MenY had significantly higher absolute numbers of $CD45RA^{+}CD25^{dim}$ cells ($p = 0.022$) as well as lower absolute numbers of natural effector ($CD27^{+}IgD^{+}$) B cells ($p = 0.008$), T cells ($p = 0.043$), CD4 TemRO intermediate cells ($p = 0.011$), CD8 TemRO cells ($p = 0.027$), and CD8 TemRO late cells ($p = 0.036$) than the high responders (**Figure 3A**; Figures S3B,D,E,H,I,K in Supplementary Material). Moreover, trends toward lower absolute numbers of total B cells ($p = 0.060$), $CD27^{+}$memory B cells (Bmem) ($p = 0.062$), CD4RO T cells ($p = 0.070$), CD4RO early T cells ($p = 0.081$), and CD8 TemRO intermediate T cells ($p = 0.090$) (**Figure 3A**; Figures S3A,C,F,G,J in Supplementary Material) as well as a trend to a lower BMI ($p = 0.053$) (**Figure 3B**; Figure S3I in Supplementary Material) were observed in the low responders.

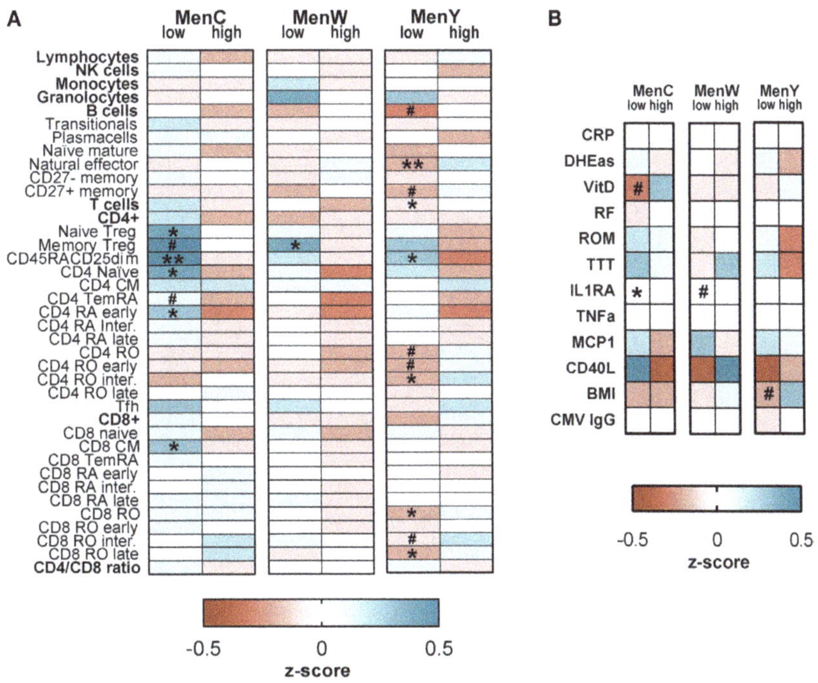

FIGURE 3 | Comparison of prevaccination immune markers between the high and low vaccine responders. Heat maps comparing the absolute immune cells numbers **(A)**, serum cytokines and biochemical markers **(B)** between the low and high vaccine responders for the different meningococcal serotypes separately. The absolute immune cell numbers as well as the concentrations of the serum markers were normalized to *z*-scores using the geometric means. The geometric means of the two groups were compared with the overall group geometric mean and standard deviation. The normalized *z*-scores are displayed on a color scale, ranging from red (below the geometric mean of the total group) to blue (above the geometric mean of the total group). The white color indicates values that are equal to the group geometric mean. The stronger the deviation from the group geometric mean, the darker the color. The different immune markers were compared between the low and high responders using the Mann–Whitney *U*-test. #$p < 0.1$, *$p < 0.05$, **$p < 0.01$. MenC: low $N = 25$, high $N = 27$; MenW: low $N = 46$, high $N = 35$; and MenY: low $N = 40$, high $N = 34$.

Multivariate RDA Revealing Significant Associations between the Prevaccination Immune Phenotype and Vaccine Responsiveness

In order to determine whether high or low vaccine responsiveness at day 28 postvaccination was significantly associated with all measured prevaccination immune markers combined, hereafter called the immune phenotype; a multivariate RDA was performed for the three meningococcal groups separately (**Figures 4A–C**). Overall the included variables (age, sex, CMV, BMI, and vaccine response) explained 14.5, 10.4, and 12.0% of the total variation in immune phenotype for MenC, MenW, and MenY, respectively.

For MenC and MenY, the variable "vaccine response" was significantly associated with the immune phenotype (MenC: $p = 0.012$, FDR = 0.07 and MenY: $p = 0.028$, FDR = 0.098) (**Figures 4A,C**). As expected, based on the heat map depicted in **Figure 3A**, for MenW no significant association between vaccine response and immune phenotype was observed ($p = 0.068$, FDR = 0.16) (**Figure 4B**).

For MenC group, higher levels of DHEA, TTT, and ROM as well as higher absolute numbers of memory Treg cells, naïve Treg cells, CD45RA^{+}CD25^{dim} cells, CD4 TemRA early cells, CD4 naïve cells, lymphocytes, and CD4 T cells were strongly associated with low responsiveness, whereas higher levels of IL-1Ra were related with high responsiveness (**Figure 4A**). For MenY group, higher levels of DHEA and higher absolute numbers of CD4 naïve, CD45RA^{+}CD25^{dim}, CD8 naïve, and naïve Treg cells were strongly associated with low vaccine responsiveness, while high absolute numbers of Bmem cells were linked to high vaccine responsiveness (**Figure 4C**).

In addition, CMV seropositivity was significantly associated with the immune phenotype (**Figure 4A**: $p = 0.098$, FDR = 0.23, **Figure 4B**, $p = 0.002$, FDR = 0.014, and **Figure 4C**, $p = 0.002$, FDR = 0.014). In these analyses, CMV seropositivity was associated with higher absolute numbers of CD4RO late, CD4RA late, and CD8RA late T cells, and not related to either low or high vaccine responsiveness. Of note, the explanatory variables BMI, age, and sex were not significantly associated with the immune phenotype.

Differences in Immune Cell Ratios in the CD4 T Cell Compartment between the High and Low Vaccine Responders

In relation to the mentioned findings of higher naïve CD4 T cells and memory Treg cells in the low vaccine responders, we determined whether the ratio of naïve to memory cells, as well as the ratio of Treg to effector cells in the CD4 T cell compartment was different between the low and high vaccine responders

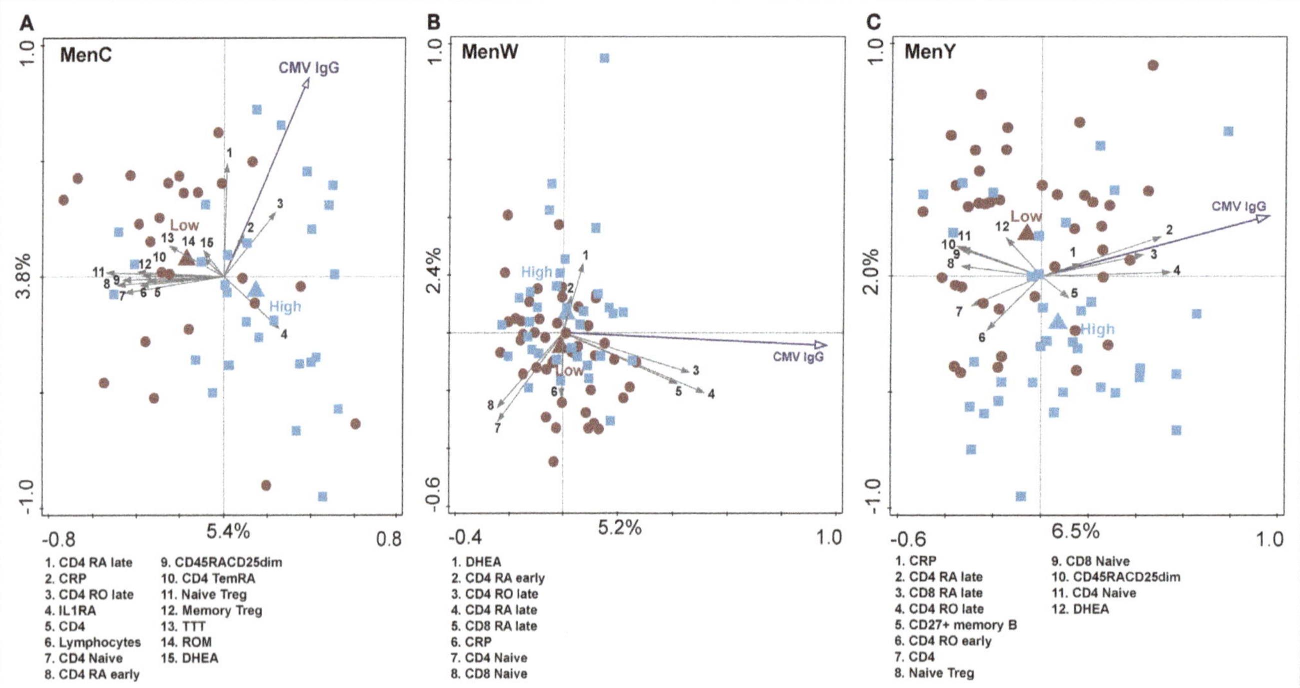

FIGURE 4 | Redundancy analysis (RDA) assessing the association between the prevaccination immune phenotype and the meningococcal vaccine response. RDA of samples collected 28 days postvaccination for MenC **(A)**, MenW **(B)**, and MenY **(C)**. Low vaccine responders are shown in red circles; High responders are shown in light blue squares. The first and second ordination axes are plotted, including the percentages of explained variation. Overall, 14.5, 10.4, and 12.0% of the variation in the datasets was explained for MenC, MenW, and MenY, respectively. The vaccine response variable (i.e., low or high responder) was significantly associated with the immune phenotype for MenC ($p = 0.012$, FDR = 0.07) and MenY ($p = 0.028$, FDR = 0.098), but not for MenW ($p = 0.068$, FDR = 0.16). CMV was significantly associated with the immune composition for MenW ($p = 0.002$, FDR = 0.014) and MenY ($p = 0.002$, FDR = 0.014) but not for MenC ($p = 0.098$, FDR = 0.23). Other environmental variables tested (i.e., BMI, age, and sex) did not significantly influence the variation in the dataset. The biological variables with the highest variation explained by the explanatory variables are depicted in the plots (FitE > 15). The length of the arrows relates to the strength of the association.

(**Figure 5**). No difference in the ratio between the total Treg cells and the number of CD4 TemRO T cells was observed (**Figure 5A**), whereas the ratio of memory Treg cells to CD4 TemRO T cells was significantly higher in the low responders for MenC and MenY as compared with the high responders (**Figure 5B**). In addition, the low responders for MenC and MenY possessed a significantly higher ratio of the naïve CD4 T cells and the total CD4 memory cells (**Figure 5C**), as well as a higher ratio of the post thymically expanded $CD45RA^{+}CD25^{dim}$ cells and the total CD4 memory cells (**Figure 5D**). Thus, the higher numbers of both naïve CD4 T cell subsets and Treg cells as seen in low responders at baseline (prevaccination) give rise to clear compositional changes in the peripheral CD4 T cell compartment.

DISCUSSION

In this explorative study, we investigated whether the prevaccination immune phenotype was significantly different between the middle-aged adults being either low or high responder after a primary meningococcal vaccination. Interestingly, the numbers of several CD4 T cell subsets differed between the low and high vaccine responders. More specifically, low vaccine responders possessed higher numbers of naïve Treg, memory Treg, naïve CD4 cells, and the subset of post thymically expanded $CD4^{+}CD45RA^{+}CD25^{dim}$ T cells, whereas high responders showed high levels of serum IL-1Ra. These results suggest that the prevaccination CD4 signature may be used to identify middle-aged adults who are potential non/low responders to a primary meningococcal vaccine. Identification of these middle-aged adults may help improve timely vaccination strategies, since vaccination schemes, doses, and adjuvant use might be adapted to improve the vaccine responsiveness in these adults.

Numbers of Treg cells are known to increase with advancing age and suggest elevated immune suppression in older adults, although the exact functionality of these Treg cells in aging individuals is still under investigation (19, 48). Accordingly, high numbers of Treg cells were previously associated with low VZV vaccine responses in nursing home elderly (18). Within our study, high absolute numbers of both naïve and memory Treg cells were associated with low vaccine responsiveness. Naïve Treg cells express CCR7 enabling these cells to migrate to lymphoid organs, whereas memory Treg cells home to the sites of inflammation along with effector T cells (49, 50). Accordingly, our results suggest enhanced suppression of the vaccine response both in the lymphoid organs as well as the site of vaccination in low responders. Elevated numbers of Treg cells might suppress T cell responses toward the tetanus carrier in this conjugated meningococcal vaccine and/or inhibit B cell responses directly (51). Our results confirm previous findings of high numbers of memory Treg cells in low vaccine responders to influenza (21), whereas we are the first showing an association between low vaccine responsiveness and high numbers of naïve Treg cells. Of importance, we observed a higher ratio of memory Treg to effector CD4 T cells in the low responders, suggesting a shift in the Treg/Teffector balance, as previously observed with advancing age (21).

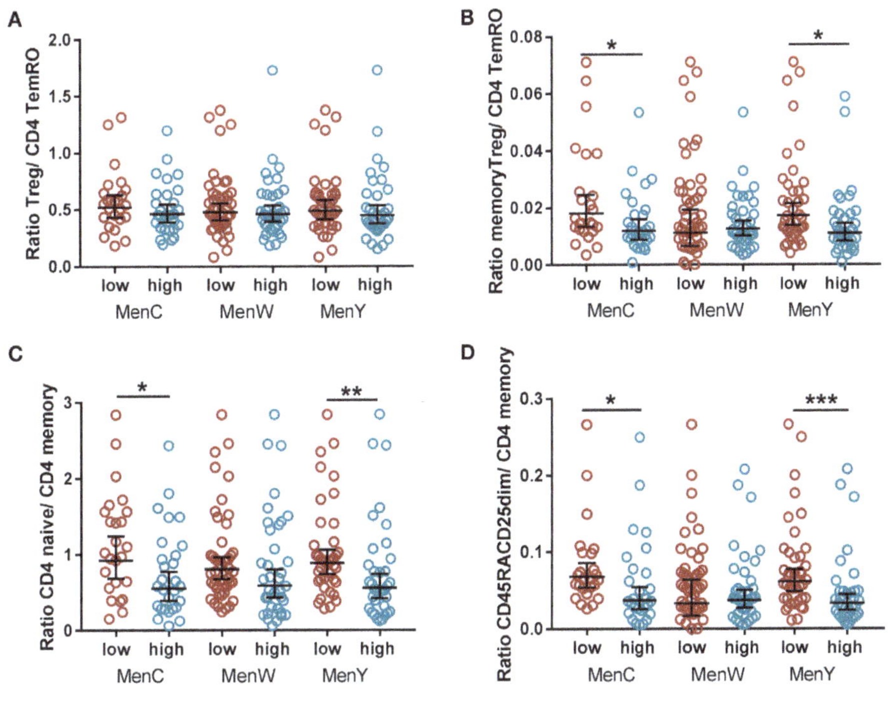

FIGURE 5 | Comparison of immune cell ratios in the CD4 T cell compartment between the high and low vaccine responders. Comparison of the Treg/TemRO ratio **(A)**, memory Treg/TemRO ratio **(B)**, CD4 naïve/CD4 memory ratio **(C)**, and $CD45RA^{+}CD25^{dim}$/CD4 memory ratio **(D)** between the low (red) and high (blue) vaccine responders for the different meningococcal groups separately. The total CD4 memory cells were determined as the sum of the CD4 CM, CD4 TemRO, and CD4 TemRA cells. The low and high responders were compared with the Mann–Whitney *U*-test. $^{*}p < 0.05$, $^{**}p < 0.01$, and $^{***}p < 0.001$.

The consistent association found between high numbers of CD4 naïve and the post thymically expanded $CD4^+CD45RA^+CD25^{dim}$ cells and a higher ratio of these naïve cells to the memory CD4 T cell compartment with low vaccine responsiveness was unexpected, since a naïve T cell repertoire is generally accepted to be beneficial in older adults (9, 11). Previously, the $CD4^+CD45RA^+CD25^{dim}$ subset was found to represent a broad and functional reservoir of naïve CD4 T cells, although some contraction in certain TCR Vβ families was observed in comparison to naïve CD4 T cells that recently left the thymus (52). Since no prior studies were available that linked the numbers of $CD4^+CD45RA^+CD25^{dim}$ cells to vaccine responses, our findings indicate the necessity for further research into repertoire size and functionality of these cells. However, the increase in memory Treg cells might be the dominant factor in predicting vaccine response, overruling the presence of a capable naïve CD4 T cell repertoire.

In line with the different studies investigating biomarkers for influenza and hepatitis B vaccine responses in the elderly (17, 23, 25), we observed trends toward lower numbers of switched memory $CD27^+$ B cells in the low responders. In contrast, we did not find increased numbers of CD27-memory B cells in the low responders, as reported by others in vaccine recipients aged over 65 years (23). In addition, low numbers of natural effector $CD27^+IgD^+$ B cells that were previously found to decrease with age (24) were observed in the low vaccine responders. Since we previously described that IgM is essential in the antibody functionality against the meningococcal groups (4), lower numbers of these natural effector cells, mainly producing IgM, likely explain the lower functional antibody titers.

Currently, effects of latent CMV infection on vaccine responses are controversial (53). Despite the clear associations between CMV seropositivity and higher numbers of late differentiated T cells, we did not find an association between CMV seropositivity and meningococcal vaccine responsiveness. As this meningococcal vaccine response is primarily B cell mediated, the effect of CMV might be limited. Hence, the effects of CMV on T cell-mediated vaccine responses, i.e., to influenza and VZV vaccination should be further elucidated. Although frequently suggested by others (54–57), we did not observe any effects of sex and BMI on the vaccine responses. Moreover, the effect of chronological age was inconsistent, although low responders to MenC were significantly older than high responders.

Of note, high levels of IL-1Ra were found in the high responders. IL-1Ra is known as the receptor antagonist of the IL-1 family, executing anti-inflammatory functions (58, 59). These results possibly suggest that IL-1Ra acts as an anti-inflammatory counterpart of the "inflammageing" process. Of note, a trend toward high levels of MCP-1 was found in the low responders. MCP-1 is classified as a pro-inflammatory cytokine, attracting monocytes to the site of inflammation, and serum levels were shown to increase with age (60). Consequently, our findings may suggest a higher pro-inflammatory state in the low responders (33, 34). Nevertheless, serum levels of other inflammatory cytokines, such as IL-6 and TFN-α were still low in all participants. Remarkably, trends toward higher levels of sCD40L were found in the low responders for MenC, as compared with lower levels in the low responders for MenW and MenY, which needs further evaluation.

Of importance, associations with the immune phenotype were primarily found between the extremes in the vaccine response, being either low or high responders. The intermediate group showed high variability of immune markers. In addition, our results may imply meningococcal group-specific associations between the prevaccination immune phenotype and vaccine responsiveness. Noteworthy, the difference in functional antibody titers between the low and high vaccine responders was largest for MenC, possibly explaining the higher numbers of immune parameters found associated with the vaccine response for this meningococcal group. Moreover, the participants that were classified as low or high responder did not completely overlap between the different meningococcal groups. This might be explained by the structural differences in the meningococcal polysaccharides by which different meningococcal epitopes will induce distinct immune responses (61), also shown previously for several pneumococcal conjugated polysaccharides (62). Possible structural differences will affect the B cell processing and subsequently the quality and quantity of the T cell help provided by the carrier, that might cause differences in antibody functionality to the various polysaccharides. Currently, differences between meningococcal group-specific polysaccharides conjugated to TT are not known (63). Furthermore despite similar prevaccination functional antibody titers in the low and high vaccine responders, differences in numbers of meningococcal group-specific memory B cells in the bone marrow could have been present due to historical contacts (64) and affect the vaccine response. Nevertheless, the finding of meningococcal group-specific associations between vaccine responsiveness and immune phenotype is remarkable and requires further research. Of note, we previously found that most participants possessed high prevaccination TT-specific antibody levels (4). Importantly, no direct correlation between the antibody responses to TT or the different polysaccharides and the strength or classification of the T cell response induced by the TT-carrier protein was observed (5). In this study, the similar prevaccination TT-specific antibody levels in the low and high responders, suggests that the prevaccination immunity against the TT carrier protein did not largely affect the immune responses.

An important strength of this study is the ability to compare multiple antigens and multiple immune parameters within the same group of participants. Also, the primary nature of the vaccination allowed us to explore the use of biomarkers, without the strong interference of prevaccination meningococcal immunity, as often seen in other studies. Unfortunately, the presence of prevaccination immunity in some participants did interfere with the long-term functional antibody titers (after 1 year). Consequently, we were not able to investigate the associations between prevaccination immune phenotype and the long-term vaccine responsiveness, since exclusion of participants with detectable prevaccination functional antibody titers dramatically reduced the power of the statistical analysis. In addition, information on the genetic background of the participants could have added to the predictive factors in our analysis, since several studies found associations between genetic signatures and vaccine responsiveness (25, 31, 32).

Future studies, analyzing large cohorts, using different vaccines, and using similar biomarker analyzing techniques are warranted to validate the use of the suggested biomarkers. Hence, systems vaccinology, combining data on genetic background, and environmental factors such as diet, stress, and infections, and even microbiome composition is a promising tool to discover these predictive biomarkers (65). Moreover, future research should compare the suitability of biomarkers in cohorts of different ages, in order to determine the predictive values of these markers over the entire lifespan.

In conclusion, our explorative biomarker analysis suggests several associations between the prevaccination immune phenotype and vaccine responsiveness after primary meningococcal vaccination in middle-aged adults. In general, an altered CD4 T cell signature, involving high absolute numbers of naïve Treg, memory Treg, naïve CD4 T cells, and $CD45RA^{+}CD25^{dim}$ T cells might be used as a predictive immune phenotype for low vaccine responsiveness in middle-aged adults. Accordingly, these findings support the development of vaccination strategies to enhance the memory immunity before reaching old age, in the rapidly aging population.

ETHICS STATEMENT

Written informed consent was obtained from all participants prior to enrollment and all procedures were in accordance with the Declaration of Helsinki. The medical ethical committee: Medical Research Ethics Committees United (MEC-U) approved the study and the study was registered at the Dutch trial register (Protocol no. NTR4636).

AUTHOR CONTRIBUTIONS

MH, GB, MZ, A-MB, and AB conceptualized the study. MH planned and performed the clinical work and executed the laboratory experiments. MH and SF performed the statistical analysis. MH, GB, MZ, MD, SF, A-MB, and AB interpreted the data and wrote the manuscript. All authors critically revised the manuscript.

ACKNOWLEDGMENTS

We thank all the middle-aged adults who participated in this study and the nurses who performed the vaccinations and blood drawings. Moreover, we thank Martijn Dolle, Eugene Jansen, and Piet Beekhof for their help with biochemical marker analysis. Furthermore, we thank Wilco de Jager from the Luminex department (UMCU) for measuring the serum cytokine levels. Moreover, we are grateful to Jan van de Kasteele for the statistical advice and Gerco den Hartog for critically reviewing the manuscript.

FUNDING

This work was supported by the Dutch Ministry of Public Health and an Erasmus MC Fellowship to MZ.

REFERENCES

1. Lang PO, Aspinall R. Immunosenescence and herd immunity: with an ever-increasing aging population do we need to rethink vaccine schedules? *Expert Rev Vaccines* (2012) 11(2):167–76. doi:10.1586/erv.11.187
2. Boraschi D, Aguado MT, Dutel C, Goronzy J, Louis J, Grubeck-Loebenstein B, et al. The gracefully aging immune system. *Sci Transl Med* (2013) 5(185):185s8. doi:10.1126/scitranslmed.3005624
3. Poland GA, Ovsyannikova IG, Kennedy RB, Lambert ND, Kirkland JL. A systems biology approach to the effect of aging, immunosenescence and vaccine response. *Curr Opin Immunol* (2014) 29:62–8. doi:10.1016/j.coi.2014.04.005
4. van der Heiden M, Boots AM, Bonacic Marinovic A, de Rond LG, van Maurik M, Tcherniaeva I, et al. Novel intervention in the aging population: a primary meningococcal vaccine inducing protective IgM responses in middle-aged adults. *Front Immunol* (2017) 8:817. doi:10.3389/fimmu.2017.00817
5. van der Heiden M, Duizendstra A, Berbers GA, Boots AM, Buisman A-M. Tetanus toxoid carrier protein induced T-helper cell responses upon vaccination of middle-aged adults. *Vaccine* (2017) 35(42):5581–8. doi:10.1016/j.vaccine.2017.08.056
6. High KP, D'Aquila RT, Fuldner RA, Gerding DN, Halter JB, Haynes L, et al. Workshop on immunizations in older adults: identifying future research agendas. *J Am Geriatr Soc* (2010) 58(4):765–76. doi:10.1111/j.1532-5415.2010.02772.x
7. Goronzy JJ, Weyand CM. Understanding immunosenescence to improve responses to vaccines. *Nat Immunol* (2013) 14(5):428–36. doi:10.1038/ni.2588
8. den Braber I, Mugwagwa T, Vrisekoop N, Westera L, Mögling R, de Boer AB, et al. Maintenance of peripheral naive T cells is sustained by thymus output in mice but not humans. *Immunity* (2012) 36(2):288–97. doi:10.1016/j.immuni.2012.02.006
9. Herndler-Brandstetter D, Ishigame H, Flavell RA. How to define biomarkers of human T cell aging and immunocompetence? *Front Immunol* (2013) 4:136. doi:10.3389/fimmu.2013.00136
10. George AJ, Ritter MA. Thymic involution with ageing: obsolescence or good housekeeping? *Immunol Today* (1996) 17(6):267–72. doi:10.1016/0167-5699(96)80543-3
11. Arnold CR, Wolf J, Brunner S, Herndler-Brandstetter D, Grubeck-Loebenstein B. Gain and loss of T cell subsets in old age – age-related reshaping of the T cell repertoire. *J Clin Immunol* (2011) 31(2):137–46. doi:10.1007/s10875-010-9499-x
12. Weng NP, Akbar AN, Goronzy J. CD28(-) T cells: their role in the age-associated decline of immune function. *Trends Immunol* (2009) 30(7):306–12. doi:10.1016/j.it.2009.03.013
13. Akbar AN, Henson SM, Lanna A. Senescence of T lymphocytes: implications for enhancing human immunity. *Trends Immunol* (2016) 37(12):866–76. doi:10.1016/j.it.2016.09.002
14. Schulz AR, Mälzer JN, Domingo C, Jürchott K, Grützkau A, Babel N, et al. Low thymic activity and dendritic cell numbers are associated with the immune response to primary viral infection in elderly humans. *J Immunol* (2015) 195(10):4699–711. doi:10.4049/jimmunol.1500598
15. Weltevrede M, Eilers R, de Melker HE, van Baarle D. Cytomegalovirus persistence and T-cell immunosenescence in people aged fifty and older: a systematic review. *Exp Gerontol* (2016) 77:87–95. doi:10.1016/j.exger.2016.02.005
16. Fülöp T, Larbi A, Pawelec G. Human T cell aging and the impact of persistent viral infections. *Front Immunol* (2013) 4:271. doi:10.3389/fimmu.2013.00271
17. Haralambieva IH, Painter SD, Kennedy RB, Ovsyannikova IG, Lambert ND, Goergen KM, et al. The impact of immunosenescence on humoral immune response variation after influenza A/H1N1 vaccination in older subjects. *PLoS One* (2015) 10(3):e0122282. doi:10.1371/journal.pone.0122282
18. Lelic A, Verschoor CP, Lau VW, Parsons R, Evelegh C, Bowdish DM, et al. Immunogenicity of varicella vaccine and immunologic predictors of response in a cohort of elderly nursing home residents. *J Infect Dis* (2016) 214(12):1905–10. doi:10.1093/infdis/jiw462
19. Gregg R, Smith CM, Clark FJ, Dunnion D, Khan N, Chakraverty R, et al. The number of human peripheral blood CD4+ CD25high

regulatory T cells increases with age. *Clin Exp Immunol* (2005) 140(3):540–6. doi:10.1111/j.1365-2249.2005.02798.x
20. Hirokawa K, Utsuyama M, Hayashi Y, Kitagawa M, Makinodan T, Fulop T. Slower immune system aging in women versus men in the Japanese population. *Immun Ageing* (2013) 10(1):19. doi:10.1186/1742-4933-10-19
21. van der Geest KS, Abdulahad WH, Tete SM, Lorencetti PG, Horst G, Bos NA, et al. Aging disturbs the balance between effector and regulatory CD4+ T cells. *Exp Gerontol* (2014) 60:190–6. doi:10.1016/j.exger.2014.11.005
22. Siegrist CA, Aspinall R. B-cell responses to vaccination at the extremes of age. *Nat Rev Immunol* (2009) 9(3):185–94. doi:10.1038/nri2508
23. Frasca D, Diaz A, Romero M, Blomberg BB. Human peripheral late/exhausted memory B cells express a senescent-associated secretory phenotype and preferentially utilize metabolic signaling pathways. *Exp Gerontol* (2017) 87:113–20. doi:10.1016/j.exger.2016.12.001
24. Dunn-Walters D. The ageing human B cell repertoire: a failure of selection? *Clin Exp Immunol* (2016) 183(1):50–6. doi:10.1111/cei.12700
25. Fourati S, Cristescu R, Loboda A, Talla A, Filali A, Railkar R, et al. Prevaccination inflammation and B-cell signalling predict age-related hyporesponse to hepatitis B vaccination. *Nat Commun* (2016) 7:10369. doi:10.1038/ncomms10369
26. Frasca D, Diaz A, Romero M, Phillips M, Mendez NV, Landin AM, et al. Unique biomarkers for B-cell function predict the serum response to pandemic H1N1 influenza vaccine. *Int Immunol* (2012) 24:175–82. doi:10.1093/intimm/dxr123
27. Tsang JS, Schwartzberg PL, Kotliarov Y, Biancotto A, Xie Z, Germain RN, et al. Global analyses of human immune variation reveal baseline predictors of postvaccination responses. *Cell* (2014) 157(2):499–513. doi:10.1016/j.cell.2014.03.031
28. Frasca D, Diaz A, Romero M, Landin AM, Blomberg BB. High TNF-α levels in resting B cells negatively correlate with their response. *Exp Gerontol* (2014) 54:116–22. doi:10.1016/j.exger.2014.01.004
29. Frasca D, Diaz A, Romero M, Mendez NV, Landin AM, Blomberg BB. Effects of age on H1N1-specific serum IgG1 and IgG3 levels evaluated during the 2011–2012 influenza vaccine season. *Immun Ageing* (2013) 10(1):14. doi:10.1186/1742-4933-10-14
30. Frasca D, Diaz A, Romero M, Landin AM, Blomberg BB. Cytomegalovirus (CMV) seropositivity decreases B cell responses to the influenza vaccine. *Vaccine* (2015) 33(12):1433–9. doi:10.1016/j.vaccine.2015.01.071
31. Furman D, Jojic V, Kidd B, Shen-Orr S, Price J, Jarrell J, et al. Apoptosis and other immune biomarkers predict influenza vaccine responsiveness. *Mol Syst Biol* (2013) 9(1):659. doi:10.1038/msb.2013.15
32. Nakaya HI, Hagan T, Duraisingham SS, Lee EK, Kwissa M, Rouphael N, et al. Systems analysis of immunity to influenza vaccination across multiple years and in diverse populations reveals shared molecular signatures. *Immunity* (2015) 43(6):1186–98. doi:10.1016/j.immuni.2015.11.012
33. Franceschi C. Inflammaging as a major characteristic of old people: can it be prevented or cured? *Nutr Rev* (2007) 65(s3):S173–6. doi:10.1301/nr.2007.dec.S173-S176
34. Pangrazzi L, Meryk A, Naismith E, Koziel R, Lair J, Krismer M, et al. "Inflamm-aging" influences immune cell survival factors in human bone marrow. *Eur J Immunol* (2017) 47:481–92. doi:10.1002/eji.201646570
35. Singh T, Newman AB. Inflammatory markers in population studies of aging. *Ageing Res Rev* (2011) 10(3):319–29. doi:10.1016/j.arr.2010.11.002
36. Sohal RS, Weindruch R. Oxidative stress, caloric restriction, and aging. *Science* (1996) 273(5271):59. doi:10.1126/science.273.5271.59
37. Orentreich N, Brind JL, Rizer RL, Vogelman JH. Age changes and sex differences in serum dehydroepiandrosterone sulfate concentrations throughout adulthood. *J Clin Endocrinol Metab* (1984) 59(3):551–5. doi:10.1210/jcem-59-3-551
38. Sakem B, Nock C, Stanga Z, Medina P, Nydegger UE, Risch M, et al. Serum concentrations of 25-hydroxyvitamin D and immunoglobulins in an older Swiss cohort: results of the senior labor study. *BMC Med* (2013) 11(1):1–9. doi:10.1186/1741-7015-11-176
39. Engelfriet PM, Jansen EH, Picavet HSJ, Dollé ME. Biochemical markers of aging for longitudinal studies in humans. *Epidemiol Rev* (2013) 35:132–51. doi:10.1093/epirev/mxs011
40. Borrow R, Balmer P, Miller E. Meningococcal surrogates of protection—serum bactericidal antibody activity. *Vaccine* (2005) 23(17):2222–7. doi:10.1016/j.vaccine.2005.01.051
41. Borrow R, Andrews N, Goldblatt D, Miller E. Serological basis for use of meningococcal serogroup C conjugate vaccines in the United Kingdom: reevaluation of correlates of protection. *Infect Immun* (2001) 69(3):1568–73. doi:10.1128/IAI.69.3.1568-1573.2001
42. van der Heiden M, van Zelm MC, Bartol SJ, de Rond LG, Berbers GA, Boots AM, et al. Differential effects of cytomegalovirus carriage on the immune phenotype of middle-aged males and females. *Sci Rep* (2016) 6:26892. doi:10.1038/srep26892
43. Van Den Heuvel D, Jansen MA, Nasserinejad K, Dik WA, van Lochem EG, Bakker-Jonges LE, et al. Effects of nongenetic factors on immune cell dynamics in early childhood: the Generation R Study. *J Allergy Clin Immunol* (2017) 139(6):1923–34.e17. doi:10.1016/j.jaci.2016.10.023
44. Heeringa JJ, Hajdarbegovic E, Thio HB, van Zelm MC. Systemic B-cell abnormalities in patients with atopic dermatitis? *J Allergy Clin Immunol* (2016) 138(1):317–8. doi:10.1016/j.jaci.2016.01.038
45. de Jager W, Prakken BJ, Bijlsma JW, Kuis W, Rijkers GT. Improved multiplex immunoassay performance in human plasma and synovial fluid following removal of interfering heterophilic antibodies. *J Immunol Methods* (2005) 300(1):124–35. doi:10.1016/j.jim.2005.03.009
46. de Jager W, Bourcier K, Rijkers GT, Prakken BJ, Seyfert-Margolis V. Prerequisites for cytokine measurements in clinical trials with multiplex immunoassays. *BMC Immunol* (2009) 10(1):52. doi:10.1186/1471-2172-10-52
47. Ter Braak C, Šmilauer P. *Canoco Reference Manual and User's Guide: Software for Ordination (Version 5.0)*. Wageningen. Ithaca, USA: Microcomputer Power (2012).
48. Jagger A, Shimojima Y, Goronzy JJ, Weyand CM. Regulatory T cells and the immune aging process: a mini-review. *Gerontology* (2014) 60(2):130–7. doi:10.1159/000355303
49. Menning A, Höpken UE, Siegmund K, Lipp M, Hamann A, Huehn J. Distinctive role of CCR7 in migration and functional activity of naïve- and effector/memory-like Treg subsets. *Eur J Immunol* (2007) 37(6):1575–83. doi:10.1002/eji.200737201
50. Duhen T, Duhen R, Lanzavecchia A, Sallusto F, Campbell DJ. Functionally distinct subsets of human FOXP3+ Treg cells that phenotypically mirror effector Th cells. *Blood* (2012) 119(19):4430–40. doi:10.1182/blood-2011-11-392324
51. Lim HW, Hillsamer P, Banham AH, Kim CH. Cutting edge: direct suppression of B cells by CD4+ CD25+ regulatory T cells. *J Immunol* (2005) 175(7):4180–3. doi:10.4049/jimmunol.175.7.4180
52. Geest KS, Abdulahad WH, Teteloshvili N, Tete SM, Peters JH, Horst G, et al. Low-affinity TCR engagement drives IL-2-dependent post-thymic maintenance of naive CD4+ T cells in aged humans. *Aging Cell* (2015) 14(5):744–53. doi:10.1111/acel.12353
53. Müller L, Hamprecht K, Pawelec G. The role of CMV in immunosenescence. *The Ageing Immune System and Health*. Springer (2017). p. 53–68.
54. Poland G, Ovsyannikova I, Kennedy R. Personalized vaccinology: a review. *Vaccine* (2017). doi:10.1016/j.vaccine.2017.07.062
55. Klein SL, Marriott I, Fish EN. Sex-based differences in immune function and responses to vaccination. *Trans R Soc Trop Med Hyg* (2015) 109(1):9–15. doi:10.1093/trstmh/tru167
56. Weber DJ, Rutala WA, Samsa GP, Santimaw JE, Lemon SM. Obesity as a predictor of poor antibody response to hepatitis B plasma vaccine. *JAMA* (1985) 254(22):3187–9. doi:10.1001/jama.254.22.3187
57. Talbot H, Coleman L, Crimin K, Zhu Y, Rock M, Meece J, et al. Association between obesity and vulnerability and serologic response to influenza vaccination in older adults. *Vaccine* (2012) 30(26):3937–43. doi:10.1016/j.vaccine.2012.03.071
58. Arend WP, Malyak M, Guthridge CJ, Gabay C. Interleukin-1 receptor antagonist: role in biology. *Annu Rev Immunol* (1998) 16(1):27–55. doi:10.1146/annurev.immunol.16.1.27
59. Gabay C, Smith MF, Eidlen D, Arend WP. Interleukin 1 receptor antagonist (IL-1Ra) is an acute-phase protein. *J Clin Invest* (1997) 99(12):2930. doi:10.1172/JCI119488
60. Mansfield A, Nevala W, Dronca RS, Leontovich A, Shuster L, Markovic SN. Normal ageing is associated with an increase in Th2 cells, MCP-1 (CCL1) and RANTES (CCL5), with differences in sCD40L and PDGF-AA between sexes. *Clin Exp Immunol* (2012) 170(2):186–93. doi:10.1111/j.1365-2249.2012.04644.x

61. Bröker M, Dull PM, Rappuoli R, Costantino P. Chemistry of a new investigational quadrivalent meningococcal conjugate vaccine that is immunogenic at all ages. *Vaccine* (2009) 27(41):5574–80. doi:10.1016/j.vaccine.2009.07.036
62. Kamboj KK, Kirchner HL, Kimmel R, Greenspan NS, Schreiber JR. Significant variation in serotype-specific immunogenicity of the seven-valent *Streptococcus pneumoniae* capsular polysaccharide-CRM197 conjugate vaccine occurs despite vigorous T cell help induced by the carrier protein. *J Infect Dis* (2003) 187(10):1629–38. doi:10.1086/374785
63. Bröker M, Berti F, Costantino P. Factors contributing to the immunogenicity of meningococcal conjugate vaccines. *Hum Vaccin Immunother* (2016) 12(7):1808–24. doi:10.1080/21645515.2016.1153206
64. Perrett KP, Jin C, Clutterbuck E, John TM, Winter AP, Kibwana E, et al. B cell memory to a serogroup C meningococcal conjugate vaccine in childhood and response to booster: little association with serum IgG antibody. *J Immunol* (2012) 189(5):2673–81. doi:10.4049/jimmunol.1200451
65. Hagan T, Nakaya HI, Subramaniam S, Pulendran B. Systems vaccinology: enabling rational vaccine design with systems biological approaches. *Vaccine* (2015) 33(40):5294–301. doi:10.1016/j.vaccine.2015.03.072

Effect of Age on NK Cell Compartment in Chronic Myeloid Leukemia Patients Treated with Tyrosine Kinase Inhibitors

Paulo Rodrigues-Santos[1,2,3†‡], *Nelson López-Sejas*[4†‡], *Jani Sofia Almeida*[2,3], *Lenka Ruzičková*[5], *Patricia Couceiro*[2,3], *Vera Alves*[1,3], *Carmen Campos*[4*], *Corona Alonso*[4], *Raquel Tarazona*[6], *Paulo Freitas-Tavares*[5], *Rafael Solana*[4*†§] *and Manuel Santos-Rosa*[1,3†§]

[1] *Faculty of Medicine, Institute of Immunology, University of Coimbra, Coimbra, Portugal,* [2] *Laboratory of Immunology and Oncology, Center for Neuroscience and Cell Biology, University of Coimbra, Coimbra, Portugal,* [3] *Faculty of Medicine, Center of Investigation in Environment, Genetics and Oncobiology - CIMAGO, University of Coimbra, Coimbra, Portugal,* [4] *Department of Immunology, Instituto Maimónides de Investigación Biomédica de Córdoba - Reina Sofia University Hospital - University of Córdoba, Córdoba, Spain,* [5] *Hematology Service, Coimbra Hospital and Universitary Centre, Coimbra, Portugal,* [6] *Immunology Unit, University of Extremadura, Cáceres, Spain*

***Correspondence:**
Carmen Campos
mccampos1977@gmail.com
Rafael Solana
rsolana@uco.es

† *These authors have contributed equally to this work*

‡ *These authors share co-first authorship*

§ *These authors share co-senior authorship*

Natural killer (NK) cells are a very important component of the innate immune response involved in the lysis of virus infected and tumor cells. Aging has a profound impact in the frequency, phenotype and function of NK cells. Chronic Myeloid Leukemia (CML) is caused by the BCR-ABL gene formation encoding aberrant oncoprotein tyrosine kinase. Treatment with tyrosine kinase inhibitors (TKIs) induces durable deep molecular response. The response to treatment and life expectancy is lower in older patients with chronic phase of CML than in younger patients. In this work we analyse NK cells from TKI-treated CML patients and healthy controls stratified according to age. We have analyzed the expression of NK receptors, activation markers, NK cell differentiation in CD56^{bright} and CD56^{dim} NK cell subsets and the expression of CD107a and IFN-γ in NK cells stimulated with K562. Whereas significant differences on the phenotype and function of NK cells were found between middle-aged (35–65 years old) and elderly (older than 65) healthy individuals, NK cells from TKI-treated CML patients do not show significant differences related with age in most parameters studied, indicating that age is not a limitation of the NK cell recovery after treatment with TKI. Our results also revealed differences in the expression of NK receptors, activation markers and functional assays in NK cells from TKI-treated CML patients compared with age-matched healthy controls. These results highlight the relevance of NK cells in TKI-treated patients and the need of an extensive analysis of the effect of aging on NK cell phenotype and function in these patients in order to define new NK-cell based strategies directed to control CML progression and achieve long-term disease remission after TKI cessation.

Keywords: aging, CML, NK receptors, activation markers, differentiation markers, cytokines, NK cell subsets, tyrosine kinase inhibitors

INTRODUCTION

Natural Killer cells (NK) are innate lymphoid cells (ILCs) that represent ~15% of peripheral blood lymphocytes (PBLs). NK cells share many features with ILC1 although they are developmentally distinct (1). NK cells can be classified in two major subpopulations according to CD56 expression. $CD56^{bright}$ NK cells are less differentiated subpopulation that represents <10% of peripheral blood NK cells and have an immune-modulatory role with high production of cytokines and chemokines. $CD56^{dim}$ NK cells, a more differentiated subpopulation that represents about 90% of NK cells, are mainly cytotoxic and interferon-gamma (IFN-γ) producers after direct contact with target cells (2, 3). A model of differentiation from immature $CD56^{bright}$ that leads to more mature $CD56^{dim}$ NK cells in the periphery has been proposed (4). Another subpopulation of NK cells, that do not express CD56 but express other NK receptors, expanded in healthy old and HIV-1 or hepatitis C infected individuals (5, 6), has been defined. NK cell function depends on a balance between activating and inhibitory signals triggered by activating and inhibitory receptors (7).

Chronic Myeloid Leukemia (CML) is an aging-associated disease (approximately half of cases are diagnosed in people older than 65) caused by reciprocal translocation between chromosomes 9 and 22 that give rise to the Philadelphia chromosome (Ph) and the BCR-ABL gene formation that encodes an oncoprotein tyrosine kinase with an aberrant activity in the hematopoietic stem cells (8, 9). Age has been included as a poor prognostic factor for survival in CML (10, 11). About half of the patients diagnosed with CML are between 60 and 65 years old (12–14) and the response to disease and life expectancy is lower in older patients with chronic phase of CML than in younger patients (15, 16). However, elderly CML patients are underrepresented in clinical studies having a reduced access to investigational therapies and median age of CML patients in cancer registries and patients included in clinical trials differs by 10–20 years (13, 14), supporting the interest to study immune parameters in elderly CML patients.

Immunosenescence is defined as age-associated dysregulation and dysfunction of the immune system characterized by impaired protective immunity and decreased efficacy of vaccines (17–20). These changes mainly affect the adaptive immune response (21) although consistent findings reveal that innate immune response is also affected (22, 23). In addition to age, situations of chronic activation of the human immune system, such as viral infections, autoimmune diseases and cancer, are involved in the development of immunosenescence (24–27).

Age-related alterations in frequency, distribution, phenotype, and function of NK cell subsets have been described, including an increased expression of CD57 (considered a marker of 'memory-like' NK) and a decreased expression of Natural Cytotoxicity Receptors (NCRs) and other NK activating receptors (22, 23, 28–31), CD69 (32), and CD94/NKG2A, and an increase of killer Ig-like receptors (KIR) (33–35) in older individuals.

Several studies have also found a decrease in the frequency and function of NK cells in CML patients at the time of diagnosis, with a progressive functional deterioration during all phases of the disease (36–39). It has been described a decreased expression of NKG2A, NKp30, and NKp46 at the time of diagnosis and changes in the NKG2C and KIR receptors (40, 41). Patients with CML also show a decrease in NKG2D expression, that mediates NK anti-CML response through its ligands MICA/B, when compared with healthy controls (42). NK cells from acute myeloid leukemia patients also have a downregulated expression of activating receptors NKp30 and NKp46 (27, 43–45) and DNAM-1 (27, 46), likely as a consequence of the interaction with their ligands in leukemic blasts.

The standard treatment for CML patients is based in the use of tyrosine kinase inhibitors (TKIs) such as imatinib, and more potent second-generation nilotinib and dasatinib, that have improved CML poor prognosis (47, 48). TKIs have a direct effect inhibiting the BCR-ABL1 kinase activity to induce a durable deep molecular response, a prelude to successful treatment-free remission that occurs in ~50% of all CML patients who cease TKI therapy (48–51). In addition to their direct anti-kinase activity, TKIs contribute to the restoration of immune cell function leading to the efficient immunological control of CML (41). Recent studies show the impact of TKIs on NK cells, finding that the expression of NK activating receptors is restored to normal levels compared to their low level at the time of diagnosis (40, 41).

Considering that both aging and CML induce changes in phenotype and function of NK cells, in this work we have studied the expression of several markers (CD11b, CD27, CD57, CD69, HLA-DR, NKG2A, NKG2C, NKG2D, NKp30, NKp44, NKp46, and NKp80) in NK cell subsets, and CD107a and IFN-γ in K562 stimulated NK cells, from CML patients and healthy controls, stratified according to age in middle-aged and elderly donors.

MATERIALS AND METHODS

Study Subjects

A total of 80 individuals were included in the study, 38 CML patients treated with first-line TKIs Imatinib, and 42 healthy controls, stratified in two groups according to age: middle-aged (35–65 years) and old-age (over 65 years) (**Table 1**). All the participants in the study were CMV-seropositive (Non-reactive IgM and reactive IgG, data not shown). Controls were excluded of the study if they had infection at the time of sample collection, suffered or had suffered cancer or autoimmune diseases, were under immunosuppressive drugs or calcium channel blockers. The Ethical Committees of the Faculty of Medicine of the University of Coimbra and the Coimbra Hospital and University Centre (Portugal) and the Ethics Committee of the Reina Sofia University Hospital of Cordoba (Spain) approved this study and all volunteers agreed and signed informed consent to participate.

Procedures of Sample Collection and Processing

Peripheral blood samples from all individuals were obtained in heparinized tubes. Flow cytometry studies were performed on freshly-obtained cells. After antibody staining, BD FACS Lysing Solution (BD Biosciences, San Jose, CA, USA) was used for lysis of red blood cells. Subsequently, cells were washed and resuspended in Dulbecco's Phosphate Buffered Saline (PBS)

TABLE 1 | Demographics characteristics of individuals ($n = 80$).

Group name	No.	Sex (male: female)	Mean (SD)[a]	p[b]
Middle age (Control)	19	8:11	51 (7.85)	0.924
Middle age (CML*)	19	12:7	51 (8.97)	
OLD (Control)	23	10:13	74 (6.17)	0.814
OLD (CML*)	19	12:7	75 (5.71)	

[a]*Average age (Standard Deviation) of the group.*
[b]*p-value for the comparison of means between controls and CML, within the same age group (t-Student test).* **TKI-treated CML patients.*

pH 7.4 (Ambion, Austin, TX, USA) for later acquisition on the cytometer. Cell suspensions were acquired in a BD FACS Canto II cytometer (BD Biosciences, San Jose, CA, USA). These procedures were performed according to the manufacturer protocols.

Flow Cytometric Analysis and Monoclonal Antibodies

Fresh blood was used for the analysis of the surface receptors by flow cytometry in different tubes. The following mouse anti-human conjugated monoclonal antibodies (mAbs) were used: anti-CD3 V500 (clone UCHT1, BD Horizon), anti-CD14 V500 (clone M5E2, BD Horizon), anti-CD19 V500 (clone HIB19, BD Horizon), anti-CD3 APC-H7 (clone SK7, BD Biosciences), anti-CD56 PerCP-Cy5.5 (clone HCD56, BD Pharmingen), anti-CD11b V450 (clone ICRF44, BD Horizon), anti-CD27 FITC (clone 0323, Biolegend), anti-CD57 Pacific Blue (clone HNK-1, Biolegend), anti-CD69 FITC (clone FN50, Biolegend), anti-HLA-DR V500 (clone G46-6, BD Pharmingen), anti-NKp30 Alexa Fluor 647 (clone P30-15, Biolegend), anti-NKp44 Alexa Fluor 647 (clone P44-8, Biolegend), anti-NKp46 PE (clone 9E2, Biolegend), anti-NKp80 PE (clone SD12, Biolegend), anti-NKG2A PE (clone 131411, R&D Systems), anti-NKG2C APC (clone 134591 R&D Systems), anti-NKG2D APC (clone 1D11, Biolegend). The expression of HLA-DR, NKp30, NKp44, NKp46, NKp80, NKG2D, (measured as Median Fluorescence Intensity, MFI) and the expression of CD11b, CD27, CD57, CD69, NKG2A, and NKG2C (measured as relative frequency) were determined in the different NK cell subpopulations and analyzed by multiparametric flow cytometry. The data were analyzed using FlowJo v10 (Tree Star, Inc.) from PBLs, selecting singlets. NK cells ($CD56^+$ and $CD3^-/CD14^-/CD19^-$) were selected and two subpopulations of NK cells were described, in relation to their expression of CD56, as $CD56^{bright}$ and $CD56^{dim}$ (**Figure S1A**). Isotype matched antibodies, labeled with the appropriate fluorochromes, were used as negative controls. Representative histograms for the NK cell markers, and the isotype and fluorochrome of the antibodies used in the studies, are shown in **Figure S1B**.

NK Cell Stimulation With K562, Degranulation Assay, and IFN-γ Staining

Effector peripheral blood mononuclear cells were isolated from heparinized blood samples by a standard density gradient procedure (Ficoll-Paque PLUS, Merck KGaA, Darmstadt, Germany) and counted to adjust the concentration to 50 × 10^6cells/mL. Target cells (K562 cell line) were prepared; viability determined and counted to adjust the concentration to 1 × 10^5cells/mL. Then, effector and target cells were mixed in a 25:1 effector-to-target ratio into 12 × 75 mm tubes with anti-CD107a PE (clone H4A3, BD Pharmingen®) antibody and brefeldin A (Merck, 10 μg/mL). Tubes were incubated in a humidified CO_2 incubator in the water reservoir at the bottom for 4 h. At the end of incubation cells were washed and resuspended in 100 μL of 1xPBS (phosphate-buffered saline) and the extracellular antibodies were added, anti-CD56 APC (clone B159, BD Pharmingen®) and anti-CD3V500 (clone UCTH1, BD Horizon®). After 15 min of incubation at RT in the dark, suspensions were treated with Fix and Perm A solution (Invitrogen®) for 15 min, in the dark at room temperature. Cells were centrifuged at 453 g for 5 min and the supernatant discarded. Next, cells were incubated with Fix and Perm B solution (Invitrogen®) and the intracellular antibody anti-IFN-γ PE-Cy7 (clone B27, BD Horizon®) for 20 min, in the dark at room temperature. After centrifugation at 453 g for 5 min and supernatant discarded cells were resuspended in 1x PBS and acquired in the flow cytometer (BD FACS Canto II).

Statistical Analysis

Shapiro-Wilk test was used for checking the normal distribution of the data. We used Kruskall-Wallis (non-parametric) test for multiple comparison and Mann-Whitney *U*-test (non-parametric) was used to compare specific groups. All tests were performed using statistical software package SPSS 18.0 (SPSS Inc., Chicago, IL, USA). Values $p < 0.05$ were considered significant. The results were shown as median with interquartile range and the graphics were performed using GraphPad Prism software version 6.0 (GraphPad Software, La Jolla, CA, USA).

RESULTS

Expression of Activating and Inhibitory Receptors on NK Cells From TKI-Treated CML Patients

We studied the expression of activating and inhibitory receptors on $CD56^{dim}$ and $CD56^{bright}$ NK cells in healthy donors and CML patients, stratified in middle age and old age. The expression of Natural Killer Group 2 (NKG2) receptors was measured as the percentage of positive cells or as MFI measured in the total of cells (**Figure 1A**). Our results showed a significant decrease in the expression of the inhibitory receptor NKG2A on $CD56^{dim}$ NK cells in middle-aged CML patients compared with middle-aged healthy donors and a decrease in the percentage of $NKG2A^+CD56^{bright}$ NK cells in old CML patients compared with old healthy donors. Age-associated changes in the expression of NKG2A were only observed in healthy donors showing an increase with age in the percentage of $NKG2A^+CD56^{bright}$ NK cells. In contrast, NKG2C receptor expression was not influenced by CML or age. Regarding the activating receptor NKG2D, we found a significant decrease in

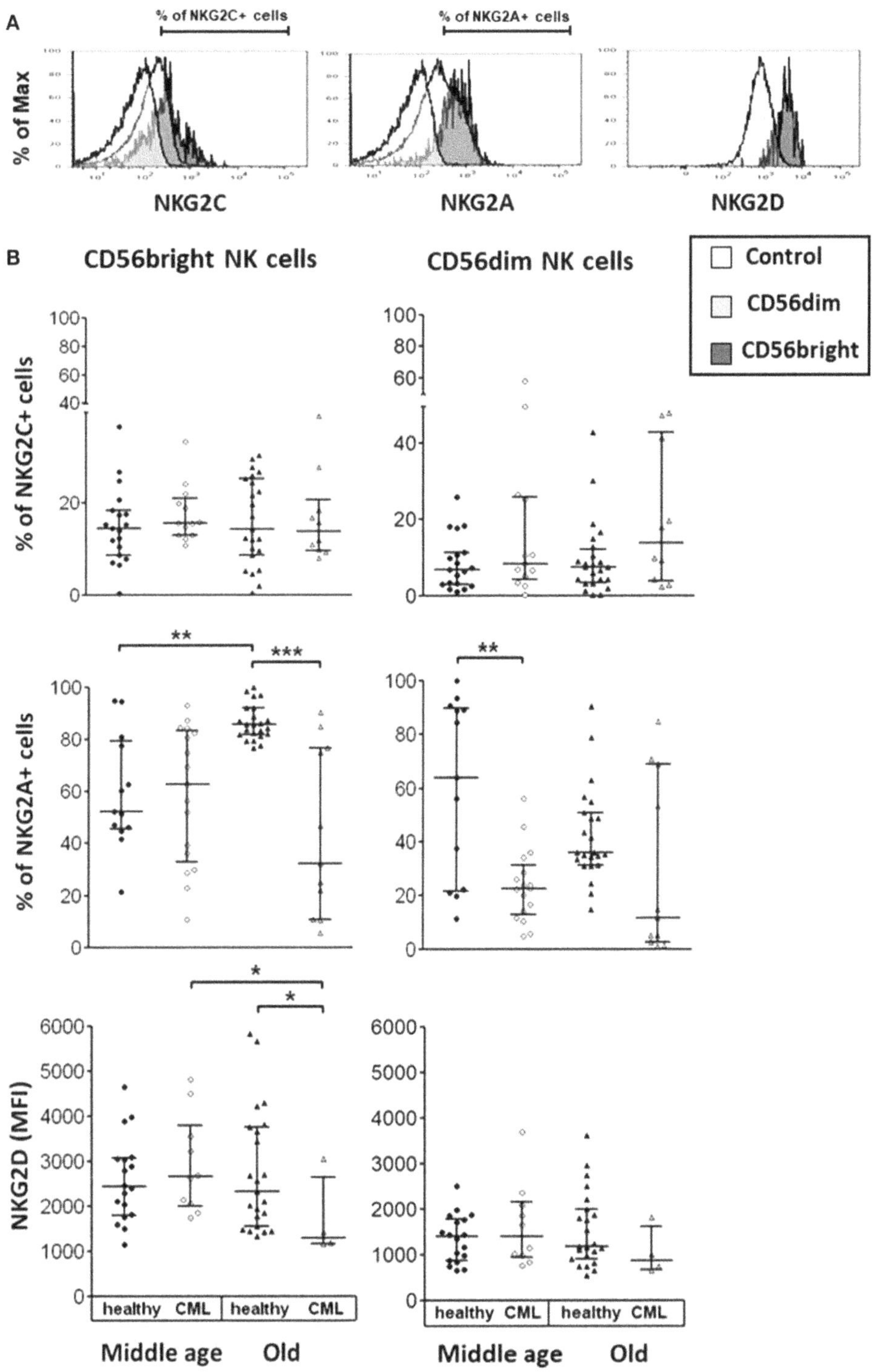

FIGURE 1 | Expression of Natural Killer Group 2 (NKG2) receptors on NK cell subpopulations. **(A)** Representative histograms for each marker are shown (the non-shaded area represents the control, the shaded area of light gray, the CD56^{dim} cells, the shaded one of gray, the CD56^{bright} cells). The percentage of cells expressing NKG2C, NKG2A, and NKG2D as (MFI) measured in the total of cells, was determined on the surface of each subset by multiparametric flow cytometry. **(B)** Expression of activating receptors (NKG2C and NKG2D) and of inhibitory receptor (NKG2A) on CD56^{bright} and CD56^{dim} NK subsets from healthy individuals and TKI-treated CML patients, stratified according to age (middle-aged 35–65 years and old >65 years). Number of donors: NKG2C middle-aged healthy $n = 19$, middle-aged CML $n = 13$, old healthy $n = 23$, and old CML $n = 10$; NKG2D middle-aged healthy $n = 18$, middle-aged CML $n = 10$, old healthy $n = 23$, and old CML $n = 4$; NKG2A middle-aged healthy $n = 13$, middle-aged CML $n = 17$, old healthy $n = 23$, and old CML $n = 11$. The results, expressed as median with interquartile range, were considered significant at $p < 0.05$. *P*-values were determined comparing middle age with old and healthy with TKI-treated CML patients. *p <0.05; **p <0.01; ***p <0.001.

the MFI of NKG2D on CD56^{bright} NK cells in old CML patients compared with old healthy donors, and a decrease with age in CML patients (**Figure 1B**).

We have also studied the expression of NCRs on NK cell subpopulations. Results were expressed as MFI measured in the total number of cells (**Figure 2A**). We have found that the expression of NKp30 and NKp80 (not a NCR) on CD56^{bright} NK cells and NKp80 on CD56^{dim} NK cells was lower in old CML patients compared with old healthy donors. NKp80 expression on CD56^{bright} cells and NKp46 expression on CD56^{dim} NK cells were significantly decreased in middle-aged CML patients compared with middle-aged healthy donors. The analysis of age-associated changes in the expression of NCRs in CML patients showed a decrease in NKp30 expression on CD56^{bright} NK cells. No significant differences associated with age (middle-aged vs. old age) were observed in healthy donors (**Figure 2B**).

Expression of Activation Markers of NK Cells From TKI-Treated CML Patients

In this study, we have analyzed the expression of several activation markers (HLA-DR, CD69, and NKp44) on the surface of NK cell subsets in resting conditions. CD56^{bright} NK cells in elderly CML patients showed a decreased expression of HLA-DR (measured as MFI) and a reduction in the percentage of CD69 and NKp44 positive cells compared with elderly healthy donors. An age-associated increase in the expression of these three markers was observed on CD56^{bright} NK cells in elderly healthy donors compared with middle-aged healthy donors. In contrast, in CML patients a decrease of CD69 expression on CD56^{bright} NK cells was associated with age (**Figure 3A**).

Regarding the expression of these activation markers on the CD56^{dim} NK cell subset, our results showed a decreased expression of these markers in elderly CML patients, as well as a decreased expression of CD69 and HLA-DR in middle-aged CML patients compared with age-matched healthy donors. Nevertheless, it is interesting to highlight the increase observed in the percentage of NKp44^{+} cells in middle-aged CML patients compared with middle-aged healthy donors. We also found an age-associated increase in the expression of HLA-DR and NKp44 in healthy individuals and a decrease of CD69 and NKp44 expression in CD56^{dim} NK cells from elderly CML patients compared with CD56^{dim} NK cells from middle-aged CML patients (**Figure 3B**).

Analysis of NK Cell Differentiation Markers on NK Cells From TKI-Treated CML Patients

The analysis of NK cell subsets in healthy donors showed a decreased percentage of CD56^{bright} that correlated with an increased percentage of CD56^{dim} NK cells in elderly donors compared with middle-aged healthy donors. In contrast, no statistical significant differences in NK cell subset distribution was observed in CML patients according to age. Percentage of total NK cells was not influenced by CML or age (**Figure 4A**). The expression of CD57 was increased on CD56^{dim} NK cells from CML patients compared with age-matched healthy donors. Moreover, in healthy individuals, CD57 expression on both CD56^{bright} and CD56^{dim} NK cells increased with age (**Figure 4B**). The co-expression of CD11b and CD27 markers was also analyzed in each NK cell subset (**Figure 4C**). Whereas, a high percentage of CD56^{bright} NK cells were CD11b^{+}CD27^{+}, the majority of CD56^{dim} NK cells from peripheral blood were CD11b^{+}CD27^{-}. Our results revealed a decrease of CD11b^{+}CD27^{+}CD56^{dim} NK cells associated with CML in middle-aged individuals and a decrease of this cell subset related to age in healthy donors (**Figure 4C**). Not significant differences were found in CD56^{bright} NK cells.

CD107a Expression and IFN-γ Production in NK Cells From TKI-Treated CML Patients Activated With K562

We analyzed the percentage of NK cells expressing CD107a or IFN-γ after stimulation with the K562 cell line. Representative analysis of middle-aged and old controls and TKI-treated CML patients are shown **Figures 5A,C**. The results did not show significant differences on CD107a expression and IFN-γ production in K562 stimulated NK cells between middle-aged healthy donors and middle-aged CML patients. NK cells from healthy elderly donors have higher expression of CD107a or IFN-γ compared with middle-aged healthy donors. In a similar way the percentage of NK cells expressing CD107a or IFN-γ was higher in healthy elderly donors than in TKI-treated CML old patients. On the contrary no significant age-associated differences on CD107a expression and IFN-γ production were observed in K562 stimulated NK cells from CML patients (**Figures 5B,D**).

As shown in **Figure S2**, the comparison of cytokine production in healthy controls vs. TKI-treated CML patients shows that the expression of IFN-γ by unstimulated NK cells is higher in middle-aged TKI-treated CML patients and lower in elderly patients compared with their age-matched controls, whereas the expression of IL-10 is higher in TKI-treated CML patients from both age groups compared with their respective controls.

DISCUSSION

A decrease in the frequency and function of NK cells in CML patients at the time of diagnosis has been demonstrated, with a progressive functional deterioration during disease progression to advanced and blast crisis phase (36–39, 52). In addition, NK cells from CML patients at diagnosis show a reduced expression of activating and inhibitory NK receptors compared to healthy donors (40, 53). NK cells play an important role in the control of CML not only during TKI treatment (40, 41) but also after TKI cessation (54, 55).

It has been shown that life expectancy is lower in older than in younger patients with chronic phase of CML and that aging is a poor prognostic factor for survival and response to treatment in CML (10, 11, 15, 16). Cumulative evidences support that aging affects NK cell subsets, phenotype and

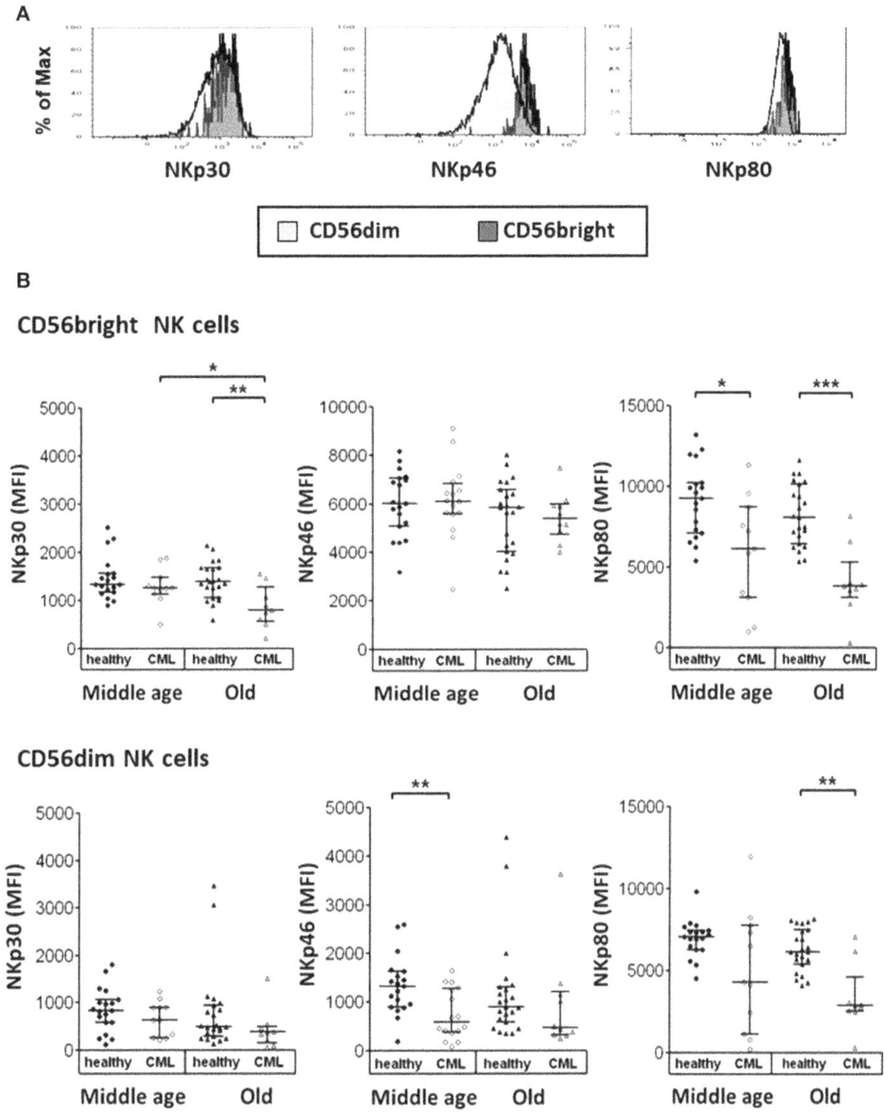

FIGURE 2 | Expression of Natural Cytotoxicity Receptors (NCRs) on CD56^{bright} and CD56^{dim} NK cells. **(A)** Representative histograms for NKp30, NKp46, and NKp80 are shown (the shaded area of light gray, the CD56^{dim} cells, the shaded one of gray, the CD56^{bright} cells). Results were expressed as Median Fluorescence Intensity (MFI), measured in the total of cells. **(B)** Expression of activating receptors NKp30, NKp46, and NKp80 on CD56^{bright} and CD56^{dim} NK subsets from healthy individuals and TKI-treated CML patients, stratified according to age (middle-aged 35–65 years and old >65 years). Number of donors: NKp30 and NKp80 middle-aged healthy $n = 19$, middle-aged CML $n = 11$, old healthy $n = 23$, and old CML $n = 9$; NKp46 middle-aged healthy $n = 19$, middle-aged CML $n = 16$, old healthy $n = 23$ and old CML $n = 10$. The results were expressed as median with interquartile range. *P*-values were determined comparing middle age with old and healthy with TKI-treated CML patients and were considered significant at $p < 0.05$. * $p < 0.05$; ** $p < 0.01$; *** $p < 0.001$.

function (22, 23, 56), including the expression of activating and inhibitory NK cell receptors (28–30, 57). The analysis of NK cells from middle-aged and elderly healthy donors, summarized in **Figure 6A**, is in line with previous data on the differences between NK cells from young and old healthy donors. Thus, there are significant differences in the frequency of NK cells subsets with different maturation stages. The percentages of more immature CD56^{bright} NK cells (2, 3), and CD11b^{+}/CD27^{+} NK cells, that represent a minor subset of immunoregulatory NK cells described as an intermediate differentiation stage (58), are lower in elderly than in middle-aged healthy donors, whereas the percentage of mature highly cytotoxic CD56^{dim}CD57^{+} NK cells is higher in the elderly (**Figure 6A**), confirming the age-associated shaping of NK cell subsets (22, 30). The expression of NK cell activation markers HLA-DR, CD69, and NKp44 is also higher in NK cells from elderly healthy donors, likely as a consequence of low grade age-associated inflammation (inflamm-aging) (59). Inflamm-aging is also consistent with the observation that NK cells from old healthy donors show higher expression of CD107a or IFN-γ in response to K562

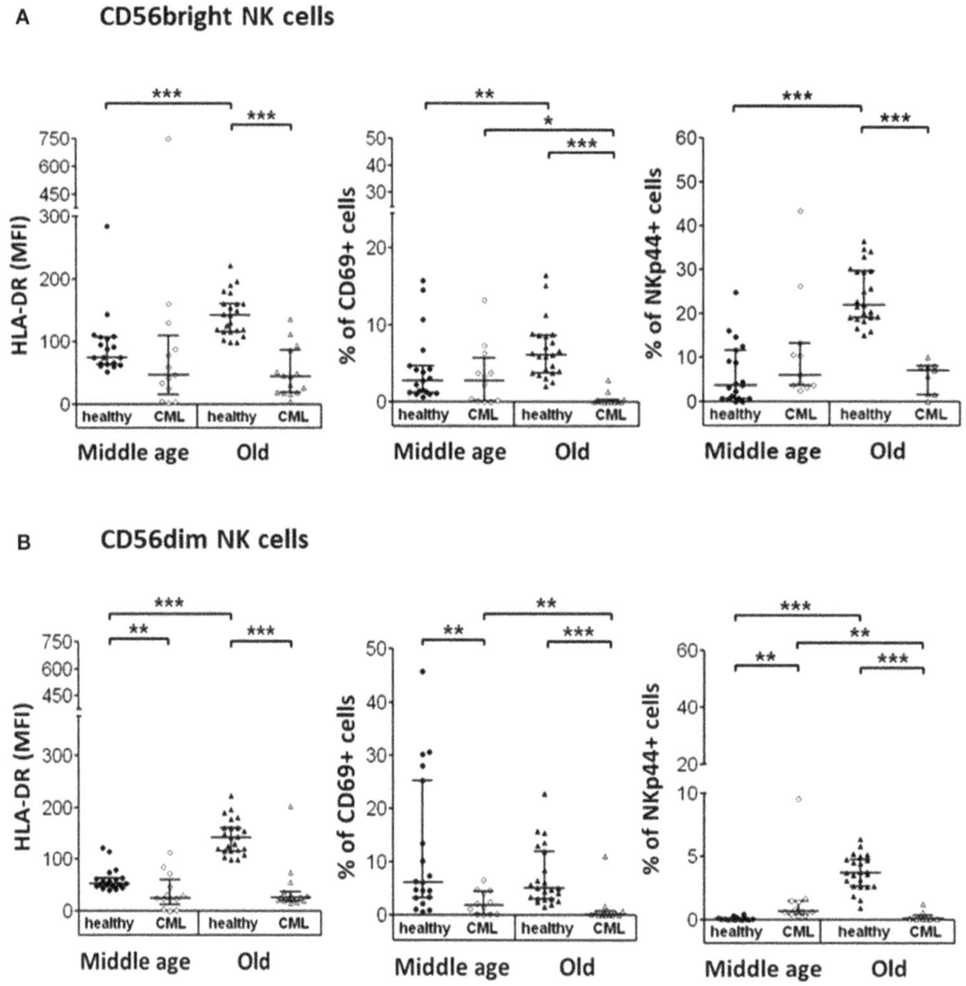

FIGURE 3 | Expression of activation markers on CD56^{bright} and CD56^{dim} NK cell subpopulations. Determination of activation markers expression (HLA-DR, CD69, and NKp44) on the surface of CD56^{bright} and CD56^{dim} NK cells from the different study groups. NK cells were not stimulated. **(A)** Expression of HLA-DR (measured as MFI), CD69 and NKp44 (in percentage) on CD56^{bright} NK cells. **(B)** Expression of HLA-DR (MFI) and percentage of CD69 and NKp44 on CD56^{dim} NK cells. Number of donors: HLA-DR middle-aged healthy $n = 19$, middle-aged CML $n = 13$, old healthy $n = 23$ and old CML $n = 15$; CD69 middle-aged healthy $n = 19$, middle-aged CML $n = 12$, old healthy $n = 23$, and old CML $n = 15$; NKp44 middle-aged healthy $n = 19$, middle-aged CML $n = 11$, old healthy $n = 23$, and old CML $n = 9$. The results, expressed as median with interquartile range, were considered significant at $p < 0.05$. *P*-values were determined comparing middle age with old and healthy with TKI-treated CML patients. *$p < 0.05$; **$p < 0.01$; ***$p < 0.001$.

stimulation than NK cells from middle-aged donors. The effect of aging on NK cell cytotoxicity and IFN-γ has been extensively analyzed in discrepant results have been found among different groups probably due to different selection age ranges, technical procedures, and health status of the individuals studied although it is generally accepted that the total number and cytotoxic function of NK cell are preserved or increased in healthy aging compared with young and middle-aged individuals (22, 23, 56).

The study of NK cells in middle-aged TKI-treated CML patients shows that the percentage of CD56^{bright} NK cells is similar to the percentage found in heathy middle-aged individuals, whereas the minor population of CD56^{dim} NK cells co-expressing CD11b and CD27 is dramatically decreased (**Figure 6B**). In addition, CD56^{dim} NK cells from TKI-treated CML patients have higher expression of CD57, a marker of highly differentiated NK cells (22, 30), and NKp44 indicating that NK cells from TKI-treated CML patients are highly differentiated activated NK cells, as it has been recently suggested (40, 54). However, there is a lower expression of NKp46, NKG2A, CD69, and HLA-DR on CD56^{dim} NK cells and of NKp80 on CD56^{bright} NK cells (**Figure 6B**). The comparison of NK cells from old TKI-treated CML patients with those from old healthy individuals shows a lower expression of NK receptors NKp44, NKp80, CD69, and HLA-DR in both CD56^{bright} and CD56^{dim} NK cells and also a reduced expression of NKp30, NKG2D, and NKG2A in CD56^{bright} NK cells (**Figure 6C**). Thus, despite the well-established observations that CML patients

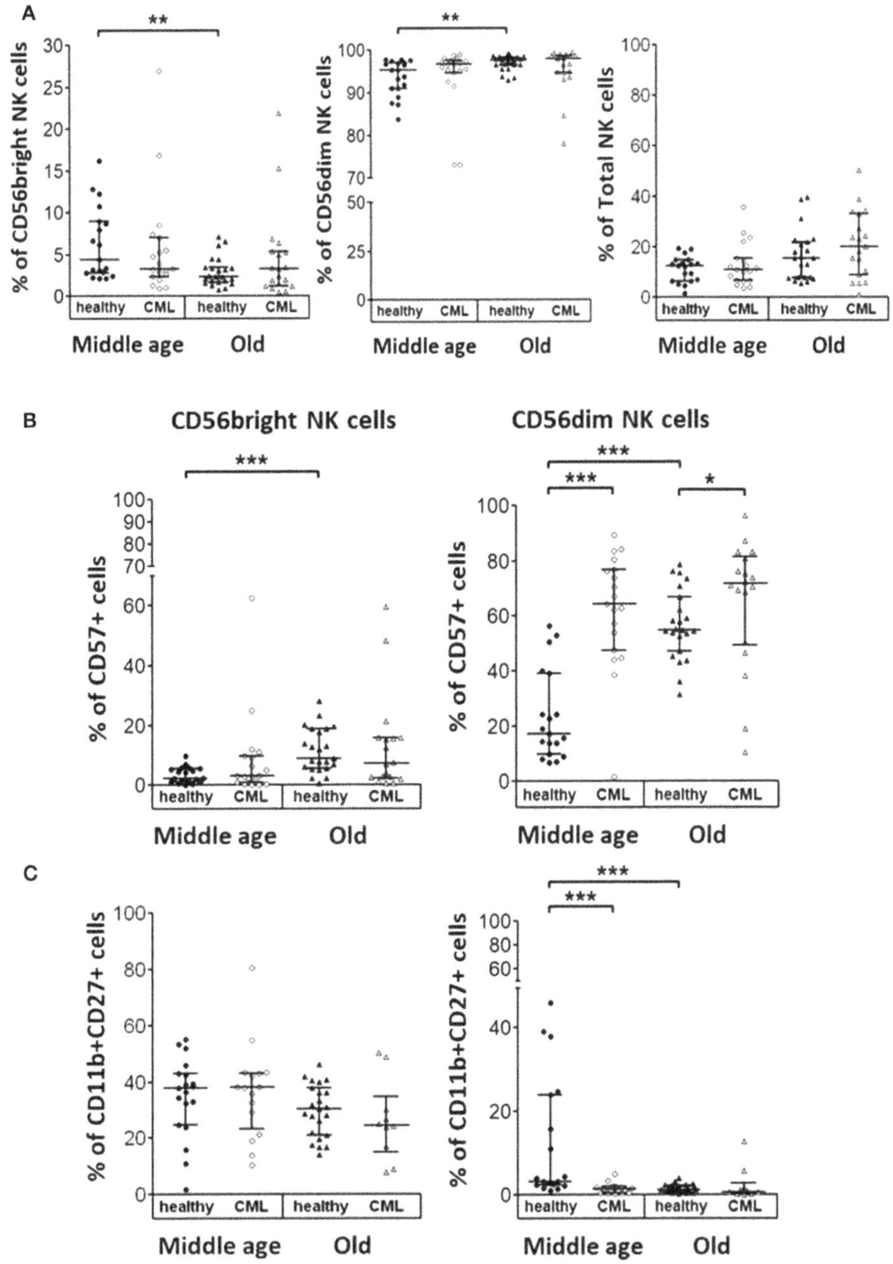

FIGURE 4 | NK cell subsets in healthy and TKI-treated CML individuals stratified by age. **(A)** Percentage of CD56^{bright} and CD56^{dim} NK cells referred to the total of CD56^{+} NK cells and NK cells referred of total Lymphocytes from healthy donors and TKI-treated CML patients. **(B)** Percentage of NK cells expressing CD57 determined in CD56^{bright} and CD56^{dim} NK cell subsets from both healthy and TKI-treated CML individuals. **(C)** Percentage of CD11b and CD27 positive cells in CD56^{bright} and CD56^{dim} NK cell subsets from both healthy and TKI-treated CML individuals. Number of donors: CD56^{bright}, CD56^{dim}, and NK cells, middle-aged healthy $n = 19$, middle-aged CML $n = 19$, old healthy $n = 23$, and old CML $n = 19$; CD57 middle-aged healthy $n = 19$, middle-aged CML $n = 19$, old healthy $n = 23$, and old CML $n = 18$; CD11b^{+}CD27^{+} middle-aged healthy $n = 19$, middle-aged CML $n = 16$, old healthy $n = 23$, and old CML $n = 10$. Graphics show the median with interquartile range. Kruskal-Wallis test was used for multiple comparisons and the Mann-Whitney *U*-test for the comparison of specific groups. The differences were considered significant in a range of $p < 0.05$. $^{*}p < 0.05$; $^{**}p < 0.01$; $^{***}p < 0.001$.

have a decreased expression of NK receptors at diagnosis (36–39), our results confirm that NK cells from TKI-treatment CML patients can express NK activating receptors (40, 41) such as NKp30, NKp46, and NKp80, although this expression is heterogeneous and in some cases their levels are lower than those found in age-matched healthy controls. NKp30 and NKp46 are NCRs involved in NK cells cytotoxicity after interaction with their ligands on target cells (60). NKp80, is

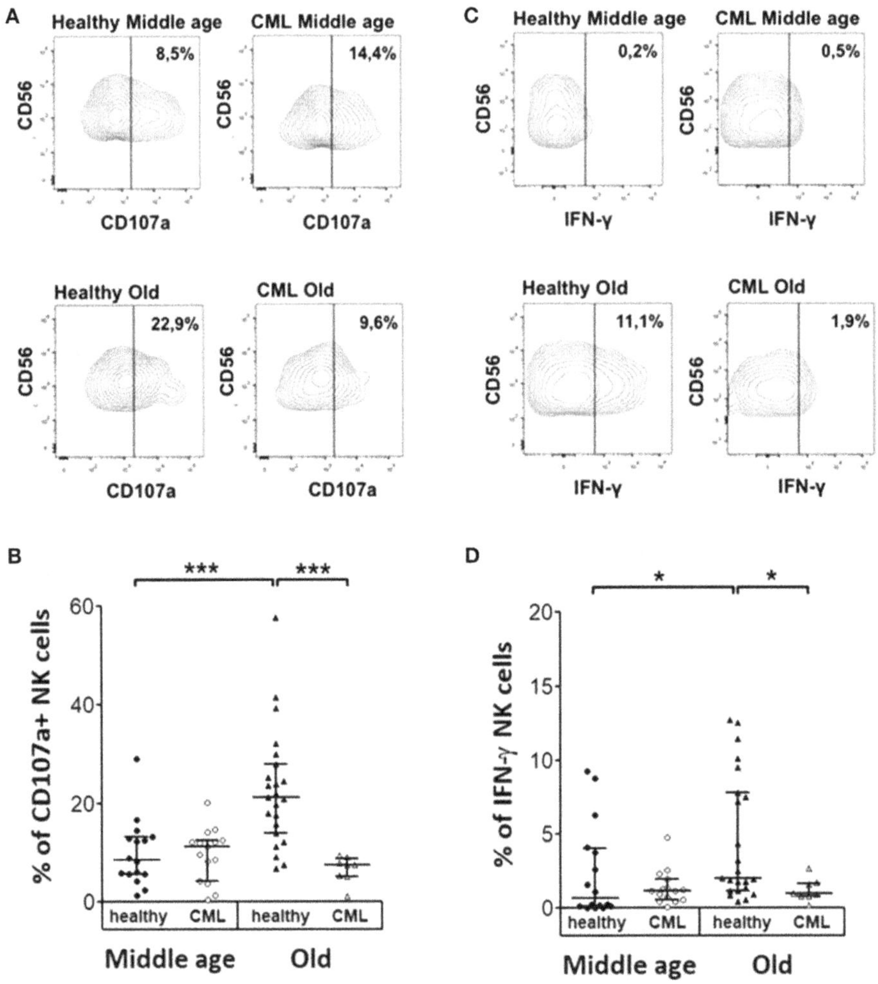

FIGURE 5 | Cytokine expression and degranulation in stimulated NK cells. Analysis of CD107a degranulation assay and IFN-γ expression by Natural killer cells following stimulation with K562 target cells. **(A)** Representative dotplots and **(B)** percentage of CD107a in NK cells from healthy donors and TKI-treated CML patients according to age and CML. **(C)** Representative dotplots and **(D)** IFN-γ expression in NK cells from healthy donors and TKI-treated CML patients according to age and CML (middle-aged healthy $n = 16$, middle-aged CML $n = 15$, old healthy $n = 23$, and old CML $n = 8$). Numbers in **(A,C)** represent the percentage of positive cells referred to the $CD56^+$ NK cells. The results in **(B,D)** were shown as median with interquartile range. Values of $p < 0.05$ were considered significant. *P*-values were determined comparing middle age with old and healthy with TKI-treated CML patients. $^*p < 0.05$; $^{***}p < 0.001$.

an activating C-type lectin-like receptor expressed on NK cells that interact with its ligand activation-induced C-type lectin (AICL) expressed on myeloid cells, including myeloid leukemia cells (61). It has been suggested that after TKI treatment NK cells are involved in the control of CML blasts (40, 41), thus the lower expression of these receptors compared with healthy controls can be the consequence of the interaction of NK cells with their ligands expressed on leukemic blasts, as suggested for NK cells from AML patients (44–46). Downregulation of NKG2D after its interactions with MICA/B ligand is a well-defined phenomenon in different tumors (62, 63). However, the expression of NKG2D is well preserved in all NK cell subsets from TKI treated CML patients, with the exception of $CD56^{bright}$ from elderly patients, confirming recent studies showing that the downregulated expression of NKG2D at the time of CML diagnosis, is restored to normal levels after TKI treatment (40, 41). The comparison of NK cell response to K562 in healthy controls vs. TKI-treated CML patients did not show significant differences on CD107a expression in K562 stimulated NK cells when middle-aged healthy donors were compared with middle-aged or old CML patients (**Figures 6B,C**) supporting previous findings that TKI treatment is associated with immune system re-activation and restoration of NK cell immune surveillance in CML patients (40, 41). On the contrary the observation that the percentage of NK cells expressing CD107a in TKI-treated CML old patients was lower than in healthy elderly donors, together with the lower expression of NK receptors in old TKI-treated CML patients compared with healthy elderly healthy donors (**Figure 6C**), support that the alterations on NK cells observed in healthy elderly donors likely associated

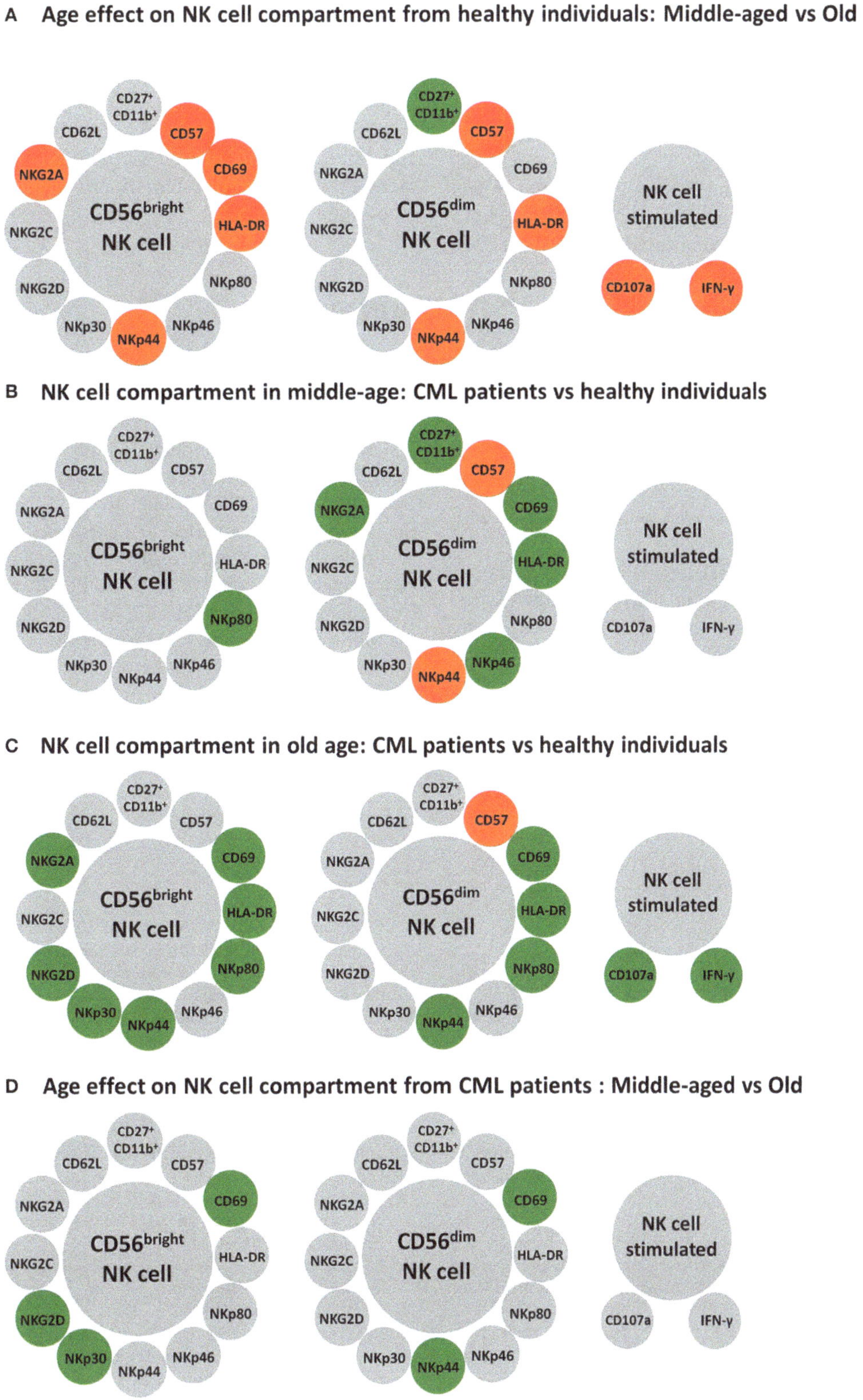

FIGURE 6 | Schematic representation of major differences in resting and K562 stimulated NK cells according to age and CML. Circles represent NK cell subpopulations expressing the indicated membrane markers in CD56^{bright} and CD56^{dim} resting NK cells and the expression of CD107a and IFN-γ in K562 stimulated NK cells. Red color was used for increased expression and green color for decreased expression of the membrane markers in NK cells from healthy old compared with healthy middle-aged individuals **(A)**, from CML patients compared with age-matched healthy donors **(B,C)**, or in old CML patients compared with middle-aged CML patients **(D)**.

with chronic virus infection, such as CMV, and inflamm-aging are not observed in old TKI-treated CML patients. The high variability observed in IFN-γ production by NK cells in response to K562 in healthy donors and the low response observed in most CML patients, represent a limitation of the study that precludes to obtain a conclusion on the significance of cytokine production in the disease control. The NK cell functional capacity and cytokine production during TKI-treatment and after TKI cessation in CML patients requires further analysis to discriminate a possible role in the long-term elimination of CML blasts (54, 55).

The analysis of the possible effect of age on NK cells from TKI-treated CML patients shows a lower expression of activation markers NKp44 and CD69 in elderly compared with middle-aged TKI-treated CML patients whereas no significant differences related with age are found in the other parameters studied, including CD107a expression and IFN-γ production in K562 stimulated NK cells from TKI-treated CML patients **(Figure 6D)**, indicating that age is not a limitation of the NK cell recovery after treatment with TKI.

In conclusion, despite the deleterious effect of aging in CML prognosis, our results showing that activating NK cell receptors can be expressed both in middle-aged and elderly TKI-treated CML patients highlight the interest to extensively analyse the effect of aging on NK cell phenotype and function in these patients. The possibility of enhancing NK cell activity by using cytokines and immunomodulating agents open new perspectives for the design of novel clinical trials aiming effective long-term treatment-free remission after TKI cessation in CML patients.

AUTHOR CONTRIBUTIONS

PR-S, NL-S, CC, RS, RT, and MS-R: research study design; PR-S, NL-S, JSA, PC, and VA: experiments conduction and data acquisition; LR and PF-T: clinical data and patient management; PR-S, NL-S, RT, JSA, CC, and CA: data analysis; PR-S, CA, and MS-R: reagents providing; PR-S, NL-S, CC, RT, and RS: manuscript writing; All authors approved the final version of the manuscript.

FUNDING

This work was supported by the FEDER Funds through the Operational Program Competitiveness Factors—COMPETE 2020 and by National Funds through the FCT—Foundation for Science and Technology within the framework of the Strategic Project with reference assigned by COMPETE: POCI-01-0145-FEDER-007440 (to PR-S and MS-R) and by the program Iberoamerica Scholarships. Santander Research Santander Universities 2016–2017 (to NL-S). This work also was supported by grants PI13/02691 and PI16/01615 (to RS and CA) from Spanish Ministry of Health, SAF2017-87538-R (to RT) from the Ministry of Economy and Competitiveness of Spain, IB16164 and GR18085 from Junta de Extremadura (to RT), cofinanced by European Regional Development Funds (FEDER).

REFERENCES

1. Spits H, Bernink JH, Lanier L. NK cells and type 1 innate lymphoid cells: partners in host defense. *Nat Immunol.* (2016) 17:758–64. doi: 10.1038/ni.3482
2. Cooper MA, Fehniger TA, Caligiuri MA. The biology of human natural killer-cell subsets. *Trends Immunol.* (2001) 22:633–40. doi: 10.1016/S1471-4906(01)02060-9
3. Fauriat C, Long EO, Ljunggren HG, Bryceson YT. Regulation of human NK-cell cytokine and chemokine production by target cell recognition. *Blood* (2010) 115:2167–76. doi: 10.1182/blood-2009-08-238469
4. Ouyang Q, Baerlocher G, Vulto I, Lansdorp PM. Telomere length in human natural killer cell subsets. *Ann N Y Acad Sci.* (2007) 1106:240–52. doi: 10.1196/annals.1392.001
5. Tarazona R, Casado JG, DelaRosa O, Torre-Cisneros J, Villanueva JL, Sanchez B et al. Selective depletion of CD56(dim) NK cell subsets and maintenance of CD56(bright) NK cells in treatment-naive HIV-1-seropositive individuals. *J Clin Immunol.* (2002) 22:176–83. doi: 10.1023/A:10154761 14409
6. Gonzalez VD, Falconer K, Bjorkstrom NK, Blom KG, Weiland O, Ljunggren HG et al. Expansion of functionally skewed CD56-negative NK cells in chronic hepatitis C virus infection: correlation with outcome of pegylated IFN-alpha and ribavirin treatment. *J Immunol.* (2009) 183:6612–8. doi: 10.4049/jimmunol.0901437
7. Moretta L, Montaldo E, Vacca P, Del ZG, Moretta F, Merli P et al. Human natural killer cells: origin, receptors, function, and clinical applications. *Int Arch Allergy Immunol.* (2014) 164:253–64. doi: 10.1159/0003 65632
8. Hehlmann R, Hochhaus A, Baccarani M. Chronic myeloid leukaemia. *Lancet* (2007) 370:342–50. doi: 10.1016/S0140-6736(07)61165-9
9. Goldman JM, Melo JV. BCR-ABL in chronic myelogenous leukemia–how does it work? *Acta Haematol.* (2008) 119:212–7. doi: 10.1159/000140633
10. Sokal JE, Cox EB, Baccarani M, Tura S, Gomez GA, Robertson JE et al. Prognostic discrimination in "good-risk" chronic granulocytic leukemia. *Blood* (1984) 63:789–99.
11. Hasford J, Pfirrmann M, Hehlmann R, Allan NC, Baccarani M, Kluin-Nelemans JC et al. A new prognostic score for survival of patients with chronic myeloid leukemia treated with interferon alfa. Writing Committee for the Collaborative CML Prognostic Factors Project Group. *J Natl Cancer Inst.* (1998) 90:850–8.
12. Phekoo KJ, Richards MA, Moller H, Schey SA. The incidence and outcome of myeloid malignancies in 2,112 adult patients in southeast England. *Haematologica* (2006) 91:1400–4.
13. Rohrbacher M, Hasford J. Epidemiology of chronic myeloid leukaemia (CML). *Best Pract Res Clin Haematol.* (2009) 22:295–302. doi: 10.1016/j.beha.2009.07.007
14. Rohrbacher M, Berger U, Hochhaus A, Metzgeroth G, Adam K, Lahaye T et al. Clinical trials underestimate the age of chronic myeloid leukemia (CML) patients. Incidence and median age of Ph/BCR-ABL-positive CML and other chronic myeloproliferative disorders in a representative area in Germany. *Leukemia* (2009) 23:602–4. doi: 10.1038/leu.2008.245
15. Kantarjian HM, Keating MJ, McCredie KB, Walters R, Talpaz M, Smith TL et al. Old age: a sign of poor prognosis in patients with chronic myelogenous leukemia. *South Med J.* (1987) 80:1228–32. doi: 10.1097/00007611-198710000-00007

16. Rodriguez J, Cortes J, Smith T, O'Brien S, Rios MB, Talpaz M et al. Determinants of prognosis in late chronic-phase chronic myelogenous leukemia. *J Clin Oncol.* (1998) 16: 3782–7. doi: 10.1200/JCO.1998.16.12.3782
17. Grubeck-Loebenstein B, Della BS, Iorio AM, Michel JP, Pawelec G, Solana R. Immunosenescence and vaccine failure in the elderly. *Aging Clin Exp Res.* (2009) 21:201–9. doi: 10.1007/BF03324904
18. Larbi A, Franceschi C, Mazzatti D, Solana R, Wikby A, Pawelec G. Aging of the immune system as a prognostic factor for human longevity. *Physiology* (2008) 23:64–74. doi: 10.1152/physiol.00040.2007
19. Goronzy JJ, Weyand CM. Understanding immunosenescence to improve responses to vaccines. *Nat Immunol.* (2013) 14:428–36. doi: 10.1038/ni.2588
20. Pera A, Campos C, Lopez N, Hassouneh F, Alonso C, Tarazona R et al. Immunosenescence: implications for response to infection and vaccination in older people. *Maturitas* (2015) 82:50–5. doi: 10.1016/j.maturitas.2015.05.004
21. Fulop T, Larbi A, Pawelec G. Human T cell aging and the impact of persistent viral infections. *Front Immunol.* (2013) 4:271. doi: 10.3389/fimmu.2013.00271
22. Solana R, Campos C, Pera A, Tarazona R. Shaping of NK cell subsets by aging. *Curr Opin Immunol.* (2014) 29:56–61. doi: 10.1016/j.coi.2014.04.002
23. Solana R, Tarazona R, Gayoso I, Lesur O, Dupuis G, Fulop T. Innate immunosenescence: Effect of aging on cells and receptors of the innate immune system in humans. *Semin Immunol.* (2012) 24:331–41. doi: 10.1016/j.smim.2012.04.008
24. Pita-Lopez ML, Pera A, Solana R. Adaptive memory of human NK-like CD8+ T-cells to aging, and viral and tumor antigens. *Front Immunol.* (2016) 7:616. doi: 10.3389/fimmu.2016.00616
25. Pita-Lopez ML, Gayoso I, DelaRosa O, Casado JG, Alonso C, Munoz-Gomariz E et al. Effect of ageing on CMV-specific CD8 T cells from CMV seropositive healthy donors. *Immun Ageing* (2009) 6:11. doi: 10.1186/1742-4933-6-11
26. Weyand CM, Yang Z, Goronzy JJ. T-cell aging in rheumatoid arthritis. *Curr Opin Rheumatol.* (2014) 26:93–100. doi: 10.1097/BOR.0000000000000011
27. Sanchez-Correa B, Campos C, Pera A, Bergua JM, Arcos MJ, Banas H et al. Natural killer cell immunosenescence in acute myeloid leukaemia patients: new targets for immunotherapeutic strategies? *Cancer Immunol Immunother.* (2016) 65:453–63. doi: 10.1007/s00262-015-1720-6
28. Lopez-Sejas N, Campos C, Hassouneh F, Sanchez-Correa B, Tarazona R, Pera A et al. Effect of CMV and aging on the differential expression of CD300a, CD161, T-bet, and eomes on NK cell subsets. *Front Immunol.* (2016) 7:476. doi: 10.3389/fimmu.2016.00476
29. Campos C, Lopez N, Pera A, Gordillo JJ, Hassouneh F, Tarazona R et al. Expression of NKp30, NKp46 and DNAM-1 activating receptors on resting and IL-2 activated NK cells from healthy donors according to CMV-serostatus and age. *Biogerontology* (2015) 16:671–83. doi: 10.1007/s10522-015-9581-0
30. Campos C, Pera A, Sanchez-Correa B, Alonso C, Lopez-Fernandez I, Morgado S et al. Effect of age and CMV on NK cell subpopulations. *Exp Gerontol.* (2014) 54:130–7. doi: 10.1016/j.exger.2014.01.008
31. Gayoso I, Sanchez-Correa B, Campos C, Alonso C, Pera A, Casado JG et al. Immunosenescence of human natural killer cells. *J Innate Immun.* (2011) 3:337–43. doi: 10.1159/000328005
32. Borrego F, Alonso MC, Galiani MD, Carracedo J, Ramirez R, Ostos B et al. NK phenotypic markers and IL2 response in NK cells from elderly people. *Exp Gerontol.* (1999) 34:253–65. doi: 10.1016/S0531-5565(98)00076-X
33. Lutz CT, Moore MB, Bradley S, Shelton BJ, Lutgendorf SK. Reciprocal age related change in natural killer cell receptors for MHC class I. *Mech Ageing Dev.* (2005) 126:722–31. doi: 10.1016/j.mad.2005.01.004
34. Almeida-Oliveira A, Smith-Carvalho M, Porto LC, Cardoso-Oliveira J, Ribeiro AS, Falcao RR et al. Age-related changes in natural killer cell receptors from childhood through old age. *Hum Immunol.* (2011) 72:319–29. doi: 10.1016/j.humimm.2011.01.009
35. Le Garff-Tavernier M, Beziat V, Decocq J, Siguret V, Gandjbakhch F, Pautas E et al. Human NK cells display major phenotypic and functional changes over the life span. *Aging Cell* (2010) 9:527–35. doi: 10.1111/j.1474-9726.2010.00584.x
36. Pierson BA, Miller JS. CD56+bright and CD56+dim natural killer cells in patients with chronic myelogenous leukemia progressively decrease in number, respond less to stimuli that recruit clonogenic natural killer cells, and exhibit decreased proliferation on a per cell basis. *Blood* (1996) 88:2279–87.
37. Nakajima H, Zhao R, Lund TC, Ward J, Dolan M, Hirsch B et al. The BCR/ABL transgene causes abnormal NK cell differentiation and can be found in circulating NK cells of advanced phase chronic myelogenous leukemia patients. *J Immunol.* (2002) 168:643–50. doi: 10.4049/jimmunol.168.2.643
38. Mellqvist UH, Hansson M, Brune M, Dahlgren C, Hermodsson S, Hellstrand K. Natural killer cell dysfunction and apoptosis induced by chronic myelogenous leukemia cells: role of reactive oxygen species and regulation by histamine. *Blood* (2000) 96:1961–8.
39. Kiladjian JJ, Bourgeois E, Lobe I, Braun T, Visentin G, Bourhis JH et al. Cytolytic function and survival of natural killer cells are severely altered in myelodysplastic syndromes. *Leukemia* (2006) 20:463–70. doi: 10.1038/sj.leu.2404080
40. Hughes A, Clarson J, Tang C, Vidovic L, White DL, Hughes TP et al. CML patients with deep molecular responses to TKI have restored immune effectors and decreased PD-1 and immune suppressors. *Blood* (2017) 129:1166–76. doi: 10.1182/blood-2016-10-745992
41. Hughes A, Yong ASM. Immune effector recovery in chronic myeloid leukemia and treatment-free remission. *Front Immunol.* (2017) 8:469. doi: 10.3389/fimmu.2017.00469
42. Sconocchia G, Lau M, Provenzano M, Rezvani K, Wongsena W, Fujiwara H et al. The antileukemia effect of HLA-matched NK and NK-T cells in chronic myelogenous leukemia involves NKG2D-target-cell interactions. *Blood* (2005) 106:3666–72. doi: 10.1182/blood-2005-02-0479
43. Costello RT, Knoblauch B, Sanchez C, Mercier D, Le TT, Sebahoun G. Expression of natural killer cell activating receptors in patients with chronic lymphocytic leukaemia. *Immunology* (2012) 135:151–7. doi: 10.1111/j.1365-2567.2011.03521.x
44. Fauriat C, Just-Landi S, Mallet F, Arnoulet C, Sainty D, Olive D et al. Deficient expression of NCR in NK cells from acute myeloid leukemia: Evolution during leukemia treatment and impact of leukemia cells in NCRdull phenotype induction. *Blood* (2007) 109:323–30. doi: 10.1182/blood-2005-08-027979
45. Sanchez-Correa B, Morgado S, Gayoso I, Bergua JM, Casado JG, Arcos MJ et al. Human NK cells in acute myeloid leukaemia patients: analysis of NK cell-activating receptors and their ligands. *Cancer Immunol Immunother.* (2011) 60:1195–205. doi: 10.1007/s00262-011-1050-2
46. Sanchez-Correa B, Gayoso I, Bergua JM, Casado JG, Morgado S, Solana R et al. Decreased expression of DNAM-1 on NK cells from acute myeloid leukemia patients. *Immunol Cell Biol.* (2012) 90: 109–115. doi: 10.1038/icb.2011.15
47. Hochhaus A, O'Brien SG, Guilhot F, Druker BJ, Branford S, Foroni L et al. Six-year follow-up of patients receiving imatinib for the first-line treatment of chronic myeloid leukemia. Leukemia (2009) 23:1054–61. doi: 10.1038/leu.2009.38
48. Hochhaus A, Larson RA, Guilhot F, Radich JP, Branford S, Hughes TP et al. Long-term outcomes of imatinib treatment for chronic myeloid leukemia. *N Engl J Med.* (2017) 376:917–27. doi: 10.1056/NEJMoa1609324
49. Ross DM, Hughes TP. How I determine if and when to recommend stopping tyrosine kinase inhibitor treatment for chronic myeloid leukaemia. *Br J Haematol.* (2014) 166:3–11. doi: 10.1111/bjh.12892
50. Saussele S, Richter J, Hochhaus A, Mahon FX. The concept of treatment-free remission in chronic myeloid leukemia. *Leukemia* (2016) 30:1638–47. doi: 10.1038/leu.2016.115
51. Imagawa J, Tanaka H, Okada M, Nakamae H, Hino M, Murai K et al. Discontinuation of dasatinib in patients with chronic myeloid leukaemia who have maintained deep molecular response for longer than 1 year (DADI trial): a multicentre phase 2 trial. *Lancet Haematol.* (2015) 2:e528–35. doi: 10.1016/S2352-3026(15)00196-9
52. Chen CI, Koschmieder S, Kerstiens L, Schemionek M, Altvater B, Pscherer S et al. NK cells are dysfunctional in human chronic myelogenous leukemia before and on imatinib treatment and in BCR-ABL-positive mice. *Leukemia* (2012) 26:465–74. doi: 10.1038/leu.2011.239
53. Boissel N, Rea D, Tieng V, Dulphy N, Brun M, Cayuela JM et al. BCR/ABL oncogene directly controls MHC class I chain-related molecule A expression in chronic myelogenous leukemia. *J Immunol.* (2006) 176:5108–16. doi: 10.4049/jimmunol.176.8.5108
54. Ilander M, Olsson-Stromberg U, Schlums H, Guilhot J, Bruck O, Lahteenmaki H et al. Increased proportion of mature NK cells is associated with successful

imatinib discontinuation in chronic myeloid leukemia. *Leukemia* (2017) 31:1108–16. doi: 10.1038/leu.2016.360
55. Kumagai T, Nakaseko C, Nishiwaki K, Yoshida C, Ohashi K, Takezako N et al. Dasatinib cessation after deep molecular response exceeding 2 years, and NK cell transition during dasatinib consolidation. *Cancer Sci.* (2017) 109:182–92. doi: 10.1111/cas.13430
56. Camous X, Pera A, Solana R, Larbi A. NK cells in healthy aging and age-associated diseases. *J Biomed Biotechnol.* (2012) 2012:195956. doi: 10.1155/2012/195956
57. Campos C, Pera A, Lopez-Fernandez I, Alonso C, Tarazona R, Solana R. Proinflammatory status influences NK cells subsets in the elderly. *Immunol Lett.* (2014) 162:298–302. doi: 10.1016/j.imlet.2014.06.015
58. Fu B, Wang F, Sun R, Ling B, Tian Z, Wei H. CD11b and CD27 reflect distinct population and functional specialization in human natural killer cells. *Immunology* (2011) 133:350–9. doi: 10.1111/j.1365-2567.2011.03446.x
59. Franceschi C, Campisi J. Chronic inflammation (inflammaging) and its potential contribution to age-associated diseases. *J Gerontol A Biol Sci Med Sci.* (2014) 69(Suppl. 1):S4–9. doi: 10.1093/gerona/glu057
60. Moretta L, Pietra G, Montaldo E, Vacca P, Pende D, Falco M et al. Human NK cells: from surface receptors to the therapy of leukemias and solid tumors. *Front Immunol.* (2014) 5:87. doi: 10.3389/fimmu.2014.00087
61. Bartel Y, Bauer B, Steinle A. Modulation of NK cell function by genetically coupled C-type lectin-like receptor/ligand pairs encoded in the human natural killer gene complex. *Front Immunol.* (2013) 4:362. doi: 10.3389/fimmu.2013.00362
62. Zhang J, Basher F, Wu JD. NKG2D Ligands in tumor immunity: two sides of a coin. *Front Immunol.* (2015) 6:97. doi: 10.3389/fimmu.2015.00097
63. Champsaur M, Lanier LL. Effect of NKG2D ligand expression on host immune responses. *Immunol Rev.* (2010) 235:267–85. doi: 10.1111/j.0105-2896.2010.00893.x

4

Impact of Aging on the Frequency, Phenotype and Function of CD161-Expressing T Cells

Kornelis S. M. van der Geest[1], Bart-Jan Kroesen[2], Gerda Horst[1], Wayel H. Abdulahad[1,3], Elisabeth Brouwer[1] and Annemieke M. H. Boots[1]*

[1] Department of Rheumatology and Clinical Immunology, University of Groningen, University Medical Center Groningen, Groningen, Netherlands, [2] Department of Laboratory Medicine, University of Groningen, University Medical Center Groningen, Groningen, Netherlands, [3] Department of Pathology and Medical Biology, University of Groningen, University Medical Center Groningen, Groningen, Netherlands

***Correspondence:**
Kornelis S. M. van der Geest
k.s.m.van.der.geest@umcg.nl

Immune-aging is associated with perturbed immune responses in the elderly. CD161-expressing T cells, i.e., the previously described subsets of CD161$^+$ CD4$^+$ T cells, CD161^{high} CD8$^+$ T cells, and CD161^{int} CD8$^+$ T cells, are highly functional, pro-inflammatory T cells. These CD161-expressing T cells are critical in immunity against microbes, while possibly contributing to autoimmune diseases. So far, little is known about the impact of aging on the frequency, phenotype, and function of these CD161-expressing T cells. In the current study, we investigated the impact of aging on CD161$^+$ CD4$^+$ T cells, CD161^{high} CD8$^+$ T cells, and CD161^{int} CD8$^+$ T cells in peripheral blood samples of 96 healthy subjects (age 20–84). Frequencies of CD161$^+$ CD4$^+$ T cells and CD161^{int} CD8$^+$ T cells were stable with aging, whereas frequencies of CD161^{high} CD8$^+$ T cells declined. Although CD161^{high} CD8$^+$ T cells were mostly T cell receptor-Vα7.2$^+$ mucosal-associated invariant T cells, CD161 expressing CD4$^+$ and CD8$^+$ T cells showed a limited expression of markers for gamma–delta T cells or invariant natural killer (NK) T cells, in both young and old subjects. In essence, CD161-expressing T cells showed a similar memory phenotype in young and old subjects. The expression of the inhibitory NK receptor KLRG1 was decreased on CD161$^+$ CD4$^+$ T cells of old subjects, whereas the expression of other NK receptors by CD161-expressing T cells was unaltered with age. The expression of cytotoxic effector molecules was similar in CD161^{high} and CD161^{int} CD8$^+$ T cells of young and old subjects. The ability to produce pro-inflammatory cytokines was preserved in CD161^{high} and CD161^{int} CD8$^+$ T cells of old subjects. However, the percentages of IFN-γ^+ and interleukin-17$^+$ cells were significantly lower in CD161$^+$ CD4$^+$ T cells of old individuals than those of young individuals. In addition, aging was associated with a decrease of nonclassic T helper 1 cells, as indicated by decreased percentages of CD161-expressing cells within the IFN-γ^+ CD4$^+$ T cell compartment of old subjects. Taken together, aging is associated with a numerical decline of circulating CD161^{high} CD8$^+$ T cells, as well as a decreased production of pro-inflammatory cytokines by CD161$^+$ CD4$^+$ T cells. These aging-associated changes could contribute to perturbed immunity in the elderly.

Keywords: aging, T lymphocytes subsets, CD161, cytokines, T helper 1 cells, T helper 17 cells, mucosal-associated invariant T cell

---

Abbreviations: CM, central memory; CMV, cytomegalovirus; DN, double negative; DNAM-1, DNAX accessory molecule-1; EM, effector memory; IL, interleukin; LLT1, lectin-like transcript 1; iNKT cell, invariant natural killer T cell; MAIT cell, mucosal-associated invariant T cell; NK, natural killer; TCR, T cell receptor; TD, terminally differentiated; Th1, T helper 1; Th17, T helper 17; TNF-α, tumor necrosis factor-α.

INTRODUCTION

Aging-associated perturbations of the immune system have been linked to increased risks for infections and autoimmune diseases in the elderly (1, 2). Insight into these immunological changes may eventually help to develop strategies to correct immunological disturbances in aged subjects.

The T cell compartment is especially affected by aging. The production of naive T cells shows a strong aging-associated decline, which starts already early in life (3). By contrast, a shift toward the memory T cell compartment develops upon antigenic stimulation by environmental stimuli (4). Consequently, the maintenance of the already existing naive and memory T cells is important to preserve immunity during adult life (5). Another aging-associated change in the T cell compartment of humans includes the acquisition of natural killer (NK) receptors and cytotoxic effector molecules by aged T cells (6, 7). In addition, the balance between pro-inflammatory and anti-inflammatory T cells is disturbed in the elderly (8). Thus, aging affects the numerical, phenotypic, and functional aspects of both the naive and memory T cell compartment in humans.

Cytomegalovirus (CMV) infection also has a broad impact on the T cell compartment (9). Latent infection with CMV is associated with skewing of the T cell receptor (TCR) repertoire (4). CMV drives the expansion of memory T cells, both in the circulation and in the peripheral tissues (10, 11). CMV-specific memory T cells may express NK receptors and are potent producers of pro-inflammatory cytokines, such as IFN-γ and tumor necrosis factor-α (TNF-α) (12–14). Furthermore, CMV has been linked to poor vaccination responses and a slightly increased mortality rate in the elderly (9, 15–17). Overall, CMV contributes to immune senescence in humans (9).

Ample evidence indicates that the expression of the C-type lectin receptor CD161 identifies subsets of $CD4^+$ and $CD8^+$ T cells with a strong pro-inflammatory phenotype (18–20). These CD161-expressing T cells are considered important for antimicrobial immunity in humans (20–24). However, CD161-expressing T cells may also contribute to the development of various autoimmune diseases (25–28). CD161 is expressed by $CD4^+$ T helper 17 (Th17) lineage cells and nonclassic T helper 1 (Th1) cells (18, 29–31). In addition, two subsets of $CD8^+$ T cells with different expression levels of CD161 have been identified (19, 20). Firstly, high expression levels of CD161 ($CD161^{high}$) are found on a subset of innate-like $CD8^+$ T cells termed mucosal-associated invariant T (MAIT) cells (32, 33). Another population of $CD8^+$ T cells is characterized by intermediate expression levels of CD161 ($CD161^{int}$) and contributes to antiviral immunity (20). Although several studies have shown that frequencies of MAIT cells decrease with age (34–36), little is known about the effect of aging on the other CD161-expressing T cell subsets.

In the current study, we assessed the impact of aging on the frequencies, phenotype, and function of CD161-expressing $CD4^+$ and $CD8^+$ T cells in the peripheral blood of humans. While taking into account CMV serostatus, we investigated the effect of age on the numbers of circulating CD161-expressing T cells in a large group of healthy subjects. Furthermore, we studied the expression of T cell differentiation markers, NK receptors, cytotoxic effector molecules, and pro-inflammatory cytokines by CD161-expressing T cells of young and old subjects. Taken together, our study provides a unique and comprehensive insight into the effect of aging on highly functional, pro-inflammatory T cell populations in humans.

MATERIALS AND METHODS

Study Subjects and Samples

Blood samples were obtained from 96 healthy individuals (age range 20–84, of which 26 were males) Subjects underwent a thorough examination of their health status, as described previously (8). Exclusion criteria included infection, malignancy, autoimmune disease, chronic liver or kidney disease, alcohol or drug abuse, diabetes mellitus, current pregnancy, or immunosuppressive treatment. Written informed consent was obtained from all study participants. The study was approved by the Medical Ethical Committee of the UMCG. All procedures were in accordance with the Declaration of Helsinki.

Flow Cytometry

Blood samples (EDTA) were stained with the following monoclonal antibodies: CD3-eFluor605, CD4-eFluor450, TCRγδ-PE (eBioscience), CD45RO-FITC, CCR7-PE-Cy7, CD4-PerCP, CD8-PerCP, CD8-APC-H7, DNAX accessory molecule-1 (DNAM-1)-FITC (BD), CD161-PE, CD161-APC (Miltenyi), 2B4-PE, NKG2D-PE-Cy7, TCR-Vα7.2-FITC, TCR-Vα24-Jα18-FITC (Biolegend), TCR-Vβ11-PE (Beckman Coulter), and KLRG1-FITC (generous gift from H. Pirchner). An overview of antibody panels is shown in Table S1 in Supplementary Material. Samples were subsequently treated with BD Lysing Solution (BD Biosciences) according to instructions of the manufacturer. Samples were measured on a LSR-II flow cytometer (BD) and analyzed with Kaluza Analysis Software (Beckman Coulter). In addition, the absolute numbers of circulating lymphocyte subsets were determined according to the MultiTest TruCount method (BD), as described by the manufacturer. Data were acquired on a FACSCanto-II flow cytometer (BD) and analyzed with FACSCanto Clinical Software (BD). The number of events for a particular T cell population needed to be more than 100 to allow for subsequent analysis of cellular markers, cytokines, and cytotoxic molecules.

Intracellular Cytokine Staining

Blood samples (heparin) were diluted 1:1 with RPMI and stimulated with 40 nM PMA and 2 nM Ca^{2+} ionophore A23187 in the presence of 3 μM brefeldin A (all Sigma) for 4 h. Subsequently, red blood cells were lysed with ammonium chloride. The remaining cells were treated with Fix/Perm reagents A and B (Invitrogen) and stained with the following antibodies: CD3-eFluor 605, CD4-eFluor450, interleukin (IL)-17-AF488, Perforin-FITC (eBioscience), CD161-APC (Miltenyi), CD8-APC-H7, Granzyme-B-PE (BD), IFN-γ-PerCP-Cy5.5, IL-4-PE, and TNF-α-PerCP-Cy5.5 (Biolegend). Samples were measured on an LSR-II flow cytometer (BD) and analyzed with Kaluza Analysis Software (Beckman Coulter).

Measurement of CMV-Specific IgG

As previously described (4), 96-well ELISA plates (Greiner) were coated overnight with lysates of CMV-infected fibroblasts. Lysates of non-infected fibroblasts were used as negative controls. Following the coating, diluted serum samples were incubated for 1 h. Goat anti-human IgG was added and incubated for 1 h. Samples were incubated with phosphatase for 15 min, and the reaction was stopped with NaOH. The plates were scanned on a Versamax reader (Molecular Devices). A pool of sera from three CMV-seropositive individuals with known concentrations of CMV-specific IgG was used to quantify CMV-specific IgG in the tested samples. Detailed information on CMV serostatus of the healthy donors is shown for experiments reporting the phenotype and function of CD161-expressing T cells in Table S2 in Supplementary Material.

Statistics

The Mann–Whitney *U*-test was used to compare continuous variables between different age groups. Correlations were determined with Spearman's rank correlation coefficient. Univariate and multivariate linear regression analyses were used to further determine the impact of age and CMV serostatus on CD161-expressing T cell counts in healthy subjects. Firstly, each variable was tested in a univariate linear regression analysis. Subsequently, variables with $p < 0.3$ in the univariate analysis were used in the multivariate analysis. Reported *B*-coefficients indicate how much cell counts (10^9/L) change with every unit increase of the tested variable. The categorical variable CMV serostatus was assigned a value of 0 or 1. CMV: 0 = seronegative, 1 = seropositive. Non-normally distributed outcome variables were transformed (i.e., log or square root). Analysis was performed with SPSS 23.0 Software and GraphPad Prism 5.0. *P*-values less than 0.05 were considered to be significant.

RESULTS

Characterization of Healthy Subjects

To investigate the impact of aging on CD161-expressing T cells, we recruited a group of healthy subjects with a wide age range. Detailed characteristics of the healthy subjects are shown in **Table 1**. Young (age 18–39), intermediate (age 40–59), and old (age ≥60) subjects showed a similar distribution of gender and CMV serostatus. Furthermore, general laboratory parameters were comparable among the different age groups.

TABLE 1 | Subject characteristics.

	Young (age 18–39)	Intermediate (age 40–59)	Old (age ≥60)
No.	22	24	50
Age, years, median (range)	27 (20–38)	57 (40–59)	69 (60–84)
No. male (%)	6 (27)	6 (25)	14 (28)
No. CMV positive (%)	12 (55)	11 (46)	27 (54)
Hemoglobin, mmol/L, median (range)[a]	8.3 (7.3–9.5)	8.5 (7.5–10.0)	8.6 (7.1–10.2)
Leukocyte count, 10^9/L, median (range)[a]	4.7 (2.8–7.5)	5.3 (3.5–8.2)	5.8 (2.9–9.1)
Thrombocyte count, 10^9/L, median (range)[a]	275 (173–422)	240 (161–381)	240 (121–350)
ESR, mm/h, median (range)[a]	6 (1–16)	8 (1–15)	8 (2–26)
Creatinine, μmol/L, median (range)[a]	62 (53–90)	71 (58–89)	69 (49–97)

No., number; ESR, erythrocyte sedimentation rate.
[a]Performed in 11/22 young individuals, 19/24 intermediate age individuals, and 50/50 aged individuals.

Aging Is Associated With a Decrease of Circulating CD161^{high} CD8$^+$ T Cells

Firstly, we determined the impact of age on total CD3$^+$, CD4$^+$, and CD8$^+$ T cell numbers in our study population. The numbers of CD3$^+$ T cells, CD4$^+$ T cells, and CD8$^+$ T cells were stable with age (**Figures 1A,B**).

Next, we studied the effect of age on the numbers of CD161-expressing T cells. In accordance with prior studies (18–20), we identified CD161$^+$ cells within the CD4$^+$ T cell compartment, as well as CD8$^+$ T cells with high and intermediate expression levels of CD161, i.e., CD161^{high} and CD161^{int} cells (**Figure 1C**). The absolute numbers of CD161$^+$ CD4$^+$ T cells showed a slight decrease with age ($p = 0.04$), whereas the absolute numbers of CD161$^-$ CD4$^+$ T cells remained stable (**Figure 1D**). The percentages of CD161$^+$ CD4$^+$ T cells showed a statistically significant inverse correlation with age (Figure S1A in Supplementary Material). The absolute numbers of CD161^{high} and CD161$^-$ CD8$^+$ T cells showed a negative correlation with age, while the absolute numbers of CD161^{int} CD8$^+$ T cells remained stable (**Figure 1E**). Percentages of CD161^{high} CD8$^+$ T cells were also negatively associated with age (Figure S1B in Supplementary Material). However, due to the absolute decrease of CD161^{high} and CD161$^-$ CD8$^+$ T cells, the percentage of CD161^{int} CD8$^+$ T cells increased with age. These findings suggest that aging might impact the numbers of CD161-expressing T cells.

Subsequently, we performed a multivariate analysis in order to evaluate the impact of both aging and CMV serostatus on the absolute numbers of CD161-expressing T cells. In this analysis, neither aging nor CMV showed an effect on the numbers of CD161$^+$ and CD161$^-$ CD4$^+$ T cells (**Table 2**). Aging was associated with declining numbers of CD161^{high} CD8$^+$ T cells, whereas CMV seropositivity was linked to a higher number of CD161^{int} CD8$^+$ T cells. Independent effects of aging and CMV serostatus were also observed on the absolute numbers of CD161$^-$ CD8$^+$ T cells. Taken together, aging is associated with a decrease of CD161^{high} CD8$^+$ T cells, whereas the absolute numbers of CD161^{int} CD8$^+$ T cells and CD161$^+$ CD4$^+$ T cells remain stable.

Aging Does Not Affect the Expression of Innate-Like T Cell Markers by CD161-Expressing T Cells

Previous studies have reported that gamma–delta T cells, invariant natural killer T (iNKT) cells, and MAIT cells may express CD161 (33, 37, 38). Therefore, we investigated if CD161-expressing T cells of young and old subjects express markers defining these innate-like T cells. Gamma–delta T cells were identified by the expression of the TCRγδ receptor (**Figure 2A**) in young and old subjects with comparable CMV-seropositivity rates (Figure S2 in Supplementary Material). The TCRγδ receptor was present on few CD161$^+$ CD4$^+$ T cells, both in young and in old subjects

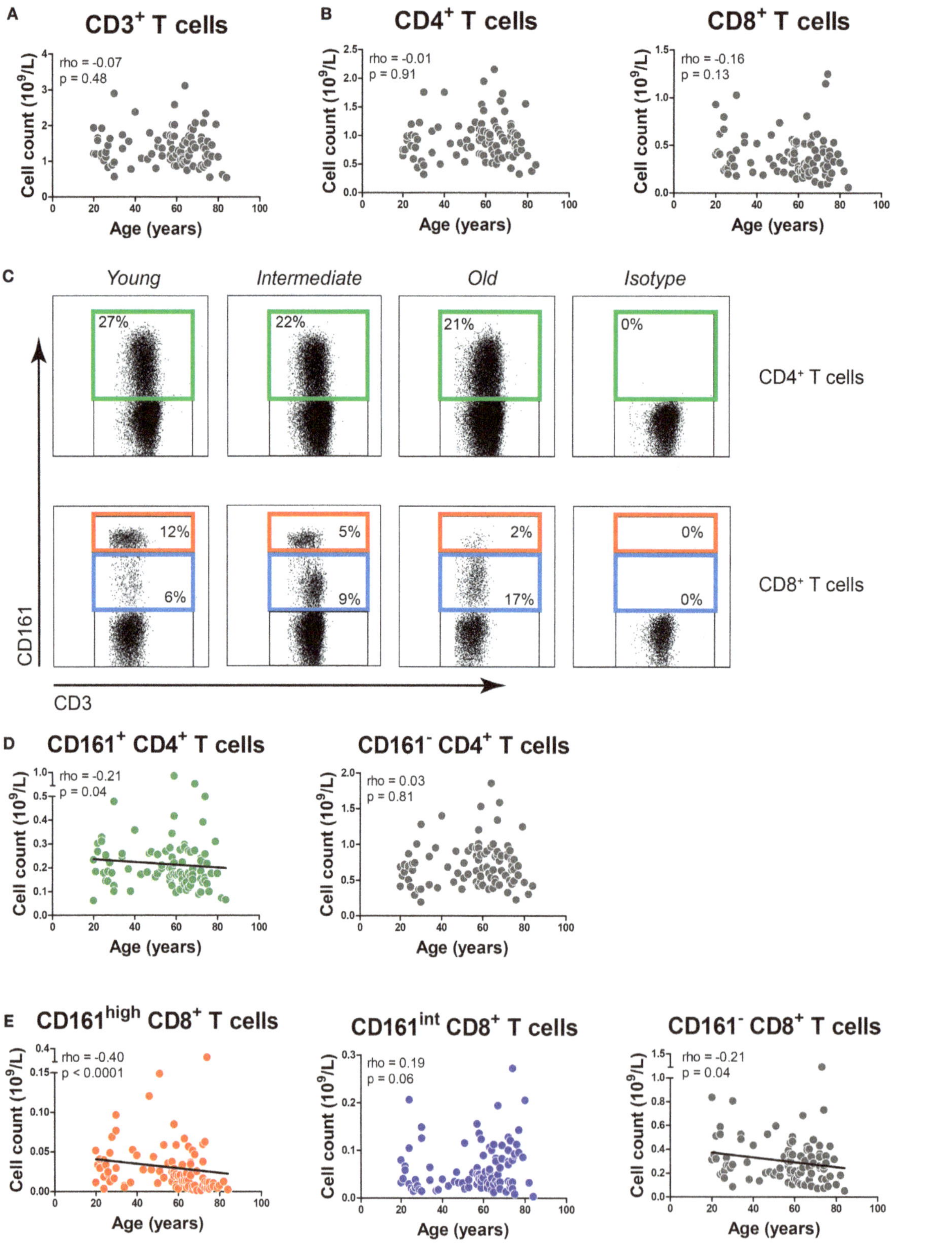

FIGURE 1 | The effect of age on the absolute numbers of CD161-expressing T cells. **(A)** The absolute numbers of $CD3^+$ T cells, as well as **(B)** $CD4^+$ T cells and $CD8^+$ T cells in the peripheral blood of 96 healthy subjects (age range 20–84). **(C)** Flow cytometric gating of $CD161^+$ $CD4^+$ T cells, $CD161^{high}$ $CD8^+$ T cells, and $CD161^{int}$ $CD8^+$ T cells in the peripheral blood of healthy young, intermediate, and old subjects. **(D)** The absolute numbers of $CD161^+$ $CD4^+$ T cells, $CD161^-$ $CD4^+$ T cells, and **(E)** $CD161^{high}$ $CD8^+$ T cells, $CD161^{int}$ $CD8^+$ T cells, and $CD161^-$ $CD8^+$ T cells in the peripheral blood of same donors as mentioned at **(A,B)**. Statistical significance by Spearman's rank test is shown.

TABLE 2 | Univariate and multivariate linear regression analysis for the absolute numbers of CD161-expressing T cell subsets.

Dependent variable	Predicting variables	Univariate analysis *B* (95% CI)	*p*-value	Multivariate analysis *B* (95% CI)	*p*-value
CD161+ CD4+ (10^9/L)	Age	−0.001 (−0.002 to 0.000)	0.176	−0.001 (−0.002 to 0.000)[a]	0.158
	CMV	0.027 (−0.008 to 0.068)	0.133	0.034 (−0.008 to 0.084)[a]	0.120
CD161− CD4+ (10^9/L)	Age	0.001 (−0.002 to 0.004)	0.426	†	
	CMV	0.030 (−0.083 to 0.152)	0.614	†	
CD161high CD8+ (10^9/L)	Age	−0.001 (−0.002 to 0.000)	0.001	−0.001 (−0.002 to 0.000)[b]	0.001
	CMV	−0.004 (−0.010 to 0.004)	0.294	−0.010 (−0.026 to 0.012)[b]	0.318
CD161int CD8+ (10^9/L)	Age	0.000 (0.000 to 0.001)	0.156	0.000 (0.000 to 0.000)[c]	0.159
	CMV	0.030 (0.014 to 0.051)	0.000	0.021 (0.010 to 0.037)[c]	0.000
CD161− CD8+ (10^9/L)	Age	−0.003 (−0.006 to −0.001)	0.016	−0.003 (−0.005 to −0.001)[d]	0.006
	CMV	0.122 (0.059 to 0.200)	0.000	0.199 (0.101 to 0.320)[d]	0.000

Data are obtained for 96 healthy individuals (age range 20–84). Firstly, each variable was tested in a univariate linear regression analysis. Subsequently, variables with $p < 0.3$ in the univariate analysis were used in the multivariate analysis. Reported B-coefficients indicate how much cell counts (10^9/L) change with every unit increase of the predicting variable. The categorical variable CMV was assigned a value of 0 or 1, where 0 = CMV seronegative and 1 = CMV seropositive. Age: in years. CI = confidence interval.

[a]Model $R^2 = 0.045$.

[b]Model $R^2 = 0.120$.

[c]Model $R^2 = 0.184$.

[d]Model $R^2 = 0.233$.

†Not tested in multivariate analysis due to $p > 0.3$ in univariate regression analysis.

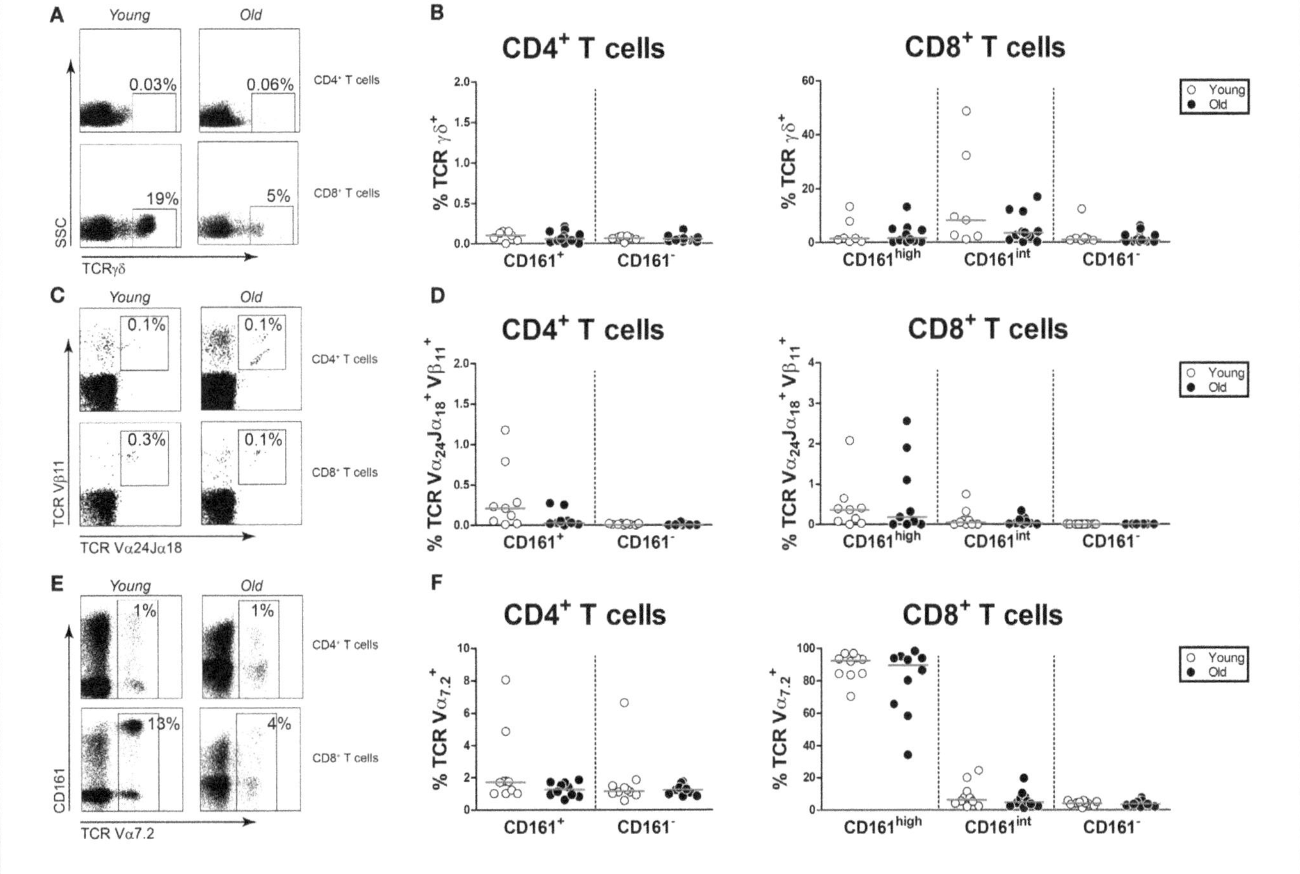

FIGURE 2 | Innate-like T cell markers on CD161-expressing T cells. **(A)** Flow cytometric gating of TCRγδ+ cells in the CD4+ and CD8+ T cell compartment of a young and old subject. **(B)** Percentages of TCRγδ+ cells within the CD161-defined CD4+ and CD8+ T cell subsets of 7 young [of which 4 were cytomegalovirus (CMV) seropositive] and 16 old (of which 8 were CMV seropositive) subjects. **(C)** Flow cytometric gating of TCR-Vα24-Jα18+TCR-Vβ11+ cells in the CD4+ and CD8+ T cell compartment of a young and old subject. **(D)** Percentages of TCR-Vα24-Jα18+ TCR-Vβ11+ cells within the CD161-defined CD4+ and CD8+ T cell subsets of nine young (of which four were CMV seropositive) and nine old (of which four were CMV seropositive) subjects. **(E)** Flow cytometric gating of TCR-Vα7.2+ cells in the CD4+ and CD8+ T cell compartment of a young and old subject. **(F)** Percentages of TCR-Vα7.2+ cells within the CD161-defined CD4+ and CD8+ T cell subsets of 10 young (of which 5 were CMV seropositive) and 10 old (of which 5 were CMV seropositive) subjects. Graphs in which CMV-seropositive young and old subjects are highlighted in the figures are shown in Figure S2 in Supplementary Material.

(**Figure 2B**). Percentages of TCRγδ⁺ cells were limited within the CD161^{high} and CD161^{int} CD8⁺ T cell subsets, and no differences were observed between young and old subjects. iNKT cells were identified as TCR-Vα24-Jα18 and TCR-Vβ11 co-expressing cells (**Figure 2C**). Overall, percentages of iNKT cells were low and similar among the CD161-expressing T cell subsets of young and old subjects (**Figure 2D**). To delineate MAIT cells, additional staining was performed for the TCR-Vα7.2 receptor (**Figure 2E**). Although limited expression of TCR-Vα7.2 was observed among all CD161-defined T cell populations, the expression of this receptor was largely restricted to CD161^{high} CD8⁺ T cells, with similar percentages observed in young and old subjects (**Figure 2F**). Overall, the expression of innate-like T cell markers by CD161-expressing CD4⁺ and CD8⁺ T cells was not affected by age.

We subsequently investigated the effect of aging on proportions of the CD161-expressing innate-like T cell subsets within the total CD3⁺ T cell compartment. Percentages of TCRγδ⁺ cells, i.e., gamma–delta T cells, were similar in young and old subjects (**Figure 3A**). The same was true for percentages of CD161⁺ TCRγδ⁺ CD8⁺ T cells (**Figure 3B**). CD161⁺ TCRγδ⁺ CD4⁺ T cells were nearly absent, both in young and in old subjects (data not shown). However, a small portion of TCRγδ⁺ cells showed a CD4/CD8 double-negative (DN) phenotype. No difference was observed for percentages of CD161⁺ TCRγδ⁺ DN T cells within the CD3⁺ T cell pool of young and old subjects (**Figure 3C**). Proportions of TCR-Vα24-Jα18 and TCR-Vβ11 co-expressing cells, i.e., iNKT cells, were comparable in young and old subjects (**Figure 3D**). The low frequencies of iNKT cells precluded any further sub-analyses of these cells. Percentages of CD161^{high}

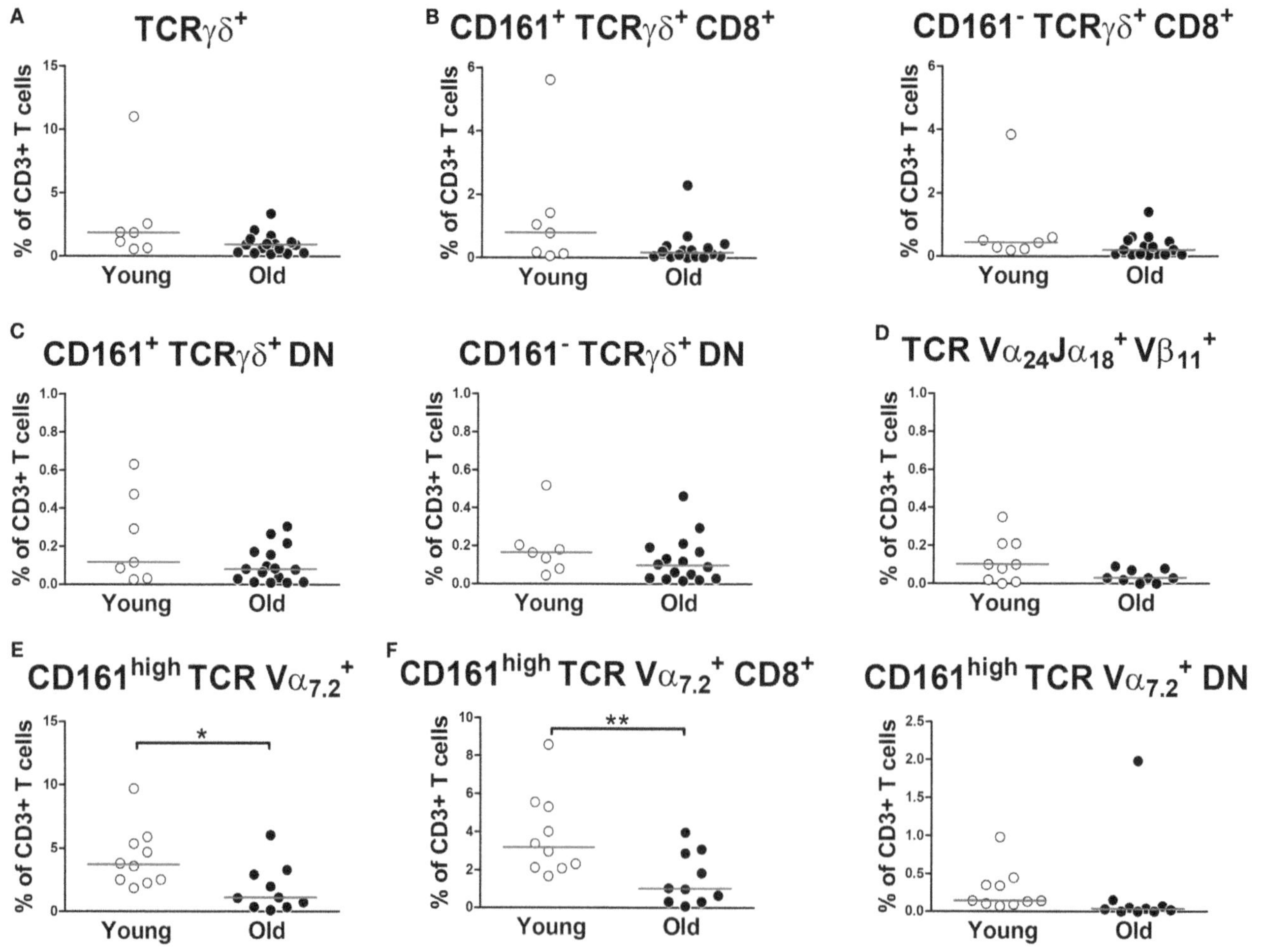

FIGURE 3 | Proportions of CD161-expressing innate-like T cells in the CD3⁺ T cell compartment **(A)** Percentages of total TCRγδ⁺ cells (i.e., gamma–delta T cells) [**(B)** left panel], CD161⁺ CD8⁺ gamma–delta T cells [**(B)** right panel], CD161⁻ CD8⁺ gamma–delta T cells [**(C)**, left panel], CD161⁺ double-negative (DN) gamma–delta T cells, and [**(C)**, right panel] CD161⁻ DN gamma–delta T cells within the CD3⁺ T cell compartment of 7 young [of which 4 were cytomegalovirus (CMV) seropositive] and 16 old (of which 8 were CMV seropositive) subjects. **(D)** Percentages of TCR-Vα24-Jα18⁺TCR-Vβ11⁺ cells (i.e., invariant natural killer T cells) within the CD3⁺ T cell compartment of nine young (of which four were CMV seropositive) and nine old (of which four were CMV seropositive) subjects. **(E)** Percentages of total CD161^{high} TCR-Vα7.2⁺ mucosal-associated invariant T (MAIT) cells, [**(F)**, left panel] CD8⁺ MAIT cells, and [**(F)**, right panel] DN MAIT cells within the CD3⁺ T cell compartment of 10 young (of which 5 were CMV seropositive) and 10 old (of which 5 were CMV seropositive) subjects. Statistical significance by Mann–Whitney *U*-test is shown as $^{*}p < 0.05$ or $^{**}p < 0.01$. Graphs in which CMV-seropositive young and old subjects are highlighted in the figures are shown in Figure S3 in Supplementary Material.

TCR-Vα7.2⁺ MAIT cells were lower in the CD3⁺ T cell compartment of old subjects than that of young subjects (**Figure 3E**). This decrease resulted from a decrease of CD8⁺ MAIT cells rather than DN MAIT cells (**Figure 3F**). As previously reported by others (32, 35), CD4⁺ MAIT cells were nearly absent (data not shown). Thus, aging is associated with a decrease of CD8⁺ MAIT cells.

Aging Is Not Associated With Major Changes in the Memory Phenotype of CD161-Expressing T Cells

Next, we questioned if aging would impact the differentiation status of CD161-expressing CD4⁺ and CD8⁺ T cells. Based on the expression of CD45RO and CCR7, we identified naive (N; CD45RO⁻CCR7⁺), central memory (CM) (CD45RO⁺CCR7⁺), effector memory (EM) (CD45RO⁺CCR7⁻), and terminally differentiated (TD) (CD45RO⁻CCR7⁻) cells in the peripheral blood of the healthy subjects (**Figure 4A**). CD161⁺ CD4⁺ T cells were predominantly CM and EM cells, irrespective of age (**Figure 4B**). Nearly all CD161^{high} CD8⁺ T cells showed an EM cell phenotype (**Figure 4C**). Similar percentages of EM cells were observed among CD161^{high} CD8⁺ T cells of young and old subjects, whereas a small increase of CM cells was observed in the old. CD161^{int} CD8⁺ T cells were mostly EM and TD cells, with similar percentages in young and old subjects. In contrast to the relatively stable differentiation phenotype of CD161-expressing T cells, a clear

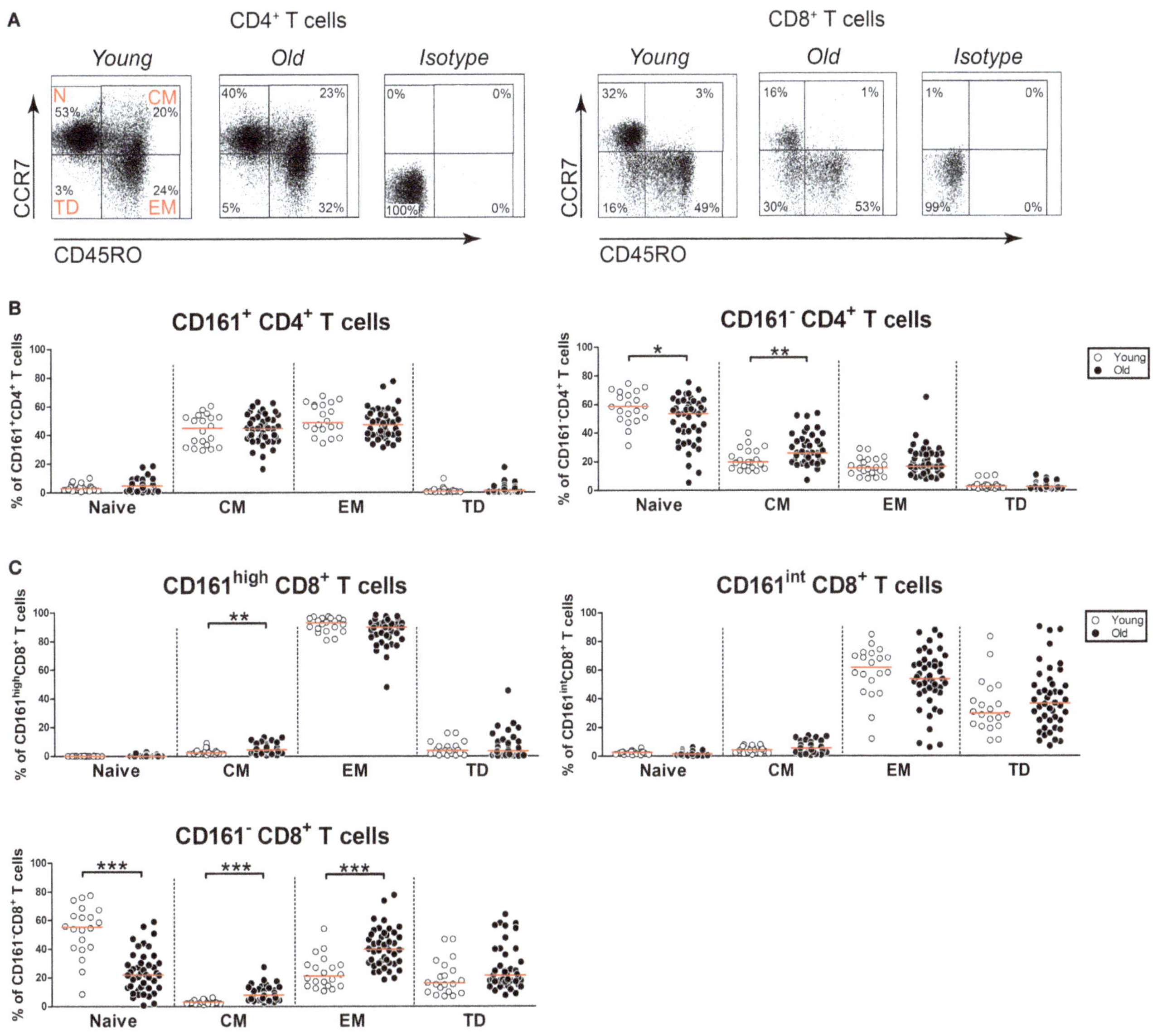

FIGURE 4 | Differentiation markers on CD161-expressing T cells. **(A)** Flow cytometric gating of naive cells (N; CD45RO⁻CCR7⁺), central memory cells (CM) (CD45RO⁺CCR7⁺), effector memory cells (EM) (CD45RO⁺CCR7⁻), and terminally differentiated cells (TD) (CD45RO⁻CCR7⁻) within the CD4⁺ and CD8⁺ T cell compartment of a young and old subject. **(B)** Percentages of differentiation subsets within the CD161-defined CD4⁺ T cell subsets of 20 young [of which 10 were cytomegalovirus (CMV) seropositive] and 44 old (of which 22 were CMV seropositive) subjects. **(C)** Percentages of differentiation subsets within the CD161-defined CD8⁺ T cell subsets of the same donors as mentioned at **(B)**. Statistical significance by Mann–Whitney *U*-test is shown as $^{*}p < 0.05$, $^{**}p < 0.01$, or $^{***}p < 0.001$. Graphs in which CMV-seropositive young and old subjects are highlighted in the figures are shown in Figure S4 in Supplementary Material.

shift from naive toward memory cells was observed among the CD161⁻ CD4⁺ and CD161⁻ CD8⁺ T cell fractions (**Figures 4B,C**). Thus, aging showed no substantial effect on the differentiation status of CD161-expressing T cells.

Aging Has Limited Effect on NK Receptor Expression by CD161-Expressing T Cells

As aging is associated with the expression of NK receptors by T cells (6, 7), we next investigated the expression of NK receptors on CD161-expressing $CD4^+$ and $CD8^+$ T cells of young and old subjects. Firstly, we evaluated the activating NK receptor 2B4 on the $CD4^+$ and $CD8^+$ T cell subsets (**Figure 5A**). Few $CD161^+$ $CD4^+$ T cells expressed 2B4, without any difference between young and old subjects (**Figure 5B**). Nearly all $CD161^{high}$ and $CD161^{int}$ $CD8^+$ T cells showed the expression of 2B4, irrespective of age. Next, we studied the activating NK receptor DNAM-1 (**Figure 5C**). The majority of $CD161^+$ $CD4^+$ T cells, $CD161^{high}$ $CD8^+$ T cells, and $CD161^{int}$ $CD8^+$ T cells expressed DNAM-1 (**Figure 5D**). Among these T cell subsets, the percentages of DNAM-1^+ cells were similar in young and old

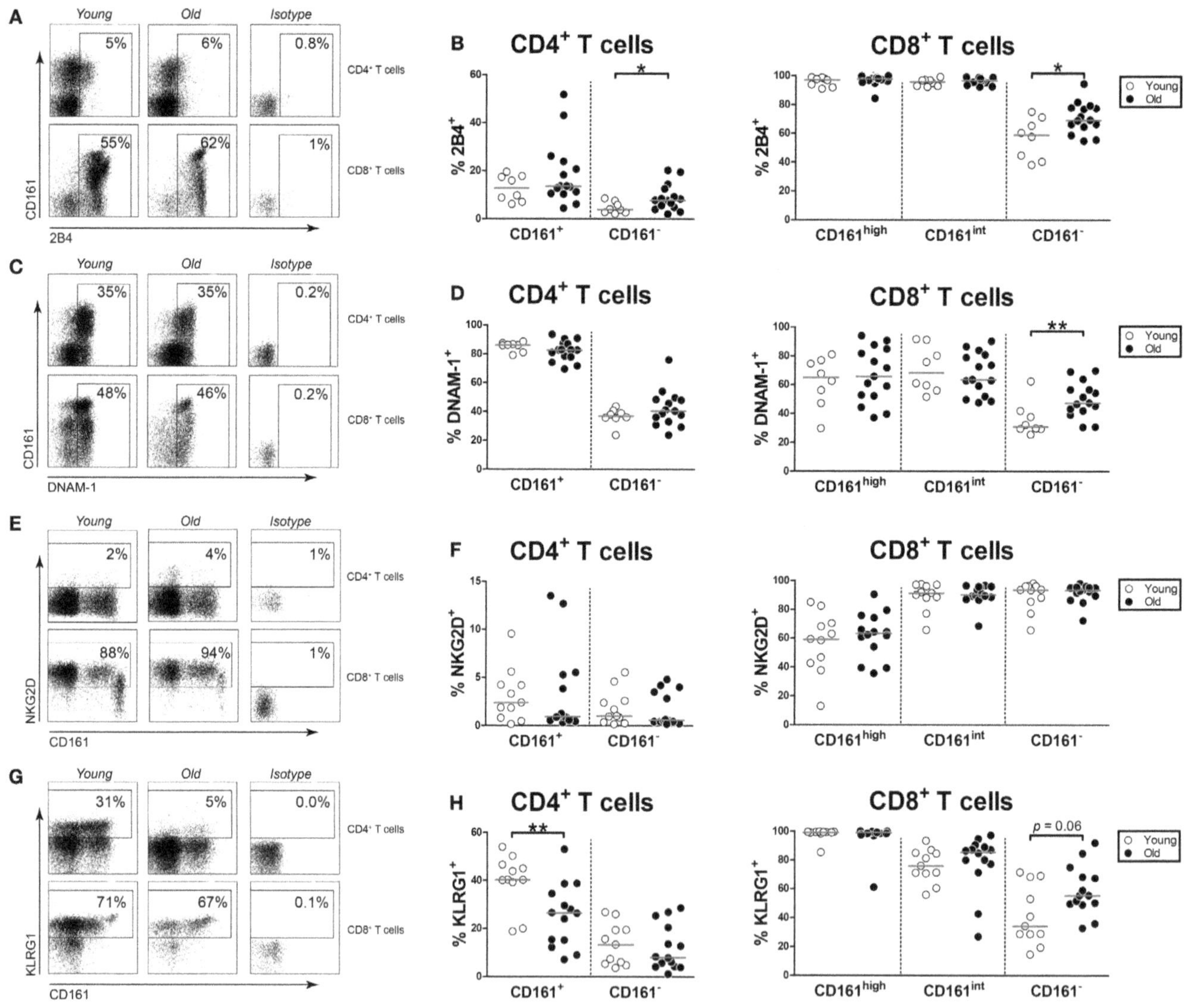

FIGURE 5 | Natural killer markers on CD161-expressing T cells. **(A)** Flow cytometric gating of $2B4^+$ cells within the $CD4^+$ and $CD8^+$ T cell compartment of a young and old subject. **(B)** Percentages of $2B4^+$ cells within the CD161-defined $CD4^+$ and $CD8^+$ T cell subsets of 8 young [of which 4 were cytomegalovirus (CMV) seropositive] and 15 old (of which 7 were CMV seropositive) subjects. **(C)** Flow cytometric gating of DNAX accessory molecule-1 (DNAM-1)⁺ cells within the $CD4^+$ and $CD8^+$ T cell compartment of a young and old subject. **(D)** Percentages of DNAM-1^+ cells within the CD161-defined $CD4^+$ and $CD8^+$ T cell subsets of the same subjects as shown in **(B)**. **(E)** Flow cytometric gating of $NKG2D^+$ cells within the $CD4^+$ and $CD8^+$ T cell compartment of a young and old subject. **(F)** Percentages of $NKG2D^+$ cells within the CD161-defined $CD4^+$ and $CD8^+$ T cell subsets of 11 young (of which 6 were CMV seropositive) and 14 old (of which 8 were CMV seropositive) subjects. **(G)** Flow cytometric gating of $KLRG1^+$ cells within the $CD4^+$ and $CD8^+$ T cell compartment of a young and old subject. **(H)** Percentages of $KLRG1^+$ cells within the CD161-defined $CD4^+$ and $CD8^+$ T cell subsets of the same subjects as shown in **(F)**. Statistical significance by Mann–Whitney *U*-test is shown as $^*p < 0.05$ or $^{**}p < 0.01$. Graphs in which CMV-seropositive young and old subjects are highlighted in the figures are shown in Figure S5 in Supplementary Material.

subjects. Subsequently, the expression of the activating receptor NKG2D was evaluated (**Figure 5E**). Equally low percentages of NKG2D$^+$ cells were observed among CD161$^+$ CD4$^+$ T cells of young and old individuals (**Figure 5F**). A significant proportion of CD161^{high} CD8$^+$ T cells and nearly all CD161^{int} CD8$^+$ T cells expressed NKG2D, with similar percentages in young and old subjects. Next, we evaluated the expression of the inhibitory receptor KLRG1 (**Figure 5G**). A significant portion of CD161$^+$ CD4$^+$ T cells expressed KLRG1 in young subjects, but the percentage of KLRG1$^+$ cells was significantly lower in CD161$^+$ CD4$^+$ T cells of old subjects (**Figure 5H**). Most CD161^{high} and CD161^{int} CD8$^+$ T cells expressed KLRG1, with similar percentages in young and old subjects. Taken together, aging was associated with a decreased expression of KLRG1 on CD161$^+$ CD4$^+$ T cells, while the expression of the other NK receptors was stable.

Aging Has Limited Effect on Cytotoxic Effector Molecule Expression by CD161-Expressing T Cells

Next, we questioned if aging would affect the expression of cytotoxic effector molecules, i.e., perforin and granzyme B, by CD161-expressing CD4$^+$ and CD8$^+$ T cells. Few CD161$^+$ CD4$^+$ T cells and approximately half of CD161^{high} and CD161^{int} CD8$^+$ T cells expressed perforin (**Figures 6A,B**). In this respect, no difference was observed between young and old subjects. The expression of granzyme B was limited in CD161$^+$ CD4$^+$ T cells and CD161^{high} CD8$^+$ T cells, whereas a significant portion of CD161^{int} CD8$^+$ T cells expressed this cytotoxic effector molecule (**Figures 6C,D**). The expression of granzyme B was similar among the CD161-expressing subsets of young and old individuals. Overall, the expression of perforin and granzyme B among CD161-expressing cells was rather stable with age.

Aging Is Associated With Decreased IFN-γ and IL-17 Expression by CD161$^+$ CD4$^+$ T Cells

As CD161-expressing T cells are potent producers of pro-inflammatory cytokines, we investigated if aging impacts this function of CD161-expressing T cells. In contrast to CD161$^-$ CD4$^+$ and CD8$^+$ T cells, a substantial portion of CD161$^+$ CD4$^+$ T cells and the vast majority of CD161^{high} and CD161^{int} CD8$^+$ T cells were capable of producing IFN-γ upon PMA/Ca^{2+}-ionophore stimulation (**Figures 7A–C**). Interestingly, percentages of IFN-γ producing cells were lower among CD161$^+$ CD4$^+$ T cells of old subjects than those of young subjects. By contrast, slightly more CD161^{int} CD8$^+$ T cells were capable of producing IFN-γ in old subjects than young subjects. IL-17 was mostly produced by CD161$^+$ CD4$^+$ T cells and CD161^{high} CD8$^+$ T cells (**Figures 7D–F**). Whereas the percentage of IL-17-producing cells was similar in CD161^{high} CD8$^+$ T cells of young and old subjects, the percentage of IL-17$^+$ cells was decreased in CD161$^+$ CD4$^+$ T cells of old individuals. A small fraction of CD161$^+$ CD4$^+$ T cells was capable of producing IL-4, with no differences between young and old subjects (**Figures 7G,H**). The expression of IL-4 was nearly absent in CD161^{high} and CD161^{int} CD8$^+$ cells, irrespective

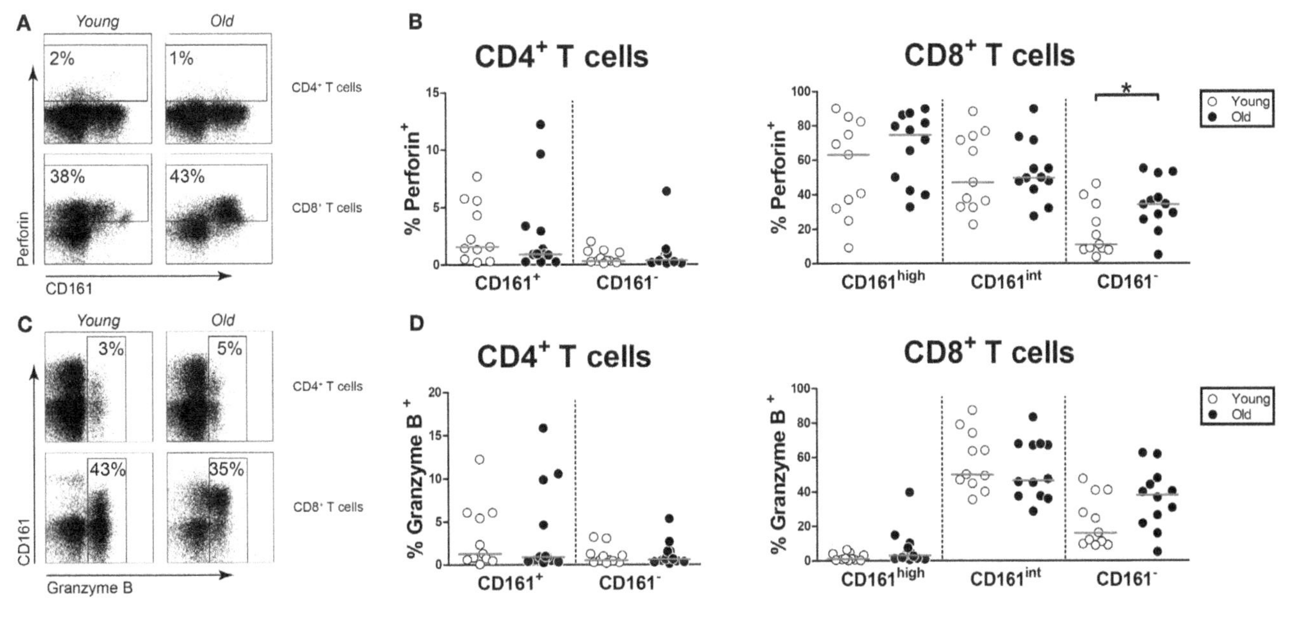

FIGURE 6 | Cytotoxic effector molecules in CD161-expressing T cells. Intracellular staining for perforin and granzyme B was performed on non-stimulated blood samples. **(A)** Flow cytometric gating of perforin$^+$ cells within the CD4$^+$ and CD8$^+$ T cell compartment of a young and old subject. **(B)** Percentages of perforin$^+$ cells within the CD161-defined CD4$^+$ and CD8$^+$ T cell subsets of 11 young [of which 7 were cytomegalovirus (CMV) seropositive] and 12 old (of which 8 were CMV seropositive) subjects. **(C)** Flow cytometric gating of granzyme B$^+$ cells within the CD4$^+$ and CD8$^+$ T cell compartment of a young and old subject. **(D)** Percentages of granzyme B$^+$ cells within the CD161-defined CD4$^+$ and CD8$^+$ T cell subsets of the same subjects as shown in **(B)**. Statistical significance by Mann–Whitney *U*-test is shown as *$p < 0.05$. Graphs in which CMV-seropositive young and old subjects are highlighted in the figures are shown in Figure S6 in Supplementary Material.

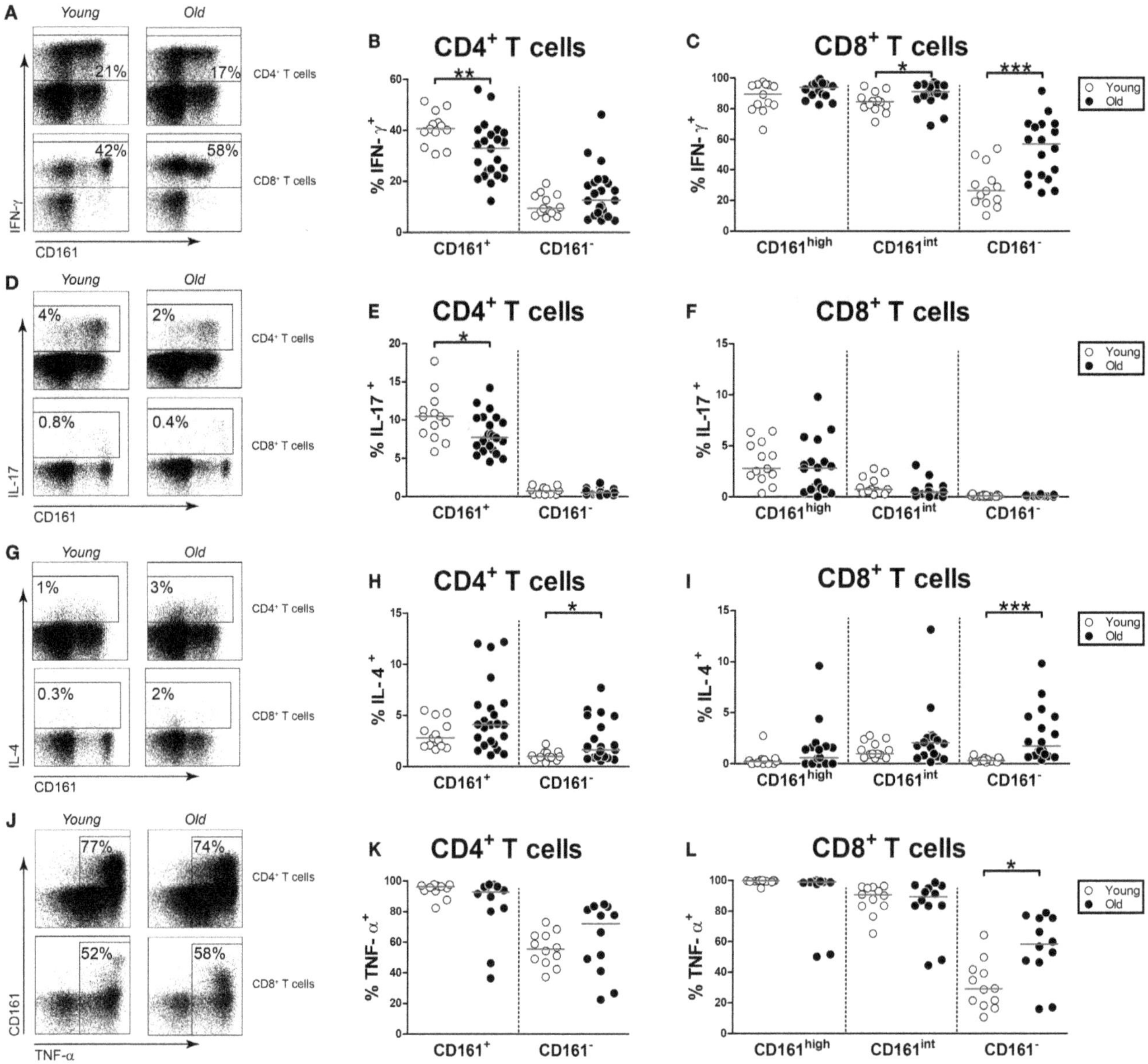

FIGURE 7 | Cytokine expression by CD161-expressing T cells. Intracellular staining for pro-inflammatory cytokines was determined on blood samples that were stimulated with PMA and calcium ionophore in the presence of brefeldin A. **(A)** Flow cytometric gating of IFN-γ+ cells within the CD4+ and CD8+ T cell compartment of a young and old subject. **(B)** Percentages of IFN-γ+ cells within the CD161-defined CD4+ T cell subsets of 13 young [of which 8 were cytomegalovirus (CMV) seropositive] and 23 old (of which 15 were CMV seropositive) subjects. **(C)** Percentages of IFN-γ+ cells within the CD161-defined CD8+ T cell subsets of 13 young (of which 8 were CMV seropositive) and 18 old (of which 12 were CMV seropositive) subjects. **(D)** Flow cytometric gating of interleukin (IL)-17+ cells within the CD4+ and CD8+ T cell compartment of a young and old subject. **(E)** Percentages of IL-17+ cells within the CD161-defined CD4+ T cell subsets of the same subjects as shown in **(B)**. **(F)** Percentages of IL-17+ cells within the CD161-defined CD8+ T cell subsets of the same subjects as shown in **(C)**. **(G)** Flow cytometric gating of IL-4+ cells within the CD4+ and CD8+ T cell compartment of a young and old subject. **(H)** Percentages of IL-4+ cells within the CD161-defined CD4+ T cell subsets of the same subjects as shown in **(B)**. **(I)** Percentages of IL-4+ cells within the CD161-defined CD8+ T cell subsets of the same subjects as shown in **(C)**. **(J)** Flow cytometric gating of TNF-α+ cells within the CD4+ and CD8+ T cell compartment of a young and old subject. **(K)** Percentages of TNF-α+ cells within the CD161-defined CD4+ T cell subsets and **(L)** CD161-defined CD8+ T cell subsets of 12 young (of which 7 were CMV seropositive) and 12 old (of which 7 were CMV seropositive) subjects. Statistical significance by Mann–Whitney *U*-test is shown as *$p < 0.05$, **$p < 0.01$, or ***$p < 0.001$. Graphs in which CMV-seropositive young and old subjects are highlighted in the figures are shown in Figure S7 in Supplementary Material.

of age (**Figures 7G,I**). Finally, we investigated CD161-expressing T cells for their ability to produce TNF-α (**Figure 7J**). Nearly all CD161+ CD4+ T cells, CD161high CD8+ T cells, and CD161int CD8+ T cells were capable of producing TNF-α (**Figures 7K,L**). Similar percentages of TNF-α+ cells were observed in these CD161-expressing T cell subsets of young and old subjects. Taken together, our findings confirm that CD161-expressing cells are potent producers of pro-inflammatory cytokines. However,

CD161⁺ CD4⁺ T cells of old subjects show a diminished capacity to produce IFN-γ and IL-17 upon stimulation.

Aging Is Associated With a Numerical Decline of Nonclassic Th1 Cells

CD4⁺ T cells may co-express pro-inflammatory cytokines such as IFN-γ, IL-17, and IL-4 (39). Therefore, we next investigated CD161⁺ and CD161⁻ CD4⁺ T cells for the co-expression of the Th1, Th17, and Th2 lineage cytokines, i.e., IFN-γ, IL-17, and IL-4, respectively. The CD161⁺ CD4⁺ T cell pool contained cells solely producing IFN-γ, IL-17, or IL-4, but also IFN-γ⁺ IL-17⁺, and IFN-γ⁺ IL-4⁺ cells (**Figure 8A**). Interestingly, the percentages of both IFN-γ⁺ and IFN-γ⁺ IL-17⁺ cells were decreased among CD161⁺ CD4⁺ T cells of old subjects when compared to those of young subjects. In essence, the CD161⁻ CD4⁺ T cell pool showed limited potential to produce pro-inflammatory cytokines, with only few cells producing solely IFN-γ or IL-4. The percentages of IL-4-producing cells were slightly higher in CD161⁻ CD4⁺ T cells of old subjects than those of young subjects. Thus, the percentages of Th1 and Th1/Th17 cells are decreased in the CD161⁺ CD4⁺ T cell compartment of aged subjects.

Prior reports indicate that Th17 cells show plasticity toward Th1/Th17 cells and ultimately Th1 cells. The latter cells have been termed nonclassic Th1 cells and are characterized by the expression of CD161 (39). To assess the impact of aging on frequencies of nonclassic Th1 cells, we next investigated CD161 expression on Th1, Th1/Th17, and Th17 cells (**Figure 8B**, left panel). Percentages of CD161-expressing cells were equally high among Th17 and Th1/Th17 cells of young and old subjects (**Figure 8B**, right panel). Percentages of CD161-expressing cells were clearly lower among Th1 cells than among Th17 and Th1/Th17 cells. Moreover, fewer Th1 cells expressed CD161 in old subjects than in young subjects. This finding suggests that aging is associated with decreased frequencies of nonclassic Th1 cells.

DISCUSSION

We here provide the first comprehensive analysis of the impact of aging on CD161-expressing T cells in humans. We show that the numbers of CD161^high CD8⁺ T cells decline with age, whereas the numbers of CD161^int CD8⁺ T cells and CD161⁺ CD4⁺ T cells remain stable. In respect to the expression of innate-like T cell markers, differentiation markers, and NK receptors, the phenotype of CD161-expressing T cell subsets appeared rather stable with age. Overall, the expression of pro-inflammatory cytokines and cytotoxic effector molecules was comparable in CD161-expressing T cells of young and old subjects. However, the ability to produce IFN-γ and IL-17 upon stimulation was

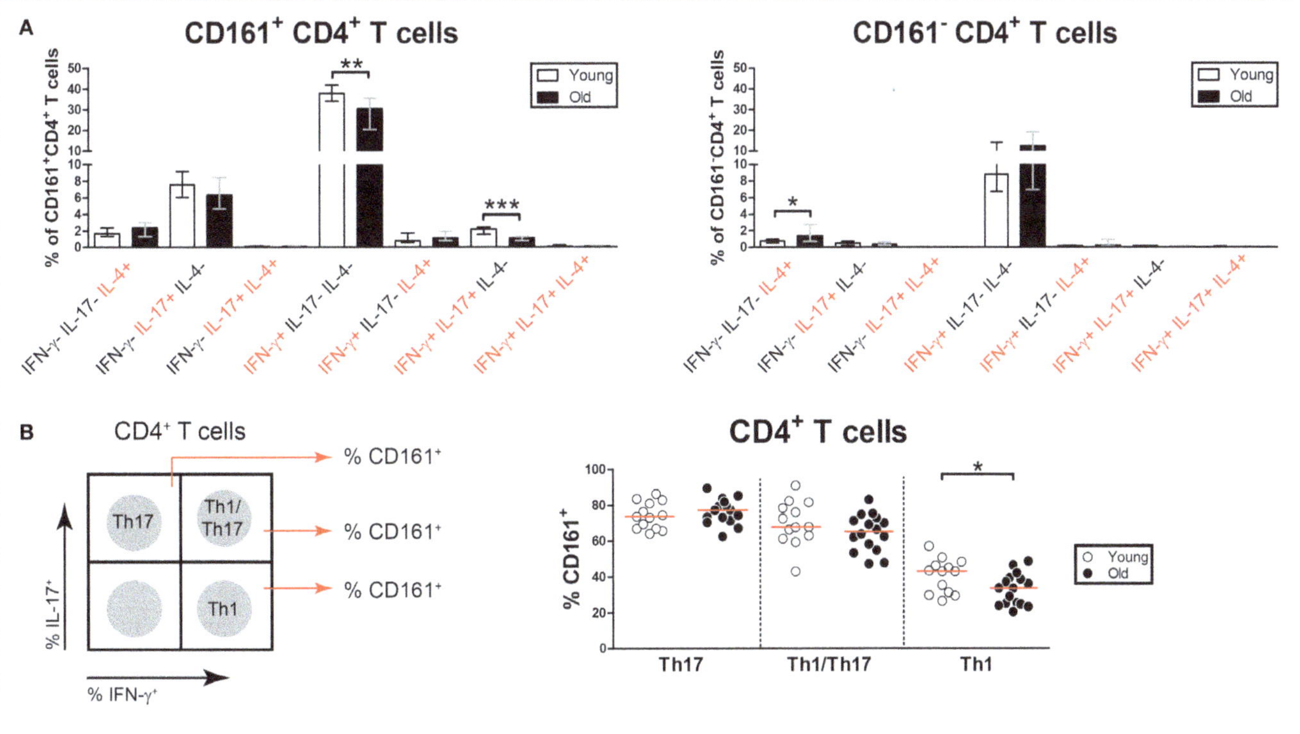

FIGURE 8 | Co-expression of pro-inflammatory cytokines by CD4⁺ T cells. Intracellular staining for pro-inflammatory cytokines was determined on blood samples that were stimulated with PMA and calcium ionophore in the presence of brefeldin A. **(A)** Analysis of co-expression of IFN-γ, interleukin (IL)-17, and IL-4 by CD161⁺ CD4⁺ T cells and CD161⁻ CD4⁺ T cells of 13 young [of which 8 were cytomegalovirus (CMV) seropositive] and 23 old (of which 15 were CMV seropositive) subjects. Percentages of cells co-expressing different combinations of these cytokines within the CD161⁺ and CD161⁻ CD4⁺ T cell pool are shown. **(B)** Analysis of CD161 expression by Th17 cells (IL-17⁺ IFN-γ⁻), Th1/Th17 cells (IL-17⁺ IFN-γ⁺), and Th1 cells (IL-17⁻ IFN-γ⁺) in 13 young (of which 8 were CMV seropositive) and 16 old (of which 11 were CMV seropositive) subjects. A schematic illustration of the gating strategy is shown in the left panel. Percentages of CD161⁺ cells among Th17, Th1/Th17, and Th1 cells are shown in the right panel. Bars and whiskers indicate median and interquartile range. Statistical significance by Mann–Whitney *U*-test is shown as $^*p < 0.05$ and $^{**}p < 0.01$.

diminished among CD161$^+$ CD4$^+$ T cells of old individuals. Thus, aging is associated with both numerical and functional changes of CD161-expressing T cells, whereas we observed no substantial phenotypic alterations of these cells.

Aging was associated with stable frequencies of circulating CD161$^+$ CD4$^+$ T cells and a diminished production of pro-inflammatory cytokines by these cells. So far, the impact of age on the numbers of CD161$^+$ CD4$^+$ T cells remained unclear. The absolute numbers of CD161$^+$ CD4$^+$ T cells were not affected by aging in our multivariate linear regression analysis. We confirmed that CD161$^+$ CD4$^+$ T cells primarily show a CM or an EM phenotype, both in young and in old subjects. In accordance with their pro-inflammatory function, CD161$^+$ CD4$^+$ T cells produced more IFN-γ, IL-17, and TNF-α than CD161$^-$ CD4$^+$ T cells. Previously, we have shown that frequencies of Th17 cells and Th1 cells are decreased within the memory CD4$^+$ T cell compartment of elderly subjects (8). In the current study, we add that the proportions of IL-17$^+$ and IFN-γ$^+$ cells are decreased among CD161$^+$ CD4$^+$ T cells of old subjects. Thus, the pro-inflammatory function of CD161$^+$ CD4$^+$ T cells declines with age.

Frequencies of nonclassic Th1 cells were found to be decreased in old subjects. Previous studies have shown that most Th17 cells are contained within the CD161$^+$ CD4$^+$ T cell compartment (18). It has been suggested that these Th17 cells show plasticity toward Th1/Th17 cells and eventually Th1 cells under pro-inflammatory conditions (30, 31). The latter Th1 cells have been termed nonclassic Th1 cells, while maintaining their expression of CD161 (39). In the current study, we show that the proportions of Th1/Th17 and Th1 cells are decreased among CD161$^+$ CD4$^+$ T cells of old subjects when compared to young subjects. Moreover, we show that fewer Th1 cells expressed CD161 in old subjects. Together, these findings suggest that aging affects the plasticity of Th17 cells toward nonclassic Th1 cells. It would be interesting to further study the mechanisms explaining this decreased plasticity in the elderly.

The numbers of circulating CD161^{high} CD8$^+$ T cells decreased with age, whereas their ability to produce pro-inflammatory cytokines remained intact. As previously shown by others (32, 33), we observed that most CD161^{high} CD8$^+$ T cells are MAIT cells, as evidenced by the expression of the TCR-Vα7.2 receptor. Proportions of MAIT cells were uniformly high among CD161^{high} CD8$^+$ T cells of young and old subjects. In accordance with prior reports (34–36), we observed that the numbers of CD161^{high} TCR-Vα7.2$^+$ CD8$^+$ T cells decline with age. We confirmed that CD161^{high} CD8$^+$ T cells are mostly contained within the EM compartment (19). Prior reports indicate that CD161^{high} CD8$^+$ T cells are strong producers of pro-inflammatory cytokines (19). In the current study, we show that this function of CD161^{high} CD8$^+$ T cells is not affected by aging. CD161^{high} CD8$^+$ T cells of young and old subjects showed similar ability to produce IFN-γ, IL-17, and TNF-α. This finding seems in agreement with a prior study showing that the percentages of IFN-γ$^+$ and IL-17$^+$ cells are comparable in the CD8$^+$ MAIT cell compartment of young and old individuals (34). Thus, only the frequency, but not the pro-inflammatory function, of CD161^{high} CD8$^+$ T cells declines with age.

Neither the numbers of CD161^{int} CD8$^+$ T cells nor their cytokine-producing potential was affected by age. The absolute numbers of CD161^{int} CD8$^+$ T cells were comparable in young and old subjects. Nevertheless, the percentages of CD161^{int} CD8$^+$ T cells showed an increase with age due to loss of CD161^{high} and CD161$^-$ CD8$^+$ T cells from the CD8$^+$ T cell compartment. CD161^{int} CD8$^+$ T cells primarily resided within the EM and TD compartments, as previously shown by others (20). In this respect, we observed no difference between CD161^{int} CD8$^+$ T cells of young and old subjects. We confirmed that most CD161^{int} CD8$^+$ T cells are able to produce IFN-γ and TNF-α (19, 20). In addition, CD161^{int} CD8$^+$ T cells of old subjects more frequently produced IFN-γ than those of young subjects, whereas no difference was observed for TNF-α. Thus, both the frequencies and cytokine-producing potential of CD161^{int} CD8$^+$ T cells are preserved on to high age.

The expression of NK receptors was comparable in CD161-expressing T cells of young and old subjects. In addition to signaling *via* the TCR and conventional co-stimulation molecules, T cell activation may be influenced by NK receptors. In particular, late-stage T cells of aged subjects may express activating and inhibitory NK receptors (6, 7). We here examined CD161-expressing T cells for the presence of three well-defined activating NK receptors (i.e., 2B4, DNAM-1, and NKG2D), as well as one inhibitory NK receptor (i.e., KLRG1). CD161^{high} and CD161^{int} CD8$^+$ T cells showed prominent expression of all four NK receptors, without any difference between young and old subjects. By contrast, CD161$^+$ CD4$^+$ T cells primarily expressed DNAM-1 and KLRG1. DNAM-1 expression was similar in CD161$^+$ CD4$^+$ T cells of young and old subjects, but the percentage of KLRG1$^+$ cells was decreased among CD161$^+$ CD4$^+$ T cells of old subjects. Although our analysis was restricted to only four NK receptors, a decreased expression of the latter inhibitory NK receptor could indicate that CD161$^+$ CD4$^+$ T cells of old subjects might be more prone to activation.

The expression of cytotoxic effector molecules by CD161-expressing T cells was not affected by age. CD161$^+$ CD4$^+$ T cells showed little expression of perforin and granzyme B, irrespective of age. Approximately half of the CD161^{int} CD8$^+$ T cells expressed perforin and granzyme B in young and old subjects. This finding underscores the prominent cytotoxic potential of these cells. Similar percentages of perforin expressing CD161^{high} CD8$^+$ T cells were observed in young and old individuals. In accordance with prior studies, few CD161^{high} CD8$^+$ T cells expressed granzyme B (19, 40), both in young and in old subjects. It has been demonstrated that CD161^{high} CD8$^+$ T cells primarily express granzymes A and K (40). Although the latter cytotoxic effector molecules were not analyzed in the current study, the stable expression of perforin by CD161^{high} CD8$^+$ T cells suggests that the cytotoxic potential of these cells remains intact with age.

Limited data suggest that CD161-mediated signaling promotes the secretion of pro-inflammatory cytokines by T cells. Lectin-like transcript 1 (LLT1) has been identified as the ligand for CD161 (41, 42). LLT1 is expressed by antigen-presenting cells, including B cells and macrophages (43, 44). It has been shown that the engagement of CD161 by LLT1 enhances the production of pro-inflammatory cytokines by T cells. For instance, the ligation of CD161 when given in addition to TCR stimulation increased the production of IFN-γ and TNF-α by MAIT cells (37). Similar experiments with CD161-expressing T cell clones also indicate that CD161 ligation in the presence of TCR stimulation promotes IFN-γ production by T cells (41). Thus, current evidence suggests that CD161 may act as a co-stimulatory receptor on T cells. An early study has also suggested that CD161 may be directly involved in transendothelial migration of T cells (45). However, this observation has not yet been confirmed by others. It would be interesting to study the effect of aging on the function of CD161 itself.

Given the broad antimicrobial functions of CD161-expressing T cells (20–24), it is likely that the aging-associated changes of $CD161^{+}$ $CD4^{+}$ T cells and $CD161^{high}$ $CD8^{+}$ T cells may compromise immunity in the elderly. The $CD161^{+}$ $CD4^{+}$ T cell compartment contains antiviral Th1-like cells (22), as well as Th17 cells promoting immunity against bacteria and yeasts (46). In patients undergoing treatment for hematological malignancies, $CD161^{+}$ $CD4^{+}$ T cells have recently been linked to preserved immunity against CMV and lower risks for neutropenic infections (22, 47). $CD161^{high}$ $CD8^{+}$ T cells, which primarily consist of MAIT cells, are critical for immunity against common bacteria and viruses, such as *Escherichia coli* and influenza, respectively (23, 48). Numerical decreases of MAIT cells might put elderly subjects at risk for infections with these microbes. Indeed, sepsis due to Gram-negative bacteria and pneumonia occurs more frequently and with a higher severity in the elderly (49). The $CD161^{int}$ $CD8^{+}$ T cell compartment has been identified as a polyclonal $CD8^{+}$ T cell population that contributes to antiviral immunity (20). The stable frequencies of $CD161^{int}$ $CD8^{+}$ T cells, and the ability to produce cytotoxic effector molecules and pro-inflammatory cytokines, likely contribute to immunity throughout adult life. Thus, not all CD161-expressing T cell subsets are compromised with age. It remains to be elucidated if the aging-related effects on $CD161^{+}$ $CD4^{+}$ T cells and $CD161^{high}$ $CD8^{+}$ T cells might be advantageous in the context of autoimmune diseases (25, 26, 50).

We precluded that CMV confounded our findings regarding the impact of aging on CD161-expressing T cells. Indeed, CMV markedly influences the T cell compartment and might potentially compromise immunity to other pathogens in the elderly (9–11, 17). Therefore, we delineated the effects of aging and CMV on the absolute numbers of CD161-expressing cells by performing multivariate linear regression analyses. We confirmed that the aging-associated decline of $CD161^{high}$ $CD8^{+}$ T cell numbers occurred independently from CMV serostatus. These analyses also demonstrated that CMV seropositivity by itself is associated with higher numbers of $CD161^{int}$ $CD8^{+}$ T cells. Interestingly, a recent report indicates that $CD161^{int}$ $CD8^{+}$ T cells are highly functional memory cells that contribute to antiviral immunity (20). Ample evidence also suggests that CMV-specific memory cells upregulate NK receptors and have a strong potential to produce cytotoxic effector molecules and pro-inflammatory cytokines (12–14). Importantly, CMV-seropositivity rates were comparable between young and old subjects in our extensive phenotypical and functional analyses of CD161-expressing T cells. Thus, CMV unlikely influenced the findings in the current study. Indeed, it would be interesting to further perform a comprehensive analysis of CMV and CD161-expressing T cells.

In conclusion, we here show that aging affects the frequencies and function of CD161-expressing T cells. Aging-associated changes of CD161-expressing T cells might potentially contribute to a decreased antimicrobial immunity in the elderly. Future studies should evaluate the mechanisms and implications of aging-associated changes of CD161-expressing T cells in humans.

ETHICS STATEMENT

Written informed consent was obtained from all study participants. The study was approved by the Medical Ethical Committee of the UMCG. All procedures were in accordance with the Declaration of Helsinki.

AUTHOR CONTRIBUTIONS

KG, B-JK, WA, EB, and AB conceived the study and designed the experiments. KG and EB recruited the study participants. KG and GH performed the experiments and acquired data. All authors were involved in data analysis and interpretation. KG and AB wrote the manuscript, and all authors revised it critically for important intellectual content. All authors approved the final version of the manuscript.

ACKNOWLEDGMENTS

We are grateful to all healthy volunteers and patients who kindly participated in the study. We also thank the members of the Medical Immunology laboratory for their technical assistance. WA, EB, and AB have received funding from the European Union's Horizon 2020 research and innovation program under grant agreement No. 668036. The opinions expressed in this article are those of the authors and do not purport to reflect the official position or views of the EC, its agencies, or officers.

FUNDING

This work was supported by unrestricted grants from NV Organon (now MSD) to AB, Foundation "De Drie Lichten" (project no. 19/11 GJF/mk), and Foundation "Jan Kornelis de Cock" to KG (project no. 2012-22). The funders had no role in study design, data collection and analysis, decision to publish, or preparation of the manuscript.

REFERENCES

1. Boots AM, Maier AB, Stinissen P, Masson P, Lories RJ, De Keyser F. The influence of ageing on the development and management of rheumatoid arthritis. *Nat Rev Rheumatol* (2013) 9:604–13. doi:10.1038/nrrheum.2013.92
2. Boraschi D, Aguado MT, Dutel C, Goronzy J, Louis J, Grubeck-Loebenstein B, et al. The gracefully aging immune system. *Sci Transl Med* (2013) 5:185ps8. doi:10.1126/scitranslmed.3005624
3. den Braber I, Mugwagwa T, Vrisekoop N, Westera L, Mogling R, de Boer AB, et al. Maintenance of peripheral naive T cells is sustained by thymus output in mice but not humans. *Immunity* (2012) 36:288–97. doi:10.1016/j.immuni.2012.02.006
4. van der Geest KS, Abdulahad WH, Horst G, Lorencetti PG, Bijzet J, Arends S, et al. Quantifying distribution of flow cytometric TCR-Vbeta usage with economic statistics. *PLoS One* (2015) 10:e0125373. doi:10.1371/journal.pone.0125373
5. van der Geest KS, Abdulahad WH, Teteloshvili N, Tete SM, Peters JH, Horst G, et al. Low-affinity TCR engagement drives IL-2-dependent post-thymic maintenance of naive CD4+ T cells in aged humans. *Aging Cell* (2015) 14:744–53. doi:10.1111/acel.12353
6. Weng NP, Akbar AN, Goronzy J. CD28(-) T cells: their role in the age-associated decline of immune function. *Trends Immunol* (2009) 30:306–12. doi:10.1016/j.it.2009.03.013
7. Akbar AN, Henson SM. Are senescence and exhaustion intertwined or unrelated processes that compromise immunity? *Nat Rev Immunol* (2011) 11:289–95. doi:10.1038/nri2959
8. van der Geest KS, Abdulahad WH, Tete SM, Lorencetti PG, Horst G, Bos NA, et al. Aging disturbs the balance between effector and regulatory CD4+ T cells. *Exp Gerontol* (2014) 60:190–6. doi:10.1016/j.exger.2014.11.005
9. Sansoni P, Vescovini R, Fagnoni FF, Akbar A, Arens R, Chiu YL, et al. New advances in CMV and immunosenescence. *Exp Gerontol* (2014) 55:54–62. doi:10.1016/j.exger.2014.03.020
10. Gordon CL, Miron M, Thome JJ, Matsuoka N, Weiner J, Rak MA, et al. Tissue reservoirs of antiviral T cell immunity in persistent human CMV infection. *J Exp Med* (2017) 214:651–67. doi:10.1084/jem.20160758
11. Wertheimer AM, Bennett MS, Park B, Uhrlaub JL, Martinez C, Pulko V, et al. Aging and cytomegalovirus infection differentially and jointly affect distinct circulating T cell subsets in humans. *J Immunol* (2014) 192:2143–55. doi:10.4049/jimmunol.1301721
12. Makwana N, Foley B, Fernandez S, Lee S, Irish A, Pircher H, et al. CMV drives the expansion of highly functional memory T cells expressing NK-cell receptors in renal transplant recipients. *Eur J Immunol* (2017) 47:1324–34. doi:10.1002/eji.201747018
13. Jackson SE, Sedikides GX, Mason GM, Okecha G, Wills MR. Human cytomegalovirus (HCMV)-specific CD4(+) T cells are polyfunctional and can respond to HCMV-infected dendritic cells *in vitro*. *J Virol* (2017) 91:e02128-16. doi:10.1128/JVI.02128-16
14. Bajwa M, Vita S, Vescovini R, Larsen M, Sansoni P, Terrazzini N, et al. CMV-specific T-cell responses at older ages: broad responses with a large central memory component may be key to long-term survival. *J Infect Dis* (2017) 215:1212–20. doi:10.1093/infdis/jix080
15. Johnstone J, Parsons R, Botelho F, Millar J, McNeil S, Fulop T, et al. T-cell phenotypes predictive of frailty and mortality in elderly nursing home residents. *J Am Geriatr Soc* (2017) 65:153–9. doi:10.1111/jgs.14507
16. Haq K, Fulop T, Tedder G, Gentleman B, Garneau H, Meneilly GS, et al. Cytomegalovirus seropositivity predicts a decline in the T cell but not the antibody response to influenza in vaccinated older adults independent of type 2 diabetes status. *J Gerontol A Biol Sci Med Sci* (2017) 72:1163–70. doi:10.1093/gerona/glw216
17. Derhovanessian E, Maier AB, Hahnel K, McElhaney JE, Slagboom EP, Pawelec G. Latent infection with cytomegalovirus is associated with poor memory CD4 responses to influenza A core proteins in the elderly. *J Immunol* (2014) 193:3624–31. doi:10.4049/jimmunol.1303361
18. Maggi L, Santarlasci V, Capone M, Peired A, Frosali F, Crome SQ, et al. CD161 is a marker of all human IL-17-producing T-cell subsets and is induced by RORC. *Eur J Immunol* (2010) 40:2174–81. doi:10.1002/eji.200940257
19. Billerbeck E, Kang YH, Walker L, Lockstone H, Grafmueller S, Fleming V, et al. Analysis of CD161 expression on human CD8+ T cells defines a distinct functional subset with tissue-homing properties. *Proc Natl Acad Sci U S A* (2010) 107:3006–11. doi:10.1073/pnas.0914839107
20. Fergusson JR, Huhn MH, Swadling L, Walker LJ, Kurioka A, Llibre A, et al. CD161(int)CD8+ T cells: a novel population of highly functional, memory CD8+ T cells enriched within the gut. *Mucosal Immunol* (2016) 9:401–13. doi:10.1038/mi.2015.69
21. Chua WJ, Truscott SM, Eickhoff CS, Blazevic A, Hoft DF, Hansen TH. Polyclonal mucosa-associated invariant T cells have unique innate functions in bacterial infection. *Infect Immun* (2012) 80:3256–67. doi:10.1128/IAI.00279-12
22. Alsuliman A, Muftuoglu M, Khoder A, Ahn YO, Basar R, Verneris MR, et al. A subset of virus-specific CD161+ T cells selectively express the multidrug transporter MDR1 and are resistant to chemotherapy in AML. *Blood* (2017) 129:740–58. doi:10.1182/blood-2016-05-713347
23. Loh L, Wang Z, Sant S, Koutsakos M, Jegaskanda S, Corbett AJ, et al. Human mucosal-associated invariant T cells contribute to antiviral influenza immunity *via* IL-18-dependent activation. *Proc Natl Acad Sci U S A* (2016) 113:10133–8. doi:10.1073/pnas.1610750113
24. Cosgrove C, Ussher JE, Rauch A, Gartner K, Kurioka A, Huhn MH, et al. Early and nonreversible decrease of CD161++/MAIT cells in HIV infection. *Blood* (2013) 121:951–61. doi:10.1182/blood-2012-06-436436
25. Chalan P, Kroesen BJ, van der Geest KS, Huitema MG, Abdulahad WH, Bijzet J, et al. Circulating CD4+CD161+ T lymphocytes are increased in seropositive arthralgia patients but decreased in patients with newly diagnosed rheumatoid arthritis. *PLoS One* (2013) 8:e79370. doi:10.1371/journal.pone.0079370
26. Annibali V, Ristori G, Angelini DF, Serafini B, Mechelli R, Cannoni S, et al. CD161(high)CD8+T cells bear pathogenetic potential in multiple sclerosis. *Brain* (2011) 134:542–54. doi:10.1093/brain/awq354
27. Kleinschek MA, Boniface K, Sadekova S, Grein J, Murphy EE, Turner SP, et al. Circulating and gut-resident human Th17 cells express CD161 and promote intestinal inflammation. *J Exp Med* (2009) 206:525–34. doi:10.1084/jem.20081712
28. Zhao L, Nocturne G, Haskett S, Boudaoud S, Lazure T, Le Pajolec C, et al. Clinical relevance of RORgamma positive and negative subsets of CD161+ CD4+ T cells in primary Sjogren's syndrome. *Rheumatology (Oxford)* (2017) 56:303–12. doi:10.1093/rheumatology/kew360
29. Cosmi L, De Palma R, Santarlasci V, Maggi L, Capone M, Frosali F, et al. Human interleukin 17-producing cells originate from a CD161+CD4+ T cell precursor. *J Exp Med* (2008) 205:1903–16. doi:10.1084/jem.20080397
30. Cosmi L, Cimaz R, Maggi L, Santarlasci V, Capone M, Borriello F, et al. Evidence of the transient nature of the Th17 phenotype of CD4+CD161+ T cells in the synovial fluid of patients with juvenile idiopathic arthritis. *Arthritis Rheum* (2011) 63:2504–15. doi:10.1002/art.30332
31. Maggi L, Cimaz R, Capone M, Santarlasci V, Querci V, Simonini G, et al. Brief report: etanercept inhibits the tumor necrosis factor alpha-driven shift of Th17 lymphocytes toward a nonclassic Th1 phenotype in juvenile idiopathic arthritis. *Arthritis Rheumatol* (2014) 66:1372–7. doi:10.1002/art.38355
32. Walker LJ, Kang YH, Smith MO, Tharmalingham H, Ramamurthy N, Fleming VM, et al. Human MAIT and CD8alphaalpha cells develop from a pool of type-17 precommitted CD8+ T cells. *Blood* (2012) 119:422–33. doi:10.1182/blood-2011-05-353789
33. Dusseaux M, Martin E, Serriari N, Peguillet I, Premel V, Louis D, et al. Human MAIT cells are xenobiotic-resistant, tissue-targeted, CD161hi IL-17-secreting T cells. *Blood* (2011) 117:1250–9. doi:10.1182/blood-2010-08-303339
34. Lee OJ, Cho YN, Kee SJ, Kim MJ, Jin HM, Lee SJ, et al. Circulating mucosal-associated invariant T cell levels and their cytokine levels in healthy adults. *Exp Gerontol* (2014) 49:47–54. doi:10.1016/j.exger.2013.11.003
35. Novak J, Dobrovolny J, Novakova L, Kozak T. The decrease in number and change in phenotype of mucosal-associated invariant T cells in the elderly and differences in men and women of reproductive age. *Scand J Immunol* (2014) 80:271–5. doi:10.1111/sji.12193
36. Walker LJ, Tharmalingam H, Klenerman P. The rise and fall of MAIT cells with age. *Scand J Immunol* (2014) 80:462–3. doi:10.1111/sji.12237
37. Fergusson JR, Smith KE, Fleming VM, Rajoriya N, Newell EW, Simmons R, et al. CD161 defines a transcriptional and functional phenotype across distinct human T cell lineages. *Cell Rep* (2014) 9:1075–88. doi:10.1016/j.celrep.2014.09.045

38. Takahashi T, Dejbakhsh-Jones S, Strober S. Expression of CD161 (NKR-P1A) defines subsets of human CD4 and CD8 T cells with different functional activities. *J Immunol* (2006) 176:211–6. doi:10.4049/jimmunol.176.1.211
39. Maggi L, Santarlasci V, Capone M, Rossi MC, Querci V, Mazzoni A, et al. Distinctive features of classic and nonclassic (Th17 derived) human Th1 cells. *Eur J Immunol* (2012) 42:3180–8. doi:10.1002/eji.201242648
40. Havenith SH, Yong SL, Henson SM, Piet B, Idu MM, Koch SD, et al. Analysis of stem-cell-like properties of human CD161++IL-18Ralpha+ memory CD8+ T cells. *Int Immunol* (2012) 24:625–36. doi:10.1093/intimm/dxs069
41. Aldemir H, Prod'homme V, Dumaurier MJ, Retiere C, Poupon G, Cazareth J, et al. Cutting edge: lectin-like transcript 1 is a ligand for the CD161 receptor. *J Immunol* (2005) 175:7791–5. doi:10.4049/jimmunol.175.12.7791
42. Rosen DB, Bettadapura J, Alsharifi M, Mathew PA, Warren HS, Lanier LL. Cutting edge: lectin-like transcript-1 is a ligand for the inhibitory human NKR-P1A receptor. *J Immunol* (2005) 175:7796–9. doi:10.4049/jimmunol.175.12.7796
43. Llibre A, Lopez-Macias C, Marafioti T, Mehta H, Partridge A, Kanzig C, et al. LLT1 and CD161 expression in human germinal centers promotes B cell activation and CXCR4 downregulation. *J Immunol* (2016) 196:2085–94. doi:10.4049/jimmunol.1502462
44. Chalan P, Bijzet J, Huitema MG, Kroesen BJ, Brouwer E, Boots AM. Expression of lectin-like transcript 1, the ligand for CD161, in rheumatoid arthritis. *PLoS One* (2015) 10:e0132436. doi:10.1371/journal.pone.0132436
45. Poggi A, Costa P, Zocchi MR, Moretta L. Phenotypic and functional analysis of CD4+ NKRP1A+ human T lymphocytes. Direct evidence that the NKRP1A molecule is involved in transendothelial migration. *Eur J Immunol* (1997) 27:2345–50. doi:10.1002/eji.1830270932
46. Zielinski CE, Mele F, Aschenbrenner D, Jarrossay D, Ronchi F, Gattorno M, et al. Pathogen-induced human TH17 cells produce IFN-gamma or IL-10 and are regulated by IL-1beta. *Nature* (2012) 484:514–8. doi:10.1038/nature10957
47. Kim TW, Lee SE, Lim JY, Ryu DB, Jeon YW, Yoon JH, et al. Clinical significance of pre-transplant circulating CD3(+) CD4(+) CD161(+) cell frequency on the occurrence of neutropenic infections after allogeneic stem cell transplantation. *Transpl Infect Dis* (2017) 19:e12643. doi:10.1111/tid.12643
48. Le Bourhis L, Guerri L, Dusseaux M, Martin E, Soudais C, Lantz O. Mucosal-associated invariant T cells: unconventional development and function. *Trends Immunol* (2011) 32:212–8. doi:10.1016/j.it.2011.02.005
49. Girard TD, Opal SM, Ely EW. Insights into severe sepsis in older patients: from epidemiology to evidence-based management. *Clin Infect Dis* (2005) 40:719–27. doi:10.1086/427876
50. Samson M, Audia S, Fraszczak J, Trad M, Ornetti P, Lakomy D, et al. Th1 and Th17 lymphocytes expressing CD161 are implicated in giant cell arteritis and polymyalgia rheumatica pathogenesis. *Arthritis Rheum* (2012) 64:3788–98. doi:10.1002/art.34647

5

Impairment of Several Immune Functions and Redox State in Blood Cells of Alzheimer's Disease Patients: Relevant Role of Neutrophils in Oxidative Stress

*Carmen Vida[1,2], Irene Martinez de Toda[1,2], Antonio Garrido[1,2], Eva Carro[2,3], José Antonio Molina[2,3] and Mónica De la Fuente[1,2]**

[1] *Facultad de Biología, Universidad Complutense de Madrid, Madrid, Spain,* [2] *Instituto de Investigación Hospital Universitario12 de Octubre (i+12), Madrid, Spain,* [3] *Centro de Investigación Biomédica en Red sobre Enfermedades Neurodegenerativas (CIBERNED), Madrid, Spain*

***Correspondence:**
Mónica De la Fuente
mondelaf@ucm.es

Since aging is considered the most risk factor for sporadic Alzheimer's Disease (AD), the age-related impairment of the immune system (immunosenescence), based on a chronic oxidative-inflammatory stress situation, could play a key role in the development and progression of AD. Although AD is accompanied by systemic disturbance, reflecting the damage in the brain, the changes in immune response and redox-state in different types of blood cells in AD patients have been scarcely studied. The aim was to analyze the variations in several immune functions and oxidative-inflammatory stress and damage parameters in both isolated peripheral neutrophils and mononuclear blood cells, as well as in whole blood cells, from patients diagnosed with mild (mAD) and severe AD, and of age-matched controls (elderly healthy subjects) as well as of adult controls. The cognitive decline of all subjects was determined by Mini-Mental State Examination (MMSE) test (mAD stage was established at $20 \leq$ MMSE ≤ 23 score; AD stage at <18 MMSE; elderly subjects >27 MMSE). The results showed an impairment of the immune functions of human peripheral blood neutrophils and mononuclear cells of mAD and AD patients in relation to healthy elderly subjects, who showed the typical immunosenescence in comparison with the adult individuals. However, several alterations were only observed in severe AD patients (lower chemotaxis, lipopolysaccharide lymphoproliferation, and interleukin (IL)-10 release; higher basal proliferation, tumor necrosis factor (TNF)-α release, and IL-10/TNF-α ratio), others only in mAD subjects (higher adherence), meanwhile others appeared in both mAD and AD patients (lower phytohemaglutinin lymphoproliferation and higher IL-6 release). This impairment of immune functions could be mediated by: (1) the higher oxidative stress and damage also observed in blood cells from mAD and AD patients and in isolated neutrophils [lower glutathione (GSH) levels, high oxidized glutathione (GSSG)/GSH ratio, and GSSG and malondialdehyde contents], and (2) the higher release of basal pro-inflammatory cytokines (IL-6 and TNF-α) found in AD patients. Because the immune system parameters studied are markers of health and rate of aging, our results supported an accelerated immunosenescence in AD patients.

We suggest the assessment of oxidative stress and function parameters in peripheral blood cells as well as in isolated neutrophils and mononuclear cells, respectively, as possible markers of AD progression.

Keywords: Alzheimer's disease, immunosenescence, immune function, oxidative stress, inflammation, blood cells, neutrophils, mononuclear cells

INTRODUCTION

Alzheimer's disease (AD) is the most common neurodegenerative disorder and one of the major causes of senile dementia in later life. Epidemiological studies have revealed that AD is a multifactorial disease, with a complex interplay of environmental and genetics factors, which helps explain its variable clinical presentation (1, 2). Traditionally, AD has been classified into hereditary and sporadic forms. The hereditary form is linked with several genes and typically presents an earlier age of onset. By contrast, the sporadic form, which is the most common cause of AD (>95% of cases), has a later age of onset and a stronger association with aging, the major risk-incurring variable (1, 2). Due to the increase in mean life span, this pathology is exponentially increasing and is estimated that the prevalence of AD may reach >115 million worldwide by 2050 (3). Despite the enormous social, economic and health care impact, public health care systems do not have the medical therapies necessary to address AD. Moreover, the diagnosis of individual with early AD is not easy, and it is usually diagnosed in late stages (even postmortem), by which time the available treatments are not effective (4). For this reason, it is crucial to identify biomarkers of early diagnosis of AD that can help in the development of effective therapeutics and prevention methods.

Neuropathologically, AD is a progressive and irreversible brain disorder characterized by the extracellular accumulation of amyloid-β (Aβ) plaques and intracellular neurofibrillary tangles (NFTs) of hyperphosphorylated tau protein, associated with neuronal cell death and synaptotoxicity (5). Additional changes such as brain atrophy, mitochondrial dysfunction, increase in oxidative stress, and neuroinflammation can also occur in the brains of people with AD (6, 7). However, the mechanism of AD pathogenesis and progression still remain unclear. During the last few years, a higher number of studies have demonstrated that AD is also accompanied by a systemic disturbance, reflecting the damage in the brain (8–10). Thus, several studies support the involvement of an immune-related systemic alteration in AD, which includes changes in both innate and adaptive immune systems (11–15). Given the bidirectional communication between the immune and the nervous systems, and due to how the mediators of peripheral immune cells can influence the central nervous system (CNS) (16), it is not surprising that the age-related immunological variations can modify this neuroimmune communication network, contributing to the progressive cognitive impairment in AD (16). Indeed, numerous studies have shown changes in the distribution and reactivity of immune cells in the blood of AD patients (12, 17–21). This seems to cause a chronic inflammation in the periphery, which can be propagated through CNS immune cells, leading to neuroinflammation, which contributes to the cognitive deficits associated with AD (16, 22, 23).

Given that aging is accompanied by a decline of the nervous and the immune systems, as well as of their communication (24), which contributes to the deterioration of homeostasis and health, AD can be understood in the context of aging (25). Since advanced age is considered the most consistent risk factor for sporadic AD (1), the age-related dysregulation of the immune system, which is denominated immunosenescence, should be considered to understand the development of this pathology (11, 16, 17, 25–27). Immunosenescence involves restructuring changes in both innate and adaptive immune functions, which negatively affect the health of older adults, increasing susceptibility to infections and mortality (24, 28). Thus, there is an age-related decrease in several leukocytes functions, such as phagocytosis, chemotaxis, or stimulated proliferation, as well as an increase in other functions, such as adherence capacity to tissues and spontaneous lymphoproliferations, among others (24, 28–30). In AD patients, several immune functions are hampered in relation to healthy individuals with the same chronological age (8, 11, 19, 31–34), suggesting that this immune deterioration may be considered as a pathogenically relevant factor in this disease (33). Thus, it is assumed the advanced immunosenescence in AD patients, with remarkable immunological changes compared to healthy elderly subjects, which could contribute to AD pathology (11, 16, 17, 26, 33). Among these changes in AD patients the most relevant have been observed in the adaptive immune system. In fact, as also occurs in immunosenescence, several authors have reported changes in T and B lymphocyte differentiation and subpopulation distribution in peripheral blood of AD subjects, as well as an altered proliferative T lymphocytes response (11, 33, 34). Nevertheless, the results are inconsistent since increased or decreased lymphoproliferation and percentages in T and B lymphocytes, as well as no alterations in these immune parameters have been detected in AD patients (11, 33, 34). Regarding innate immunity, abnormalities in the function of natural killer (NK) cells (31, 32), a decreased phagocytosis of Aβ in peripheral macrophages (19), and an altered release of pro-inflammatory cytokines [e.g. interleukin-(IL)-6, tumor necrosis factor (TNF)-α, etc.] (8) have been shown in AD patients in relation to age-matched controls. However, the data of human studies are still scarce, preliminary, and contradictory.

According to the oxidation–inflammation theory of aging, the basis of immunosenescence is a chronic oxidative-inflammatory stress situation (a progressive imbalance between higher endogenous levels of oxidant and inflammatory compounds and lower antioxidant and anti-inflammatory defenses) (24, 28). In fact, immune cells continuously generate oxidants and inflammatory compounds to carry out their defensive functions; however, if the overproduction of oxidant compounds is not well-controlled by the antioxidant defenses, an alteration occurs in the redox balance, leading to an oxidative stress situation, which causes oxidative damage in biomolecules (e.g., lipids, proteins, etc.), inducing remarkable negative consequences on cellular functioning (24, 28). In addition, the chronic inflammation, which is characterized by excessive production and release of pro-inflammatory cytokines and chemokines, also leads to signaling cascades that trigger the production of oxidant compounds and depletion of antioxidants (35, 36). Therefore, since oxidation and inflammation are interlinked processes, an active inflammatory response by immune cells can lead to cellular damage due to oxidant overproduction, which can also recruit other inflammatory cells amplifying the cellular damage (35, 36). In this context, there is much evidence that indicates the strong involvement of inflammation and oxidative stress and damage in the onset, progression, and pathogenesis of AD (37–40). Thus, as occurs in aging, an enhanced oxidative stress has been observed in the brain (39, 40), as well as in peripheral tissues and cells (e.g., blood cells) (27, 41, 42) from AD patients. Indeed, many studies show both overproduction of oxidant compounds and impairment of antioxidant systems, as well as increased of oxidative damage (e.g., lipid peroxidation, proteins and DNA oxidation) in several brain regions of patients with both severe AD and mild cognitive impairment (MCI) (40, 43, 44). These markers of oxidative damage were also detected in high levels in peripheral blood and cerebrospinal fluid (CSF) obtained from both MCI and AD patients, together with decreased plasma levels of non-enzymatic antioxidants and impaired activity of antioxidant enzymes. Moreover, peripheral levels of the pro-inflammatory cytokines (e.g., IL-6 or TNF-α) have been described to be higher, whereas anti-inflammatory cytokine levels (e.g., IL-10 and IL-4) are lower in patients with AD compared to age-matched controls (27, 42, 43, 45–47). Interestingly, the fact that high levels of peripheral markers of oxidative-inflammatory stress were also detected in individuals with MCI, support the hypothesis that oxidative stress and inflammation are early events in the pathogenesis of AD, and precede Aβ deposit and onset of AD symptoms, as has been seen in experimental models of AD (48, 49). However, although several studies have evaluated oxidative stress parameters in both the early and advanced stages of human AD, the findings are controversial, as well as the relation between oxidative stress and cognitive performance, in mild and severe AD subjects, not yet being fully understood.

The use of animal models is particularly useful to study the molecular mechanisms involved in the development of AD and to identify potential therapeutic targets. In the last few decades, several transgenic animal models of AD have been developed to reproduce the neuronal pathology and behavioral symptomatology of human AD. The triple-transgenic mouse model (3xTg-AD) represents a unique animal model that closely mimics neuropathological manifestations, Aβ-plaques, and NFTs, in an age-dependent and region-specific manner like those in the human AD brain (50). Interestingly, as occurs in aging, it has been described that 3xTg-AD mice also suffer a pronounced and accelerated impairment in the neuroimmune network (16, 26), as well as a marked deterioration of several immune functions and an increased oxidative stress in different types of immune cells (e.g., peritoneal leukocytes) in comparison to control mice (16, 26, 51, 52). These alterations were observed in both early and advanced stages of the AD neuropathology, as well as before the onset establishment of AD (16, 26, 51, 52). Given that these changes are characteristics of prematurely and chronologically aged subjects (28, 30, 53), the premature immunosenescence observed in the 3xTg-AD mice at early stages of AD could explain the shorter life span also observed in these animals (52). Interestingly, the immune functions of peritoneal leukocytes of mice have been found to possess similar age-related evolutions to those observed in human circulating immune cells (30). Therefore, since immune functions are good markers of the rate of aging, and their analysis allows the early identification of premature and accelerated aging in humans (28, 30), the assessment of these parameters could be useful peripheral markers of the prodromal and preclinical states of AD (52).

It is also important to note that the most of studies performed in peripheral blood cells, have been carried out using mainly isolated peripheral mononuclear cells (95% lymphocytes and 5% monocytes), which are the most commonly used cells in the clinical setting. However, there are a few studies in which changes in immune function and redox status have been assessed in isolated phagocytes. Since these cells (e.g., neutrophils and macrophages) have been suggested to be the main cells responsible for the chronic oxidative-inflammatory stress associated with immunosenescence (28, 54), they could provide a helpful sample to clarify the molecular mechanisms underlying the impairment of the immune system throughout of AD progression. Moreover, blood, and particularly circulating leukocytes, reflects the major physiological changes in various body organs and systems (47). Therefore, the use of blood cells seems to be more useful in assessing markers that are analyzed in CSF, as well as identifying new markers that could be predictive of AD. Thus, it is possible that the assessment of these immune function parameters in the different types of peripheral blood immune cells, together with the evaluation of their oxidative-inflammatory state, could be useful early peripheral markers of the progression of AD in humans. However, this kind of study in different stages of human AD is still a subject that has scarcely been explored.

With the above in mind, the aim of the present work was to study the changes in several immune functions and inflammatory-oxidative stress and damage parameters in different types of human blood immune cells at early and advance stages of AD progression. To address this study, we performed assays on both isolated peripheral polymorphonuclear (PMN) and mononuclear blood leukocytes, as well as in whole blood (WB) cells, from patients diagnosed with mild and severe AD, and age-matched controls (elderly healthy subjects) as well as adult controls.

MATERIALS AND METHODS

Subjects and Clinical Classification

For this cross-sectional study, a total of 102 volunteers were selected and divided into four experimental groups: adult healthy subjects ($n = 20$), elderly healthy individuals ($n = 38$), mild AD (mAD) patients ($n = 26$), and severe AD patients ($n = 18$). All subjects were recruited by the Neurology Department of the Hospital, 12

Octubre of Madrid, and were tested by a standardized neuropsychological battery. The AD diagnosis was established according to the guidelines of the National Institute on Neurological Disorders and Stroke and the Alzheimer's Disease and Related Disorders Association (55). Disease severity and normal cognitive function was determined by a clinician's judgment based on a structured interview with the patient and the results of the Clinical Dementia Rating and the Mini-Mental State Examination (MMSE) tests (56). The mAD stage was established at 20 ≤ MMSE ≤ 23 score and AD stage at <18 MMSE score. Inclusion criteria for cognitively normal elderly healthy subjects were MMSE scores > 27, no history or clinical signs of neurological or psychiatric disease or cognitive symptoms. Demographic details and MMSE test results of the different study groups are summarized in **Table 1**. All subjects were subjected to a clinical survey and physical examination. Those with a history of cardiovascular disease, cancer, or chronic inflammatory diseases, as well as individuals with current inflammatory alterations (findings of clinical significance in general laboratory parameters) were not included in this study. The consent of the subjects was obtained according to the Declaration of Helsinki, and approval was obtained from the corresponding Research Ethic Committees. Written informed consent was obtained from all participants or representatives.

Collection of Peripheral WB Cells and Isolation of Blood Neutrophil and Lymphocytes Cells

Human samples (10 mL) of peripheral blood were collected using vein puncture and sodium citrate-buffered Vacutainer tubes (BD Diagnostic, Spain). Blood extraction was performed between 9:00 a.m. and 10:00 a.m. to avoid circadian variations in immune parameters. On the one hand, 8 mL of peripheral blood was used for isolation of both PMNs (mainly neutrophils) and mononuclear (mainly lymphocytes) leukocytes following a previously described method (57). Thus, neutrophil and lymphocyte cells were isolated using 1.119 and 1.077 g/cm³ density Histopaque (Sigma-Aldrich, Spain) separation, respectively. Collected cells were counted (95% of viability determined using trypan blue staining) and adjusted to the corresponding final concentrations for the development of the different assays of redox state and immune functions. The immune functions assays were performed with fresh cells, whereas the redox state assays were assessed in aliquots of frozen cells. These aliquots were stored at −80°C until used. On the other hand, samples of WB cells, which contain the total red blood cells (RBC) together with the total leukocyte populations, were obtained following a previously described procedure (58). For this, 500 µL of the peripheral blood sample was diluted with 500 µL of RPMI 1640 medium without glutamine (Gibco, Burlington, ON, Canada) and 10 µL of gentamicin (0.1 mg/mL in tube). The samples were incubated for 4 h at 37°C in a saturated atmosphere of CO_2 and humidity. Then, samples were centrifuged at 900 × *g* for 10 min to obtain the WB cell pellets after plasma removal. RPMI 1640 with glutamine (Gibco) was added to the blood cells to make 1 mL, and then several aliquots were prepared for the determination of redox state parameters. These aliquots were stored at −80°C until used.

TABLE 1 | Demographic data and neuropsychological test results of adult and elderly healthy subjects, as well as of mild Alzheimer's disease (mAD) and severe Alzheimer's disease (AD) patients.

	Adult	Elderly	mAD	AD
n (F/M)	20 (10/10)	38 (28/10)	26 (15/11)	18 (13/5)
Age (years)	40.32 ± 8.54	74.34 ± 9.22	76.08 ± 7.46	79.10 ± 6.53
MMSE	n.e.	29.02 ± 0.7	21.02 ± 0.86	16.44 ± 0.84
CDR	n.e.	0	2	3

F, female; M, male; MMSE, Mini-Mental State Examination Score; CDR, Clinical Dementia Rating; n.e., not evaluated.
The data of age and of MMSE score are expressed as mean ± SD, but those of CDR scores are presented as range values.

Adherent Capacity Assay

For the measurement of adherence capacity of human peripheral blood neutrophils and lymphocytes, we followed a method previously described (59) with some slight modifications. This method mimics, *in vitro*, cellular adherence to endothelium *in vivo*. Briefly, 500 µL of WB diluted 1:1with Hank's medium was placed in adherence columns consisting of a Pasteur pipet, in which 50 mg of nylon fibers was packed to a height of 1.25 cm. After 10 min, the effluent had drained by gravity, and neutrophils and lymphocytes were counted in this effluent using the Neubauer hemocytometer (microscope, 40×). Aliquots of 100 µL of 50% diluted WB effluent were mixed with 900 µL of Türk's solution, which has the ability to lyse RBC and differentiate the morphology of PMNs and mononuclear leukocytes. Results were expressed as the number of cells per mm³. In addition, another aliquot of 500 µL of WB diluted 1:1 with Hank's medium was used to count the total number of neutrophils and lymphocytes present in WB, as described earlier. The difference between the number of leukocytes present in the initial mixture and in the effluent, after passing through the adherence column, gives the number of adherent cells. The percentage of adherent neutrophils and lymphocytes, expressed as Adherence Index (AI), was calculated according to the equation:

$$\text{IA} = [(\text{leukocytes}/\text{mm}^3\text{total} - \text{leukocytes}/\text{mm}^3\text{effluent}) / (\text{leukocytes}/\text{mm}^3\text{total}] \times 100.$$

Chemotaxis Assay

The induced mobility or chemotaxis of peripheral blood isolated neutrophils and lymphocytes was carried out following a method previously described (57). Boyden chambers with two compartments separated by a polycarbonate filter (3 µm of diameter; Millipore, Ireland) were used to evaluate the chemotactic index (CI). Aliquots of 300 µL of neutrophil and lymphocyte suspensions (10^6 cells/mL) in Hank's medium were deposited in the upper compartment, and aliquots of 400 µL of the chemoattractant agent *N*-formylmethionine-leucyl-phenylalanine (Sigma-Aldrich) at a concentration of 10^{-8} M in the lower compartment of the chambers. The chambers were incubated for 3 h at 37°C, and the filters were fixed and stained with Giemsa's solution (Sigma-Aldrich). The number of neutrophils and lymphocytes on the lower face of the filter was counted in 20 microscope fields using an immersion objective (×100) and recorded as CI.

Phagocytosis Assay

Phagocytosis of inert particles (latex beads, 1.1 μm diameter, Sigma-Aldrich) was assayed in phagocytes (isolated blood neutrophils) following a method previously described (57). Neutrophils adjusted to 10^6 cells/mL were incubated on migration inhibition factor plates (Kartell, Noviglio, Italy) for 30 min at 37°C in a humidified atmosphere. The adherent monolayers obtained were washed with prewarmed PBS solution, and then 200 μL of Hank's solution and 20 μL of latex beads (1.1 μm diluted to 1% PBS, Sigma-Aldrich) were added. After 30 min of incubation under the same conditions, the plates were washed, fixed with methanol (50%), and stained with Giemsa's solution (Sigma-Aldrich). The number of particles ingested by 100 neutrophils was counted using an immersion objective (×100) and this was expressed as phagocytic index, while the number of ingesting neutrophils per 100 neutrophils was expressed as phagocytic efficiency.

NK Cytotoxicity Assay

The NK cell cytotoxicity, which is the main antitumoral protection of the organism, was measured by an enzymatic colorimetric assay (Cytotox 96 TM Promega, Boehringer Ingelheim, Germany) based on the determination of lactate dehydrogenase (LDH) released by the cytolysis of targets cells (human K562 lymphoma cells), using tetrazolium salts (57). Briefly, target cells were seeded in 96-well U-bottom culture plates (Nunclon, Denmark) at 10^4 cells/well in 1640 RPMI without phenol red (Gibco). Effector cells (mononuclear leukocyte suspensions adjusted to 10^6 cells/mL) were added at 10^5 cells/well, obtaining an effector/target rate of 10/1. The plates were centrifuged at 250 × *g* for 5 min to facilitate cell-to-cell contacts and were incubated for 4 h at 37°C. After incubation, LDH activity was measured in 50 μL/well by addition of the enzyme substrate with absorbance recording at 490 nm. The results were expressed as the percentage of tumor cells killed (% lysis).

Lymphoproliferation Assay

The proliferation capacity of lymphocytes was evaluated by a standard method, previously described (57). The assay was assessed in basal and stimulated conditions using the mitogens phytohemaglutinin (PHA) and lipopolysaccharide (LPS). Aliquots of 200 μL of isolated mononuclear leukocyte suspensions adjusted to 10^6 cells/mL of complete medium [containing RPMI 1640 enriched with L-glutamine and phenol red and supplemented with 10% heat-inactivated (56°C, 30 min) fetal calf serum (Hyclone, GE Healthcare, USA) and gentamicin (100 mg/mL, Sigma-Aldrich)] were dispensed into 96-well plates (Nunclon, Denmark). 20 μL of complete medium (basal lymphoproliferation), PHA, or LPS (1 μg/mL, Sigma-Aldrich) was added to each well. After 48 h of incubation at 37°C in a sterile and humidified atmosphere of 5% CO_2, 2.5 μCi ^{3}H-thymidine (Hartmann Analytic, Germany) was added to each well. Previously, 100 μL of culture supernatant from each well was collected and stored at −80°C until used for cytokine analysis. After another incubation of 24 h, cells were harvested in a semiautomatic harvester (Skatron Instruments, Norway), and thymidine uptake was measured in a beta counter (LKB, Uppsala, Sweden) for 1 min. The results were calculated as ^{3}H-thymidine uptake (counts per minute, cpm) for basal and stimulated (with mitogens) conditions and also were expressed as lymphoproliferation capacity (%) giving 100% to the cpm in basal conditions.

Glutathione Content Assay

Both reduced [glutathione (GSH)], the main non-enzymatic reducing agent of the organism, and oxidized [oxidized glutathione (GSSG)] forms of glutathione were determined using a fluorometric assay previously described (60). This method is based on the capacity of reaction that GSSG and GSH show with *o*-phthalaldehyde (OPT, Sigma-Aldrich), at pH 12 and pH 8, respectively, resulting in the formation of a fluorescent compound. The assay was evaluated in WB cells (containing total RBC and leukocyte populations), as well as in isolated peripheral blood neutrophils and mononuclear leukocytes. For this, aliquots of frozen WB cells (50 μL) were resuspended in phosphate buffer 0.1 M, pH 7.4 (200 μL) (Sigma-Aldrich), whereas aliquots of isolated neutrophils and lymphocytes adjusted to 10^6 cells/mL in Hank's solution were centrifuged at 1,200 × *g* for 10 min at 4°C. All samples were resuspended in phosphate buffer 50 mM containing EDTA 0.1 M, pH 8 (600 μL) (Sigma-Aldrich). Then, samples were sonicated, and after the addition of $HClO_4$ (60%, Sigma-Aldrich; 7.5 μL), they were centrifuged at 9,500 × *g* for 10 min at 4°C. Aliquots of supernatants (10 μL) were dispensed into 96-well black plates (Nunc). For GSH measurement, 190 μL of phosphate buffer and 20 μL of OPT (1 mg/mL in methanol) were dispensed in the wells, and the plate was incubated for 15 min in the dark and at room temperature. For the measurement of GSSG, 8 μL of *N*-ethylmaleimide (0.04 M; Sigma-Aldrich) was added to each well to prevent interference of GSH with GSSG. The plate was incubated for 30 min under the same conditions. Then, 186 μL of NaOH (0.1 N) and 20 μL of OPT were incorporated, and the plate was incubated for 15 min in similar conditions. In both GSH and GSSG measurements, the fluorescence emitted by each well was measured at 350 nm excitation and 420 nm emission. Protein content of the samples was determined following the bicinchoninic acid protein assay kit protocol (Sigma-Aldrich), using serum albumin (BSA, Sigma-Aldrich) as standard. Results were expressed as nanomoles of GSH or GSSG per milligram of protein. Moreover, the GSSG/GSH ratio was calculated for each sample.

Lipid Peroxidation (MDA) Assay

The estimation of MDA, in both blood cells and isolated peripheral blood neutrophils and mononuclear leukocytes, was evaluated using the commercial kit "MDA Assay Kit" (Biovision, Mountain View, CA, USA), which measures the reaction of MDA with thiobarbituric acid (TBA) and the MDA-TBA adduct formation. For this, aliquots of frozen WB cells (100 μL) were resuspended in phosphate buffer 0.05 M, pH 7.4 (200 μL), whereas aliquots of isolated neutrophils and lymphocytes adjusted to 10^6 cells/mL in Hank's solution were centrifuged at 1,200 × *g* for 10 min at 4°C. All samples were resuspended in lysis buffer (300 μL) containing butylated hydroxytoluene (0.1 mM, 3 μL), sonicated, and centrifuged again at 13,000 × *g* for 10 min. The supernatants (200 μL) from each sample were added to TBA (600 μL) and incubated at 95°C for 60 min. Samples were cooled in ice for 10 min, and 200 μL of reaction mixture was mixed with 300 μL of *n*-butanol (Sigma-Aldrich) to create an organic phase in which the MDA molecules were to be placed. Samples were centrifuged 10 min at 13,000 × *g* at room temperature, and 200 μL of the supernatants (upper organic phase) was collected and dispensed into a 96-well microplate for spectrophotometric measurement at 532 nm. MDA supplied in the kit was used as standard, and MDA levels were determined by comparing the absorbance of samples with that of the standards. Protein concentration of the samples was measured as described earlier. Results were expressed as nanomoles of MDA per milligram of protein.

Cytokine Measurement

The IL-6, TNF-α, and IL-10 release was measured in culture supernatants of WB in the absence or presence of LPS following a method previously described (58). Briefly, 500 μL of blood was diluted 1:1 with RPMI 1640 medium without L-glutamine (Gibco) and incubated for 4 h with 10 μL gentamicin (1 mg/mL, Sigma-Aldrich) and 10 μL LPS (250 ng/mL, Sigma-Aldrich) or 10 μL RPMI 1640 medium (basal conditions). Samples were centrifuged, and supernatants were collected and frozen at −20°C until assay. Levels of IL-6, TNF-α, and IL-10 were measured simultaneously by multiplex luminometry (Beadlyte human multiplex cytokine detection system, HCYTOMAG-60K, Millipore, Billerica, MA, USA), with minimum detectable doses of IL-6, TNF-α, and IL-10 under 0.9, 0.7, and 1.1 pg/mL, respectively. The results were expressed as picograms per milliliter.

Statistical Analysis

Statistical analysis was performed in SPSS IBM, version 21.0 (SPSS, Chicago, USA). All tests were two-tailed, with a significant level of $\alpha = 0.05$. Data are presented as mean ± standard deviation (SD). Normality of the samples and homogeneity of the variances were checked by the Kolmogorov–Smirnov test and Levene test, respectively. Differences due to age and AD pathology were studied using a one-way analysis of variance followed by *post hoc* tests analysis or the non-parametric Kruskal–Wallis test. The Tukey test was used for *post hoc* comparisons when variances were homogeneous, whereas its counterpart analysis Games-Howell was used with unequal variances when they were not homogeneous. Figures were built using GraphPad Prism 6.

RESULTS

Immune Functions in Peripheral Blood Neutrophils and Mononuclear Leukocytes of mAD and AD Patients As Well As Healthy Controls

The results obtained in the immune functions studied in isolated human blood neutrophils and mononuclear cells obtained from adult and older healthy subjects, as well as from mAD and AD patients are shown in **Figure 1** and **Table 2**. In general, all the immune parameters analyzed in the present work (adherence, chemotaxis, and phagocytosis of neutrophils as well as adherence, chemotaxis and proliferative response of lymphocytes in both basal and stimulated conditions, and the antitumor cytotoxic activity of NK cells) have been shown to deteriorate in aging and AD pathology. However, a different pattern of impaired immune function has been observed between the early and advanced stages of AD.

In elderly healthy subjects, in comparison with healthy adults, statistically significant lower values in neutrophil chemotaxis ($P < 0.001$; **Figure 1C**) and phagocytosis (176 ± 13 and 488 ± 25 P.I., older vs adult, respectively; $P < 0.001$), as well as in the activity of NK cells ($P < 0.01$; **Figure 1E**), lymphocyte chemotaxis ($P < 0.05$; **Figure 1D**) and PHA- and LPS-lymphoproliferative response ($P < 0.001$; **Figures 1G,H**; **Table 2**) were obtained. In contrast, higher values were also shown in old subjects in neutrophil and lymphocyte adherence ($P < 0.01$; **Figures 1A,B**), as well as in basal proliferation ($P < 0.01$; **Figure 1F**).

Regarding AD pathology, there were significant differences in AD patients relative to elderly healthy controls of the same chronological age, as well as in mAD compared to the same controls. Thus, AD patients exhibited higher basal proliferation ($P < 0.05$; **Figure 1F**) and lower neutrophil and lymphocyte chemotaxis ($P < 0.05$; **Figures 1C,D**), as well as PHA- and LPS-lymphoproliferative response ($P < 0.05$; **Figures 1G,H**; **Table 2**) in comparison to elderly subjects. Interestingly, at the early stage of the disease, mAD patients also showed lower PHA-lymphoproliferation ($P < 0.01$; **Figure 1G**; **Table 2**) than elderly subjects. However, mAD exhibited a significant increase in neutrophil ($P < 0.01$; **Figure 1A**) and lymphocyte ($P < 0.001$; **Figure 1B**) adherence in relation to elderly subjects, which was not observed at the advanced stage of AD. Finally, it should be noted that immune function differences between the early and advanced stages of AD were also observed. Thus, AD patients showed significantly lower neutrophil and lymphocyte adherence ($P < 0.05$; **Figures 1A,B**), as well as lower chemotaxis of lymphocytes and lower NK cytotoxic activity ($P < 0.05$; **Figures 1D,E**) than mAD patients.

Cytokine Production in Response to LPS Stimulation in Blood Leukocytes of mAD and AD Patients As Well As Healthy Controls

Cytokines are major mediators of the complex interactions among immune cells, being responsible for the development and resolve of immune response. Aging is characterized by a chronic low-grade inflammatory state (61), and the maintenance of health relies on the adequate balance of anti-inflammatory and pro-inflammatory compounds (28). For this reason, we analyzed the levels of pro-inflammatory (IL-6 and TNF-α) and anti-inflammatory (IL-10) cytokines secreted *ex vivo* by blood cells incubated for 4 h under LPS-stimulated conditions, in mAD and AD patients, as well as in adult and elderly healthy subjects. The IL-10/TNF-α ratios, which are a good indicator of successful aging and longevity (30), were also calculated.

In general, the results of our study showed that the release of these cytokines suffers impairments with aging. Moreover,

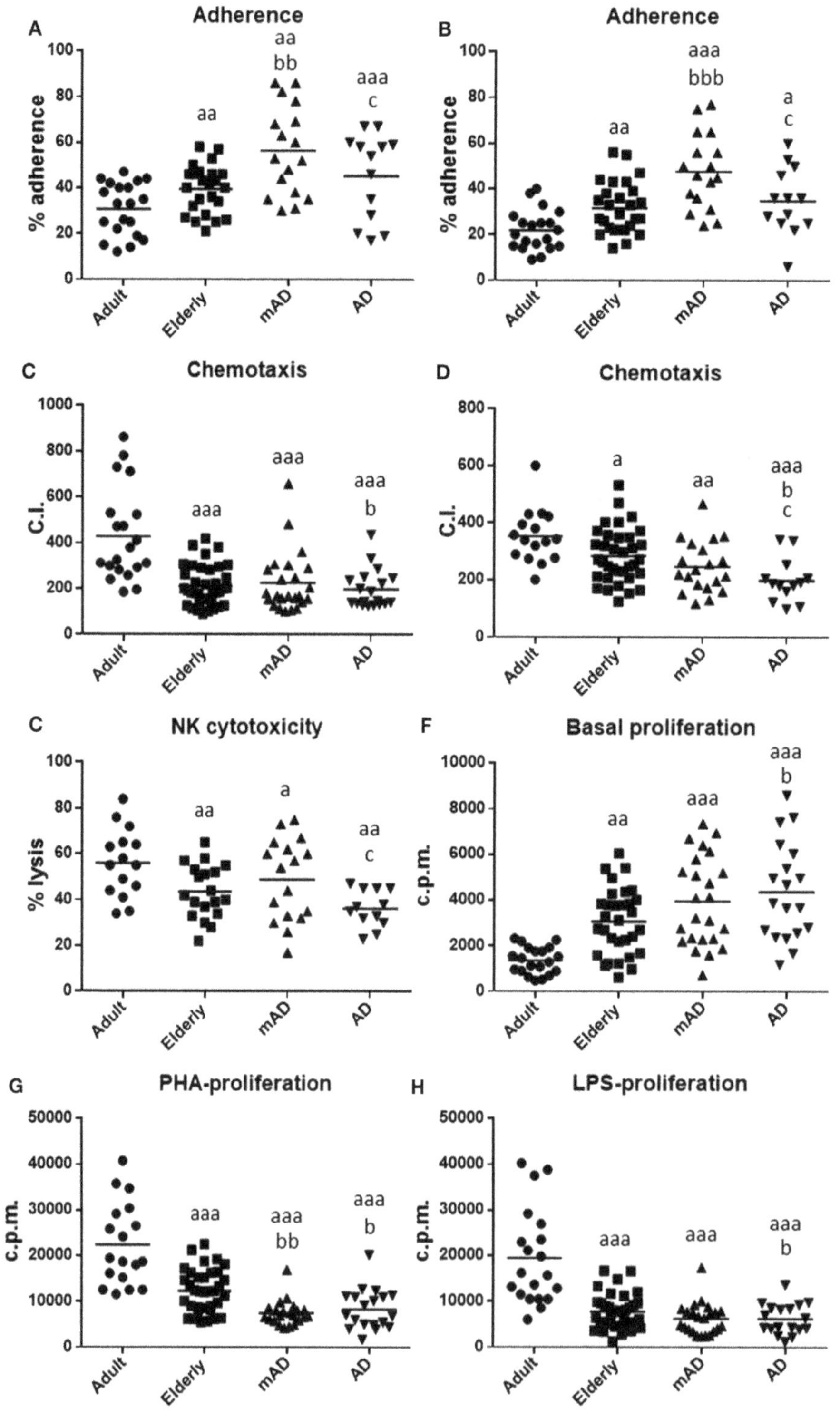

FIGURE 1 | Function parameters in isolated peripheral blood neutrophils and mononuclear cells of mild Alzheimer's disease (mAD) and Alzheimer's disease (AD) patients, as well as of adult and elderly healthy subjects. Adherence (%) of neutrophils **(A)** and lymphocytes **(B)**; chemotaxis index (C.I.) of neutrophils **(C)** and lymphocytes **(D)**; natural killer (NK) cytotoxicity (% lysis) **(E)**; proliferation of lymphocytes in basal conditions [48 h incubation; counts per minute (cpm)] **(F)**; proliferation of lymphocytes (48 h incubation; cpm) in response to phytohemagglutinin (PHA, 1 μg/mL) **(G)** and in response to lipopolysaccharide (LPS, 1 μg/mL) **(H)**. Data are shown as the mean (horizontal bar) of 18–38 values corresponding to the number of subjects analyzed in each group (20 adult, 38 elderly, 26 mAD, and 18 AD). Each value is the mean of duplicate assays. a: $P < 0.05$, aa: $P < 0.01$, and aaa: $P < 0.001$ with respect to the value in adult subjects; b: $P < 0.05$, bb: $P < 0.01$, and bbb: $P < 0.001$ with respect to the value in elderly subjects; c: $P < 0.05$ with respect to the value in mAD patients.

a similar pattern of altered secretion was observed for all investigated cytokines, in AD patients. As shown in **Figure 2**, under LPS-stimulated conditions, increased levels of IL-6 and TNF-α ($P < 0.05$ and $P < 0.001$, respectively; **Figures 2A,B**) were observed in the elderly subjects in comparison to adults. This was also accompanied by a marked decrease in IL-10 and the IL-10/TNF-α ratio ($P < 0.001$; **Figures 2C,D**). A similar cytokine profile was also observed in AD patients in relation to older subjects. Thus, AD patients had higher levels of IL-6 and TNF-α ($P < 0.01$; **Figures 2A,B**), as well as lower IL-10 release and IL-10/TNF-α ratios ($P < 0.05$; **Figures 2C,D**) than elderly controls. However, mAD patients only showed a significant increase in the levels of IL-6 ($P < 0.05$; **Figure 2A**). No differences were observed in TNF-α and IL-10 release and IL-10/TNF-α ratios between mAD and older subjects. Regarding the differences between the different stages of AD, it is important to note that AD patient exhibited a higher IL-6 LPS-induced release ($P < 0.05$; **Figure 2A**) and a lower IL-10/TNF-α ratio ($P < 0.05$; **Figure 4D**) than mAD patients.

TABLE 2 | Stimulation of proliferation (%) in response to phytohemagglutinin and lipopolysaccharide (1 µg/mL), in isolated peripheral mononuclear cells of adult and elderly healthy subjects, as well as of mild Alzheimer's disease (mAD) and severe Alzheimer's disease (AD) patients.

Lymphoproliferation (% stimulation)	Adult	Elderly	mAD	AD
PHA (%)	1,950 ± 232	391 ± 56[a]	198 ± 19[a,b]	218 ± 36[a,c]
LPS (%)	346 ± 25	176 ± 13[d]	156 ± 12[c,e]	167 ± 17[e]

Data are expressed as mean ± SD of the values corresponding to 20 adult, 38 elderly, 26 mAD, and 18 AD subjects. Each value is the mean of duplicate assays.
[a]$P < 0.001$ with respect to the value in adult subjects.
[b]$P < 0.01$ with respect to the value in elderly subjects.
[c]$P < 0.05$ with respect to the value in elderly subjects.
[d]$P < 0.05$ with respect to the value in adult subjects.
[e]$P < 0.01$ with respect to the value in adult subjects.

Oxidative Stress and Damage Parameters in Isolated Peripheral Blood Neutrophils and Mononuclear Cells of mAD and AD Patients As Well As Healthy Controls

A good maintenance of the redox state is vital for the proper functioning of immune cells, and thus the oxidative stress, which

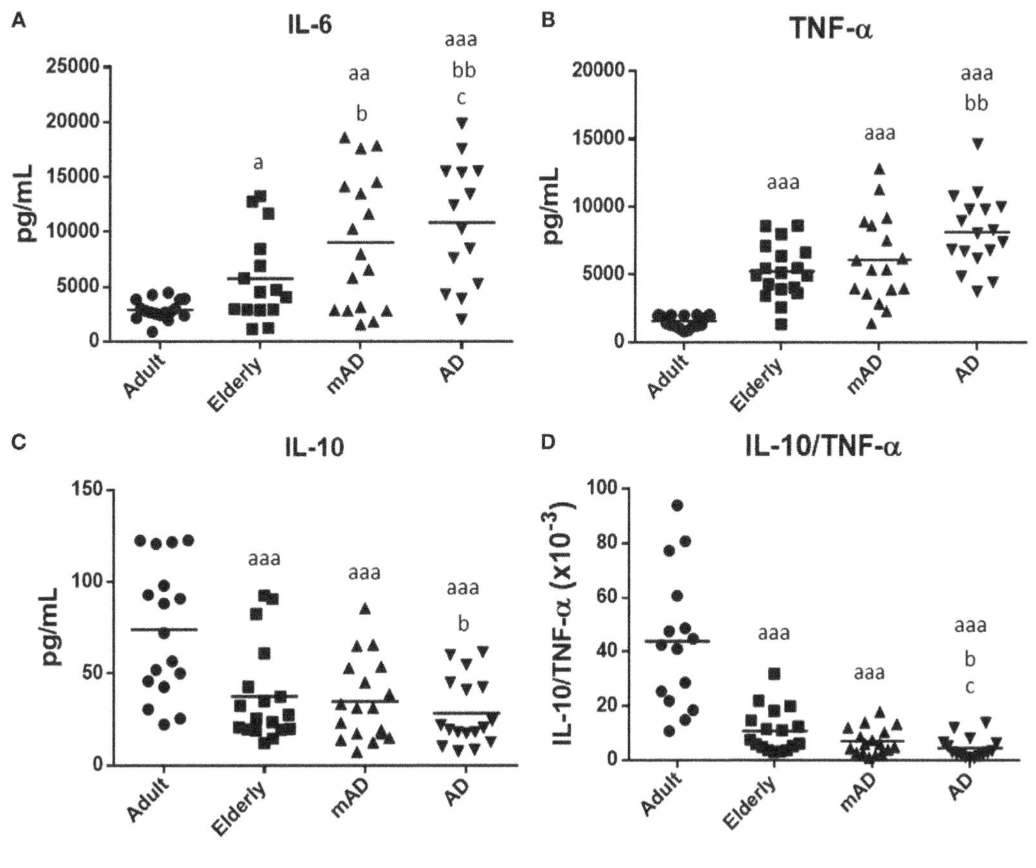

FIGURE 2 | Levels (pg/mL) of cytokines released after 4 h of culture in the presence of lipopolysaccharide (1 µg/mL) by peripheral whole blood cells of mild Alzheimer's disease (mAD) and Alzheimer's disease (AD) patients, as well as of adult and elderly healthy subjects. Interleukin (IL)-6 **(A)**, tumor necrosis factor (TNF)-α **(B)**, and IL-10 **(C)**, as well as IL-10/TNF-α ratios **(D)**. Data are shown as the mean (horizontal bar) of the values corresponding to the number of subjects analyzed in each group (20 adult, 18 elderly, 18 mAD, and 18 AD). Each value is the mean of duplicate assays. a: $P < 0.05$, aa: $P < 0.01$, and aaa: $P < 0.001$ with respect to the value in adult subjects; b: $P < 0.05$ and bb: $P < 0.01$ with respect to the value in elderly subjects; and c: $P < 0.05$ and cc: $P < 0.01$ with respect to the value in mAD patients.

is the basis of aging and age-related diseases, is detrimental for leukocyte functions (28). Hence, the decline in immune response observed in mAD and AD patients could be mediated by an increase in oxidative stress and the consequent oxidative damage. To test this possibility, the intracellular content of GSH and GSSG, the GSSG/GSH ratio (one of the best markers of oxidative stress), as well as the MDA levels (one of the major lipid peroxidation products) were assessed in isolated human blood neutrophils and mononuclear cells obtained from mAD and AD patients, as well as from adult and elderly healthy subjects. The results are shown in **Figure 3**. In general, in both leukocyte populations a higher oxidative stress and damage have been shown in elderly subjects and AD patients than in adult controls. However, a different pattern of impaired redox state has been observed between the early and advanced stages of AD, the neutrophils showing a greater oxidative stress and damage than the lymphocytes.

Regarding aging, elderly healthy controls showed in their neutrophils and lymphocytes significantly lower GSH contents ($P < 0.05$ and $P < 0.01$, respectively; **Figures 3A,B**), as well as higher GSSG amounts ($P < 0.01$; **Figures 3C,D**), higher GSSG/GSH ratios ($P < 0.01$ and $P < 0.05$, respectively; **Figures 3E,F**), and MDA levels ($P < 0.01$ and $P < 0.05$, respectively; **Figures 3G,H**) in relation to adult subjects.

Regarding the AD pathology, AD patients had in their neutrophils a marked increase in both GSSG and MDA contents ($P < 0.01$; **Figures 3C,G**), as well as in GSSG/GSH ratios ($P < 0.05$; **Figure 3E**) in comparison to elderly subjects, accompanied also by a marked decrease in the levels of GSH ($P < 0.05$; **Figure 3A**). However, in the case of lymphocytes, AD patients showed higher GSH contents ($P < 0.05$; **Figure 3B**) than elderly controls, whereas no differences were observed in the other parameters analyzed. Likewise, similar results were observed in mAD patients, who showed higher GSSG contents, GSSG/GSH ratios, and MDA levels ($P < 0.05$; **Figures 3C,E,G**) in neutrophils as well as higher GSH contents ($P < 0.01$; **Figure 3B**) in lymphocytes, than the corresponding values in elderly controls. In relation to the different stages of AD, it is important to note that AD patients had in their neutrophils markedly increased GSSG/GSH ratios and MDA levels ($P < 0.05$; **Figures 3E,G**) as well as decreased GSH contents in their lymphocytes ($P < 0.05$; **Figure 3B**) in relation to mAD patients.

Oxidative Stress and Damage Parameters in Human Peripheral Blood Cells of mAD and AD Patients as well as of Healthy Controls

It is known that there is a significant difference between the use of WB and purified and isolated PMNs and mononuclear leukocytes (62). Moreover, various peripheral blood cell types and their proportions can affect the immune response, as well as the inflammatory and oxidative stress conditions (54, 62). For this reason, the same parameters of oxidative stress and damage analyzed in isolated neutrophils and lymphocytes from mAD and AD patients, and adult and elderly healthy subjects, were also evaluated using samples of WB cells, containing both total RBC and leukocyte populations. This kind of sample better reproduces the *in vivo* conditions. The results are shown in **Figure 4**. There were higher values of oxidative stress and damage in blood cells of elderly subjects than in those of adults. Thus, GSH values were lower ($P < 0.001$; **Figure 4A**) and GSSG/GSH ratios higher ($P < 0.05$; **Figure 4C**), as well as both GSSG ($P < 0.01$; **Figure 4B** and MDA ($P < 0.001$; **Figure 4D**) levels, than those in adult subjects.

Regarding AD pathology, AD patients exhibited, in their blood cells, significantly lower GSH contents ($P < 0.05$; **Figure 4A**), higher GSSG and MDA contents ($P < 0.05$ and $P < 0.001$, respectively; **Figures 4B,D**), and GSSG/GSH ratios ($P < 0.05$; **Figure 4C**) than elderly subjects. Similar results were also observed in mAD patients in relation to elderly subjects, which also showed lower GSH levels ($P < 0.01$; **Figure 4A**) and higher GSSG/GSH ratios ($P < 0.05$; **Figure 4C**) and MDA contents ($P < 0.01$; **Figure 4D**) than elderly controls. However, no differences were observed in GSSG contents between mAD and elderly subjects. Finally, regarding the differences between early and advanced stages of AD, it is important to note that AD patients showed higher levels of GSSG and MDA ($P < 0.05$ and $P < 0.01$, respectively; **Figures 4B,D**) than mAD patients.

Basal Cytokine Production in Blood Leukocytes of mAD and AD Patients as well as of Healthy Controls

Since an age-related increase in release of pro-inflammatory cytokines in resting cells leads to a sterile inflammation (30), and this alteration of the inflammatory status in aging ("inflamm-aging") could lead to a chronic situation causing neuronal impairment and loss associated with AD (63), we also assessed extracellular release of IL-6, TNF-α, and IL-10 secreted *ex vivo* by blood cells cultured (4 h) under resting conditions, from mAD and AD patients, as well as from adult and elderly healthy controls.

As shown in **Table 3**, under basal conditions, in elderly subjects the values of IL-6 and TNF-α released were higher ($P < 0.01$ and $P < 0.05$, respectively) than in adults. Regarding AD pathology, a similar cytokine profile was also observed in AD patients in relation to both adults and elderly subjects. Thus, AD patients showed higher levels of IL-6 and TNF-α ($P < 0.05$) than elderly controls, whereas mAD patients only showed statistically significant higher values ($P < 0.05$) in the TNF-α levels. Basal IL-10 release was not detectable by the multiplex, so the IL-10/TNF-α ratio could not be calculated. Interestingly, regarding differences between early and advanced stages of AD, AD patients showed higher basal IL-6 release ($P < 0.05$) than the individuals with mAD.

DISCUSSION

To our knowledge, this is the first study that analyzed the changes in several parameters of function and oxidative-inflammatory stress state in different types of peripheral blood immune cells, such as neutrophils and mononuclear cells, from patients with mild and severe AD, compared with a healthy age-matched control group of subjects without cognitive impairment. Additionally, all these parameters were also studied in healthy adult subjects to evaluate

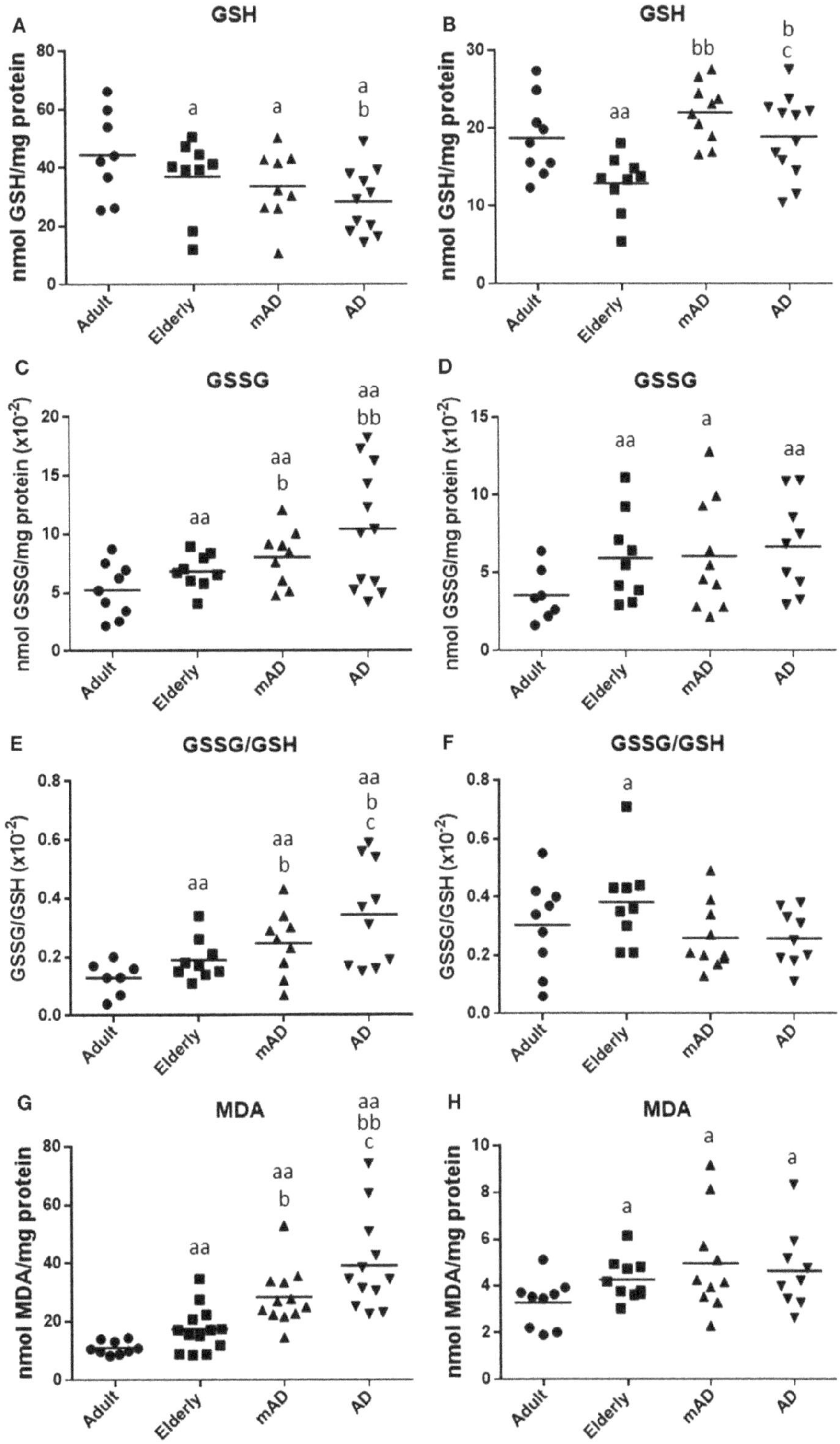

FIGURE 3 | Oxidative stress parameters and lipid peroxidation in isolated peripheral blood neutrophils and mononuclear cells of mild Alzheimer's disease (mAD) and Alzheimer's disease (AD) patients, as well as of adult and elderly healthy subjects. Intracellular reduced glutathione (GSH) contents (nmol/mg protein) in neutrophils **(A)** and lymphocytes **(B)**; intracellular oxidized glutathione (GSSG) contents (nmol/mg protein) in neutrophils **(C)** and lymphocytes **(D)**; GSSG/GSH ratios in neutrophils **(E)** and lymphocytes **(F)**; and intracellular malondialdehyde (MDA) contents (nmol/mg protein) in neutrophils **(G)** and lymphocytes **(H)**. Data are shown as the mean (horizontal bar) of 9–12 values corresponding to the number of subjects analyzed in each group (9 adult, 10 elderly, 11 mAD, and 12 AD). Each value is the mean of duplicate assays. a: $P < 0.05$ and aa: $P < 0.01$ with respect to the value in adult subjects; b: $P < 0.05$ and bb: $P < 0.01$ with respect to the value in elderly subjects; and c: $P < 0.05$ with respect to the value in mAD patients.

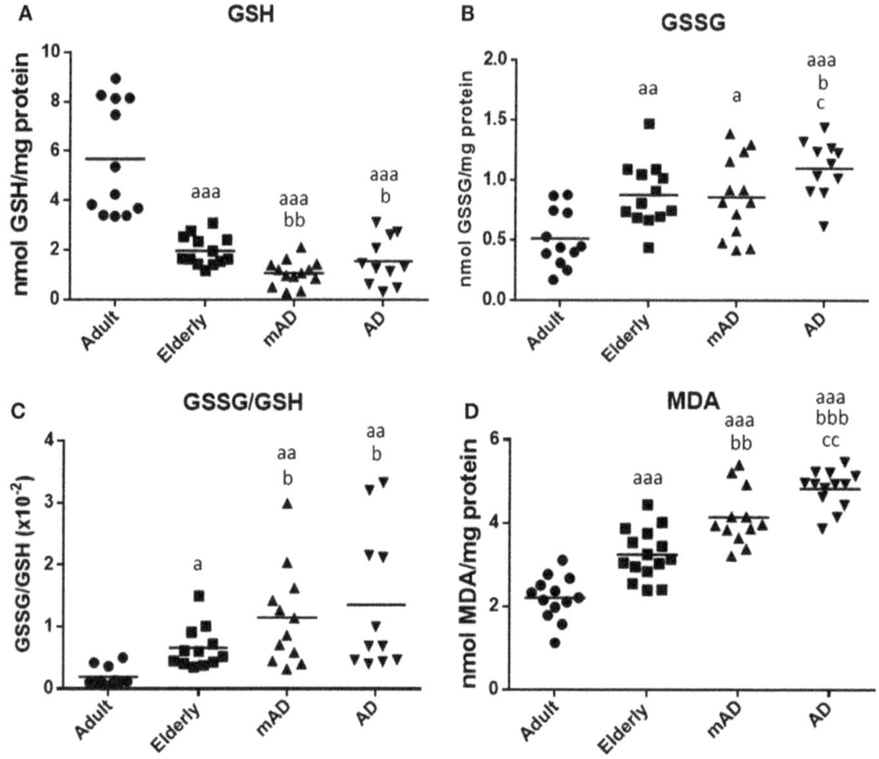

FIGURE 4 | Oxidative stress parameters and lipid peroxidation in whole blood cells (containing both total red blood cells and leukocyte populations) of mild Alzheimer's disease (mAD) and Alzheimer's disease (AD) patients, as well as of adult and elderly healthy subjects. Intracellular reduced glutathione (GSH) contents (nmol/mg protein) **(A)**; intracellular oxidized glutathione (GSSG) contents (nmol/mg protein) **(B)**; GSSG/GSH ratios **(C)**; and intracellular malondialdehyde (MDA) contents (nmol/mg protein) **(D)**. Data are shown as the mean (horizontal bar) of 11–15 values corresponding to the number of subjects analyzed in each group (13 adult, 15 elderly, 13 mAD, and 13 AD). Each value is the mean of duplicate assays. a: $P < 0.05$, aa: $P < 0.01$, and aaa: $P < 0.001$ with respect to the value in adult subjects; b: $P < 0.05$, bb: $P < 0.01$, and bbb: $P < 0.001$ with respect to the value in elderly subjects; and c: $P < 0.05$ and cc: $P < 0.01$ with respect to the value in mAD patients.

TABLE 3 | Levels of interleukin (IL)-6 and tumor necrosis factor (TNF)-α (pg/mL) released by peripheral whole blood cells of adult and elderly healthy subjects, as well as of mild Alzheimer's disease (mAD) and severe Alzheimer's disease (AD) patients, after 4 h of culture in basal conditions.

Basal cytokines	Adult	Elderly	mAD	AD
IL-6 (pg/mL)	8.89 ± 1.93	16.23 ± 4.72[a]	16.21 ± 3.84[a]	21.60 ± 5.17[b,c,d]
TNF-α (pg/mL)	24.76 ± 6.14	40.30 ± 14.89[e]	90.76 ± 26[a,c]	105.8 ± 22.5[a,c]

Data are expressed as mean ± SD of the values corresponding to 10 adult, 10 elderly, 8 mAD, and 8 AD subjects. Each value is the mean of duplicate assays.
[a]P < 0.01 with respect to the value in adult subjects.
[b]P < 0.001 with respect to the value in adult subjects.
[c]P < 0.05 with respect to the value in elderly subjects.
[d]P < 0.05 with respect to the value in mAD patients.
[e]P < 0.05 with respect to the value in adult subjects.

the differences due to the aging process. Our results revealed an impairment of the immune functions of both neutrophils and mononuclear cells at different stages of AD. Several alterations were only observed in severe AD patients and some only in mAD patients. Furthermore, our results also demonstrated that immune blood cells from mAD and AD patients, and especially neutrophils, showed an increased oxidative stress and oxidative damage in relation to elderly subjects. This altered redox balance could be mediated by the higher production of pro-inflammatory cytokines, which has been also observed in AD patients.

The immune system has a profound implication in the pathology of AD, not only at the central level but also at the peripheral level (8–10, 17, 19). Although several studies have reported alteration of both innate and acquired immunity at different stages of AD (12), there are many contradictory results (11–15, 17). Moreover, most of these studies in human and animal models have focused on the alteration of the adaptive immune response. However, little is known about the changes in innate immunity, especially those carried out by phagocytes (e.g., neutrophils). Our findings revealed that severe AD patients show lower neutrophil and lymphocyte chemotaxis, PHA- and LPS-lymphoproliferation, as well as higher basal lymphoproliferation in comparison to elderly healthy subjects. These AD-related changes are similar to those with aging (28, 30), which was also observed in the present study, although more exacerbated. This shows the presence of a lesser competent immune system in severe AD patients than in elderly subjects, which could contribute to the high mortality of these individuals. Our results agree with some of those observed in humans and experimental animals with AD (11, 16, 17, 26, 33, 52). Thus, leukocytes of 3xTg-AD mice presented an impairment of chemotaxis capacity (16, 26, 52). In relation to lymphoproliferative response in stimulated conditions some studies also report a decrease in this function in cells obtained from patients with severe AD (11, 17, 33, 64).

Surprisingly, mAD patients, but not severe AD patients, showed higher values in neutrophil and lymphocyte adherence than elderly subjects. This increase in adherence is a characteristic of aging (24, 28). Although at this moment we cannot explain the possible regulation mechanisms that severe AD patients use to present similar values to age-matched controls, this parameter could be an early marker of the appearance of AD. In mAD patients, a lower proliferative response of lymphocytes to the mitogen PHA than in elderly subjects also occurred. Thus, this function of lymphoproliferative response to mitogens, which typically decreases with aging (24, 28, 30) appeared even lower in cells of mAD and AD.

Alzheimer's disease patients in comparison to mAD showed lower lymphocyte chemotaxis and antitumoral NK activity. In this regard, although limited in number, several studies in human and 3xTg-AD mice revealed that these immune function parameters were altered in AD (16, 26, 32, 52). Thus, NK cell activity, which has been proposed as one biomarker of immune alterations in the progression of AD (32) and which was decreased in cells of 3xTg-AD mice in advanced stages of AD (16, 26), was lower in severe AD than in mAD patients. In the case of chemotaxis of lymphocytes, a function that decreases with aging (28, 30), our results reflect a clear deterioration of this activity in AD patients, even higher than shown by cells of elderly subjects and of mAD. Thus, this parameter could be considered as a possible marker of the progression of the disease.

Interestingly, it should be noted that although the decline of the immune functions showed with aging were also observed in mAD and AD patients, several of these immunological alterations were greatly exacerbated in individuals with severe AD in comparison to healthy elderly subjects of the same chronological age. This suggests that AD patients suffer an accelerated immunosenescence. Thus, since these immune function parameters are good markers of health and predictors of longevity (28, 30), these could be used as peripheral biomarkers of the progression of AD.

A chronic oxidative-inflammatory stress, a condition in which oxidant and pro-inflammatory compounds overwhelm antioxidant and anti-inflammatory defenses, is associated with aging and several age-related pathologies (26, 28). Indeed, several studies in human and animal models, including some by our group, have demonstrated that increased peripheral oxidative stress markers are associated with aging and, more specifically, with AD (16, 26, 30, 47, 52, 54). In AD, oxidative stress has been recognized as an essential contributor to the pathogenesis and progression of the disease (38, 40, 52, 65). As occurs in the brain (7, 40), an enhanced oxidative stress during AD is also present in peripheral blood cells (27, 41–43). Most studies have focused on mononuclear cells, mainly in lymphocytes, which reflect the pathological oxidative stress conditions observed in the brains of AD patients. These studies found an elevated production of oxidative compounds, lipid oxidation, DNA damage, mitochondrial susceptibility, basal apoptosis as well as altered levels of antioxidant enzymes in lymphocytes of AD patients, as well as even in those of MCI subjects, in comparison with these cells of healthy subjects (27, 66–68). These results suggest that some of these parameters could be prodromal markers of AD. However, little is known about the changes in the redox balance of neutrophils during the progression of AD. Therefore, since phagocytes may be the immune cells that contribute most to the oxidative stress and damage associated with immunosenescence (28, 54), we also analyzed different redox state and oxidative damage parameters in both isolated peripheral blood neutrophils and mononuclear cells, in order to elucidate possible differences between them. Interestingly, our results showed that neutrophils suffer a marked increased oxidative stress and damage during the progression of AD. In particular, the neutrophils of both mAD and AD patients had lower antioxidant GSH contents and higher oxidant markers, such as GSSG and MDA contents, as well as GSSG/GSH ratios, than elderly subjects. Nevertheless, this redox state alteration was not observed in mononuclear cells, which paradoxically showed higher GSH levels in individuals with mild and severe AD than those observed in age-matched controls. In this context, it has been suggested that in early states of the disease, individuals developing AD can suffer a situation of "reductive stress" as a result of the activation of a compensatory response to cope with a high exposure of oxidant compounds (40). Therefore, targeting reductive stress may be a strategy to delay and prevent the onset and progression of AD (69). Thus, it is plausible that an overexpression and high levels of GSH could be induced by an increased oxidant production in lymphocytes of mAD patients. Nevertheless, these levels were lower in severe AD patients in comparison to mAD subjects. The glutathione cycle is one of the main intracellular mechanisms to preserve a competent intracellular redox state (70). The role of this has been extensively studied in AD, in both humans and animal models, where a depletion in GSH contents and an imbalance in GSSG/GSH ratios in favor of GSSG have been noted at central (39) and peripheral levels, such as in plasma, peritoneal leukocytes, and blood cells (47, 52, 71). Moreover, it has been described that the altered levels of these circulating compounds are also directly related to the severity of cognitive impairment (47, 67). The imbalance in GSSG/GSH ratios could be the result of a defective respiratory chain caused by the activation of Aβ peptide on its complexes, which leads to overproduction of oxidant compounds, which has also been observed in peripheral leukocytes (72). In addition, an adequate immune response will require optimal levels of GSH (70). Therefore, the lower GSH observed in neutrophils of AD could contribute to the impairment of the functions of these cells.

Since the brain is very susceptible to oxidative damage (36), lipid peroxidation is one of the most promising procedures in AD diagnosis (47). Thus, higher MDA content has been reported in the brain and the peripheral levels (e.g., plasma/serum, erythrocytes, and peripheral leukocytes) of not only AD patients but also MCI subjects (42, 46, 47). Some authors suggested that lipid peroxidation could be one of the main factors responsible for cognitive deterioration and that there was a negative correlation between MDA and MMSE scores (43). Others reported that the differences depended on the stage of AD (42, 43, 47). However, although no difference between moderate and advanced AD was detected (46), our results showed that MDA levels in neutrophils were higher in patients at the advanced stage of the disease than in elderly controls and even in mAD. Thus, this parameter could be a useful marker of early stage of AD as well as progression of the disease.

Given the different pattern observed in the oxidative stress and damage parameters between neutrophils and mononuclear cells in the progression of AD, we have also analyzed these parameters in WB cells. This kind of sample better reproduces the *in vivo* conditions of immune response. Interestingly, a similarly altered redox state and oxidative damage pattern were observed in WB cells to that in neutrophils. Thus, mAD and AD patients, in general, showed lower GSH and higher GSSG contents and GSSG/GSH ratios, together with a marked increase in MDA levels, than cells from elderly subjects. Moreover, it is important to highlight that AD patients had a higher GSSG/GSH ratios, as well as GSSG and MDA contents, in their neutrophils and WB cells than mAD patients. The results suggest that the estimation of these parameters in WB cells would be a useful biomarker in the assessment of AD progression. Moreover, WB samples are clinically more feasible, reproducible, cost effective, easy to implement and apply, compared to purified and isolated neutrophils and mononuclear blood leukocytes.

In addition, since oxidation and inflammation processes are able to induce and exacerbate one another (36), the higher oxidative stress and damage observed in WB cells from mAD and AD patients could also be triggered by an increase in basal inflammation. Given that previous works supported the importance of cytokines in mediating the activity of peripheral immune cells in AD (73, 74), we also assessed the release of IL-6, TNF-α, and IL-10 *ex vivo* by blood cells cultured under resting conditions. Our results showed that mAD and AD patients had a higher basal TNF-α than elderly subjects, whereas basal IL-6 levels only were significantly higher in severe AD. Basal IL-10 release was not detectable. Even though cytokine levels are hard to detect at basal conditions, due to their short half-life, several studies also investigated these inflammatory markers in CSF, serum and plasma at different stages of the AD patients (73–76). Although the results are controversial, a strong upregulation of pro-inflammatory cytokines has been observed in these patients, but also in MCI (73, 74, 76, 77). Furthermore, these patients showed higher plasma levels of IL-6 than those at an early stage of disease and healthy controls (77). This agrees with our results, in which severe AD patients also showed higher IL-6 release than mAD. Interestingly, given that increased basal IL-6 levels in plasma have been shown to be a risk for decline in cognitive functions (73), as well as being described as one the most powerful predictors of morbidity and mortality in the elderly (30), these results suggest the possibility of using peripheral IL-6 production as a helpful tool to characterize immune dysfunction during AD progression.

The chronic oxidative-inflammatory stress situation observed in blood cells of AD patients could be involved in the impairment of their functions. Thus, the higher oxidative stress in severe AD patients could be the underlying mechanism for the decrease in PHA- and LPS-induced lymphoproliferation, as well as for the increase in the basal proliferation. This basal proliferation, which has scarcely been studied, was also increased with aging (30), as well as in the leukocytes of 3xTg-AD mice (52). The higher levels of basal proliferation in AD lymphocytes show an overactivation of these cells. This could be due to the increase age-related accumulation of damage-associated molecular patterns, which, through the production of pro-inflammatory cytokines, may be responsible for the activation of the immune system and the establishment of "sterile inflammation" (78). In addition, after a mitogenic LPS-stimulus, immune blood cells from AD patients also produced a higher release of IL-6 and TNF-α, as well as lower IL-10 levels and, consequently, a lower IL-10/TNF-α ratio, compared to age-matched controls. This reaffirms the existence of an altered immune response in advanced stages of AD. Although data on peripheral cytokines in AD patients are controversial (73, 74), several authors also found an upregulation of these cytokines in LPS-stimulated WB in AD patients in relation to elderly controls (75), as also occurred in samples of brain, serum, and other cell cultures (79). A possible explanation would be that βA peptide, which can activate the overproduction of pro-inflammatory cytokines (e.g., TNF-α, IL-1β, etc.) in peripheral blood monocytes (80, 81), could lead to an abnormal inflammatory response. This could be attributed either to an adaptive control on innate immunity and/or a compensatory mechanism for the lack of effectiveness of adaptive immunity (81). Our results also demonstrated an altered balance in the IL-10/TNF-α ratios, which showed similar values in mAD patients and elderly subjects, whereas the values were lower in AD patients. Since this IL-10/TNF-α ratio has been proposed as an indicator of successful aging and longevity (30), its determination also may be a helpful parameter for evaluating the progression of AD. Since the decline in PHA-lymphoproliferation and the high release of IL-6 after LPS stimulation not only occur in severe AD patients but also begin to decline in mAD patients, this suggests that both parameters could be used as possible early peripheral biomarkers of AD.

In conclusion, the present study shows the impairment of several immune functions of human peripheral blood neutrophils and mononuclear cells at different stages of AD. However, a different pattern of altered immune response was observed between mild and severe AD patients. Thus, several alterations were only observed in severe AD patients (e.g., chemotaxis, basal, and LPS lymphoproliferation) and others (e.g., adherence) only in individuals with mAD. Other alterations detected in the mild stage of the disease increased in the late stage (e.g., PHA lymphoproliferation and IL-6 release). As occurs in aging, this impairment of immune cell functions could have as their basis an oxidative-inflammatory stress situation. Thus, our findings also demonstrated that several peripheral oxidative stress and damage markers were increased in immune blood cells from mAD and AD patients, especially in neutrophils (e.g., low GSH levels, high GSSG/GSH ratios, and GSSG and MDA contents), in relation to elderly subjects. However, this increased oxidative stress and damage were higher in severe AD patients than in mAD and could be mediated by the higher production of peripheral pro-inflammatory cytokines in these patients. Furthermore, the fact that neutrophils showed higher oxidative stress and damage than mononuclear leukocytes supports the idea that phagocytes are the immune cells that most contribute to the peripheral chronic oxidative stress and damage associated with AD, especially in the advance stages of the disease. Therefore, our results support the idea that severe AD patients show an accelerated immunosenescence due to the parameters of function and redox state studied, these being greatly deteriorated in these patients in comparison to elderly subjects of the same chronological age. Therefore, since WB cells are very easy to obtain and reproduce the results observed in neutrophils, the assessment of oxidative stress and damage parameters, as well as peripheral cytokine release, together with the analysis of several functions in isolated neutrophils and mononuclear cells, would be useful markers of AD progression. Nevertheless, additional studies are needed to identify function and oxidative-inflammatory stress alterations in peripheral blood phagocytes and lymphocytes, especially in subjects with mild cognitive deterioration in order to identify potential prodromal and preclinical biomarkers of AD.

ETHICS STATEMENT

All procedures were carried out according to the Declaration of Helsinki, and approval was obtained from the corresponding Research Ethic Committees.

AUTHOR CONTRIBUTIONS

MF—formulated the original problem, designed the work, provided direction and guidance, wrote the manuscript and critically reviewed the final version of the manuscript. CV—provided input for experimental design, carried out experiments with patient samples, analyzed data results, and wrote the manuscript; IT—provided input for experimental design and carried out experiments with patient samples; AG—carried out experiments with patient samples; EC and JM provided the samples for the experimental study; and JM made the clinical diagnosis of Alzheimer's disease patients and control's selection.

ACKNOWLEDGMENTS

We gratefully acknowledge the participants in this study and the medical staff at Neurology Service Hospital Universitario 12 de Octubre.

FUNDING

This work was supported by the grants of the Research group of UCM (910379) and FIS (PI15/01787) and FIS (PI15/00780) from the ISCIII-FEDER of the European Union, as well as was partially supported by "Fundación Neurociencias y Envejecimiento".

REFERENCES

1. Mattson MP. Pathways towards and away from Alzheimer's disease. *Nature* (2004) 430:631–9. doi:10.1038/nature02621
2. Gatz M, Reynolds CA, Fratiglioni L, Johansson B, Mortimer JA, Berg S, et al. Role of genes and environments for explaining Alzheimer disease. *Arch Gen Psychiatry* (2006) 63:168–74. doi:10.1001/archpsyc.63.2.168
3. Prince M, Bryce R, Albanese E, Wimo A, Ribeiro W, Ferrt CP. The global prevalence of dementia: a systematic review and metaanalysis. *Alzheimers Dement* (2013) 9:63–75. doi:10.1016/j.jalz.2012.11.007
4. García-Blanco A, Baquero M, Vento M, Gil E, Bataller L, Cháfer-Pericás C. Potential oxidative stress biomarkers of mild cognitive impairment due to Alzheimer disease. *J Neurol Sci* (2017) 373:295–302. doi:10.1016/j.jns.2017.01.020
5. Selkoe DJ. Alzheimer's disease: genes, proteins, and therapy. *Physiol Rev* (2001) 81(2):741–66. doi:10.1152/physrev.2001.81.2.741
6. Ghiso J, Frangion B. Amyloidosis and Alzheimer's disease. *Adv Drug Deliv Rev* (2002) 54:1539–51. doi:10.1016/S0169-409X(02)00149-7
7. Gibson GE, Huang HM. Oxidative stress in Alzheimer's disease. *Neurobiol Aging* (2005) 26:575–8. doi:10.1016/j.neurobiolaging.2004.07.017
8. Bonotis K, Krikki E, Holeva V, Aggouridaki C, Costa V. Systemic immune aberrations in Alzheimer's disease patients. *J Neuroimmunol* (2008) 193:183–7. doi:10.1016/j.jneuroim.2007.10.020
9. Holmes C. Review: systemic inflammation and Alzheimer's disease. *Neuropathol Appl Neurobiol* (2013) 39:51–68. doi:10.1111/j.1365-2990.2012.01307.x
10. Morris JK, Honea RA, Vidoni ED, Swerdlow RH, Burns JM. Is Alzheimer's disease a systemic disease? *Biochim Biophys Acta* (2014) 1842:1340–9. doi:10.1016/j.bbadis.2014.04.012
11. Richartz E, Stransky E, Batra A, Simon P, Lewczuk P, Buchkremer G, et al. Decline of immune responsiveness: a pathogenic factor in Alzheimer's disease? *J Psychiatr Res* (2005) 39:535–43. doi:10.1016/j.jpsychires.2004.12.005
12. Britschgi M, Wyss-Coray T. Systemic and acquired immune responses in Alzheimer's disease. *Int Rev Neurobiol* (2007) 82:205–33. doi:10.1016/S0074-7742(07)82011-3
13. Boutajangout A, Wisniewski T. The innate immune system in Alzheimer's disease. *Int J Cell Biol* (2013) 2013:576383. doi:10.1155/2013/576383
14. Heneka MT, Kummer MP, Latz E. Innate immune activation in neurodegenerative disease. *Nat Rev Immunol* (2014) 14:463–77. doi:10.1038/nri3705
15. Marsha SE, Abuda EM, Lakatosc A, Karimzadehb A, Yeungc ST, Davtyane H, et al. The adaptive immune system restrains Alzheimer's disease pathogenesis by modulating microglial function. *PNAS* (2016) 113(9):E1316–25. doi:10.1073/pnas.1525466113
16. Giménez-Llort L, Maté I, Manassra R, Vida C, De la Fuente M. Peripheral immune system and neuroimmune communication impairment in a mouse model of Alzheimer's disease. *Ann N Y Acad Sci* (2012) 1262:74–84. doi:10.1111/j.1749-6632.2012.06639.x
17. Martorana A, Bulati M, Buffa S, Pellicanò M, Caruso C, Candore G, et al. Immunosenescence, inflammation and Alzheimer's disease. *Longev Healthspan* (2012) 1:8. doi:10.1186/2046-2395-1-8
18. Monsonego A, Zota V, Karni A, Krieger JI, Bar-Or A, Bitan G, et al. Increased T cell reactivity to amyloid beta protein in older humans and patients with Alzheimer's disease. *J Clin Invest* (2003) 112:415–22. doi:10.1172/JCI200318104
19. Fiala M, Lin J, Ringman J, Kermani-Arab V, Tsao G, Patel A, et al. Ineffective phagocytosis of amyloid-beta by macrophages of Alzheimer's disease patients. *J Alzheimers Dis* (2005) 7:221–32. doi:10.3233/JAD-2005-7304
20. Man SM, Ma YR, Shang DS, Zhao WD, Li B, Guo DW, et al. Peripheral T cells overexpress MIP-1α to enhance its transendothelial migration in Alzheimer's disease. *Neurobiol Aging* (2007) 28:485–96. doi:10.1016/j.neurobiolaging.2006.02.013
21. Liu YJ, Guo DW, Tian L, Shang DS, Zhao WD. Peripheral T cells derived from Alzheimer's disease patients overexpress CXCR2 contributing to its transendothelial migration, which is microglial TNF-α-dependent. *Neurobiol Aging* (2010) 31:175–88. doi:10.1016/j.neurobiolaging.2008.03.024
22. Von Bernhardi R. Glial cell dysregulation: a new perspective on Alzheimer disease. *Neurotox Res* (2007) 12:215–32. doi:10.1007/BF03033906
23. Corona AW, Fenn AM, Godbout JP. Cognitive and behavioural consequences of impaired immunoregulation in aging. *J Neuroimmune Pharmacol* (2009) 7:7–23. doi:10.1007/s11481-011-9313-4

24. De la Fuente M. Role of neuroimmunomodulation in aging. *Neuroimmunomodulation* (2008) 15:213–23. doi:10.1159/000156465
25. Giménez-Llort L, Torres-Lista V, De la Fuente M. Crosstalk between behavior and immune system during the prodromal stages of Alzheimer's disease. *Curr Pharm Des* (2014) 20(29):4723–32. doi:10.2174/1381612820666140130205500
26. Giménez-Llort L, Arranz L, Maté I, De la Fuente M. Gender-specific neuroimmunoendocrine aging in a triple-transgenic 3xTgAD mouse model for Alzheimer's disease and its relation with longevity. *Neuroimmunomodulation* (2008) 15:331–43. doi:10.1159/000156475
27. Chen SH, Bu XL, Jin WS, Shen LL, Wang J, Zhuang ZQ, et al. Altered peripheral profile of blood cells in Alzheimer disease. A hospital-based case-control study. *Medicine (Baltimore)* (2017) 96(21):e6843. doi:10.1097/MD.0000000000006843
28. De la Fuente M, Miquel J. An update of the oxidation-Inflammation theory of aging: the involvement of the immune system in oxi-inflamm-aging. *Curr Pharm Des* (2009) 15:3003–26. doi:10.2174/138161209789058110
29. De la Fuente M. Crosstalk between the nervous and the immune systems in health and sickness. *Curr Pharm Des* (2014) 20(29):4605–7. doi:10.2174/1381612820666140130213734
30. Martínez de Toda I, Maté I, Vida C, Cruces J, De la Fuente M. Immune function parameters as markers of biological age and predictors of longevity. *Aging (Albany NY)* (2017) 28(11):3110–9. doi:10.18632/aging.101116
31. Araga S, Kagimoto H, Funamoto K, Takahashi K. Reduced natural killer cell activity in patients with dementia of Alzheimer type. *Acta Neurol Scand* (1991) 844:259–63. doi:10.1111/j.1600-0404.1991.tb04948.x
32. Le Page A, Bourgade K, Lamoureux J, Frost E, Pawelec G, Larbi A, et al. NK cells are activated in amnestic mild cognitive impairment but not in mild Alzheimer's disease patients. *J Alzheimers Dis* (2015) 46(1):93–107. doi:10.3233/JAD-143054
33. Richartz-Salzburger E, Batra A, Stransky E, Laske C, Köhler N, Bartels M, et al. Altered lymphocyte distribution in Alzheimer's disease. *J Psychiatr Res* (2007) 41(1–2):174–8. doi:10.1016/j.jpsychires.2006.01.010
34. Rezai-Zadeh K, Gate D, Szekely CA, Town T. Can peripheral leukocytes be used as Alzheimer's disease biomarkers? *Expert Rev Neurother* (2009) 9(11):1623–33. doi:10.1586/ern.09.118
35. Khansari N, Shakiba Y, Mahmoudi M. Chronic inflammation and oxidative stress as a major cause of age-related diseases and cancer. *Recent Pat Inflamm Allergy Drug Discov* (2009) 3:73–80. doi:10.2174/187221309787158371
36. Vida C, González EM, De la Fuente M. Increase of oxidation and inflammation in nervous and immune systems with aging and anxiety. *Curr Pharm Des* (2014) 20(29):4656–78. doi:10.2174/1381612820666140130201734
37. Butterfield DA. B-Amiloid-associated free radical oxidative stress and neurotoxicity: implications for Alzheimer's disease. *Chem Res Toxicol* (1997) 10:495–506. doi:10.1021/tx960130e
38. Zhu X, Su B, Wang X, Smith MA, Perry G. Causes of oxidative stress in Alzheimer disease. *Cell Mol Life Sci* (2007) 64:2202–10. doi:10.1007/s00018-007-7218-4
39. Venkateshappa C, Harish G, Mahadevan A. Elevated oxidative stress and decreased antioxidant function in the human hippocampus and frontal cortex with increasing age: implications for neurodegeneration in Alzheimer's disease. *Neurochem Res* (2012) 37:1601–14. doi:10.1007/s11064-012-0755-8
40. Luca M, Luca A, Calandra C. The role of oxidative damage in the pathogenesis and progression of Alzheimer's disease and vascular dementia. *Oxid Med Cell Longev* (2015) 2015:504678. doi:10.1155/2015/504678
41. Leutner S, Schindowski K, Frölich L, Maurer K, Kratzsch T, Eckert A, et al. Enhanced ROS-generation in lymphocytes from Alzheimer's patients. *Pharmacopsychiatry* (2005) 38:312–5. doi:10.1055/s-2005-916186
42. Skoumalova A, Hort J. Blood markers of oxidative stress in Alzheimer's disease. *J Cell Mol Med* (2012) 16:2291–300. doi:10.1111/j.1582-4934.2012.01585.x
43. Torres LL, Quaglio NB, de Souza GT, Garcia RT, Dati LM, Moreira WL, et al. Peripheral oxidative stress biomarkers in mild cognitive impairment and Alzheimer's disease. *J Alzheimers Dis* (2011) 26:59–68. doi:10.3233/JAD-2011-110284
44. Sliwinska A, Kwiatkowski D, Czarny P, Toma M, Wigner P, Drzewoski J, et al. The levels of 7,8-dihydrodeoxyguanosine (8-oxoG) and 8-oxoguanine DNA glycosylase 1 (OGG1) – a potential diagnostic biomarkers of Alzheimer's disease. *J Neurol Sci* (2016) 368:155–9. doi:10.1016/j.jns.2016.07.008
45. Migliore L, Fontana I, Trippi F, Colognato R, Coppedè F, Tognoni G, et al. Oxidative DNA damage in peripheral leukocytes of mild cognitive impairment and AD patients. *Neurobiol Aging* (2005) 26:567–73. doi:10.1016/j.neurobiolaging.2004.07.016
46. Marcourakis T, Camarini R, Kawamoto EK, Rodrigue-Scorsi L, Scavone C. Peripheral biomarkers of oxidative stress in aging and Alzheimer's disease. *Dement Neuropsychol* (2008) 2(1):2–8. doi:10.1590/S1980-57642009DN20100002
47. Rani P, Krishnan S, Rani C. Study on analysis of peripheral biomarkers for Alzheimer's disease diagnosis. *Front Neurol* (2017) 8:328. doi:10.3389/fneur.2017.00328
48. Ferretti MT, Bruno MA, Ducatenzeiler A, Klein WL, Cuello AC. Intracellular Abeta-oligomers and early inflammation in a model of Alzheimer's disease. *Neurobiol Aging* (2012) 33:1329–42. doi:10.1016/j.neurobiolaging.2011.01.007
49. Wright AL, Zinn R, Hohensinn B, Konen LM, Beynon SB, Tan RP, et al. Neuroinflammation and neuronal loss precede Abeta plaque deposition in the hAPP-J20 mouse model of Alzheimer's disease. *PLoS One* (2013) 8:e59586. doi:10.1371/journal.pone.0059586
50. Oddo S, Caccamo A, Shepherd JD, Murphy MP, Golde TE, Kayed R. Tripletransgenic model of Alzheimer's disease with plaques and tangles: intracelular Aβ and synaptic dysfunction. *Neuron* (2003) 39:409–21. doi:10.1016/S0896-6273(03)00434-3
51. Arranz L, De Castro NM, Baeza I, Giménez-Llort L, De la Fuente M. Effect of environmental enrichment on the immunoendocrine aging of male and female triple-transgenic 3xTg-AD mice for Alzheimer's disease. *J Alzheimers Dis* (2011) 25(4):727–37. doi:10.3233/JAD-2011-110236
52. Maté I, Cruces J, Giménez-Llort L, De la Fuente M. Function and redox state of peritoneal leukocytes as preclinical and prodromic markers in a longitudinal study of triple-transgenic mice for Alzheimer's disease. *J Alzheimers Dis* (2015) 43(1):213–26. doi:10.3233/JAD-140861
53. Arranz L, Caamaño JH, Lord JM, De la Fuente M. Preserved immune functions and controlled leukocyte oxidative stress in naturally long-lived mice: possible role of nuclear factor kappa B. *J Gerontol A Biol Sci Med Sci* (2010) 65(9):941–50. doi:10.1093/gerona/glq101
54. Vida C, de Toda IM, Cruces J, Garrido A, Gónzalez-Sánchez M, De la Fuente M. Role of macrophages in age-related oxidative stress and lipofuscin accumulation in mice. *Redox Biol* (2017) 12:423–37. doi:10.1016/j.redox.2017.03.005
55. McKhanna GM, Knopman DS, Chertkow H, Hyman BT, Jack CR, Kawas CH, et al. The diagnosis of dementia due to Alzheimer's disease: recommendations from the National Institute on Aging-Alzheimer's Association workgroups on diagnostic guidelines for Alzheimer's disease. *Alzheimers Dement* (2011) 7:263–9. doi:10.1016/j.jalz.2011.03.005
56. Folstein MF, Folstein SE, McHugh PR. Mini-mental state. A practical method for grading the cognitive state of patients for the clinician. *J Psychiatr Res* (1975) 12:189–98. doi:10.1016/0022-3956(75)90026-6
57. De la Fuente M, Hernanz A, Guayerbas N, Victor VM, Arnalich F. Vitamin E ingestion improves several immune functions in elderly men and women. *Free Radic Res* (2008) 42:272–80. doi:10.1080/10715760801898838
58. Hernanz A, Tato E, De la Fuente M, De Miguel E, Arnalich F. Differential effects of gastrin-releasing peptide, neuropeptide Y, somatostatin and vasoactive intestinal peptide on interleukin-1β, interleukin-6 and tumour necrosis factor-α production by whole blood cells from healthy young and old subjects. *J Neuroimmunol* (1996) 71:25–30. doi:10.1016/S0165-5728(96)00118-X
59. De la Fuente M, Carrasco M, Hernanz A. Modulation of human neutrophil function in vitro by gastrin. *J Endocrinol* (1997) 153:475–83. doi:10.1677/joe.0.1530475
60. Hissin PJ, Hilf R. A fluorometric method for determination of oxidized and reduced glutathione in tissues. *Anal Biochem* (1976) 74:214–26. doi:10.1016/0003-2697(76)90326-2
61. Franceschi C, Bonafé M, Valensin S, Olivieri F, De Luca M, Ottaviani E, et al. Inflamm-aging. An evolutionary perspective on immunosenescence. *Ann N Y Acad Sci* (2000) 908:244–54. doi:10.1111/j.1749-6632.2000.tb06651.x
62. Bondar G, Cadeiras M, Wisniewski N, Maque J, Chittoor J, Chang E, et al. Comparison of whole blood and peripheral blood mononuclear cell gene expression for evaluation of the perioperative inflammatory response in patients with advanced heart failure. *PLoS One* (2014) 9(12):e115097. doi:10.1371/journal.pone.0115097

63. Deleidi M, Jäggle M, Rubino G. Immune aging, dysmetabolism, and inflammation in neurological diseases. *Front Neurosci* (2015) 9:172. doi:10.3389/fnins.2015.00172
64. Yoon SC, Kwon YA, Kim H, Kim S, Ahn Jo S, Kim DK. Altered cell viability and proliferation activity of peripheral lymphocytes in patients with Alzheimer's disease. *Psychiatry Investig* (2010) 7(1):68–71. doi:10.4306/pi.2010.7.1.68
65. Nunomura A, Perry G, Aliev G, Hirai K, Takeda A, Balraj EK, et al. Oxidative damage is the earliest event in Alzheimer disease. *J Neuropathol Exp Neurol* (2001) 60:759–67. doi:10.1093/jnen/60.8.759
66. Wojda U. Alzheimer's disease lymphocytes: potential for biomarkers? *Biomark Med* (2016) 10:1–4. doi:10.2217/bmm.15.79
67. Ponce PD, Felipe Salech F, San Martín C, Silva M, Xiong C, Roe CM, et al. Increased susceptibility to oxidative death of lymphocytes from Alzheimer patients correlates with dementia severity. *Curr Alzheimer Res* (2014) 11(9):892–8. doi:10.2174/1567205011666141001113135
68. Mecocci P, Polidori MC, Ingegni T, Cherubini A, Chionne F, Cecchetti R, et al. Oxidative damage to DNA in lymphocytes from AD patients. *Neurology* (1998) 51(4):1014–7. doi:10.1212/WNL.51.4.1014
69. Badía MC, Giraldo E, Dasí F, Alonso D, Lainez JM, Lloret A, et al. Reductive stress in young healthy individuals at risk of Alzheimer disease. *Free Radic Biol Med* (2013) 63:274–9. doi:10.1016/j.freeradbiomed.2013.05.003
70. Drögue W, Breitkreutz R. Glutathione and immune function. *Proc Nutr Soc* (2000) 59(4):595–600. doi:10.1017/S0029665100000847
71. Bermejo P, Martín-Aragón S, Benedí J, Susín C, Felici E, Gil P, et al. Peripheral levels of glutathione and protein oxidation as markers in the development of Alzheimer's disease from mild cognitive impairment. *Free Radic Res* (2008) 42:162–70. doi:10.1080/10715760701861373
72. Leuner K, Schulz K, Schütt T, Pantel J, Prvulovic D, Rhein V, et al. Peripheral mitochondrial dysfuncion in Alzheimer's disease: focus on lymphocytes. *Mol Neurobiol* (2012) 46:194–204. doi:10.1007/s12035-012-8300-y
73. Sala G, Galimberti G, Canevari C, Raggi ME, Isella V, Facheris M, et al. Peripheral cytokine release in Alzheimer patients: correlation with disease severity. *Neurobiol Aging* (2003) 24(7):909–14. doi:10.1016/S0197-4580(03)00010-1
74. Guerreiro RJ, Santana I, Brás JM, Santiago B, Paiva A, Oliveira C. Peripheral inflammatory cytokines as biomarkers in Alzheimer's disease and mil cognitive impairment. *Neurodegener Dis* (2007) 4(6):406–12. doi:10.1159/000107700
75. Lombardi VR, García M, Rey L, Cacabelos R. Characterization of cytokine production, screening of lymphocyte subset patterns and in vitro apoptosis in healthy and Alzheimer's disease (AD) individuals. *J Neuroimmunol* (1999) 97(1/2):163–71. doi:10.1016/S0165-5728(99)00046-6
76. Licastro F, Pedrini S, Caputo L, Annoni G, Davis LJ, Ferri C, et al. Increased plasma levels of interleukin-1, interleukin-6 and alpha-1-antichymotrypsin in patients with Alzheimer's disease: peripheral inflammation or signals from the brain? *J Neuroimmunol* (2000) 103:97–102. doi:10.1016/S0165-5728(99)00226-X
77. Kálmán J, Juhásh A, Laird G, Dickens P, Járdánházy T, Rimanóczy A, et al. Serum interleukin-6 levels correlate with the severity of dementia in Down syndrome and in Alzheimer's disease. *Acta Neurol Scand* (1997) 96(4):236–40. doi:10.1111/j.1600-0404.1997.tb00275.x
78. Martínez de Toda I, Vida C, De la Fuente M. An appropriate modulation of lymphoproliferative response and cytokine release as possible contributors to longevity. *Int J Mol Sci* (2017) 18(7):E1598. doi:10.3390/ijms18071598
79. Akiyama H, Barger S, Barnum S, Bradt B, Bauer J, Cole GM, et al. Inflammation and Alzheimer's disease. *Neurobiol Aging* (2000) 21:383–421. doi:10.1016/S0197-4580(00)00124-X
80. Meda L, Bonaiuto C, Szendrei GI, Ceska M, Rossi F, Cassatella MA. B-Amyloid(25-35) induces the production of interleukin-8 from human monocytes. *J Neuroimmunol* (1995) 59:29–33. doi:10.1016/0165-5728(95)00021-S
81. Rocha NP, Teixeira AL, Coelho FM, Caramelli P, Guimaraes HC, Barbosa IG, et al. Peripheral blood mono-nuclear cells derived from Alzheimer's disease patients show elevated baseline levels of secreted cytokines but resist stimulation with β-amyloid peptide. *Mol Cell Neurosci* (2012) 49(1):77–84.

6

End-Stage Renal Disease Causes Skewing in the TCR Vβ-Repertoire Primarily within CD8⁺ T Cell Subsets

*Ling Huang[1], Michiel G. H. Betjes[1], Mariska Klepper[1], Anton W. Langerak[2], Carla C. Baan[1] and Nicolle H. R. Litjens[1]**

[1] Department of Internal Medicine, Erasmus MC, University Medical Center Rotterdam, Nephrology and Transplantation, Rotterdam, Netherlands, [2] Department of Immunology, Erasmus MC, University Medical Center Rotterdam, Rotterdam, Netherlands

***Correspondence:**
Nicolle H. R. Litjens
n.litjens@erasmusmc.nl

A broad T cell receptor (TCR-) repertoire is required for an effective immune response. TCR-repertoire diversity declines with age. End-stage renal disease (ESRD) patients have a prematurely aged T cell system which is associated with defective T cell-mediated immunity. Recently, we showed that ESRD may significantly skew the TCR Vβ-repertoire. Here, we assessed the impact of ESRD on the TCR Vβ-repertoire within different T cell subsets using a multiparameter flow-cytometry-based assay, controlling for effects of aging and CMV latency. Percentages of 24 different TCR Vβ-families were tested in circulating naive and memory T cell subsets of 10 ESRD patients and 10 age- and CMV-serostatus-matched healthy individuals (HI). The Gini-index, a parameter used in economics to describe the distribution of income, was calculated to determine the extent of skewing at the subset level taking into account frequencies of all 24 TCR Vβ-families. In addition, using HI as reference population, the differential impact of ESRD was assessed on clonal expansion at the level of an individual TCR Vβ-family. $CD8^+$, but not $CD4^+$, T cell differentiation was associated with higher Gini-TCR indices. Gini-TCR indices were already significantly higher for different $CD8^+$ memory T cell subsets of younger ESRD patients compared to their age-matched HI. ESRD induced expansions of not one TCR Vβ-family in particular and expansions were predominantly observed within the $CD8^+$ T cell compartment. All ESRD patients had expanded TCR Vβ-families within total $CD8^+$ T cells and the median (IQ range) number of expanded TCR Vβ-families/patient amounted to 2 (1–4). Interestingly, ESRD also induced clonal expansions of TCR Vβ-families within naive $CD8^+$ T cells as 8 out of 10 patients had expanded TCR Vβ-families. The median (IQ range) number of expanded families/patient amounted to 1 (1–1) within naive $CD8^+$ T cells. In conclusion, loss of renal function skews the TCR Vβ-repertoire already in younger patients by inducing expansions of different TCR Vβ-families within the various T cell subsets, primarily affecting the $CD8^+$ T cell compartment. This skewed TCR Vβ-repertoire may be associated with a less broad and diverse T cell-mediated immunity.

Keywords: TCR-repertoire, T cell subsets, end-stage renal disease, ageing (aging), CMV-latency

INTRODUCTION

End-stage renal disease (ESRD) patients have a decreased vaccination efficacy (1–4), an increased susceptibility for infection (5–7) and a higher risk for the development of tumors (8–11). Loss of renal function is associated with a prematurely aged T cell system (12), most likely caused by the uremia-induced proinflammatory environment (13). These uremia-induced effects on T cells are expressed as a decline in thymic output, a severe depletion of naive T cell compartment, a shift to more highly differentiated memory T cell subsets, attrition of T cell telomeres (14) and a defective T cell receptor (TCR)-induced ERK phosphorylation (15).

A broad TCR-repertoire capable of recognizing a wide range of foreign antigens is crucial for adequate T cell-mediated immune responses (16). Most TCRs consist of an α and β chain and each chain is composed of a variable (V) and a constant (C) region (17). The TCR Vβ-repertoire can be assessed using several approaches such as gene scan spectratyping *via* a DNA-based PCR (18), Vβ-family phenotyping by flow-cytometry (19–21), and assessment of clonal diversity *via* next generation sequencing (NGS) (22, 23). Gene scan spectratyping of the TCR Vβ-repertoire is at best a semiquantitative measurement. Both flow-cytometry and NGS result in a more accurate quantitative assessment of the TCR Vβ-repertoire. As NGS is more labor-intensive and sorting of highly pure T cells or their subsets is required, many researchers prefer to use flow-cytometry. Flow-cytometry allows for measuring percentages of TCR Vβ-families at the T cell-subset level obviating the need for cell sorting.

We recently examined the TCR Vβ-repertoire in ESRD patients using multiplex DNA-based spectratyping. We showed ESRD to significantly and independently skew the TCR Vβ-repertoire in older individuals and this skewing was predominantly present within the $CD8^+$ memory T cell compartment (24). However, details of this skewed TCR Vβ-repertoire in ESRD patients are still lacking and quantitative data related to the impact of ESRD on TCR Vβ-repertoire in the various T cell populations is rare.

During aging, the TCR Vβ-repertoire has been reported to contract (25). Aging is associated with a decline in the naive T cell compartment which possess the broadest TCR repertoire (26), and a shift toward memory T cells, developing upon encountering of an antigen and having a skewed repertoire toward particular specificities (27, 28). The prevalence of CMV-seropositivity is high amongst ESRD patients, varying from 30 to 100%, depending on socioeconomic and ethnic background (29). CMV latency profoundly affects circulating T cells resembling features of aging, including increased frequencies of more differentiated memory T cells (30, 31) and loss of telomere length (32). CMV latency may also induce contraction of the TCR Vβ-repertoire as it induces expansion of CMV-specific T cells immunocompetent donors (33) and these CMV-specific clones are stably maintained for 5 years (34). Thus, TCR Vβ-repertoire diversity may be affected by various factors.

In this study, we assessed the TCR Vβ-repertoire diversity within different T cell subsets in ESRD patients using a flow-cytometry-based taking into account the effects of aging and CMV latency.

MATERIALS AND METHODS

Study Population

A cohort of 10 stable ESRD patients, either younger individuals ($n = 5$, age < 45 years) or older individuals ($n = 5$, age $\geq$ 65 years) with an oligoclonal TCR Vβ-repertoire, as determined by DNA-based spectratyping earlier (24) were studied in more detail at the T cell-subset level using a flow-cytometry based assay for TCR Vβ-repertoire analysis. Patients having a glomerular filtration rate below 15 mL/min and either or not receiving renal replacement therapy (RRT) were included. Patients were excluded from the study when having a bacterial or viral infection, malignancy, a previous transplantation or taking immunosuppressive medication (except for glucocorticoids). The patient data are compared to those generated from 10 age- and CMV-matched healthy individuals (HIs) with a polyclonal TCR Vβ-repertoire, as determined by DNA-based spectratyping (24). Lithium-heparinized blood was drawn from ESRD patients and HI. Written informed consent was obtained from all individuals included. The study was approved by the local medical ethical committee (METC number: 2012-022) and conducted according to the principles of Declaration of Helsinki and in compliance with International Conference on Harmonization/Good Clinical Practice regulations.

Sample Preparation

Peripheral blood mononuclear cells (PBMCs) were isolated from 35 mL of lithium-heparinized blood by density centrifugation as described previously (35) and then frozen at 10×10^6 PBMC per vial at −190°C until further use.

Cryopreserved PBMCs (1 vial of 10×10^6 PBMCs) were thawed, counted, washed and resuspended in Isoflow™ Sheath Fluid (Beckman Coulter B.V., Woerden, Netherlands). The PBMCs were stained with Brilliant Violet 510-labeled anti-CD3 (BioLegend, Uithoorn, Netherlands), Alexa Fluor (AF)700-labeled anti-CD4 (Beckman Coulter B.V.) and Allophycocyanin (APC)-Cy7-labeled anti-CD8 (BioLegend) to identify $CD4^+$ and $CD8^+$ within $CD3^+$ T cells. ECD-labeled anti-CD45RO (Beckman Coulter B.V.), PE-Cy7-labeled anti-CCR7 (BD, Erembodegem, Belgium), V450-labeled anti-CD31 (BD; clone WM59), peridinin chlorophyll-A protein-Cy5.5-labeled anti-CD28 (BD) and APC-labeled anti-CD57 (BioLegend) as well as fluorescence minus one controls were used to appropriately identify the different T cell subsets (illustrated in Figures S1B–D in Supplementary Material). As shown in Figure S1B in Supplementary Material, CCR7 and CD45RO are used to distinguish the different naive and memory T cell subsets, i.e., naive ($CD45RO^-CCR7^+$), central memory (CM, $CD45RO^+CCR7^+$), effector memory (EM, $CD45RO^+CCR7^-$), and terminally differentiated effector memory $CD45RA^+$ T cells subsets (EMRA, $CD45RO^-CCR7^-$). CD31-expression within naive T cells (Figure S1C in Supplementary Material) identifies T cells that recently have left the thymus, also referred to as recent thymic emigrants (RTEs) (36). Loss of CD28 ($CD28^-$ T cells) and gain of CD57 ($CD57^+$ T cells) expression is observed in relation to increased replicative history (37, 38) and allows for identification of more differentiated T cells (Figure S1D in Supplementary Material).

Subsequently, the cell suspension was divided into eight tubes (100 μL/tube) labeled A-H, corresponding to the different antibody cocktails to stain for the 24 TCR Vβ-families (IOTest® Beta Mark TCR V beta repertoire kit, Beckman Coulter B.V.). Each cocktail contains antibodies directed to three different Vβ-families, i.e., one is fluorescein isothiocyanate (FITC-), one is PE-labeled and one is labeled with both FITC and PE. **Table 1** shows the description of the antibodies directed to the different TCR Vβ-families in tube A to H. A typical example of the proportions of several TCR Vβ-families within $CD3^+$ T cells from tube

TABLE 1 | TCR Vβ-families in tube A-H.

Tube	Vβ family	Fluorochrome	Clone
A	Vβ 5.3	PE	3D11
	Vβ 3	FITC	CH92
	Vβ 7.1	PE + FITC	ZOE
B	Vβ 9	PE	FIN9
	Vβ 16	FITC	TAMAYA1.2
	Vβ 17	PE + FITC	E17.5F3
C	Vβ 18	PE	BA62.6
	Vβ 20	FITC	ELL1.4
	Vβ 5.1	PE + FITC	IMMU157
D	Vβ 13.1	PE	IMMU222
	Vβ 8	FITC	56C5.2
	Vβ 13.6	PE + FITC	JU74.3
E	Vβ 5.2	PE	36213
	Vβ 12	FITC	VER2.32
	Vβ 2	PE + FITC	MPB2D5
F	Vβ 23	PE	AF23
	Vβ 21.3	FITC	IG125
	Vβ 1	PE + FITC	BL37.2
G	Vβ 11	PE	C21
	Vβ 14	FITC	CAS1.1.3
	Vβ 22	PE + FITC	IMMU546
H	Vβ 13.2	PE	H132
	Vβ 7.2	FITC	ZIZOU4
	Vβ 4	PE + FITC	WJF24

Detailed information with respect to the different TCR Vβ-family antibodies in tube A-H, labels and clones (IOTest® Beta Mark TCR V beta repertoire kit, Beckman Coulter).

A, tube B and tube C is depicted in Figure S1A in Supplementary Material, the last three plots.

The samples were measured on a Navios flow cytometer (10-color configuration; Beckman Coulter B.V.) and at least 0.5 million CD3$^+$ T cells were acquired for each tube. Data were analyzed by Kaluza™ software (Beckman Coulter B.V.). The number of events acquired for a specific T cell subset needed to be more than 100 to allow for reliable analysis of frequencies of TCR Vβ-families within this population. The only subset that did not meet this criterion was the EMRA population within the CD4$^+$ T cells.

Gini-TCR Index and Calculation of Expanded TCR Vβ–Families

The Gini index is used to describe the distribution of income in economic statistics. As the distribution of TCR Vβ–families shows similarities to that of income, the Gini index can also be applied in TCR Vβ-repertoire analysis by flow-cytometry. It has already been used in TCR-sequencing studies (39, 40), and was recently also introduced as an accurate and reliable way for analyzing TCR Vβ-repertoire data obtained by flow-cytometry (41). The TCR (Vβ)-Gini index with scores ranging from low to high indicates TCR Vβ-families from equal distribution (broad repertoire; i.e., low score) to unequal distribution (skewed repertoire; i.e., high score). A Microsoft excel file allowing for automatic calculation of the Gini-TCR index using percentages of 24 TCR-Vβ families is provided in the supporting file (41).

An expansion in a TCR Vβ-family in ESRD patients is defined as a frequency above the mean percentage + 2 times the SD of a certain TCR Vβ-family obtained using the HI as reference population. By using this approach, finding an expansion by chance is lower than 2.5%.

TABLE 2 | Demographic and clinical characteristics of the study population.

	Healthy individuals	ESRD patients	*P*-value
Number of individuals	10	10	
Age (years; range)			
younger group (<45 years)	36 (26–42)	28 (20–29)	0.06
older group (>65 years)	68 (65–73)	70 (65–73)	0.92
Sex (% male)	60	40	0.66
CMV IgG serostatus (% pos)	60	60	1.00
RRT (%)	n.a.	70	n.a.
Duration of RRT (months; median/range)		20 (7–68)	
Hemodialysis (%)		85.7	
Peritoneal dialysis (%)		14.3	
Underlying kidney disease			
Primary glomerulopathy (%)		20	
Diabetic nephropathy (%)		30	
Reflux nephropathy (%)		10	
Polycystic kidney disease (%)		20	
Lupus nephritis (%)		10	
Unknown (%)		10	

ESRD, end-stage renal disease; CMV, cytomegalovirus; pos, positive; RRT, renal replacement therapy; n.a., not applicable.

Statistical Analyses

Gini-TCR indices or median number of expanded TCR Vβ-families/individual between two different T cell subsets within individuals were compared with Wilcoxon signed rank test and Friedman test followed by Dunn's multiple comparison *T*-test was used for comparing more than two different T cell subsets. Trend analyses were performed using two-way ANOVA, comparing different subsets between individuals or CD4$^+$ and CD8$^+$ T cells. In addition, the effect of ESRD with respect to numbers of expanded TCR Vβ-families within different T cell subsets is done using Fisher's exact test. Two-sided *P*-values <0.05 were considered statistically significant. All statistical analyses were performed with GraphPad Prism 5.

RESULTS

Study Population

Detailed information of the study population is given in **Table 2**. Ten ESRD patients (5 younger individuals: age 20–29 years and 5 older individuals: age 65–73 years) and 10 age-matched HI (5 younger individuals age 26–42 years and 5 older individuals: age 65–73 years) were recruited into this study. Sixty percent of the ESRD and HI study population is CMV-seropositive. Seven out of 10 ESRD patients received RRT.

Gini-TCR Indices Increase with T Cell Differentiation

Naive T cells expressing CD31 are considered to be RTEs and the least-differentiated T cell subset. In ESRD patients, CD31-expressing naive T cells tended to or have a lower Gini-TCR index when compared to their CD31$^-$ counterparts within CD4$^+$ (**Figure 1B**) and CD8$^+$ T cells (**Figure 1D**), respectively. For HI,

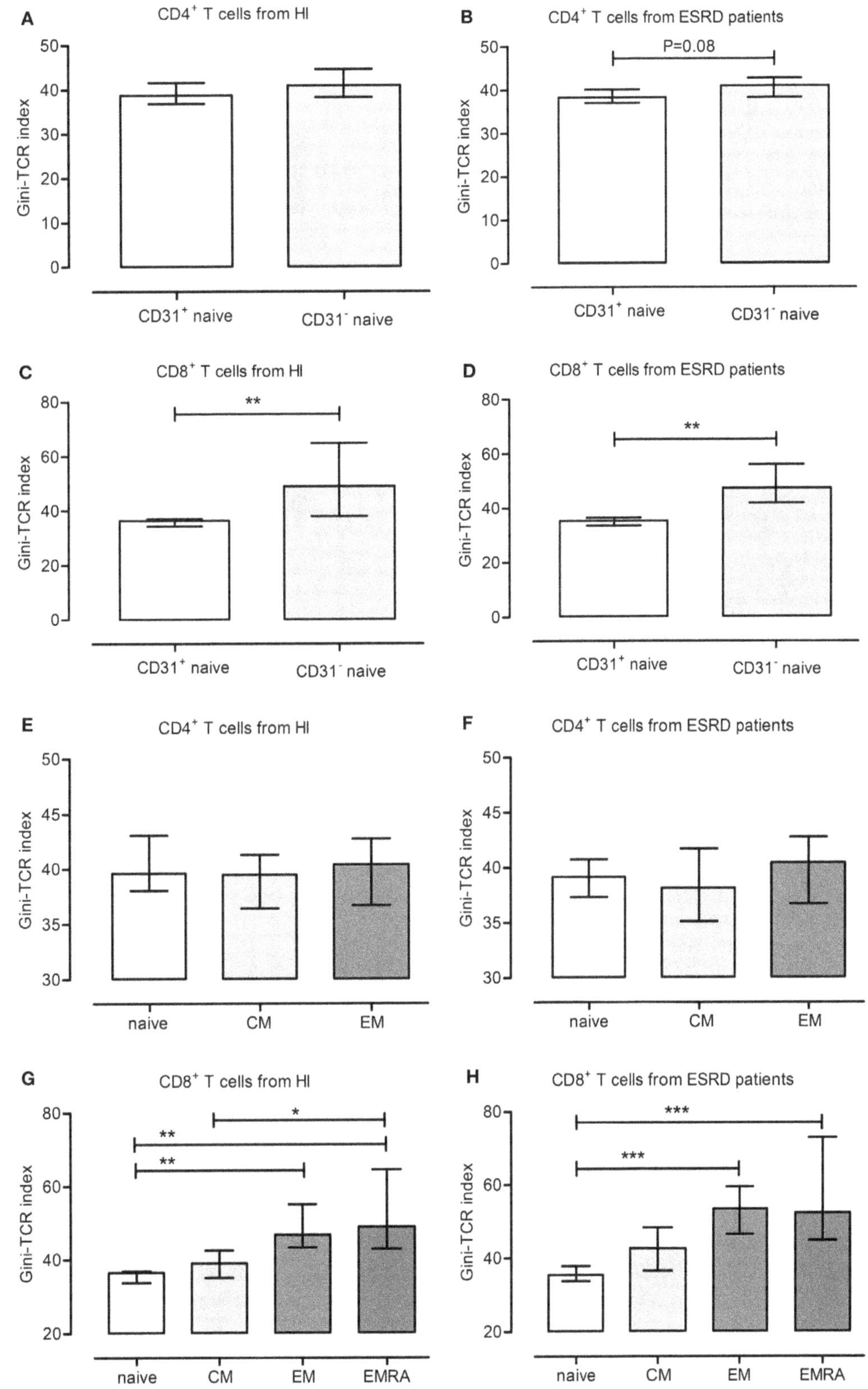

FIGURE 1 | Gini-T cell receptor (TCR) indices for different T cell subsets. The different Gini-TCR indices are depicted for healthy individual (HI) **(A,C,E,G)** and end-stage renal disease (ESRD) patients **(B,D,F,H)**. First, the Gini-TCR indices for recent thymic emigrant (CD31+ naive) and CD31− naive CD4+ **(A,B)** and CD8+ T **(C,D)** cells are given, respectively. Next, the differentiation-associated effects on Gini-TCR indices are depicted for CD4+ **(E,F)** and CD8+ **(G,H)** T cell subsets, including naive, central memory, effector memory, and terminally differentiated effector memory CD45RA+ (EMRA) T cells. *, **, and *** reflect *P*-values <0.05, 0.01, and 0.001, respectively. Data from 10 HI and 10 ESRD patients are given as median with interquartile range.

a significant lower Gini-TCR index was only observed for CD31-expressing naive CD8+ (**Figure 1C**) but not CD4+ (**Figure 1A**) T cells when compared to CD31− naive T cells. Furthermore, a T cell differentiation-associated increase in Gini-TCR indices was noted for CD8+ (**Figures 1G,H**), but not CD4+ (**Figures 1E,F**), T cells. The median value (IQ range) increased significantly ($P < 0.001$) from 36.5 (33.7–37) and 35.5 (33.8–37.9) in naive T cells to 49 (43–64.6) and 52.4 (44.9–72.8) in the highly differentiated EMRA CD8+ T cells for HI and ESRD patients, respectively.

ESRD Patients Have Increased Gini-TCR Indices within Memory CD8+ T Cell Subsets

We next analyzed the influence of ESRD, aging, and CMV latency on skewing of the TCR Vβ-repertoire by comparing Gini-TCR indices for different T cell subsets including total CD3+ T cells, as well as naive, CD31+ naive, total memory (MEM), CM, EM, EMRA, CD28−, and CD57+ populations within both the CD4+ and CD8+ T cell subsets. ESRD effects with respect to Gini-TCR indices were limited to the CD8+ T cell compartment as it tended to induce higher Gini-TCR indices ($P = 0.06$) in CD8+ memory T cells when compared to HI (**Figure 2A**). The median (IQ range) value for Gini-TCR index in CD8+ memory T cells amounted to 48.4 (45.8–63.3) and 43.8 (41.1–51.2) for ESRD patients and HI, respectively. Younger (**Figure 2B**), but not older (**Figure 2C**), ESRD patients had significantly higher Gini-TCR indices within the CD8+ CM ($P < 0.05$), EM ($P < 0.05$) and CD57+ T cell compartment when compared to age-matched HI. The median (IQ range) for Gini-TCR in CD8+ CM, EM and CD57+ T cells amounted to 47.4 (40.8–54.2) versus 35.3 (34.0–39.2), 54.4 (49.6–68.5) versus 43.7 (42.4–50.8) and 77.6 (65.8–78.4) versus 59.2 (57.2–67.1) for younger ESRD patients versus younger HI.

The following results, describing Tables S1 and S2 in Supplementary Material need to be interpreted with caution as the P-values were not adjusted for the number of parameters compared.

Aging effects were not visible when comparing Gini-TCR indices for the different T cell subsets between younger and older ESRD patients (Table S1 in Supplementary Material). In HI, aging effects were confined to the CD8+ T cell compartment and an aging-related increasing trend in Gini-TCR index was observed for CD8+ CM T cells ($P = 0.06$), as the median (IQ range) for Gini-TCR amounted to 40.1 (39.1–44.1) in older HI versus 35.3 (34.0–39.2) in younger HI. An increased Gini-TCR index ($P = 0.03$) was observed for older HI, within CD8+CD28− T cells (Table S1 in Supplementary Material). The median (IQ range) value for Gini-TCR in CD8+CD28− T cells amounted to 42.0 (40.6–47.4) versus 57.8 (43.7–63.7) for younger and older HI, respectively.

CMV latency did not significantly affect Gini-TCR indices apart from a CMV-related increasing trend within CD4+CD57+ T cells ($P = 0.07$) of HI, but not ESRD patients, i.e., the median (IQ range) Gini-TCR index amounted to 67.0 (57.4–72.2) for CMV-seropositive HI versus 45.6 (35.5–58.0) for CMV-seronegative ones (Table S2 in Supplementary Material). No differences were observed when comparing CMV-seronegative and CMV-seropositive ESRD patients to their CMV-serostatus matched HI with respect to Gini-TCR indices for the different T cell subsets (data not shown).

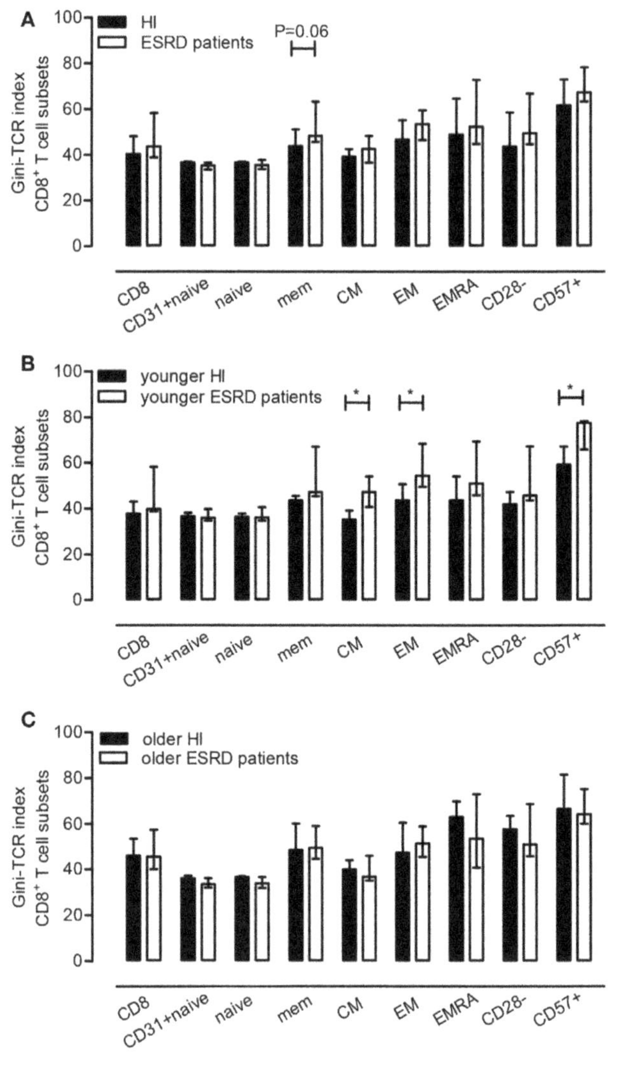

FIGURE 2 | Effect of end-stage renal disease (ESRD) on Gini-T cell receptor (TCR) indices of CD8+ T cell subsets. In **(A)**, the median and IQ range of the Gini-TCR indices for healthy individuals ($N = 10$) and ESRD patients ($N = 10$) for different CD8+ T cell subsets is depicted, whereas in **(B,C)** those for the younger and older group ($N = 5$) are given, respectively. P value: *<0.05.

Clonal Expansions of TCR Vβ-Families in Different T Cell Subsets

Apart from characterizing the impact of ESRD on Gini-TCR indices for the different T cell subsets, we also evaluated the impact of ESRD on clonal expansions of TCR Vβ-families by comparing frequencies to the average + 2SD obtained using HI as reference population. **Figure 3** shows a typical example of expanded TCR Vβ-families within CD8+ memory T cells of ESRD patients.

Clonal expansions of TCR Vβ-families were observed within the CD3+ T cells in 7 out of 10 ESRD patients (**Table 3**). Half versus all of the ESRD patients showed expanded TCR Vβ-families

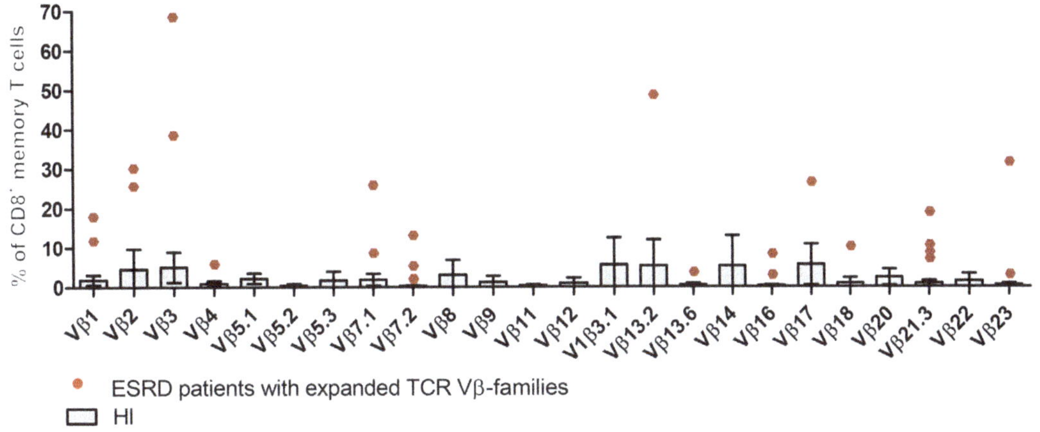

FIGURE 3 | Expansions of T cell receptor (TCR) Vβ-families within CD8⁺ memory T cells from end-stage renal disease (ESRD) patients. Boxes and error bars represent the mean and 95% confidence interval (mean ± 2SD) of 24 TCR-Vβ families from 10 healthy individuals (HI). Red dots correspond to expanded TCR Vβ-families from ESRD patients (frequencies > mean + 2SD from HI).

TABLE 3 | Effect of ESRD on expansions of TCR Vβ-families.

	# of ESRD patients with/without expansions	Median # of expanded TCR Vβ-families (IQ range)	Total # of expanded TCR Vβ-families
$CD3^+$	7/3	1 (0–2)	15
$CD4^+$	5/5	1 (0–2)	10
$CD31^+$ naive	6/4	1 (0–1)	9
Naive	3/7	0 (0–1)	5
MEM	9/1	1 (1–3)	16
CM	6/4	1 (0–2)	11
EM	6/4	1 (0–2)	13
$CD28^-$	9/1	1 (1–1)	12
$CD57^+$	9/1	1 (0–2)	11
$CD8^+$	10/0	2 (1–4)	26
$CD31^+$ naive	7/3	1 (0–2)	15
Naive	8/2	1 (1–1)	12
MEM	10/0	2 (2–4)	28
CM	7/3	2 (0–3)	20
EM	9/1	4 (2–4)	32
EMRA	10/0	2 (1–3)	26
$CD28^-$	10/0	3 (1–3)	28
$CD57^+$	9/1	3 (1–4)	25

within $CD4^+$ and $CD8^+$ T cells ($P < 0.05$), respectively. The median (IQ range) number of expanded TCR Vβ-families per patient amounted to 1 (0–2) and 2 (1–4) families for $CD4^+$ and $CD8^+$ T cells ($P < 0.05$), respectively (**Figure 4A**). Interestingly, expansions were also detected within the naive T cell compartment, as 3 out of 10 and 8 out of 10 patients had expansions of TCR Vβ-families within the naive $CD4^+$ and $CD8^+$ T cell compartment, respectively (**Table 3**). Most clonal expansions were observed within the (more differentiated) memory $CD8^+$ T cell subsets (**Figure 4A**). The median (IQ range) number of expanded TCR Vβ-families amounted to 1 (1–1) versus 2 (2–4) for naive and memory $CD8^+$ T cells, respectively ($P < 0.05$). Moreover, ESRD affected different TCR Vβ-families as illustrated in **Figure 3** for $CD8^+$ memory T cells. ESRD induced expansions within both younger (**Figure 4B**) and older (**Figure 4C**) ESRD patients when compared to their age-matched HI.

DISCUSSION

The main finding of this study is that the multiparameter flow-cytometry-based approach for evaluating the skewed TCR Vβ-repertoire diversity in ESRD patients showed that TCR skewing can be observed primarily in $CD8^+$ T cell subsets, including naive T cells. However, higher Gini-TCR indices, indicative for an enhanced TCR Vβ-repertoire skewing, were specifically associated with more differentiated $CD8^+$, but not $CD4^+$, T cell subsets in both ESRD patients and HI.

Our previous data showed that ESRD may lead to a skewed TCR Vβ-repertoire as assessed by DNA spectratyping, providing at best semiquantitative information about TCR Vβ-clonality (24). The current study provided more quantitative details with respect to this skewed TCR Vβ-repertoire at the T cell-subset level using the Gini-TCR index as a tool for calculating skewness (41) and evaluating number/type of expanded TCR Vβ-families. Higher Gini-TCR indices are indicative of a more skewed TCR Vβ-repertoire. The current study confirmed several of our previous findings. Increased skewing of the TCR Vβ-repertoire was observed for more differentiated $CD8^+$, but not $CD4^+$, T cells, corresponding to our spectratyping data as well as findings described by others (27, 42). In addition to the Gini-TCR index, we calculated the number of TCR Vβ-families per patient that were expanded beyond the mean + 2SD values of HI. This approach yielded similar results as the Gini-index but gives detailed information at the individual patient level for the different T cell subsets. For instance some patients have a large number of expanded TCR Vβ-families while others show only a few. Moreover, ESRD did not seem to affect one TCR Vβ-family in particular, indicative of expansions of different clonal origin. Altogether, using both Gini-TCR indices as well as the number of expanded TCR Vβ-families, revealed skewing to mainly occur

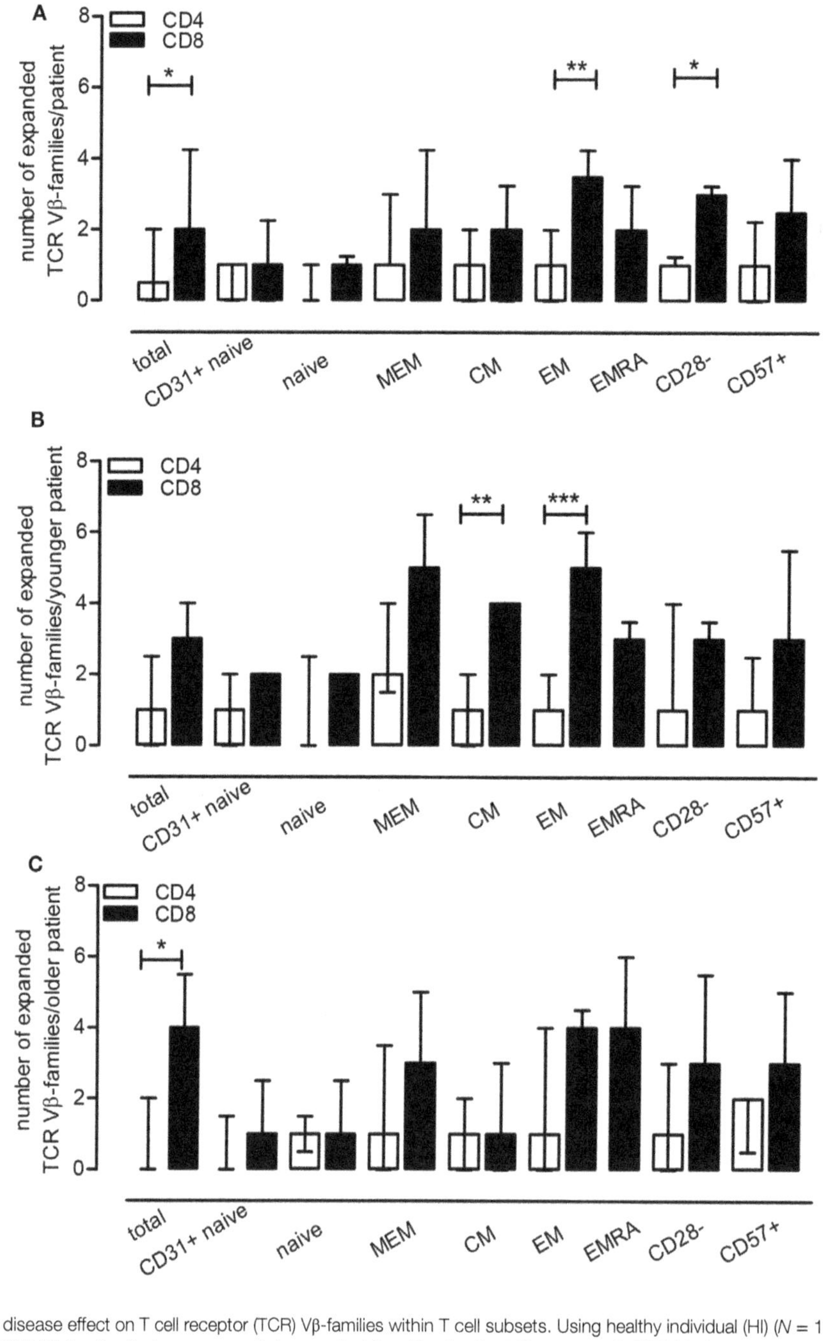

FIGURE 4 | End-stage renal disease effect on T cell receptor (TCR) Vβ-families within T cell subsets. Using healthy individual (HI) ($N = 10$) as a reference population, we evaluated the number of TCR Vβ-families that were expanded per patient for a T cell subset (frequency of a TCR Vβ-family exceeding the mean + 2SD value obtained for HI) **(A)**. In **(B,C)**, the median (IQ range) of expansions per younger and older patient for a T cell subset is depicted using the younger ($N = 5$) and older HI ($N = 5$) as a reference, respectively. The open bars represent the median and IQ range for the different $CD4^+$ T cell subsets, whereas the closed bars represent that for the different $CD8^+$ T cell subsets.

within the $CD8^+$ and in particular within the $CD8^+$ memory T cell subset similar to what was observed before using DNA-based spectratyping on sorted T cell subsets (24).

The commercially available flow-cytometry-based assay, used to characterize the TCR Vβ-repertoire, is composed of 24 different TCR Vβ-antibodies covering about 70% of the normal human TCR Vβ-repertoire (brochure Beckman Coulter). Evaluating other TCR Vβ-families as well as TCR Vα and TCR Vγ/Vδ families may contribute to a better understanding of the whole TCR-repertoire. In this respect, $\gamma\delta^+$ T cells account for approximately 8% of $CD3^+$ peripheral blood T cells and around 6% of $\gamma\delta^+$ T cells were observed within $CD3^+CD8^+$, but not $CD4^+$ T cells in HI (19). As frequencies of $\gamma\delta^+$ T cells may also vary amongst individuals, it might be more accurate to evaluate the TCR Vβ-repertoire not within total $CD3^+$, like performed in the current study, but within $\alpha\beta^+$ $CD3^+$ T cells.

Interestingly, using this multiparameter flow-cytometry-based approach, we were also able to detect expanded TCR Vβ-families within the naive T cell compartment. This characteristic has, to our knowledge never been described for ESRD patients. Uremia induces a proinflammatory environment significantly affecting T cell-mediated immunity characterized by increased risk for infections (5) and decreased vaccination efficacy (1, 43). We have observed that progressive loss of renal function is accompanied by a severe depletion of the naive T cell compartment and a relative shift toward more differentiated memory T cells (44). Naive T cells employ a mechanism referred to as homeostatic proliferation in order to maintain the naive T cell pool that is not replenished by newly developed naive T cells from the thymus due to thymic involution. Homeostatic proliferation occurs in response to homeostatic cytokines, e.g., IL-7, or low affinity self antigens presented by antigen-presenting cells (26). This mechanism has been described to be associated with a decline in TCR Vβ-repertoire diversity within naive T cells with increasing age (27, 45). ESRD enhanced homeostatic proliferation of naive T cells to a similar extent as observed in older HI (12) and as a consequence of this compensatory mechanism, loss of TCR Vβ-repertoire diversity may also be induced by ESRD within naive $CD8^+$ and/or $CD4^+$ T cells.

Naive T cells are required to mount adequate immune responses to newly encountered antigens (46, 47). ESRD patients, with a severely depleted naive T cell compartment (44), are hampered in inducing adequate protection to, for example, HBV vaccination as a result of defective generation of antigen-specific memory T cells (43). The ESRD-associated defects in T cell composition as well as function, reminiscent of aging-associated T cell defects, led to the concept of premature T cell aging introduced in 2011 (12). ESRD patients have a T cell compartment that is aged by 15–20 years compared to their chronologic age, using age-matched HI as a reference. Consistent with premature T cell aging (12), we observed ESRD-associated increases in Gini-TCR indices and TCR Vβ expansions to occur already at young age.

Aging is known to affect TCR Vβ-repertoire diversity toward a more skewed pattern, starting from roughly 600×10^3 clonotypes detected per 10^6 T cells in childhood, declining by 5×10^3 clonotypes per year (25). Age-related effects were limited within our cohort of HI and this may be a consequence of the selection procedure applied. We did select HI with a polyclonal (i.e., non-skewed) TCR Vβ-repertoire using DNA-based spectratyping (24), to ensure a relatively standard healthy population to be used as reference for comparison to ESRD patients. The ESRD patient population however only consisted of individuals with an oligoclonal (skewed) TCR Vβ-repertoire. This might have resulted in an underestimation of the effect of aging on TCR Vβ-families. Likewise, our selection procedure may also explain the minimal effects of CMV in both cohorts.

CMV latency is known to introduce skewing of the TCR Vβ-repertoire induced by expanded CMV-specific T cell clones in both HI (33, 34, 48) and ESRD patients (24). CMV latency may result in a vast and long-lasting expansion of CMV-specific T cells (33, 34). Moreover, CMV latency has additional effects mainly on circulating $CD8^+$ T cells of ESRD patients (49).

End-stage renal disease, aging, and CMV all influenced the TCR-Vβ repertoire diversity to a different extent (24), however, because of different factors present in the environment, they all have their specific effect on clonotype selection. Even though these findings need to be verified in a larger cohort without preselection using DNA-based spectratyping of TCR-Vβ-repertoire, our study already shed some light on this altered TCR-Vβ repertoire at the T cell-subset level in particular with respect to ESRD.

Relating TCR-repertoire data to functional capacities of T cells is warranted to increase knowledge on uremia-induced T cell defects in ESRD patients. Moreover, tracking TCR clones in whole blood or tissue infiltrates may provide additional information on antigen specificity important for diagnosis of infection and allograft rejection after transplantation (50–52).

In conclusion, ESRD is associated with a skewed TCR Vβ-repertoire as a result of variable TCR Vβ-family expansions, but not one TCR Vβ-family in particular. ESRD, aging and CMV latency exert their effects by influencing different TCR Vβ-families. This altered repertoire may be associated with a less broad and less diverse T cell-mediated immunity.

ETHICS STATEMENT

All individuals included gave informed consent and the Erasmus medical center medical ethical committee approved the study (METC number: 2012-022). It was conducted according to the principles of Declaration of Helsinki and in compliance with International Conference on Harmonization/Good Clinical Practice regulations.

AUTHOR CONTRIBUTIONS

LH participated in the design of the study, analyzed the data, and wrote the manuscript. MB participated in the design of the study, interpreted the data, and revised the manuscript. MK established the experimental protocol, conducted the experiments, and analyzed the data. AL participated in the design of the study, interpreted the data, and revised the manuscript. CB participated in design of the study and revised the manuscript. NL designed the study, interpreted the data, and revised the manuscript. All authors have read and approved the final manuscript.

FUNDING

The research was supported by the China Scholarship Council for funding PhD fellowship to Ling Huang (File No. 201307720043).

REFERENCES

1. Janus N, Vacher LV, Karie S, Ledneva E, Deray G. Vaccination and chronic kidney disease. *Nephrol Dial Transplant* (2008) 23(3):800–7. doi:10.1093/ndt/gfm851
2. Fabrizi F, Martin P. Hepatitis B vaccine and dialysis: current issues. *Int J Artif Organs* (2001) 24(10):683–94.
3. Remschmidt C, Wichmann O, Harder T. Influenza vaccination in patients with end-stage renal disease: systematic review and assessment of quality of evidence related to vaccine efficacy, effectiveness, and safety. *BMC Med* (2014) 12:244. doi:10.1186/s12916-014-0244-9
4. Principi N, Esposito S, Group EVS. Influenza vaccination in patients with end-stage renal disease. *Expert Opin Drug Saf* (2015) 14(8):1249–58. doi:10.1517/14740338.2015.1053459
5. Dalrymple LS, Go AS. Epidemiology of acute infections among patients with chronic kidney disease. *Clin J Am Soc Nephrol* (2008) 3(5):1487–93. doi:10.2215/CJN.01290308
6. Betjes MG. Immune cell dysfunction and inflammation in end-stage renal disease. *Nat Rev Nephrol* (2013) 9(5):255–65. doi:10.1038/nrneph.2013.44
7. Sarnak MJ, Jaber BL. Mortality caused by sepsis in patients with end-stage renal disease compared with the general population. *Kidney Int* (2000) 58(4):1758–64. doi:10.1111/j.1523-1755.2000.00337.x
8. Maisonneuve P, Agodoa L, Gellert R, Stewart JH, Buccianti G, Lowenfels AB, et al. Cancer in patients on dialysis for end-stage renal disease: an international collaborative study. *Lancet* (1999) 354(9173):93–9. doi:10.1016/S0140-6736(99)06154-1
9. Vajdic CM, McDonald SP, McCredie MR, van Leeuwen MT, Stewart JH, Law M, et al. Cancer incidence before and after kidney transplantation. *JAMA* (2006) 296(23):2823–31. doi:10.1001/jama.296.23.2823
10. Wong G, Hayen A, Chapman JR, Webster AC, Wang JJ, Mitchell P, et al. Association of CKD and cancer risk in older people. *J Am Soc Nephrol* (2009) 20(6):1341–50. doi:10.1681/ASN.2008090998
11. Butler AM, Olshan AF, Kshirsagar AV, Edwards JK, Nielsen ME, Wheeler SB, et al. Cancer incidence among US Medicare ESRD patients receiving hemodialysis, 1996-2009. *Am J Kidney Dis* (2015) 65(5):763–72. doi:10.1053/j.ajkd.2014.12.013
12. Betjes MG, Langerak AW, van der Spek A, de Wit EA, Litjens NH. Premature aging of circulating T cells in patients with end-stage renal disease. *Kidney Int* (2011) 80(2):208–17. doi:10.1038/ki.2011.110
13. Betjes MG, Litjens NH. Chronic kidney disease and premature ageing of the adaptive immune response. *Curr Urol Rep* (2015) 16(1):471. doi:10.1007/s11934-014-0471-9
14. Meijers RW, Litjens NH, de Wit EA, Langerak AW, van der Spek A, Baan CC, et al. Uremia causes premature ageing of the T cell compartment in end-stage renal disease patients. *Immun Ageing* (2012) 9(1):19. doi:10.1186/1742-4933-9-19
15. Huang L, Litjens NHR, Kannegieter NM, Klepper M, Baan CC, Betjes MGH. pERK-dependent defective TCR-mediated activation of CD4+ T cells in end-stage renal disease patients. *Immun Ageing* (2017) 14:14. doi:10.1186/s12979-017-0096-196
16. Turner SJ, La Gruta NL, Kedzierska K, Thomas PG, Doherty PC. Functional implications of T cell receptor diversity. *Curr Opin Immunol* (2009) 21(3):286–90. doi:10.1016/j.coi.2009.05.004
17. Garcia KC, Teyton L, Wilson IA. Structural basis of T cell recognition. *Annu Rev Immunol* (1999) 17:369–97. doi:10.1146/annurev.immunol.17.1.369
18. van Dongen JJ, Langerak AW, Bruggemann M, Evans PA, Hummel M, Lavender FL, et al. Design and standardization of PCR primers and protocols for detection of clonal immunoglobulin and T-cell receptor gene recombinations in suspect lymphoproliferations: report of the BIOMED-2 concerted action BMH4-CT98-3936. *Leukemia* (2003) 17(12):2257–317. doi:10.1038/sj.leu.2403202
19. van den Beemd R, Boor PP, van Lochem EG, Hop WC, Langerak AW, Wolvers-Tettero IL, et al. Flow cytometric analysis of the Vbeta repertoire in healthy controls. *Cytometry* (2000) 40(4):336–45. doi:10.1002/1097-0320(20000801)40:4<336:AID-CYTO9>3.0.CO;2-0
20. Tzifi F, Kanariou M, Tzanoudaki M, Mihas C, Paschali E, Chrousos G, et al. Flow cytometric analysis of the CD4+ TCR Vbeta repertoire in the peripheral blood of children with type 1 diabetes mellitus, systemic lupus erythematosus and age-matched healthy controls. *BMC Immunol* (2013) 14:33. doi:10.1186/1471-2172-14-33
21. Langerak AW, van Den Beemd R, Wolvers-Tettero IL, Boor PP, van Lochem EG, Hooijkaas H, et al. Molecular and flow cytometric analysis of the Vbeta repertoire for clonality assessment in mature TCRalphabeta T-cell proliferations. *Blood* (2001) 98(1):165–73. doi:10.1182/blood.V98.1.165
22. Britanova OV, Shugay M, Merzlyak EM, Staroverov DB, Putintseva EV, Turchaninova MA, et al. Dynamics of individual T cell repertoires: from cord blood to centenarians. *J Immunol* (2016) 196(12):5005–13. doi:10.4049/jimmunol.1600005
23. Yoshida K, Cologne JB, Cordova K, Misumi M, Yamaoka M, Kyoizumi S, et al. Aging-related changes in human T-cell repertoire over 20years delineated by deep sequencing of peripheral T-cell receptors. *Exp Gerontol* (2017) 96:29–37. doi:10.1016/j.exger.2017.05.015
24. Huang L, Langerak AW, Wolvers-Tettero IL, Meijers RW, Baan CC, Litjens NH, et al. End stage renal disease patients have a skewed T cell receptor Vbeta repertoire. *Immun Ageing* (2015) 12:28. doi:10.1186/s12979-015-0055-7
25. Britanova OV, Putintseva EV, Shugay M, Merzlyak EM, Turchaninova MA, Staroverov DB, et al. Age-related decrease in TCR repertoire diversity measured with deep and normalized sequence profiling. *J Immunol* (2014) 192(6):2689–98. doi:10.4049/jimmunol.1302064
26. Kohler S, Wagner U, Pierer M, Kimmig S, Oppmann B, Mowes B, et al. Post-thymic in vivo proliferation of naive CD4(+) T cells constrains the TCR repertoire in healthy human adults. *Eur J Immunol* (2005) 35(6):1987–94. doi:10.1002/eji.200526181
27. Qi Q, Liu Y, Cheng Y, Glanville J, Zhang D, Lee JY, et al. Diversity and clonal selection in the human T-cell repertoire. *Proc Natl Acad Sci U S A* (2014) 111(36):13139–44. doi:10.1073/pnas.1409155111
28. Tu W, Rao S. Mechanisms underlying T cell immunosenescence: aging and cytomegalovirus infection. *Front Microbiol* (2016) 7:2111. doi:10.3389/fmicb.2016.02111
29. Litjens NH, de Wit EA, Betjes MG. Differential effects of age, cytomegalovirus-seropositivity and end-stage renal disease (ESRD) on circulating T lymphocyte subsets. *Immun Ageing* (2011) 8(1):2. doi:10.1186/1742-4933-8-2
30. Hooper M, Kallas EG, Coffin D, Campbell D, Evans TG, Looney RJ. Cytomegalovirus seropositivity is associated with the expansion of CD4+CD28- and CD8+CD28- T cells in rheumatoid arthritis. *J Rheumatol* (1999) 26(7):1452–7.
31. Wikby A, Johansson B, Olsson J, Lofgren S, Nilsson BO, Ferguson F. Expansions of peripheral blood CD8 T-lymphocyte subpopulations and an association with cytomegalovirus seropositivity in the elderly: the Swedish NONA immune study. *Exp Gerontol* (2002) 37(2–3):445–53. doi:10.1016/S0531-5565(01)00212-1
32. van de Berg PJ, Griffiths SJ, Yong SL, Macaulay R, Bemelman FJ, Jackson S, et al. Cytomegalovirus infection reduces telomere length of the circulating T cell pool. *J Immunol* (2010) 184(7):3417–23. doi:10.4049/jimmunol.0903442
33. Gillespie GM, Wills MR, Appay V, O'Callaghan C, Murphy M, Smith N, et al. Functional heterogeneity and high frequencies of cytomegalovirus-specific CD8(+) T lymphocytes in healthy seropositive donors. *J Virol* (2000) 74(17):8140–50. doi:10.1128/JVI.74.17.8140-8150.2000
34. Klarenbeek PL, Remmerswaal EB, ten Berge IJ, Doorenspleet ME, van Schaik BD, Esveldt RE, et al. Deep sequencing of antiviral T-cell responses to HCMV and EBV in humans reveals a stable repertoire that is maintained for many years. *PLoS Pathog* (2012) 8(9):e1002889. doi:10.1371/journal.ppat.1002889
35. Litjens NH, Huisman M, Baan CC, van Druningen CJ, Betjes MG. Hepatitis B vaccine-specific CD4(+) T cells can be detected and characterised at the single cell level: limited usefulness of dendritic cells as signal enhancers. *J Immunol Methods* (2008) 330(1–2):1–11. doi:10.1016/j.jim.2007.10.013
36. Kohler S, Thiel A. Life after the thymus: CD31+ and CD31- human naive CD4+ T-cell subsets. *Blood* (2009) 113(4):769–74. doi:10.1182/blood-2008-02-139154
37. Merino J, Martinez-Gonzalez MA, Rubio M, Inoges S, Sanchez-Ibarrola A, Subira ML. Progressive decrease of CD8high+ CD28+ CD57- cells with ageing. *Clin Exp Immunol* (1998) 112(1):48–51. doi:10.1046/j.1365-2249.1998.00551.x
38. Bandres E, Merino J, Vazquez B, Inoges S, Moreno C, Subira ML, et al. The increase of IFN-gamma production through aging correlates with the expanded CD8(+high)CD28(-)CD57(+) subpopulation. *Clin Immunol* (2000) 96(3):230–5. doi:10.1006/clim.2000.4894

39. Laydon DJ, Melamed A, Sim A, Gillet NA, Sim K, Darko S, et al. Quantification of HTLV-1 clonality and TCR diversity. *PLoS Comput Biol* (2014) 10(6): e1003646. doi:10.1371/journal.pcbi.1003646
40. Thomas PG, Handel A, Doherty PC, La Gruta NL. Ecological analysis of antigen-specific CTL repertoires defines the relationship between naive and immune T-cell populations. *Proc Natl Acad Sci U S A* (2013) 110(5):1839–44. doi:10.1073/pnas.1222149110
41. van der Geest KS, Abdulahad WH, Horst G, Lorencetti PG, Bijzet J, Arends S, et al. Quantifying distribution of flow cytometric TCR-Vbeta usage with economic statistics. *PLoS One* (2015) 10(4):e0125373. doi:10.1371/journal.pone.0125373
42. Robins HS, Campregher PV, Srivastava SK, Wacher A, Turtle CJ, Kahsai O, et al. Comprehensive assessment of T-cell receptor beta-chain diversity in alphabeta T cells. *Blood* (2009) 114(19):4099–107. doi:10.1182/blood-2009-04-217604
43. Litjens NH, Huisman M, van den Dorpel M, Betjes MG. Impaired immune responses and antigen-specific memory CD4+ T cells in hemodialysis patients. *J Am Soc Nephrol* (2008) 19(8):1483–90. doi:10.1681/ASN.2007090971
44. Litjens NH, van Druningen CJ, Betjes MG. Progressive loss of renal function is associated with activation and depletion of naive T lymphocytes. *Clin Immunol* (2006) 118(1):83–91. doi:10.1016/j.clim.2005.09.007
45. Ahmed M, Lanzer KG, Yager EJ, Adams PS, Johnson LL, Blackman MA. Clonal expansions and loss of receptor diversity in the naive CD8 T cell repertoire of aged mice. *J Immunol* (2009) 182(2):784–92. doi:10.4049/jimmunol.182.2.784
46. Ramirez LA, Daniel A, Frank I, Tebas P, Boyer JD. Seroprotection of HIV-infected subjects after influenza A(H1N1) vaccination is directly associated with baseline frequency of naive T cells. *J Infect Dis* (2014) 210(4):646–50. doi:10.1093/infdis/jiu132
47. Schulz AR, Malzer JN, Domingo C, Jurchott K, Grutzkau A, Babel N, et al. Low thymic activity and dendritic cell numbers are associated with the immune response to primary viral infection in elderly humans. *J Immunol* (2015) 195(10):4699–711. doi:10.4049/jimmunol.1500598
48. Wang EC, Moss PA, Frodsham P, Lehner PJ, Bell JI, Borysiewicz LK. CD8highCD57+ T lymphocytes in normal, healthy individuals are oligoclonal and respond to human cytomegalovirus. *J Immunol* (1995) 155(10):5046–56.
49. Meijers RW, Litjens NH, de Wit EA, Langerak AW, van der Spek A, Baan CC, et al. Cytomegalovirus contributes partly to uraemia-associated premature immunological ageing of the T cell compartment. *Clin Exp Immunol* (2013) 174(3):424–32. doi:10.1111/cei.12188
50. Dziubianau M, Hecht J, Kuchenbecker L, Sattler A, Stervbo U, Rodelsperger C, et al. TCR repertoire analysis by next generation sequencing allows complex differential diagnosis of T cell-related pathology. *Am J Transplant* (2013) 13(11):2842–54. doi:10.1111/ajt.12431
51. Alachkar H, Mutonga M, Kato T, Kalluri S, Kakuta Y, Uemura M, et al. Quantitative characterization of T-cell repertoire and biomarkers in kidney transplant rejection. *BMC Nephrol* (2016) 17(1):181. doi:10.1186/s12882-016-0395-3
52. Morris H, DeWolf S, Robins H, Sprangers B, LoCascio SA, Shonts BA, et al. Tracking donor-reactive T cells: evidence for clonal deletion in tolerant kidney transplant patients. *Sci Transl Med* (2015) 7(272):272ra10. doi:10.1126/scitranslmed.3010760

7

CD8$^+$HLADR$^+$ Regulatory T Cells Change with Aging: They Increase in Number, but Lose Checkpoint Inhibitory Molecules and Suppressive Function

*Stella Lukas Yani[1], Michael Keller[1], Franz Leonard Melzer[1], Birgit Weinberger[1], Luca Pangrazzi[1], Sieghart Sopper[2], Klemens Trieb[3], Monia Lobina[4], Valeria Orrù[4], Edoardo Fiorillo[4], Francesco Cucca[4] and Beatrix Grubeck-Loebenstein[1]**

[1] Department of Immunology, Institute for Biomedical Aging Research, University of Innsbruck, Innsbruck, Austria, [2] Clinic for Haematology and Oncology, Tyrolean Cancer Research Institute, Medical University of Innsbruck, Innsbruck, Austria, [3] Department of Orthopedic Surgery, Hospital Wels-Grieskirchen, Wels, Austria, [4] Istituto di Ricerca Genetica e Biomedica (IRGB), Consiglio Nazionale delle Ricerche (CNR), Monserrato, Italy

***Correspondence:**
Beatrix Grubeck-Loebenstein
beatrix.grubeck@uibk.ac.at

CD4$^+$ regulatory T cells have been intensively studied during aging, but little is still known about age-related changes of other regulatory T cell subsets. It was, therefore, the goal of the present study to analyze CD8$^+$human leukocyte antigen–antigen D related (HLADR)$^+$ T cells in old age, a cell population reported to have suppressive activity and to be connected to specific genetic variants. We demonstrate a strong increase in the number of CD8$^+$HLADR$^+$ T cells with age in a cohort of female Sardinians as well as in elderly male and female persons from Austria. We also show that CD8$^+$HLADR$^+$ T cells lack classical activation molecules, such as CD69 and CD25, but contain increased numbers of checkpoint inhibitory molecules, such as cytotoxic T lymphocyte-associated antigen 4, T cell immunoglobulin and mucin protein-3, LAG-3, and PD-1, when compared with their HLADR$^-$ counterparts. They also have the capacity to inhibit the proliferation of autologous peripheral blood mononuclear cells. This suppressive activity is, however, decreased when CD8$^+$HLADR$^+$ T cells from elderly persons are analyzed. In accordance with this finding, CD8$^+$HLADR$^+$ T cells from persons of old age contain lower percentages of checkpoint inhibitory molecules than young controls. We conclude that in spite of high abundance of a CD8$^+$ regulatory T cell subset in old age its expression of checkpoint inhibitory molecules and its suppressive function on a per cell basis are reduced. Reduction of suppressive capacity may support uncontrolled subclinical inflammatory processes referred to as "inflamm-aging."

Keywords: CD8$^+$ T cells, CD8$^+$human leukocyte antigen–antigen D related$^+$, aging, checkpoint inhibitory molecules, regulatory T cells

---

Abbreviations: BM, bone marrow; BMMCs, bone marrow mononuclear cells; CTLA-4, cytotoxic T-lymphocyte-associated antigen 4; CXCR3, C-X-C motif chemokine receptor 3; FMO, fluorescence minus one; FOXP3, forkhead box protein P3; HLADR, human leukocyte antigen–antigen D related; LAG-3, lymphocyte activation gene-3; PB, peripheral blood; PBMCs, peripheral blood mononuclear cells; PD-1, programmed death 1; TIM-3, T cell immunoglobulin and mucin protein-3; Tregs, regulatory T cells.

INTRODUCTION

We have recently reported genetic contributions to quantitative levels of 95 immune cell types encompassing 272 immune traits in a cohort of 1,629 individuals from four clustered Sardinian villages (1). One of these 95 cell types are human leukocyte antigen–antigen D related (HLADR)$^+$ T cells. In the past, the expression of HLADR on human T cells has mainly been regarded as a marker of activated T cells (2–4). However, HLADR expression on CD4$^+$ regulatory T cells (Tregs) has also been interpreted as a marker of a functionally distinct population of mature Tregs (5). Recently, HLADR expression on CD8$^+$ T cells has been suggested to represent a marker of a natural human CD8$^+$ regulatory T cell subset (6). This subset was shown to suppress the proliferation of autologous peripheral blood mononuclear cells (PBMCs) presumably by cell-to-cell contact with cytotoxic T-lymphocyte-associated antigen 4 (CTLA-4) signaling playing an essential role in this process. In the past, CD8$^+$ T cells were the first to be described to have immunosuppressive properties (7, 8). However, difficulties in characterizing these "suppressor" CD8$^+$ T cells and lack of specific markers delimited this area noticeably. Only when CD4$^+$CD25$^+$FOXP3$^+$ T cells were shown to be strongly immunosuppressive (9–13), a global interest in the downregulation of immune activity by T cells re-emerged. Apart from the description of many interesting specific properties, CD4$^+$ Tregs were shown to increase in number in some important conditions, such as in patients with tumors (14) or during aging [reviewed in Ref. (15)]. In the latter context it was of interest that some Treg populations, specifically naturally occurring Tregs, seemed to accumulate in old age, whereas inducible Tregs decrease in elderly persons. Little information is, however, still available on the functional competence of CD4$^+$ Tregs in old age. The worldwide strong interest in CD4 Tregs also stimulated new research efforts in the analysis of potential CD8$^+$ suppressor cells. Different subsets were defined, such as CD8$^+$CD28 low cells (16–20), CD8$^+$CD122$^+$ cells in mice (21–23), CD8$^+$C-X-C motif chemokine receptor 3$^+$ cells in humans (24) and CD8$^+$CD39$^+$FOXP3$^+$ cells (25). CD8$^+$HLADR$^+$ T cells were therefore just one of several CD8$^+$ T cell subsets believed to have regulatory properties (6). In view of the clear genetic regulation of this population exerted by a genetic variant in the *CIITA* gene region (1) and the fact that the composition of the CD8$^+$ population characteristically changes with age (26), we became interested in elucidating potential age-related changes in the number and function of CD8$^+$HLADR$^+$ T cells. We now demonstrate that CD8$^+$HLADR$^+$ T cells increase in number with aging, but lose suppressive activity on a per cell basis. This may challenge the homeostatic balance between immune cell sub-populations in old age and support the development of inflammation.

MATERIALS AND METHODS

Study Subjects

Samples from three different cohorts were used for this study. Details regarding the probands' characteristics are summarized in **Table 1**.

Cohort A

Peripheral blood (PB) samples were obtained from 91 healthy females recruited in Lanusei, Sardinia, Italy. The exclusion criteria were the following:

Persons who experienced significant variation of body temperature or received vaccination in the 2 weeks before the blood draw, as well as persons under antimicrobial treatment were excluded from the study. Persons with pathological conditions were also excluded.

Cohort B

Peripheral blood samples were obtained from healthy Austrian individuals who did not receive immunomodulatory drugs or suffer from diseases known to influence the immune system, such as autoimmune diseases and cancer. None of them was frail or had symptoms of cognitive impairment.

Cohort C

Bone marrow (BM) and PB-paired samples were obtained from patients who underwent hip replacement surgery in Wels, Austria. The patients did not receive immunomodulatory drugs or suffer from diseases known to influence the immune system, such as autoimmune diseases and cancer.

Mononuclear Cell Isolation

Peripheral blood mononuclear cells from heparinized blood were purified by Ficoll-Hypaque density gradient centrifugation (GE Healthcare Life Sciences). Cells were washed with complete RPMI medium (RPMI 1640 supplemented with 10% FCS, 100 U/ml penicillin, and 100 μg/ml streptomycin; Invitrogen). PBMCs from cohort A were frozen according to a standard protocol using 10% DMSO as cryoprotective agent. PBMCs from Cohort B and C were freshly used.

Bone marrow samples (cohort C) were obtained from the femur shaft of patients of varying age (**Table 1**) during hip replacement surgery. A biopsy of *Substantia spongiosa ossium*, which would otherwise have been discarded, was used to isolate BM mononuclear cells (BMMCs). BM biopsies were fragmented, washed once with complete RPMI medium (RPMI 1640 supplemented with 10% FCS, 100 U/ml penicillin, and 100 μg/ml streptomycin; Invitrogen), and treated with purified collagenase (CLSPA, Worthington Biochemical; 20 U/ml in complete RPMI medium) for 1 h at 37°C. BM biopsies were then centrifuged and BMMCs purified by density gradient centrifugation (Ficoll-Hypaque). BMMCs were freshly used.

Cell Sorting

T cells were isolated from fresh PBMCs by magnetic cell sorting using the MACS human Pan T cell isolation kit (Miltenyi Biotech) following manufacturer's protocol. Purified T cells were then stained with anti-CD8 PerCP (RPA-T8), anti-CD28 BV421 (L293), anti-HLADR PeCy7 (G46-6) Abs, all from BD Biosciences. Labeled cells were sorted with a FACSAria II flow cytometer (BD Biosciences). Cells were either sorted into CD8$^+$HLADR$^+$, CD8$^+$HLADR$^-$ or into CD8$^+$CD28$^+$HLADR$^+$, CD8$^+$CD28$^+$HLADR$^-$, CD8$^+$CD28$^-$HLADR$^+$ or CD8$^+$CD28$^-$

TABLE 1 | Demographic data on the cohorts used.

Cohort	Material	*n*	*n* Female	Age (median)	Age (range)	Site of recruitment
A	Peripheral blood (PB)	91	91 (100%)	49 years	18–89 years	Lanusei, Sardinia, Italy
B	PB	26	16 (61%)	26 years	21–29 years	Innsbruck, Austria
B	PB	22	13 (59%)	77 years	71–88 years	Innsbruck, Austria
C	Bone marrow	29	17 (58%)	68 years	39–87 years	Wels, Austria
C	PB	29	17 (58%)	68 years	39–87 years	Wels, Austria

HLADR$^-$ T cells. Fluorescence minus one (FMO) was used as control. The cells were collected into RPMI 1640 medium containing 15% FCS and washed once prior to further studies. The purity of each subset was >95% as determined by flow cytometry.

Flow Cytometric Analyses

Peripheral blood mononuclear cells and BMMCs were stained with anti-CD4 VioGreen (REA623), anti-CD3 Vio770 (REA613) from Miltenyi Biotech, anti-CD45RA PerCp (HI100), anti-CD28 APC (28.2), anti-CTLA-4 PE (BNI3), anti-T cell immunoglobulin and mucin protein-3 (TIM-3) PerCP (F38-2E2), anti-programmed death 1 (PD-1) FITC (EH12.2H7), anti-lymphocyte activation gene-3 (LAG-3) APC (7H2C65) from Biolegend, anti-HLADR PeCy7 (G46-6), anti-CD28 BV421 (28.2), anti-CD25 APC (2A3), and anti-CD69 PE (FN 50) from BD Biosciences. Intracellular detection of FOXP3 with anti-FOXP3 FITC Abs was performed using fixed and permeabilized cells following the manufacturer's instructions. FMO was used as control. Dead cells were excluded by forward and side scatter characteristics and by using either 7-AAD or fixable viability dye Zombie violet (Biolegend).

For each sample at least 2×10^6 total events were acquired using a FACScanto II and FACSSymphony (BD Biosciences). The data were analyzed using FlowJo software.

Suppression Assay

The capacity of sorted CD8$^+$HLADR$^+$, CD8$^+$HLADR$^-$, CD8$^+$CD28$^+$HLADR$^+$, CD8$^+$CD28$^+$HLADR$^-$, CD8$^+$CD28$^-$HLADR$^+$, and of CD8$^+$CD28$^-$HLADR$^-$ T cells to suppress the proliferation of responder autologous PBMCs was analyzed by CFSE dilution.

CFSE dilution method: responder autologous PBMCs (1×10^5) labeled with 1 µM CFSE (Invitrogen) were cultured with highly purified unlabeled CD8$^+$HLADR$^+$, CD8$^+$HLADR$^-$, CD8$^+$CD28$^+$HLADR$^+$, CD8$^+$CD28$^+$HLADR$^-$, CD8$^+$CD28$^-$HLADR$^+$, and CD8$^+$CD28$^-$HLADR$^-$ T cells at different responder: suppressor cell ratios (2:1, 4:1, and 8:1). Cells were stimulated with 1 µg/ml anti-CD3 (BD Pharmingen) and 0.5 µg/ml anti-CD28 (BD Pharmingen) Abs in 96-well round-bottom plate and cultured in complete medium. After 4 days of culture cells were stained with anti-CD4 BV 510 (BD Pharmingen), anti-CD8 PeCy7 (BD Pharmingen) and proliferation of CFSE-labeled cells was assessed by flow cytometry. Percentage of suppression was calculated as 100 minus the percentage of responder PBMCs, which underwent one or more cell divisions (proliferated PBMCs) in the presence of suppressor cells divided by the percentage of proliferated PBMCs when cultured alone, and multiplied by 100 as shown in the following formula:

$$\%\ \text{suppression} = 100 - \frac{\left(\begin{array}{c}\text{proliferated PBMCs cultured}\\ \text{with suppressor cells}\end{array}\right)}{\text{proliferated PBMCs cultured alone}} \times 100$$

The following controls for the suppression assay were used:

- CFSE-unlabeled and unstimulated (in the absence of stimulatory antibodies) cells,
- CFSE-labeled and unstimulated cells,
- CFSE-labeled and stimulated cells in the absence of suppressor cells.

Neutralization Assay

To test the involvement of the checkpoint inhibitory molecules in the suppression mediated by CD8$^+$HLADR$^+$CD28$^+$ T cells, neutralizing Abs against CTLA-4 (BD Biosciences), TIM-3 (Invitrogen), LAG-3 (Adipogen Life Sciences), and PD-1 (Invitrogen) were added to the co-cultures. All neutralization assays were performed under the culture conditions described above. The corresponding isotype-matched mAb IgG1 (Biozym) was used as control. Optimal neutralizing Ab concentrations were determined in pilot experiments.

Statistical Analysis

Statistical significance was assessed by Spearman correlation analysis, Mann–Whitney *U*-test and Wilcoxon matched pairs test. *p*-Values below 0.05 were considered as significant.

Study Approval

Cohort A

The study was approved by the Research Ethics and Bioethics Committee of the Consiglio Nazionale delle Ricerche (Italy). Written informed consent was received from participants prior to their inclusion in the study.

Cohort B

The study was approved by the Ethics Committees of the Medical University of Innsbruck (Austria). Written informed consent was received from participants prior to their inclusion in the study.

Cohort C

The study was approved by the Ethics Committees of the "Klinikum Wels-Grieskirchen" (Austria). Written informed consent was received from participants prior to their inclusion in the study.

RESULTS

CD8$^+$HLADR$^+$ T Cells Increase With Age

The percentage of HLADR$^+$ cells within the CD8 T cell fraction was analyzed by FACS (**Figure 1**), first in a cohort of 91 female Sardinians (**Figure 1A**) who had previously been recruited and genotyped (1) and second in a young (<30 years) and an elderly (≥70 years) cohort of Austrian males and females (**Figure 1B**). When HLADR$^+$ T cells were correlated with age, there was a highly significant positive correlation in the Sardinian cohort. In the Austrian cohort, CD8$^+$HLADR$^+$ T cells were compared in young and elderly persons and there was a significant difference between the groups, the elderly persons having a higher percentage of CD8$^+$HLADR$^+$ T cells. In order to define whether the phenotype of HLADR$^+$ T cells corresponded to previous reports (6), FACS analysis of HLADR$^+$ cells from young persons was performed (**Figure 2**). The gating strategy for HLADR$^+$ cells and the assessment of CD28 and CD45RA on HLADR$^+$ T cells are shown in **Figure 2A**. The percentages of CD28$^+$CD45RA$^+$, CD28$^+$CD45RA$^-$, CD28$^-$CD45RA$^-$, and CD28$^-$CD45RA$^+$ cells indicating different differentiation stages from naïve to T_{EMRA}-like cells are shown in CD8$^+$HLADR$^+$ and in CD8$^+$HLADR$^-$ cells in **Figure 2B**. **Figures 2C,D** demonstrate the gating strategy as well as the expression of CD28, FOXP3, CD25, and CD69 in the CD8$^+$HLADR$^+$ as well as in the CD8$^+$HLADR$^-$ cell populations. The figures show that CD8$^+$HLADR$^+$ and CD8$^+$HLADR$^-$ cells contained cells of every CD8 T cell subset when defined according to the expression of CD28 and CD45RA, although there were fewer cells in the CD28$^+$CD45RA$^+$ (naïve) subset and more cells in the CD28$^+$CD45RA$^-$ and the CD28$^-$CD45RA$^-$ (memory) subsets (**Figures 2A,B**). In accordance with previous reports (6) neither CD8$^+$HLADR$^+$ nor CD8$^+$HLADR$^-$ T cells expressed the classical activation markers CD69 and CD25 and they were negative for FOXP3. The percentage of CD28$^+$ cells was identical in the two T cell subsets (**Figures 2C,D**).

Expression of Checkpoint Inhibitory Molecules in CD8$^+$HLADR$^+$ and CD8$^+$HLADR$^-$ T Cells

The checkpoint inhibitory molecules CTLA-4, TIM-3, LAG-3, and PD-1 were analyzed in CD8$^+$HLADR$^+$ and CD8$^+$HLADR$^-$ T cells in the resting state (**Figures 3A,C**). The HLADR$^+$ subset contained between 7% (LAG-3) and 28% (PD-1) cells which carried the inhibitory molecules. In contrast, CD8$^+$HLADR$^-$ cells did not contain checkpoint inhibitory molecules in the resting state. Following stimulation with anti-CD3 and anti-CD28, the percentage of total HLADR$^+$ cells expectedly increased (**Figure 3B**; $p < 0.0001$). The percentage of inhibitory molecule-expressing cells also increased in the stimulated CD8$^+$HLADR$^+$ as well as in the CD8$^+$HLADR$^-$ subsets, but there was always a difference between the two populations. CD8$^+$HLADR$^+$ cells contained more cells expressing inhibitory molecules than CD8$^+$HLADR$^-$ cells (**Figures 3B,D**). When one assessed the percentage of cells positive for checkpoint inhibitory molecules in HLADR$^+$CD28$^+$ and HLADR$^+$CD28$^-$ T cells, the CD28$^+$ subset always contained more cells expressing inhibitory molecules than the CD28$^-$ subset (**Figure 3E**). The same pattern was observed following stimulation of the cells with anti-CD3 and anti-CD28 antibodies (**Figure 3F**). When we assessed the percentage of cells positive for checkpoint inhibitory molecules in the four populations defined by divergent expression of CD45RA and CD28 (**Figure 2**) in CD8$^+$HLADR$^+$ T cells, the CD28$^+$CD45RA$^+$ population contained more cells expressing CTLA-4, TIM-3, and LAG-3 than the CD28$^+$CD45RA$^-$, CD28$^-$CD45RA$^-$, and CD28$^-$CD45RA$^+$ populations (Figure S1 in Supplementary Material). In contrast, PD1$^+$HLADR$^+$ cells were more frequent in CD45RA$^-$ than in CD45RA$^+$ cells. A similar marker profile was observed following stimulation (Figure S1B in Supplementary Material). In CD8$^+$HLADR$^-$ cells the expression of checkpoint inhibitory molecules was generally very low even after stimulation (Figures S1C,D in Supplementary Material).

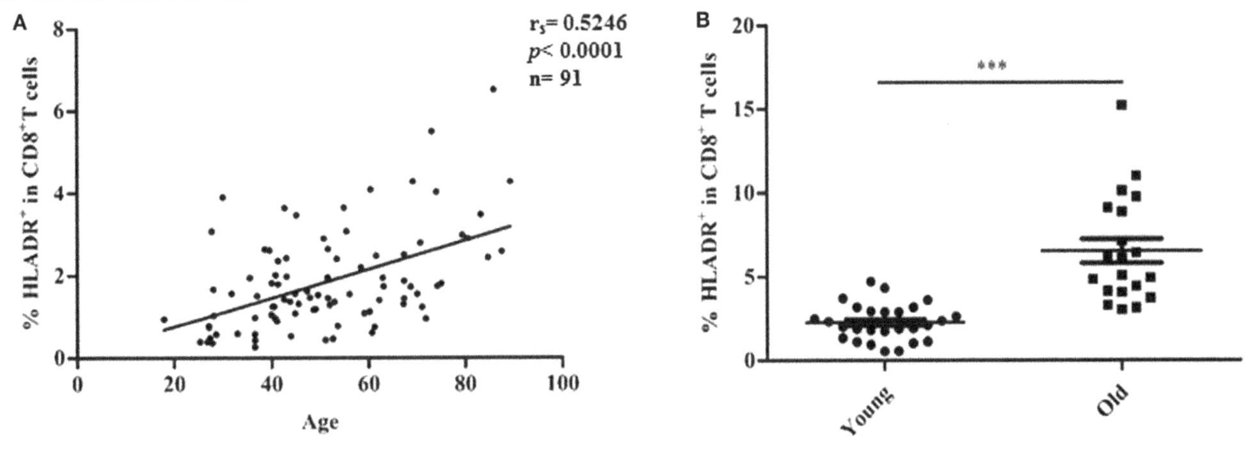

FIGURE 1 | CD8$^+$human leukocyte antigen–antigen D related (HLADR)$^+$ T cells increase with age. HLADR$^+$ cells (%) within CD3$^+$CD8$^+$ (100%) were measured by FACS analysis. **(A)** Correlation of CD8$^+$HLADR$^+$ cells in 91 female donors from Sardinia with age. Relationship between CD8$^+$HLADR$^+$ T cells (%) and age was assessed by Spearman correlation analysis; (r_s), p value, and sample size (n) are indicated in **(B)** CD8$^+$HLADR$^+$ T cells in young vs elderly donors from Austria. Mean ± SEM are indicated for each group; young (<30 years), n = 26, old (≥70 years), n = 20. Statistical significance was assessed by Mann–Whitney test, ***p < 0.0001.

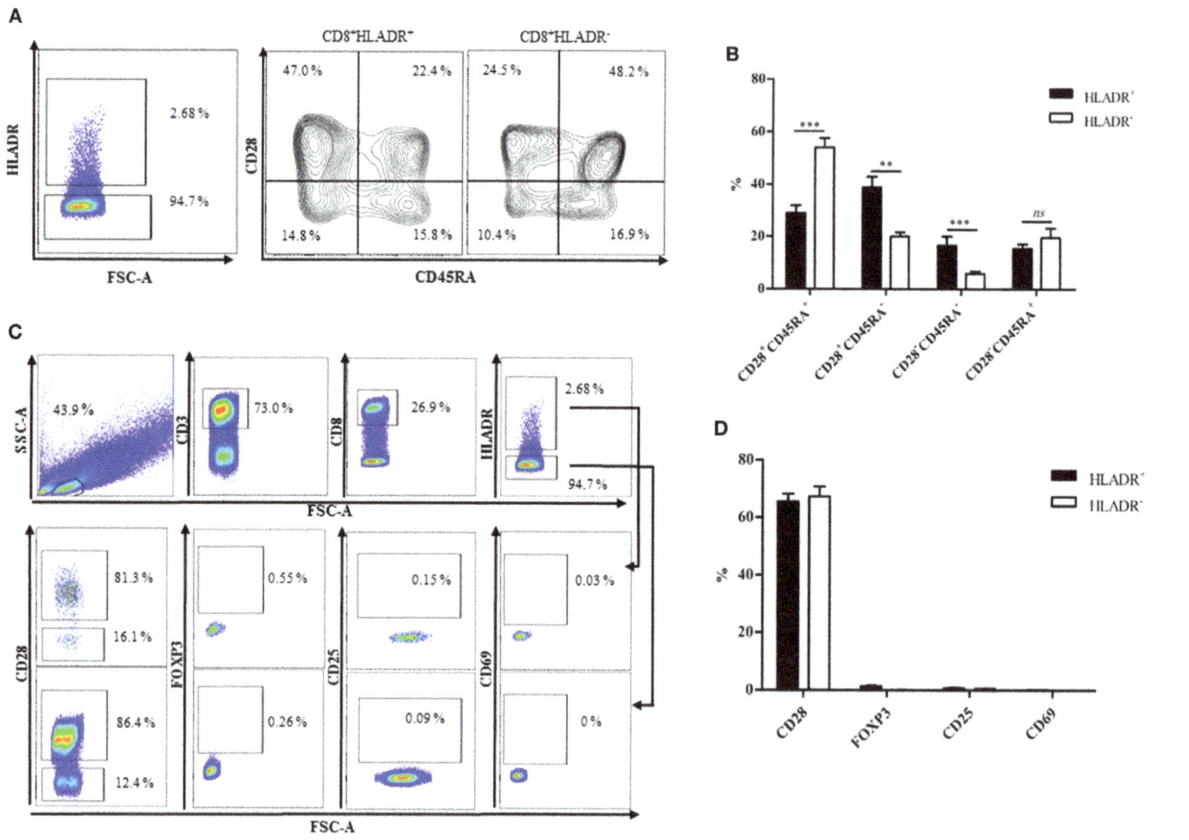

FIGURE 2 | Phenotypical characterization of CD8+human leukocyte antigen–antigen D related (HLADR)+ and CD8+HLADR− T cells. **(A)** Representative FACS plots demonstrating the expression of CD45RA and CD28 in HLADR+ and HLADR− cells from a young donor. **(B)** Percentages of HLADR+ and HLADR− cells (CD28+CD45RA+, CD28+CD45RA−, CD28−CD45RA−, and CD28−CD45RA+ cells), young donors $n = 24$ (<30 years), mean ± SEM, $^{**}p < 0.001$, $^{***}p < 0.0001$, ns, not significant. **(C)** Representative FACS plots of activation markers and other molecules in CD8+HLADR+ and CD8+HLADR− cells. The upper panel represents the gating strategy. **(D)** Percentages of CD28, FOXP3, CD25, and CD69 in CD8+HLADR+ vs CD8+HLADR− cells; mean ± SEM, young donors $n = 22$ (<30 years).

CD8+HLADR+ T Cells Have Suppressive Activity Toward the Proliferation of Autologous Stimulated PBMCs

CD8+HLADR+ T cells have been referred to as "suppressor cells" (6). It was, therefore, our next goal to confirm this assumption in cells from young persons. CD3+ cells were purified with magnetic beads and CD8+HLADR+ T cells were sorted according to a strategy depicted in Figure S2A in Supplementary Material. CD8+HLADR+ T cells were additionally sub-divided into CD28+ and CD28− T cells. The purity of the different fractions was always >95%. The purified subsets were then co-cultured with CFSE- labeled autologous PBMCs and the proliferation of the labeled cells was measured 4 days after stimulation with anti-CD3 and anti-CD28 (Figures S2B–E in Supplementary Material). In the first set of experiments, HLADR+ cells were compared with HLADR− cells without considering the expression of CD28 (Figures S2A–D in Supplementary Material). CD8+HLADR+ T cells suppressed the proliferation of autologous PBMCs in a dose-dependent manner. At a ratio of 4:1 they were still suppressive (Figures S2C,D in Supplementary Material). In Figure S2D in Supplementary Material mean suppressive activities of CD8+HLADR+ and CD8+HLADR− T cells on PBMC proliferation are shown. In spite of a minor not dose-dependent suppressive effect of the CD8+HLADR− population, suppression of the CD8+HLADR+ subset was always higher. In view of the difference in the expression of inhibitory molecules on HLADR+CD28+ and HLADR+CD28− T cells we were interested whether these two subsets had the same suppressive activity. For this reason, the purified HLADR+CD28+ and HLADR+CD28− T cells were added to CFSE-labeled autologous PBMCs. At least at a ratio of 1:2, HLADR+CD28+ cells had a more pronounced suppressive effect than their CD28− counterparts. At lower cell concentrations there was still a tendency toward increased suppression, but this did not reach statistical significance.

CD8+HLADR+ T Cells Occur Also in the BM Where They Have a Similar Phenotype as in the PB

In order to define whether CD8+HLADR+ T cells occur only in the PB or in other lymphatic organs, we investigated BM samples

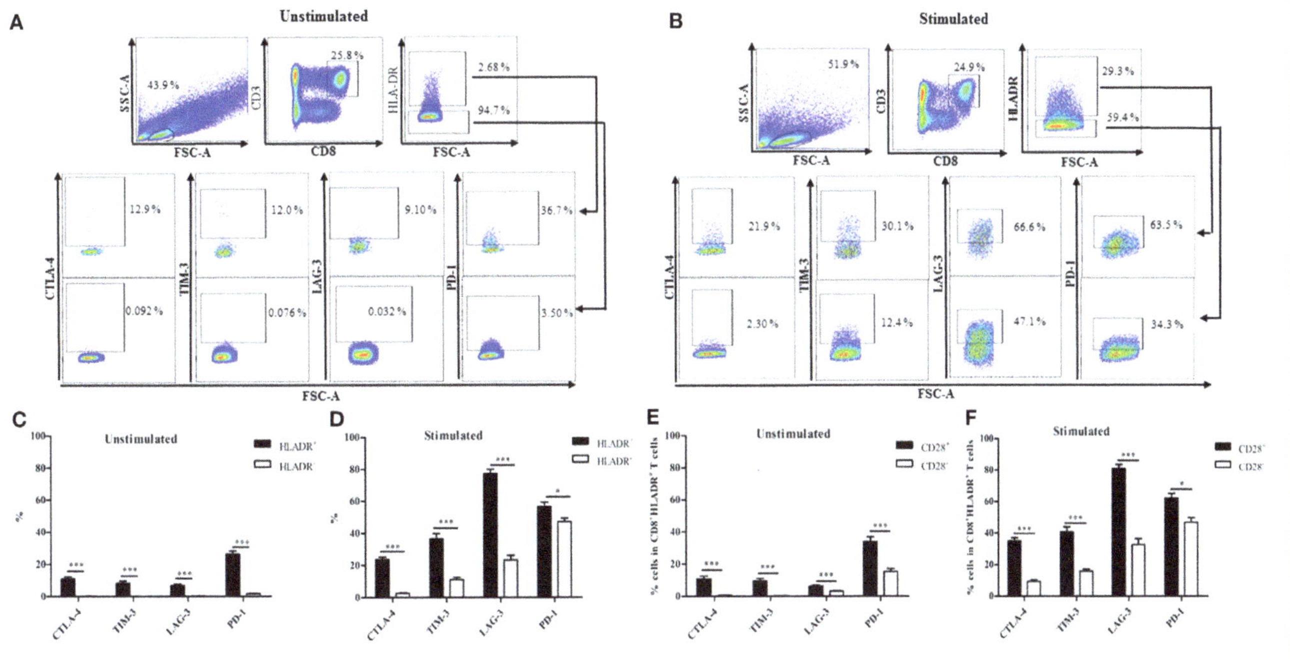

FIGURE 3 | Expression of checkpoint inhibitory molecules on CD8⁺human leukocyte antigen–antigen D related (HLADR)⁺ and on CD8⁺HLADR⁻ T cells. **(A)** Representative FACS plots of inhibitory molecules in the CD8⁺HLADR⁺ (upper panel) and the CD8⁺HLADR⁻ population (lower panel) using cells from a young donor. **(B)** Representative FACS plots of inhibitory molecules in the CD8⁺HLADR⁺ and the CD8⁺HLADR⁻ population using cells from a young donor following stimulation with anti-CD3 (1 µg/ml) and anti-CD28 (0.5 µg/ml) for 24 h. **(C)** Expression of checkpoint inhibitory molecules in CD8⁺HLADR⁺ vs CD8⁺HLADR⁻ T cells in unstimulated cells; young donors $n = 22$ (<30 years), mean ± SEM, $^{***}p < 0.0001$. **(D)** Expression of checkpoint inhibitory molecules in CD8⁺HLADR⁺ vs CD8⁺HLADR⁻ T cells following stimulation; young donors $n = 9$ (<30 years), mean ± SEM, $^{***}p < 0.0001$, $^{*}p < 0.05$. **(E)** Expression of checkpoint inhibitory molecules in CD8⁺HLADR⁺CD28⁺ vs CD8⁺HLADR⁺CD28⁻ T cells in unstimulated cells; young donors $n = 22$ (<30 years), mean ± SEM, $^{***}p < 0.0001$. **(F)** Expression of checkpoint inhibitory molecules CD8⁺HLADR⁺CD28⁺ vs CD8⁺HLADR⁺CD28⁻ T cells following stimulation; young donors $n = 9$ (<30 years), mean ± SEM, $^{***}p < 0.0001$, $^{*}p < 0.05$.

from the femur of patients of varying age (**Table 1**) after hip replacement surgery. We and others have recently studied the immunological memory in the human BM in depth (27–31). We were, therefore, interested whether a CD8 regulatory T cell type was also present in this organ. We compared CD8⁺HLADR⁺ T cells in BMMCs and PBMCs (**Figure 4**) and found that the proportions of this specific cell type were even higher in the BM than in the PB (**Figure 4B**). As in the PB, BM CD8⁺HLADR⁺ T cells are frequently CD28⁺ and do not express FOXP3 or CD25 (**Figure 4C**). In contrast to PBMCs, they contain a small proportion of CD69⁺ T cells (**Figure 4C**), but this is a characteristic feature of BM resting T cells and not of activation (27). The difference between CD8⁺HLADR⁺CD69⁺ T cells in the BM and the PB was also not significant (**Figure 4D**). As in the PB, cells expressing checkpoint inhibitory molecules were more frequent in the HLADR⁺ than in the HLADR⁻ population and more frequent in HLADR⁺CD28⁺ than in HLADR⁺CD28⁻ cells (**Figures 5A–C**). When CD8⁺HLADR⁺ T cells were compared in BMMCs and PBMCs there was no significant difference in the number of cells (**Figure 5D**). However, when only the CD28⁺ population of CD8⁺HLADR⁺ cells was analyzed, checkpoint inhibitory molecules were with the exception of LAG-3 more frequently expressed in BMMCs than in PBMCs (**Figure 5E**). As the number of samples available from the BM was relatively small and age greatly varied, no correlations with age could be made.

CD8⁺HLADR⁺ T Cells Have a Lower Expression of Checkpoint Inhibitory Molecules in Old Age

We compared CD8⁺HLADR⁺ T cells in the PB from young and elderly persons. Having found that there were more CD8⁺HLADR⁺ T cells in the PB from elderly persons than from young ones (**Figure 1**), we were now interested to define their phenotype and function. As in samples from young donors, CD8⁺HLADR⁺ T cells were more frequently CD28⁺CD45RA⁻ memory-like T cells than CD28⁺CD45RA⁺ naïve (**Figures 6A,B**). Decreased percentages of CD28⁺CD45RA⁺ naïve T cells in the CD8⁺HLADR⁺ population combined with increased percentages of CD28⁻CD45RA⁺ T_{EMRA}-like cells in the old compared to the young cohort reflected age-related changes typical for the total CD8 T cell pool in old age (26). This suggests that CD8⁺HLADR⁺ T cells do not necessarily represent a separate lineage, but are subject to differentiation such as the CD8⁺HLADR⁻ T cell population. As in the young population, FOXP3, CD25, and CD69 were not expressed in PB CD8⁺HLADR⁺ T cells from elderly persons (**Figures 6C,D**).

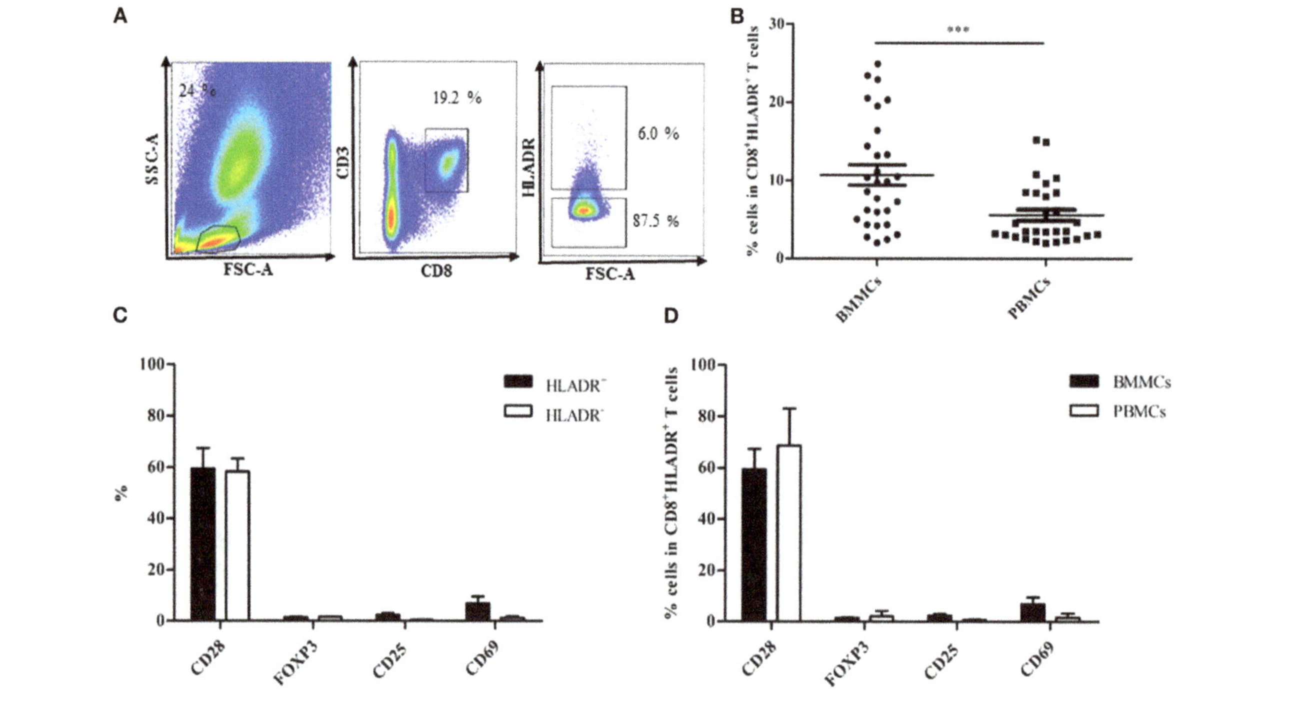

FIGURE 4 | Phenotypical characterization of CD8+human leukocyte antigen–antigen D related (HLADR)+ and CD8+HLADR− T cells in bone marrow mononuclear cells (BMMCs) and peripheral blood mononuclear cells (PBMCs) paired samples. **(A)** Representative FACS plots of the gating strategy in the bone marow. **(B)** Percentages of HLADR+ cells in CD8+ T cells in BMMCs vs PBMCs; $n = 29$; mean ± SEM, ***$p < 0.0001$. **(C)** Percentages of CD28, FOXP3, CD25, and CD69 in CD8+HLADR+ and CD8+HLADR− cells in BMMCs; $n = 5$; mean ± SEM. **(D)** Percentages of CD28, FOXP3, CD25, and CD69 in CD8+HLADR+ cells in BMMCs and PBMCs; $n = 5$; mean ± SEM.

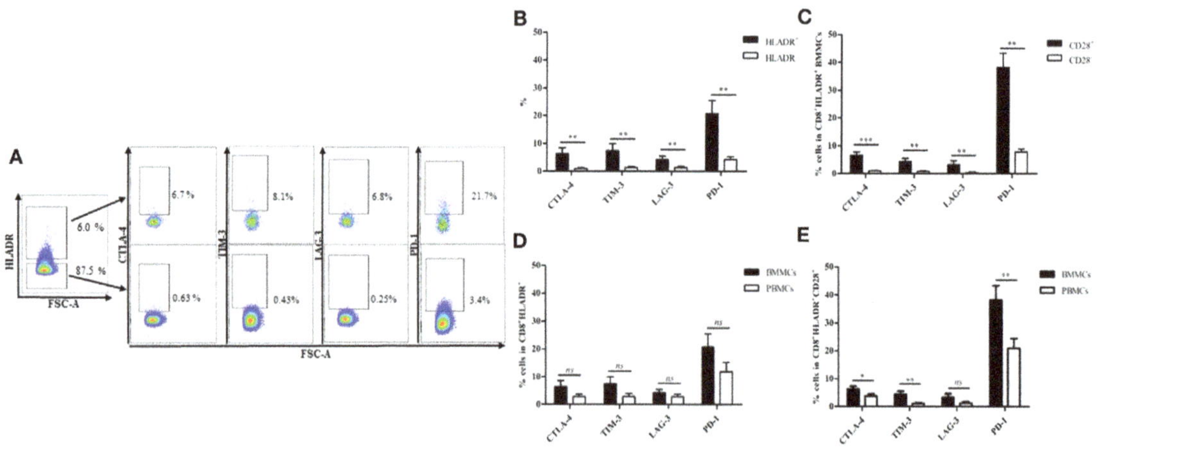

FIGURE 5 | Expression of checkpoint inhibitory molecules on CD8+human leukocyte antigen–antigen D related (HLADR)+ and on CD8+HLADR+CD28+ T cells in bone marrow mononuclear cells (BMMCs). **(A)** Representative FACS plots of inhibitory molecules in the CD8+HLADR+ (upper panel) and in CD8+HLADR− (lower panel) T cell population in BMMCs. **(B)** Expression of checkpoint inhibitory molecules in CD8+HLADR+ vs CD8+HLADR− cells in BMMCs; $n = 8$; mean ± SEM, **$p < 0.001$. **(C)** Expression of checkpoint inhibitory molecules in CD8+HLADR+CD28+ vs CD8+HLADR+CD28− cells in BMMCs; $n = 8$; mean ± SEM, ***$p < 0.0001$, **$p < 0.001$. **(D)** Expression of checkpoint inhibitory molecules in CD8+HLADR+ in BMMCs and in PBMCs; $n = 8$; mean ± SEM, ns, not significant. **(E)** Expression of checkpoint inhibitory molecules in CD8+HLADR+CD28+ in BMMCs and in PBMCs; $n = 8$; mean ± SEM, **$p < 0.001$ *$p < 0.05$.

When we compared the number of checkpoint inhibitory molecule positive cells in the CD8+HLADR+ T cell population from young and elderly persons, we found lower percentages of cells expressing CTLA-4+, TIM-3+, LAG-3+, and PD-1+ in the old than in the young group (**Figures 7A,B**). The mean fluorescence intensity of CTLA-4+, TIM-3+, LAG-3+, and PD-1+ (MFI) on CD8+HLADR+ T cells was also lower in the old than in the young group (**Figure 7C**). This was the case when the total

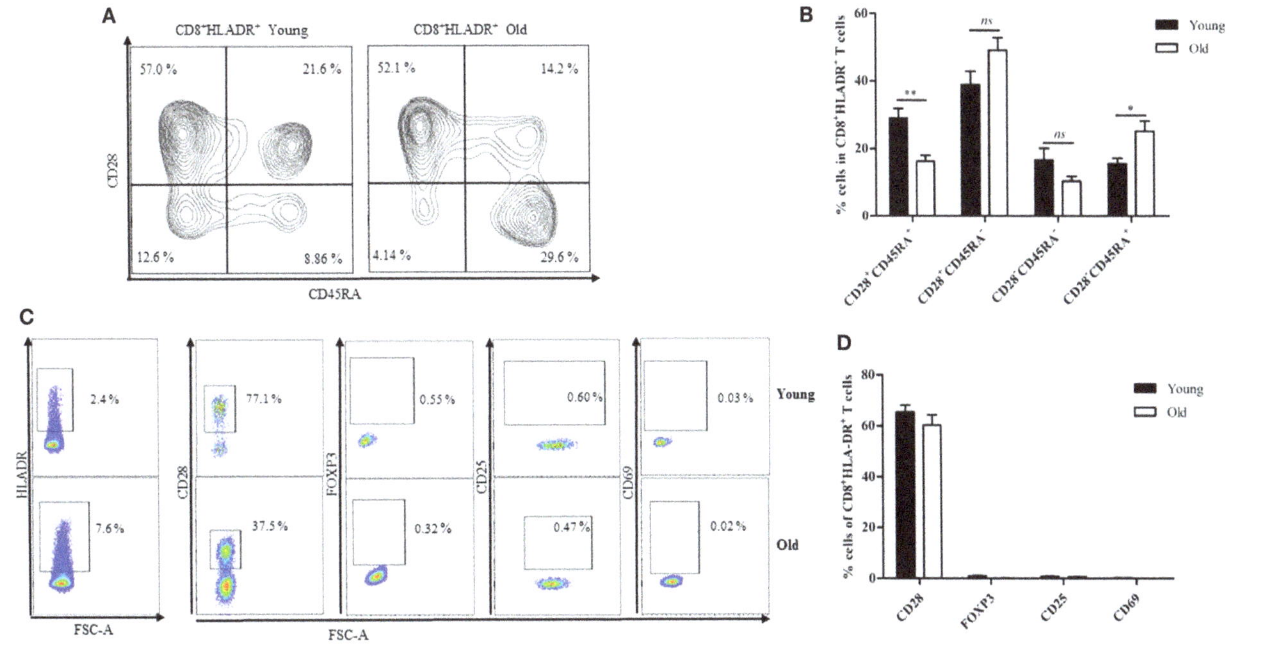

FIGURE 6 | Phenotypical characterization of CD8+human leukocyte antigen–antigen D related (HLADR)+ T cells from young and old donors. **(A)** Representative FACS plots demonstrating the expression of CD45RA and CD28 in CD8+HLADR+ cells from a young and an old donor. **(B)** Expression of CD45RA and CD28 in CD8+HLADR+ cells from young and old donors, CD28+CD45RA+, CD28+CD45RA−, CD28−CD45RA−, CD28−CD45RA+ cells are shown, young donors $n = 18–21$ (<30 years) and old donors $n = 18–21$ (≥70 years), mean ± SEM, $^{**}p < 0.001$, $^{*}p < 0.05$, ns, not significant. **(C)** Representative FACS plots of activation markers and other molecules in CD8+HLADR+ T cells from a young (upper panel) and an old donor (lower panel). **(D)** Percentages of CD28, FOXP3, CD25, and CD69 cells in the CD8+ HLADR+ population from young and old donors, young $n = 18–21$ (<30 years) and old donors $n = 18–21$ (≥70 years), mean ± SEM.

CD8+HLADR+ population was analyzed (**Figures 7B,C**) as well as in CD8+HLADR+CD28+ cells (Figures S3A,B in Supplementary Material). The number of checkpoint inhibitory molecule positive cells was low in both groups when cells were unstimulated (**Figures 7A–C**; Figures S3A,B in Supplementary Material), but increased following stimulation with anti-CD3 and anti-CD28 (**Figures 7D–F**; Figures S3C,D in Supplementary Material). As in unstimulated cells, the percentage of checkpoint inhibitory positive cells in CD8+HLADR+ and in CD8+HLADR+CD28+ cells was always higher in the young than in the old cohort following stimulation.

CD8+HLADR+ T Cells From Elderly Persons Have Reduced Suppressive Function Toward the Proliferation of Autologous PBMCs

In view of the reduced expression of checkpoint inhibitory molecules on CD8+HLADR+ T cells in old age, we were interested in the question whether this cell population also had a decreased suppressive function. We, therefore, purified CD8+HLADR+CD28+ T cells from young and elderly persons by cell sorting and co-cultured them with autologous PBMCs labeled with CFSE. In view of low cell numbers available, the co-culture experiment was only performed at a PBMC: HLADR+ T cell population ratio of 2:1 (**Figure 8**). We found that CD8+HLADR+CD28+ T cells from elderly persons had indeed lost most of their suppressive function. Whereas CD8+HLADR+CD28+ T cells from young persons had a suppressive activity of around 40%, suppression was below 20% in cells from elderly persons (**Figure 8B**). Considering that the number of cells of the different subsets of PBMCs may vary with age, we looked at the proliferation of CD4+ and CD8+ T cells within the PBMCs. We found no significant differences when we compared the suppression of CD4+ T cells vs the suppression of CD8+ T cells in both young and old persons (**Figure 8C**).

Checkpoint Inhibitory Molecules Mediate the Suppression of CD8+HLADR+CD28+ T Cells

Checkpoint inhibitory molecules are expressed at a higher level in the CD8+HLADR+ than in the CD8+HLADR− subset. They are also expressed at a higher level in young than in old donors. This may explain the higher suppressive effect of CD8+HLADR+ T cells of young donors. To check this possibility, we investigated the involvement of these molecules in mediating the suppressive effect of HLADR+ cells in neutralizing Ab experiments (**Figure 9**). We showed that the suppressive effect induced by CD8+HLADR+CD28+ Tregs at a PBMCs: suppressor cell ratio of 2:1 was distinctly inhibited by anti-CTLA-4, anti-TIM-3, anti-LAG-3 and slightly, but still significantly by anti-PD-1. The isotype control had no effect on suppression.

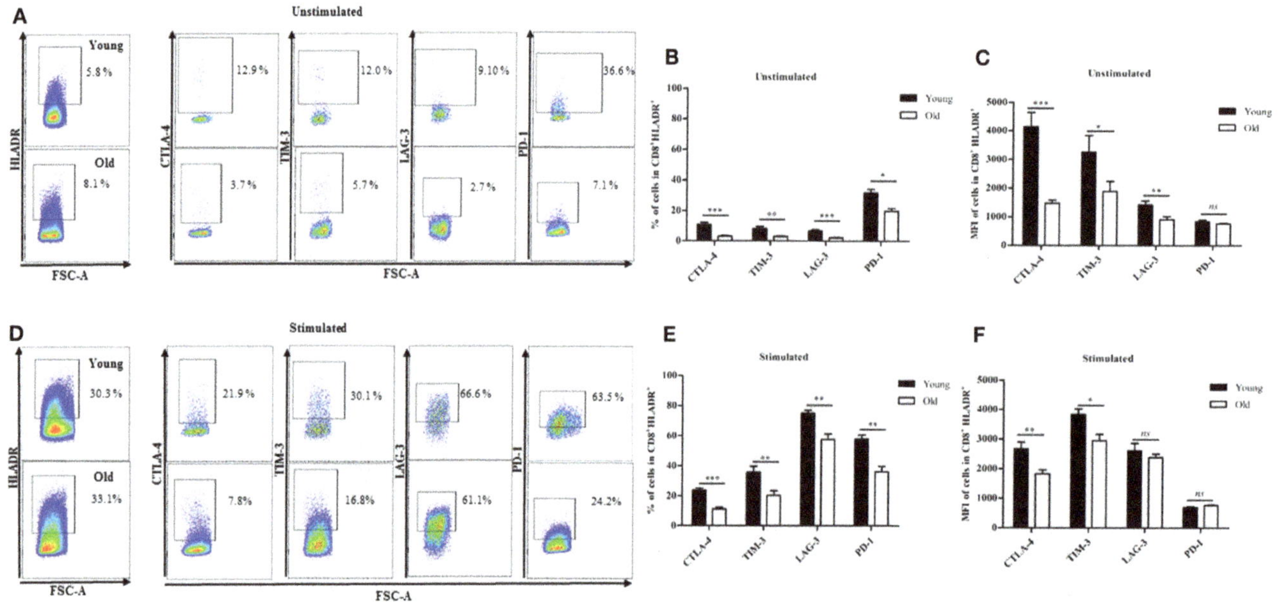

FIGURE 7 | Expression of checkpoint inhibitory molecules on CD8+human leukocyte antigen–antigen D related (HLADR)+ T cells in young and old persons. **(A)** Representative FACS plots of inhibitory molecules in the CD8+HLADR+ population from one young (upper panel) and one old (lower panel) donor before stimulation. **(B)** Expression of checkpoint inhibitory molecules (percentages) in CD8+HLADR+ cells from young and old donors before stimulation; young donors $n = 22$ (<30 years) and old donors $n = 20$ (>70 years), mean ± SEM, ***$p < 0.0001$, **$p < 0.001$, *$p < 0.05$. **(C)** Expression of checkpoint inhibitory molecules (MFI) in CD8+HLADR+ cells from young and old donors before stimulation; young donors $n = 20$ (<30 years) and old donors $n = 18$ (>70 years), mean ± SEM, ***$p < 0.0001$, **$p < 0.001$, *$p < 0.05$. **(D)** Representative FACS plots of inhibitory molecules in the CD8+HLADR+ population from one young (upper panel) and one old (lower panel) donor following stimulation with anti-CD3 (1 µg/ml) and anti-CD28 (0.5 µg/ml) for 24 h. **(E)** Expression of checkpoint inhibitory molecules (percentages) in the CD8+HLADR+ population from young and old donors following stimulation; young donors $n = 9$ (<30 years) and old donors $n = 7$ (>70 years), mean ± SEM, ***$p < 0.0001$, **$p < 0.001$. **(F)** Expression of checkpoint inhibitory molecules (MFI) in the CD8+HLADR+ population from young and old donors; young donors $n = 9$ (<30 years) and old donors $n = 7$ (>70 years), mean ± SEM, ***$p < 0.0001$, **$p < 0.001$ *$p < 0.05$.

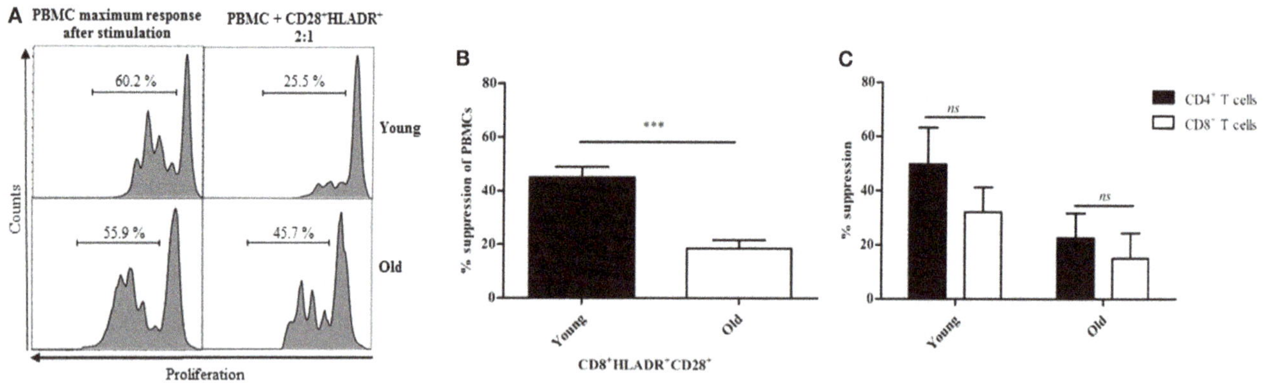

FIGURE 8 | CD8+human leukocyte antigen–antigen D related (HLADR)+CD28+ T cells suppressor properties decrease with age. **(A)** Representative histograms showing the suppressive activity of sorted CD8+HLADR+CD28+ T cells from one young and one old donor on CFSE-labeled peripheral blood mononuclear cells (PBMCs) assessed in co-culture 4 days after stimulation with anti-CD3 (1 µg/ml) and anti-CD28 (0.5 µg/ml). **(B)** Suppressive effect of CD8+HLADR+CD28+ T cells on the proliferation of CFSE-labeled autologous PBMCs (ratio 2:1); mean ± SEM, young donors $n = 5$ (<30 years), old donors $n = 6$ (≥70 years); ***$p < 0.001$. **(C)** Suppressive effect of CD8+HLADR+CD28+ T cells on the proliferation of CD4+ vs CD8+ T cells within the CFSE-labeled PBMCs (ratio 2:1); mean ± SEM, young donors $n = 2$ (<30 years), old donors $n = 4$ (≥70 years).

DISCUSSION

We here show increased numbers of CD8+HLADR+ T cells in old age in a female Sardinian cohort previously genotyped and described (1) and in a smaller population of young and elderly Austrians. As the number of HLADR+ T cells has been demonstrated to be genetically linked (1), it is possible that at least in the Sardinian population the increased numbers of this specific cell

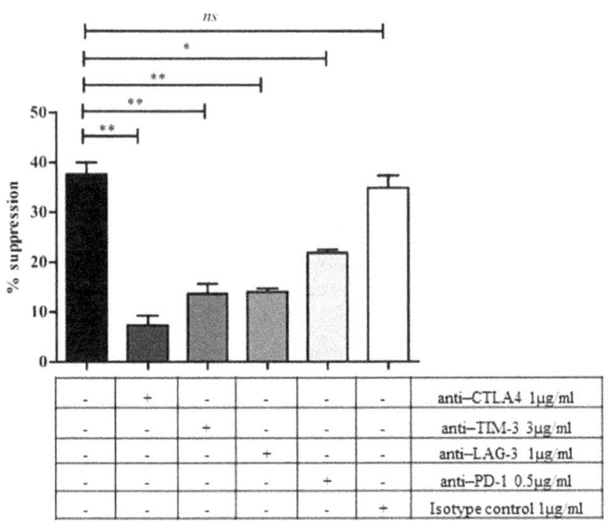

FIGURE 9 | Checkpoint inhibitory molecules are involved in the suppressive activity of CD8⁺human leukocyte antigen–antigen D related (HLADR)⁺CD28⁺ T cells. CFSE-labeled peripheral blood mononuclear cells (PBMCs) were analyzed following a 4 days co-culture after stimulation with anti-CD3 (1 µg/ml) and anti-CD28 (0.5 µg/ml) in the absence or presence of anti-cytotoxic T-lymphocyte-associated antigen 4 (1 µg/ml), anti-T cell immunoglobulin and mucin protein-3 (3 µg/ml), anti-lymphocyte activation gene-3 (1 µg/ml), or anti-programmed death 1 (0.5 µg/ml). Mouse IgG1 isotype Ab was used as control. PBMCs: suppressor cell ratio of 2:1. Young donors $n = 2–3$ (<30 years); mean ± SEM, $^{**}p < 0.001$, $^{*}p < 0.05$, ns, not significant.

type may be driven by the influence of certain genes. However, this is not likely to be the case in the Austrian population. We show here that $CD8^+HLADR^+$ cells most frequently have a $CD28^+$ memory phenotype. As elderly persons have more memory than naïve cells (26), it seems plausible that the increased numbers of $CD8^+HLADR^+$ T cells in old age reflect an enlarged $CD8^+$ memory T cell pool. In this context, it is also of interest that there are even more $CD8^+HLADR^+$ cells in the BM than in the PB, which may reflect the fact that the BM is known to be a reservoir for memory T cells (27–29, 32). $CD8^+HLADR^+$ T cells have been suggested to represent a separate lineage of T cells, as they occur also in cord blood (6). This possibility cannot be excluded, as we find $CD8^+HLADR^+$ T cells in the naïve cell population in our study. They may still be primed as naïve cells. In consequence they seem to persevere with differentiation, as $CD8^+HLADR^+$ cells occur also in memory as well as effector cell subsets. There is presently no information what the trigger for the induction of a $CD8^+HLADR^+$ phenotype is, but it may on the one hand be antigenic stimulation or also stimulation with cytokines, as suggested by the fact that high numbers are found in the BM, where BM niche cytokines such as IL-7 and IL-15 are prominent (31, 33). Experiments trying to analyze whether *in vitro* stimulation of naïve cells with various BM cytokines can induce this specific phenotype and function are presently underway.

In accordance with previous reports, we demonstrate that $CD8^+HLADR^+$ T cells can inhibit the proliferation of autologous PBMCs and can, therefore, be regarded as Tregs cells (6). As such, they may be an important cell type to maintain homeostatic equilibrium within the immune system. Suppression has previously been suggested to be due to cellular interactions mediated by CTLA-4. We now show that $CD8^+HLADR^+$ cells not only express increased amounts of CTLA-4 but also of other checkpoint inhibitory molecules such as TIM-3, LAG-3, and PD-1. It seems likely that suppression of other cells is not only mediated by one but also by a whole panel of inhibitory molecules. Our results using neutralizing Abs are in favor of this possibility. It was of interest that inhibitory molecules were stronger expressed on the $CD28^+$ than the $CD28^-$ fraction, which may indicate that pre-stimulation *via* the antigen receptor may be one possible requirement for the induction of inhibitory molecules and their regulatory function.

In this context, it is remarkable that inhibitory molecule expression and regulatory function were decreased in $CD8^+HLADR^+$ T cells from elderly persons in spite of high cell numbers. Decreased T cell receptor signaling is known to be a characteristic feature of old age (34, 35). If inhibitory molecule levels reflect previous antigenic stimulation, checkpoint inhibitory molecule expression would be low in old age as a consequence. In how far high cell numbers could neutralize a decrease in function on a per cell basis is not clear. A similar situation is being discussed for natural killer (NK) cells (36, 37). In the case of $CD8^+HLADR^+$ T cells it seems imaginable that the synergy of a whole panel of different checkpoint inhibitory molecules on the cell surface is needed to trigger the full regulatory capacity of the cells. If these molecules are expressed at low concentrations even after antigenic stimulation, there might be no guarantee that suppressive function is maintained and decreased stimulatory activity would be the consequence.

From our data it is not yet clear toward which cell types the regulatory effect of $CD8^+HLADR^+$ T cells is directed. We can presently only show inhibition of the proliferation of autologous PBMCs as well as $CD4^+$ and $CD8^+$ T cells. It would be of major interest to define which cell types are target cells of the inhibitory effect and which functions other than proliferation can be influenced. This topic is difficult to study, as purified $CD8^+HLADR^+$ T cells are needed and it is hard to obtain sufficiently high numbers of pure cells after sorting. Isolation of purified cells from the BM is even more difficult. We keep trying to analyze whether BM niche cells (38), monocytes/macrophages, or dendritic cells (DCs) are affected in their stimulatory function. This would influence inflammatory processes. If $CD8^+HLADR^+$ Tregs cells do not function properly in old age, this could then support age-associated subclinical inflammation referred to as "inflamm-aging" (39, 40). As we have recently shown that "inflamm-aging" affects the BM in old age leading to increased levels of oxygen radicals, IL-15, TNF-α, and IFN-γ (31, 33), it is tempting to speculate that lack of regulatory function by $CD8^+HLADR^+$ T cells is a cause of this phenomenon.

In conclusion, we demonstrate for the first time that a decreased expression of checkpoint inhibitory molecules and consecutive lack of suppressive function of the $CD8^+HLADR^+$ T cell type is a characteristic feature of the immune system in old age. It will be of interest to learn more about the functional properties of this specific cell type in regard to inflammation and a possible imbalance between the different types of immune cells.

ETHICS STATEMENT

Cohort A: the study was approved by the Research Ethics and Bioethics Committee of the Consiglio Nazionale delle Ricerche (Italy). Written informed consent was received from participants prior to their inclusion in the study. Cohort B: the study was approved by the Ethics Committees of the Medical University of Innsbruck (Austria). Written informed consent was received from participants prior to their inclusion in the study. Cohort C: the study was approved by the Ethics Committees of the "Klinikum Wels-Grieskirchen" (Austria). Written informed consent was received from participants prior to their inclusion in the study.

AUTHOR CONTRIBUTIONS

SY, BG-L, BW, EF, FC, and SS: study design, interpretation of data, critical appraisal, final approval of the version to be published. ML and VO: recruitment of the Sardinian cohort. KT: recruitment of Austrian probands, sample collection, and study design. SY: method design. SS: study design and sorting of cells. SY, MK, FM, and LP: experimental work.

FUNDING

This study was supported by the European Union's Horizon 2020 Research and Innovation Programme under grant agreement 633964 (ImmunoAgeing). Innovation Programme under grant agreement 633964 (ImmunoAgeing) and by the Austrian Research Promotion Agency's (FFG) grant #858057 "HD FACS." The Austrian Research Promotion Agency's (FFG) grant #858057 "HD FACS." The authors are grateful to Anita Hohenegger for the help in the manuscript preparation and to Brigitte Jenewein for helping with blood draws.

REFERENCES

1. Orru V, Steri M, Sole G, Sidore C, Virdis F, Dei M, et al. Genetic variants regulating immune cell levels in health and disease. *Cell* (2013) 155(1): 242–56. doi:10.1016/j.cell.2013.08.041
2. Evans RL, Faldetta TJ, Humphreys RE, Pratt DM, Yunis EJ, Schlossman SF. Peripheral human T cells sensitized in mixed leukocyte culture synthesize and express Ia-like antigens. *J Exp Med* (1978) 148(5):1440–5. doi:10.1084/jem.148.5.1440
3. Ko HS, Fu SM, Winchester RJ, Yu DT, Kunkel HG. Ia determinants on stimulated human T lymphocytes. Occurrence on mitogen- and antigen-activated T cells. *J Exp Med* (1979) 150(2):246–55. doi:10.1084/jem.150.2.246
4. Oshima S, Eckels DD. Selective signal transduction through the CD3 or CD2 complex is required for class II MHC expression by human T cells. *J Immunol* (1990) 145(12):4018–25.
5. Baecher-Allan C, Wolf E, Hafler DA. MHC class II expression identifies functionally distinct human regulatory T cells. *J Immunol* (2006) 176(8):4622–31. doi:10.4049/jimmunol.176.8.4622
6. Arruvito L, Payaslian F, Baz P, Podhorzer A, Billordo A, Pandolfi J, et al. Identification and clinical relevance of naturally occurring human CD8+HLA-DR+ regulatory T cells. *J Immunol* (2014) 193(9):4469–76. doi:10.4049/jimmunol.1401490
7. Cantor H, Shen FW, Boyse EA. Separation of helper T cells from suppressor T cells expressing different Ly components. II. Activation by antigen: after immunization, antigen-specific suppressor and helper activities are mediated by distinct T-cell subclasses. *J Exp Med* (1976) 143(6):1391–1340. doi:10.1084/jem.143.6.1391
8. Gershon RK, Kondo K. Cell interactions in the induction of tolerance: the role of thymic lymphocytes. *Immunology* (1970) 18(5):723–37.
9. Baecher-Allan C, Brown JA, Freeman GJ, Hafler DA. CD4+CD25high regulatory cells in human peripheral blood. *J Immunol* (2001) 167(3):1245–53. doi:10.4049/jimmunol.167.3.1245
10. Levings MK, Sangregorio R, Roncarolo MG. Human cd25(+)cd4(+) t regulatory cells suppress naive and memory T cell proliferation and can be expanded in vitro without loss of function. *J Exp Med* (2001) 193(11):1295–302. doi:10.1084/jem.193.11.1295
11. Ng WF, Duggan PJ, Ponchel F, Matarese G, Lombardi G, Edwards AD, et al. Human CD4(+)CD25(+) cells: a naturally occurring population of regulatory T cells. *Blood* (2001) 98(9):2736–44. doi:10.1182/blood.V98.9.2736
12. Fontenot JD, Gavin MA, Rudensky AY. Foxp3 programs the development and function of CD4+CD25+ regulatory T cells. *Nat Immunol* (2003) 4(4):330–6. doi:10.1038/ni904
13. Hori S, Nomura T, Sakaguchi S. Control of regulatory T cell development by the transcription factor Foxp3. *Science* (2003) 299(5609):1057–61. doi:10.1126/science.1079490
14. Wolf AM, Wolf D, Steurer M, Gastl G, Gunsilius E, Grubeck-Loebenstein B. Increase of regulatory T cells in the peripheral blood of cancer patients. *Clin Cancer Res* (2003) 9(2):606–12.
15. Jagger A, Shimojima Y, Goronzy JJ, Weyand CM. Regulatory T cells and the immune aging process: a mini-review. *Gerontology* (2014) 60(2):130–7. doi:10.1159/000355303
16. Colovai AI, Liu Z, Ciubotariu R, Lederman S, Cortesini R, Suciu-Foca N. Induction of xenoreactive CD4+ T-cell anergy by suppressor CD8+CD28- T cells. *Transplantation* (2000) 69(7):1304–10. doi:10.1097/00007890-200004150-00016
17. Najafian N, Chitnis T, Salama AD, Zhu B, Benou C, Yuan X, et al. Regulatory functions of CD8+CD28- T cells in an autoimmune disease model. *J Clin Invest* (2003) 112(7):1037–48. doi:10.1172/JCI17935
18. Strioga M, Pasukoniene V, Characiejus D. CD8+ CD28- and CD8+ CD57+ T cells and their role in health and disease. *Immunology* (2011) 134(1):17–32. doi:10.1111/j.1365-2567.2011.03470.x
19. Ciubotariu R, Colovai AI, Pennesi G, Liu Z, Smith D, Berlocco P, et al. Specific suppression of human CD4+ Th cell responses to pig MHC antigens by CD8+CD28- regulatory T cells. *J Immunol* (1998) 161(10):5193–202.
20. Liu Z, Tugulea S, Cortesini R, Suciu-Foca N. Specific suppression of T helper alloreactivity by allo-MHC class I-restricted CD8+CD28- T cells. *Int Immunol* (1998) 10(6):775–83. doi:10.1093/intimm/10.6.775
21. Lu L, Cantor H. Generation and regulation of CD8(+) regulatory T cells. *Cell Mol Immunol* (2008) 5(6):401–6. doi:10.1038/cmi.2008.50
22. Endharti AT, Rifa IM, Shi Z, Fukuoka Y, Nakahara Y, Kawamoto Y, et al. Cutting edge: CD8+CD122+ regulatory T cells produce IL-10 to suppress IFN-gamma production and proliferation of CD8+ T cells. *J Immunol* (2005) 175(11):7093–7. doi:10.4049/jimmunol.175.11.7093
23. Rifa'i M, Kawamoto Y, Nakashima I, Suzuki H. Essential roles of CD8+CD122+ regulatory T cells in the maintenance of T cell homeostasis. *J Exp Med* (2004) 200(9):1123–34. doi:10.1084/jem.20040395
24. Shi Z, Okuno Y, Rifa'i M, Endharti AT, Akane K, Isobe K, et al. Human CD8+CXCR3+ T cells have the same function as murine CD8+CD122+ Treg. *Eur J Immunol* (2009) 39(8):2106–19. doi:10.1002/eji.200939314
25. Boer MC, van Meijgaarden KE, Bastid J, Ottenhoff TH, Joosten SA. CD39 is involved in mediating suppression by *Mycobacterium bovis* BCG-activated human CD8(+) CD39(+) regulatory T cells. *Eur J Immunol* (2013) 43(7):1925–32. doi:10.1002/eji.201243286

26. Arnold CR, Wolf J, Brunner S, Herndler-Brandstetter D, Grubeck-Loebenstein B. Gain and loss of T cell subsets in old age – age-related reshaping of the T cell repertoire. *J Clin Immunol* (2011) 31(2):137–46. doi:10.1007/s10875-010-9499-x
27. Herndler-Brandstetter D, Landgraf K, Jenewein B, Tzankov A, Brunauer R, Brunner S, et al. Human bone marrow hosts polyfunctional memory CD4+ and CD8+ T cells with close contact to IL-15-producing cells. *J Immunol* (2011) 186(12):6965–71. doi:10.4049/jimmunol.1100243
28. Palendira U, Chinn R, Raza W, Piper K, Pratt G, Machado L, et al. Selective accumulation of virus-specific CD8+ T cells with unique homing phenotype within the human bone marrow. *Blood* (2008) 112(8):3293–302. doi:10.1182/blood-2008-02-138040
29. Tokoyoda K, Zehentmeier S, Hegazy AN, Albrecht I, Grun JR, Lohning M, et al. Professional memory CD4+ T lymphocytes preferentially reside and rest in the bone marrow. *Immunity* (2009) 30(5):721–30. doi:10.1016/j.immuni.2009.03.015
30. Pritz T, Lair J, Ban M, Keller M, Weinberger B, Krismer M, et al. Plasma cell numbers decrease in bone marrow of old patients. *Eur J Immunol* (2015) 45(3):738–46. doi:10.1002/eji.201444878
31. Pangrazzi L, Meryk A, Naismith E, Koziel R, Lair J, Krismer M, et al. "Inflamm-aging" influences immune cell survival factors in human bone marrow. *Eur J Immunol* (2017) 47(3):481–92. doi:10.1002/eji.201646570
32. Herndler-Brandstetter D, Landgraf K, Tzankov A, Jenewein B, Brunauer R, Laschober GT, et al. The impact of aging on memory T cell phenotype and function in the human bone marrow. *J Leukoc Biol* (2012) 91(2):197–205. doi:10.1189/jlb.0611299
33. Pangrazzi L, Naismith E, Meryk A, Keller M, Jenewein B, Trieb K, et al. Increased IL-15 production and accumulation of highly differentiated CD8(+) effector/memory T Cells in the bone marrow of persons with cytomegalovirus. *Front Immunol* (2017) 8:715. doi:10.3389/fimmu.2017.00715
34. Larbi A, Pawelec G, Wong SC, Goldeck D, Tai JJ, Fulop T. Impact of age on T cell signaling: a general defect or specific alterations? *Ageing Res Rev* (2011) 10(3):370–8. doi:10.1016/j.arr.2010.09.008
35. Larbi A, Douziech N, Dupuis G, Khalil A, Pelletier H, Guerard KP, et al. Age-associated alterations in the recruitment of signal-transduction proteins to lipid rafts in human T lymphocytes. *J Leukoc Biol* (2004) 75(2):373–81. doi:10.1189/jlb.0703319
36. Camous X, Pera A, Solana R, Larbi A. NK cells in healthy aging and age-associated diseases. *J Biomed Biotechnol* (2012) 2012:195956. doi:10.1155/2012/195956
37. Pita-Lopez ML, Pera A, Solana R. Adaptive memory of human NK-like CD8(+) T-cells to aging, and viral and tumor antigens. *Front Immunol* (2016) 7:616. doi:10.3389/fimmu.2016.00616
38. Tokoyoda K, Hauser AE, Nakayama T, Radbruch A. Organization of immunological memory by bone marrow stroma. *Nat Rev Immunol* (2010) 10(3):193–200. doi:10.1038/nri2727
39. Franceschi C, Bonafe M, Valensin S, Olivieri F, De Luca M, Ottaviani E, et al. Inflamm-aging. An evolutionary perspective on immunosenescence. *Ann N Y Acad Sci* (2000) 908:244–54. doi:10.1111/j.1749-6632.2000.tb06651.x
40. Franceschi C, Campisi J. Chronic inflammation (inflammaging) and its potential contribution to age-associated diseases. *J Gerontol A Biol Sci Med Sci* (2014) 69(Suppl 1):S4–9. doi:10.1093/gerona/glu057

8

Age and Age-Related Diseases: Role of Inflammation Triggers and Cytokines

Irene Maeve Rea[1,2,3], David S. Gibson[2], Victoria McGilligan[2], Susan E. McNerlan[4], H. Denis Alexander[2] and Owen A. Ross[5,6,7]*

[1] School of Medicine, Dentistry and Biomedical Science, Queens University Belfast, Belfast, United Kingdom, [2] Northern Ireland Centre for Stratified Medicine, Biomedical Sciences Research Institute, University of Ulster, C-TRIC Building, Altnagelvin Area Hospital, Londonderry, United Kingdom, [3] Care of Elderly Medicine, Belfast Health and Social Care Trust, Belfast, United Kingdom, [4] Regional Genetics Service, Belfast Health and Social Care Trust, Belfast, United Kingdom, [5] Department of Neuroscience, Mayo Clinic, Jacksonville, FL, United States, [6] Department of Clinical Genomics, Mayo Clinic, Jacksonville, FL, United States, [7] School of Medicine and Medical Science, University College Dublin, Dublin, Ireland

***Correspondence:**
Irene Maeve Rea
i.rea@qub.ac.uk

Cytokine dysregulation is believed to play a key role in the remodeling of the immune system at older age, with evidence pointing to an inability to fine-control systemic inflammation, which seems to be a marker of unsuccessful aging. This reshaping of cytokine expression pattern, with a progressive tendency toward a pro-inflammatory phenotype has been called "inflamm-aging." Despite research there is no clear understanding about the causes of "inflamm-aging" that underpin most major age-related diseases, including atherosclerosis, diabetes, Alzheimer's disease, rheumatoid arthritis, cancer, and aging itself. While inflammation is part of the normal repair response for healing, and essential in keeping us safe from bacterial and viral infections and noxious environmental agents, not all inflammation is good. When inflammation becomes prolonged and persists, it can become damaging and destructive. Several common molecular pathways have been identified that are associated with both aging and low-grade inflammation. The age-related change in redox balance, the increase in age-related senescent cells, the senescence-associated secretory phenotype (SASP) and the decline in effective autophagy that can trigger the inflammasome, suggest that it may be possible to delay age-related diseases and aging itself by suppressing pro-inflammatory molecular mechanisms or improving the timely resolution of inflammation. Conversely there may be learning from molecular or genetic pathways from long-lived cohorts who exemplify good quality aging. Here, we will discuss some of the current ideas and highlight molecular pathways that appear to contribute to the immune imbalance and the cytokine dysregulation, which is associated with "inflammageing" or parainflammation. Evidence of these findings will be drawn from research in cardiovascular disease, cancer, neurological inflammation and rheumatoid arthritis.

Keywords: aging, age-related diseases, inflamm-aging, redox, SASP, autophagy, cytokine dysregulation, inflammation resolution

INTRODUCTION

The inflammatory response must be tightly regulated to ensure effective immune protection. It is a dynamic network that is continuously remodeling throughout each person's life as a result of the interaction between our genes, lifestyles, and environments (1–3). Infections and tissue damage from the external environment and our personal internal response to stress can act as triggers to initiate the inflammatory defense response. While inflammation is part of the normal repair response for healing, and essential in keeping us safe from bacterial and viral infections and noxious environmental agents, not all inflammation is good. When inflammation becomes prolonged and persists, it can become damaging and destructive (4). It is essential that inflammation is tailored to the initiating stress and resolves in a timely and controlled way, to avoid pathology associated with chronicity.

The cytokine network is a highly complex system of immune molecular messengers, with multiple layers of activation and control mediated through soluble receptors, receptor antagonists, diverse serum mediators, as well as gene polymorphisms (5). Proteomic methods measuring cytokine production and expression have demonstrated further layers of complexity and control in cytokine production and expression involving long coding RNAs, siRNAs, and miRNAs, which make for challenging interpretation of cytokine production and control in the inflammatory process (6). Many cytokines are able to act in more than one-way or paradoxically at different times and many act in feedback loops with the ability to auto-control their own production (7). Cytokine expression is also influenced by local cellular microenvironments, suggesting that multiple pathways exist to achieve homeostatic immunologic control and effectiveness, or to conversely accentuate chronic immune activation. However, what seems clear is that mirroring other body systems, the homeostatic control, titration, and modulation of immune responsiveness becomes more fragile and less tightly focused with increasing age. This loosening of the cytokine balance between the pro-inflammatory and anti-inflammatory control or resolving mechanisms, or inflamm-aging (8, 9), is a characteristic feature of both aging and aging-related diseases. This kind of inflammation is similar to that originally described as "parainflammation" by Medzhitov (10).

Today there is increasing recognition that inflammation is a common molecular pathway that underlies in part, the pathogenesis of diverse human diseases ranging from infection, to immune-mediated disorders, cardiovascular pathology, diabetes, metabolic syndrome, neurodegeneration, and cancer, to aging itself (4, 11, 12). Although there is no exact understanding about the causes of "inflamm-aging", a common finding seems to involve a dysregulation of the cytokine network and its homeostasis. Several common molecular pathways have been identified that seem to be associated with both aging and low-grade inflammation. Excess oxidative stress and DNA damage trigger the inflammasome, stimulating NF-κB and the IL-1β-mediated inflammatory cascade. Autophagy, the cell machinery process that removes damaged proteins and large aggregates, is also slowed up at older age and in age-related disease, causing damaged material to accumulate and reduce cellular efficiency. Senescent cells increase with age and in age-related diseases, and the associated secretome or senescence-associated secretory phenotype (SASP) produces a self-perpetuating intracellular signaling loop and inflammatory cascade involving the NF-κB, IL-1α, TGF-β, IL-6 pathway that participates in the pro-inflammatory milieu. The molecular processes that damp down inflammation include the resolvin family of bioactive molecules, which have been much less evaluated in aging or age-related disease, but are important participants in effective and timely inflammation resolution.

Here, we will discuss some of the current ideas and highlight molecular pathways that appear to contribute to the immune imbalance and the cytokine dysregulation, which is associated with "inflamm-aging" or parainflammation. Evidence of these findings will be drawn from research in several age-related diseases, including cardiovascular and neurodegenerative disease, rheumatoid arthritis (RA), and cancers.

THE INFLAMMATION PATHWAY TO RESOLUTION

Inflammation is classically induced when innate cells detect infection or tissue injury. The pattern-recognition receptors (PRRs) on immune cells sense "danger" from protein-associated molecular patterns (PAMPs) associated with pathogens, or from danger-associated molecular patterns (DAMPs) triggered by a wide range of host-derived endogenous stress signals. DAMPs are molecules, such as ATP, the cytokine IL-1α, uric acid, and some cytoplasmic and nuclear proteins, which are released from damaged cells during necrosis and contribute to sterile inflammation (**Figure 1**). There have been suggestions that the extended IL-1 cytokine family (IL-1α, IL-1β, IL-18, IL-33, IL-36α, IL-36β, and IL-36γ) might also act as DAMPs and stimulate necrosis-initiated sterile inflammation, as well as amplify inflammation in response to infection-associated tissue injury (13).

Members of the toll-like receptor (TLR) family are the major PRRs. They are expressed on monocytes, macrophages, neutrophils, and dendritic cells, and on some lymphocytes and they respond rapidly to the "danger" response. The cyclooxygenase (COX) and 5-lipoxygenase (5-LOX) pathways of arachidonic acid (AA) metabolism (14, 15) produce highly pro-inflammatory lipid mediators responsible for the classical signs of inflammation—redness, heat, pain, swelling, and loss of function, with the aim of removing the injurious and noxious stimuli. A third pathway involves the cytochrome 450 pathway of AA metabolism and P450 epoxygenases and hydroxylases that produce both vasoconstrictor and vasodilatory effects in blood vessels and other tissues (**Figure 2**). The reactive biolipid molecules synthesized from AA are; the prostanoids—prostaglandins (PGs), prostacyclins, and thromboxanes produced by the action of COX 1 and 2 (COX 1 and 2); the leukotrienes (LTs), hydroxyeicosatetraenoids (HETEs), and lipoxins (LXs) produced by the action of the 5-, 12-, and 15-lypooxygenase (5/12/15-LOX) enzymes and; the P450 epoxygenase generates HETEs and depoxyeicosatrienoids (epoxides) (16). PGs act to amplify the inflammatory response through enhancing the inflammatory cytokine cascade, upregulating the innate response to DAMPs and PAMPs, activating subsets of T helper cells, recruiting macrophages associated with chronic inflammation, and increasing cytokine expression from cytokine inflammatory genes. Additional factors, such as histamine, pro-inflammatory cytokines, and chemokines amplify the response further and make the vascular endothelium increasingly leaky. The increase in vascular permeability combined with the expression of cellular adhesion molecules (i.e., selectins and integrins)

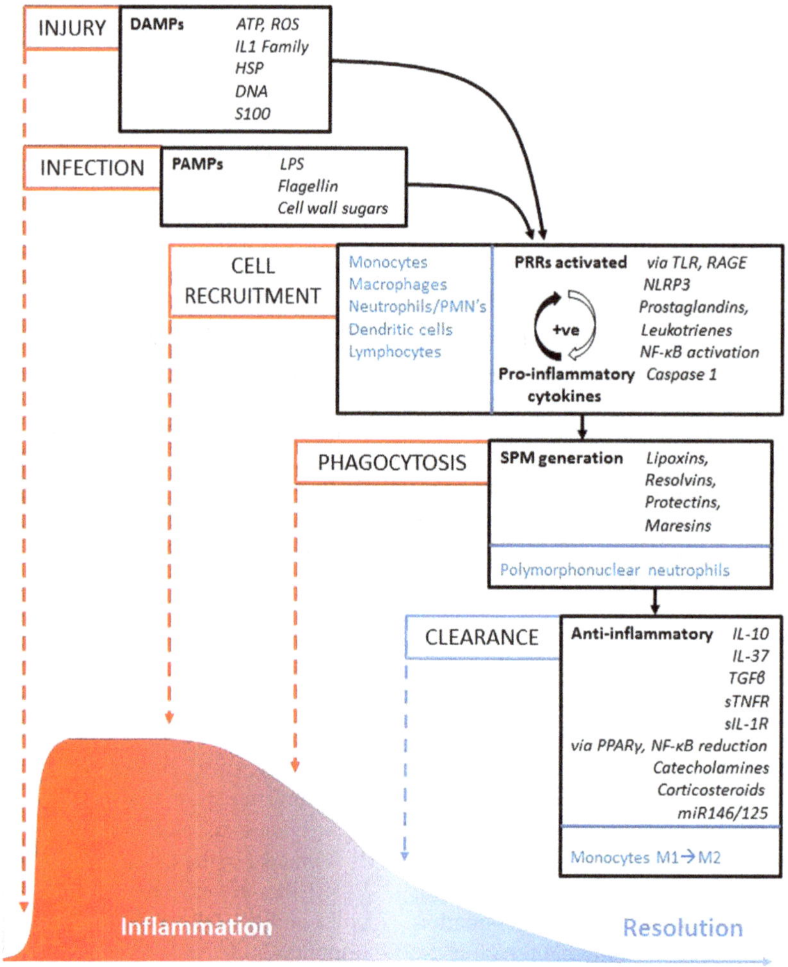

FIGURE 1 | Inflammation pathway to resolution. An illustration of the sequence of key processes (in capitalized text), cells and molecules involved in reaction to injury or infection, and how the inflammatory episode is resolved over time (from left to right). Cells from the innate and adaptive immune system that are involved in cell recruitment, phagocytosis, and clearance processes are highlighted in blue text; key molecules are in italic text.

allows neutrophils, the first responders, to transmigrate across post-capillary venules to the sites of injury or microbial invasion. Together this increases polymorphonuclear (PMN) neutrophil chemotaxis and allows PMNs to transmigrate along chemotactic gradients in order to maximize phagocytosis and killing of pathogens, and deal with the "danger" signal effectively.

As the acute inflammatory cascade develops to manage the "danger" signal, it is essential that a controlled resolution commences, so that immune homeostasis returns in an organized manner. If the inflammatory response does not shut down in a timely way, the inflammation cascade becomes chronic and smoldering. Lipid mediators derived from polyunsaturated fatty acids are now recognized to orchestrate the resolution of inflammation (17). At the peak of inflammation, the eicosanoids that initiated the inflammation undergo a class-switch so that they become the molecules that activate resolution, demonstrable through the clinical signs of removal of symptoms, relief of pain, restoration of function, regeneration of damaged tissues, and return to health. The so-called specialized pro-resolving mediators (SPMs) are key to resolving inflammation and include lipoxins derived from the 5-LOX arm of the AA pathway; the E-group of resolvins derived from dietary-derived eicosapentaenoic acid (EPA); the D-group of resolvins from dietary–derived docosahexaenoic acid (DHA); and protectins (PD), and maresins (MaR) (17–19) (**Figure 2**). The lipid class-switch starts early in inflammation and is initiated by lipoxins LXA4 and LXB4, and considered to be produced by platelets when they begin to aggregate with PMNs at the sites of inflammation (18).

After class-switching of the lipid molecules has occurred, SPMs are produced. Pro-resolving monocyte-derived macrophages begin to clear PMNs from the site of injury by a process called efferocytosis that removes apoptotic neutrophils, microbes, and necrotic debris. As resolution progresses, monocytes and macrophages, change from a pro-inflammatory (M1) to a pro-resolving phenotype (M2) by genetic and epigenetic reprogramming (20–22). Recent investigations suggest that SPMs, particularly the D-series resolvins (resolving D1 and resolving D2) and MaR 1 modulate adaptive immune responses in human peripheral blood

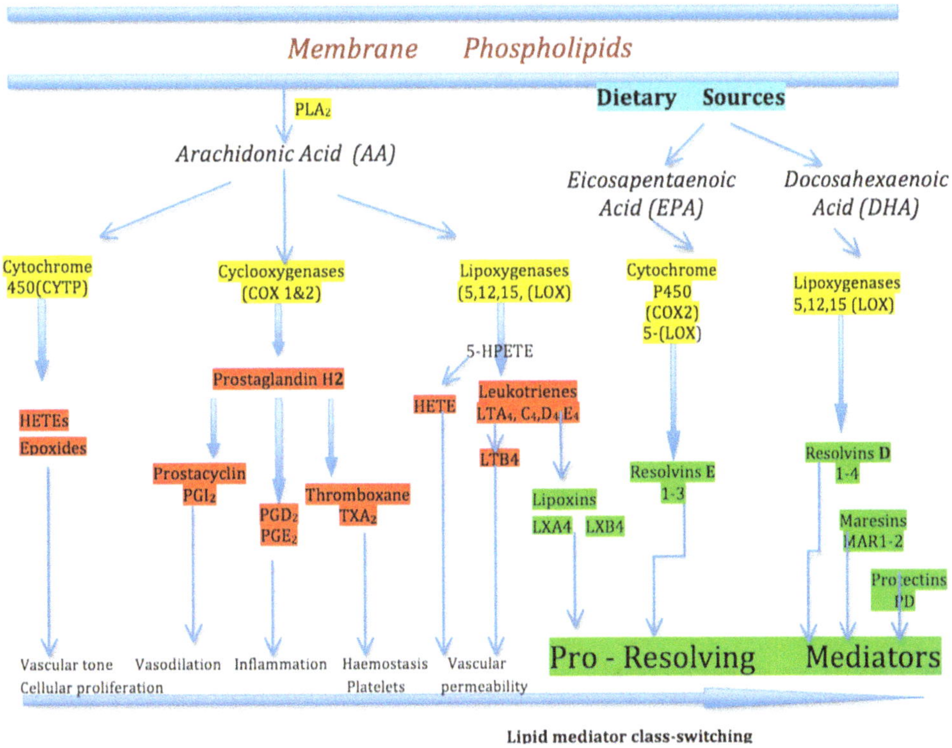

FIGURE 2 | The arachidonic acid (AA) pathway of inflammation mediators. In the simplified pathway for the eicosanoid metabolic pathway, AA is released from membrane stores by phospholipase 2 (PLA_2). AA is metabolized to biological mediators by three enzymatic pathways: cyclooxygenase, lipoxygenase, and cytochrome P450. Each pathway contains enzyme-specific steps that result in a wide variety of bioactive compounds that drive the pro-inflammatory (prostaglandins) response. After lipid mediator class-switching at the height of inflammation, the pro-resolving mediators-lipoxins begin to drive inflammation resolution. Eicosapentaenoic acid and docosahexaenoic acid-derived from dietary sources produce the E-series of resolvins and D-series of resolvins, maresins, and protectins, respectively, which are important pro-resolving mediators in progressing the resolution of inflammation.

lymphocytes. These lipid mediators reduce cytokine production by activated CD8+ T cells and CD4+ T helper 1 (TH1) and TH 17 cells, but do no modulate T cell inhibitory receptors or reduce their ability to proliferate (23, 24). Other reports show an increase in plasma cell differentiation and antibody production that supports the involvement of SPMs in the humoral response during late stages of inflammation and pathogen clearance (25). The anti-inflammatory cytokines interleukin 10 (IL-10), and IL-37 a member of the IL-1 family, together with TGF-β that is released from monocytes and platelets, are important contributors to damping down the inflammation. The soluble receptors, TNFR and IL-1 receptor (IL-1R) also limit inflammation in acting as decoy receptors, by binding to and neutralizing their respective cytokines, and inhibiting the biological activity. Additional anti-inflammatory mechanisms, include stress hormones, particularly corticosteroids and catecholamines and negative regulators, such as microRNAs—MiR-146 and MiR-125 (26).

The local environment and context also play an important role in the production and function of SPMs, which have both autocrine and paracrine actions. Inflammation resolution is likely to depend on prompt class-switching to pro-resolving lipid mediators, effective apoptosis, and efferocytic clearance of inflammatory cells and debris, timely damping down of pro-inflammatory signals and integrated repair of collateral damage. An imbalance between pro-inflammatory and pro-resolving mediators has been linked to a number of chronic inflammatory diseases (27).

In normal inflammation SPMs do not compromise host immune competence with examples of pro-resolving mediators increasing survival from infections in mouse models (28, 29). The common mechanism by which this occurs appears to be through suppression of the NF-κB activation in a partly PPAR-γ-dependent manner, with associated downstream signaling and alteration in transcriptomics pathways (30, 31). A maresin mediator has been shown to have potent anti-inflammatory and pro-resolving actions in a model of colitis, and attenuated inflammation in vascular smooth muscle and endothelial cells (32, 33). In human studies, the role of SPMs are being explored in chronic inflammatory diseases, such as RA (34), atherosclerosis (27), and cancer (35). In Alzheimer's disease, several SPMs promoted neuronal survival and β-amyloid uptake by microglia in "*in vitro*" models in Alzheimer's disease (36, 37). However, little is known about the pro-resolving mediators in aging itself. Studies are needed to assess whether pro-resolving molecules, such as E and D-resolvins, and maresins decrease or are less effective in damping down inflammation with increasing age and whether they could contribute to the pro-inflammatory phenotype associated with aging. Already synthetic analogs are in process of development, and so the design of pharmacological mimetics of naturally occurring pro-resolving mediators and their receptors offers new potential targets for drug design and the opportunity to investigate the underpinning molecular mechanisms of inflammation resolution.

Could life-style factors play a role in the epidemic of non-communicable and age-related diseases and the associated pro-inflammatory phenotype? Evidence exists that suggests that the Mediterranean diet which includes olive oil and some omega-3 lipids, can ameliorate RA (38), may give some protection from atrial fibrillation and myocardial infarction (MI) (39), and improves diabetic control (40). Research has also demonstrated a protective role of the Mediterranean diet in gene/Mediterranean diet interactions for the risk TT allele of the TCF7L2-rs7903146 gene in stroke risk and mortality (41, 42). Improving knowledge about how inflammation shuts down in a timely way is crucial to the understanding of how chronic inflammation contributes to aging and age-related diseases. Further studies are likely to be needed to advise if dietary modifications with omega-3 lipids or whether synthetic resolving mimetics are part of the answer.

TRIGGERS OF THE INFLAMMATION PATHWAY

Several common molecular pathways have been identified that seem to be associated with both aging and low-grade inflammation. These pathways trigger the inflammasome, stimulating NF-κB, and the IL-1β-mediated inflammatory cascade.

Age-Related Redox Imbalance

A redox imbalance has long been associated with aging and led to the development of the redox stress hypothesis of aging (43). Redox stress is caused by an imbalance between unregulated and overproduced reactive oxygen species (ROS) that are produced secondary to mitochondrial energy production, active immunological phagocytic processes, and the prostaglandin pathway through COX enzyme production. While ROS are important molecules regulating numerous physiological and pathological processes in the cell, there is now clear evidence that overproduction of ROS is involved in the development of a number of diseases, such as Alzheimer's disease, rheumatoid, and cardiovascular diseases. Increasing evidence supports the notion that low concentrations of ROS or "primary ROS" are involved in well controlled processes (44), where their effect on reactive target molecules can be reversible, suggesting that "primary" ROS acts as an important intracellular signaling molecule (45). In contrast, the very active OH ROS is less effectively controlled and forms the main damaging type of ROS that is able to react with many macromolecules, such as lipids, proteins, and nucleic acids. This results in DNA oxidation and cell membrane damage, which contributes to the burden of damaged molecules related to aging and age-related diseases.

Mitochondrial ROS

Mitochondria are highly efficient producers of energy, but in doing so they produce ROS. It is estimated that about 90% of intracellular ROS is generated in the mitochondria through the mitochondrial transport chain. The chain of electron flow is considered to leak prematurely between complexes 1, 11, and 111 leading to the formation of damaging oxidants like O_2^-. This ROS has been considered to cause damaging mutations in the mitochondrial genes with increasing age (43). With increasing age, mitochondrial function becomes sluggish and this compromises energy production, which in turn further contributes to mitochondrial dysfunction (46). A vicious cycle develops with age-reduced physical activity producing muscles that become weaker, are infiltrated with fat cells, and show less efficient mitochondria energy production (47). Ischemia and apoptosis can trigger O_2^-, and mitochondria themselves can be damaged by ROS production. Mitophagy, the removal of damaged mitochondria is also reduced as age increases (48). A reduced age-related capacity of the body's anti-oxidative defense systems to mop up free radicals also plays an important role in maintaining the inflammatory background of chronic inflammation (49).

The Nicotamide Adenine Dinucleotide Phosphate (NADPH) Pathway of ROS

One of the other main producers of ROS is the specialized enzyme group of the NADPH oxidases of the NOX family—(NOX1, NOX2, NOX3 NOX4, NOX5, DUOX1, and DUOX2). The NOX family or NADPH oxidases' generate O_2^- or H_2O_2 radicals by transferring electrons from cytoplasmic NADPH or the "NOX" catalytic subunit to molecular oxygen (50). The ROS produced by these enzymes has an essential function in neutrophils and macrophages as a mechanism for effective bacterial killing and host defense (51, 52). When the phagocytes sense an endogenous or exogenous danger signal, the NADPH-oxidase unit translocates to fuse with the plasma membrane to form the phagosome. This generates large amounts of highly reactive ROS called the phagocytic burst that is very effective in killing microbes, though phagosomal pH and ion concentration are also likely to be contributors.

Although NOX family of isoenzymes was initially associated with the ROS produced in phagocytes, other members of the NOX family are now known to be involved in a wide range of regulatory functions in many tissues and seem likely to play a role in aging and age-related diseases. Studies in the human vascular system suggest that NOX1, NOX2, and NOX5 promote endothelial dysfunction, inflammation, and apoptosis in the vessel walls, whereas NOX4 by contrast is vasoprotective, by increasing nitric oxide bioavailability (53). NOX enzymes, therefore, appear to play a role in vascular pathology as well as in the maintenance of normal physiological vascular function. Activation of NOX2 and NOX4 occurs in humans with atrial fibrillation and inhibition of NOX by angiotension converting enzyme inhibitor drugs or statins has proved helpful in preventing post-operative atrial fibrillation (54).

COX Pathways of ROS

The biolipids are highly reactive substances that contribute to both inflammation and healing and their pathways produce and use ROS signaling. The reaction that converts AA through COX2 into prostaglandin H2 (PGH_2) by a two-stage free radical mechanism (55) involves superoxide and can contribute to cellular oxidative stress as well as signaling. Other enzymes that generate ROS during AA metabolism include the arachidonic 12-lipoxygenase (LOX-12 or ALOX12) and arachidonic 5-lipoxygenase (LOX5 or ALOX5), both of which also activate and induce NADPH-oxidases (56).

While mitochondrial ROS are traditionally seen as the main source of intracellular ROS and, therefore, major mediators of ROS-induced damage, the relative contribution of mitochondrial and non-mitochondrial sources of ROS to induction of cellular senescence remain unclear. Both mitochondrial ROS and NADPH-produced ROS appear to be able to cross signal between each other and mitochondria have significant antioxidant capacity, which may act as a cellular redox buffer for NADPH-produced ROS, suggesting there is tight control and integration of ROS signaling within the cell.

The cellular systems that protect against ROS, include the anti-oxidative defense enzymes, superoxidase dismutase, glutathione peroxidase, and catalase (57), oxidant scavengers (vitamin E, vitamin C, carotenoids, uric acid, and polyphenols), and mechanisms to repair oxidant damage to lipids, proteins, or DNA. Despite these protective mechanisms, uncontrolled ROS can overwhelm the antioxidant capacity of the cell causing mitochondrial dysfunction (49). Increased ROS production from the various cellular sources stimulates intracellular danger-sensing multi-protein platforms called inflammasomes (58–60). Through the inflammasome, the ROS activates NF-κB which sets in motion the transcription of a cascade of pro-inflammatory cytokines—tumor necrosis factor-alpha (TNF-α), IL-1β, IL-2, and IL-6, chemokines—IL-8 and RANTES, and adhesion molecules, such as ICAM-1, VCAM, and E-selectin, that are central mediators in the inflammatory response.

Autophagy Slowing and Aging

Approximately a third of all newly synthesized proteins are formed in the endoplasmic reticulum (ER), where they are folded, modified, sorted, and transported to sites where they perform specialized roles. Stressors, such as low glucose as in fasting, alterations in calcium levels, low oxygen states, viruses, cytokines, and nutrient excess or deficiency can trigger the autophagy pathway with the aim of returning normal homeostasis to the cell.

Autophagy is a cellular process whereby cellular waste, such as modified proteins, protein aggregates, and damaged organelles are removed from the cell. It is a tightly controlled process that plays a role in growth and development and maintains a balance between the synthesis, degradation, and subsequent recycling of cellular products. Autophagy can be considered a protein and organelle quality control mechanism that maintains normal cellular homeostasis.

Two major pathways degrade cellular proteins. The ubiquitin-proteasome system (UPS) degrades 80–90% of denatured and damaged proteins. In the ATP-dependent UPS, damaged or misfolded proteins are tagged with a small protein called ubiquitin. Three different sets of enzymes—E1, E2, and E3, identify and categorize proteins in order to link ubiquitin or ubiquitin complexes to the damaged proteins. The ubiquitin-protein complexes pass through the proteasome, where they are degraded and discharged as free amino acids into the cytoplasm (**Figure 3A**).

The other main pathway is the autophagy system that degrades cystolic components, including larger aggregated proteins and cellular organelles, such as mitochondria, peroxisomes, and infectious organisms (61). This process involves membrane formation, fusion, and degradation (**Figure 3B**). When autophagy is induced, a small separate membrane structure called a phagophore arises in the cytoplasm, which gradually expands to form the autophagosome. The outer membrane of the autophagosome fuses with the lysosome and the autophagosome contents are degraded by lysosomal hydrolases (62). Like the proteasome, the macroautophagy system is stimulated by intracellular and extracellular stress-related signals, including oxidative stress. Both proteasome and autophagy produce small polypeptides that help maintain a pool of amino acids and control energy balance in starvation, since recycling amino acids is more energy efficient than *de novo* amino acid synthesis.

In aging and age-related disease there are gradual reductions of cellular repair mechanisms that lead to the accumulation of damaged molecules, proteins, DNA, and lipids leading to loss of efficient cellular function. The cell's capacity for autophagic degradation also declines with age and this in itself may contribute to the aging process (63). While both major systems for intracellular protein degradation are slowed up with increasing age, a physical reduction of autophagy-related proteins also contributes to the accumulation of misfolded proteins and damaged macromolecules in the cell. Diseases associated with increased oxidative stress, such as cardiovascular and Crohn's disease and obesity also slow up cellular clearing and reduce autophagy, further contributing to disease (64–66).

The lysosome–autophagy system carries out a wide range of non-specific intracellular degradation and cleaning processes, which include managing pathogens, damaged intra-cellular macromolecules, and surface receptors (67–69). Lysosomal dysfunction is associated with age-related pathology that reduce lifespan, such as Parkinson's and Alzheimer's diseases (70, 71). Senescent cells accumulate abnormal protein aggregates in the cytoplasm, and contribute to neurodegenerative disease (72).

The dysregulation in autophagy has important effects in the innate immune response, in aging and age-related diseases by influencing inflammasome activity, cytokine secretion, antigen presentation, and lymphocyte function (73, 74). Under normal circumstances the nod-like receptor 3 (NLRP3) inflammasome fine-tunes the progression of the innate immune response that it has initiated, by upregulating autophagy activity so that the removal of immune mediators is expedited (74). In aging and age-related diseases, the autophagy response becomes blunted, the immune mediators remain active and prolong the inflammatory response (75).

The UPS and autophagy act synergistically and cooperatively to maintain cellular homeostasis (76). Effective autophagic uptake of dysfunctional mitochondria and efficient lysosomal degradation of damaged aggregated proteins and macromolecules are crucial elements in maintaining tissue homeostasis and good health (77). The decline in the autophagy capacity, that impairs cellular housekeeping in aging, seems to be an

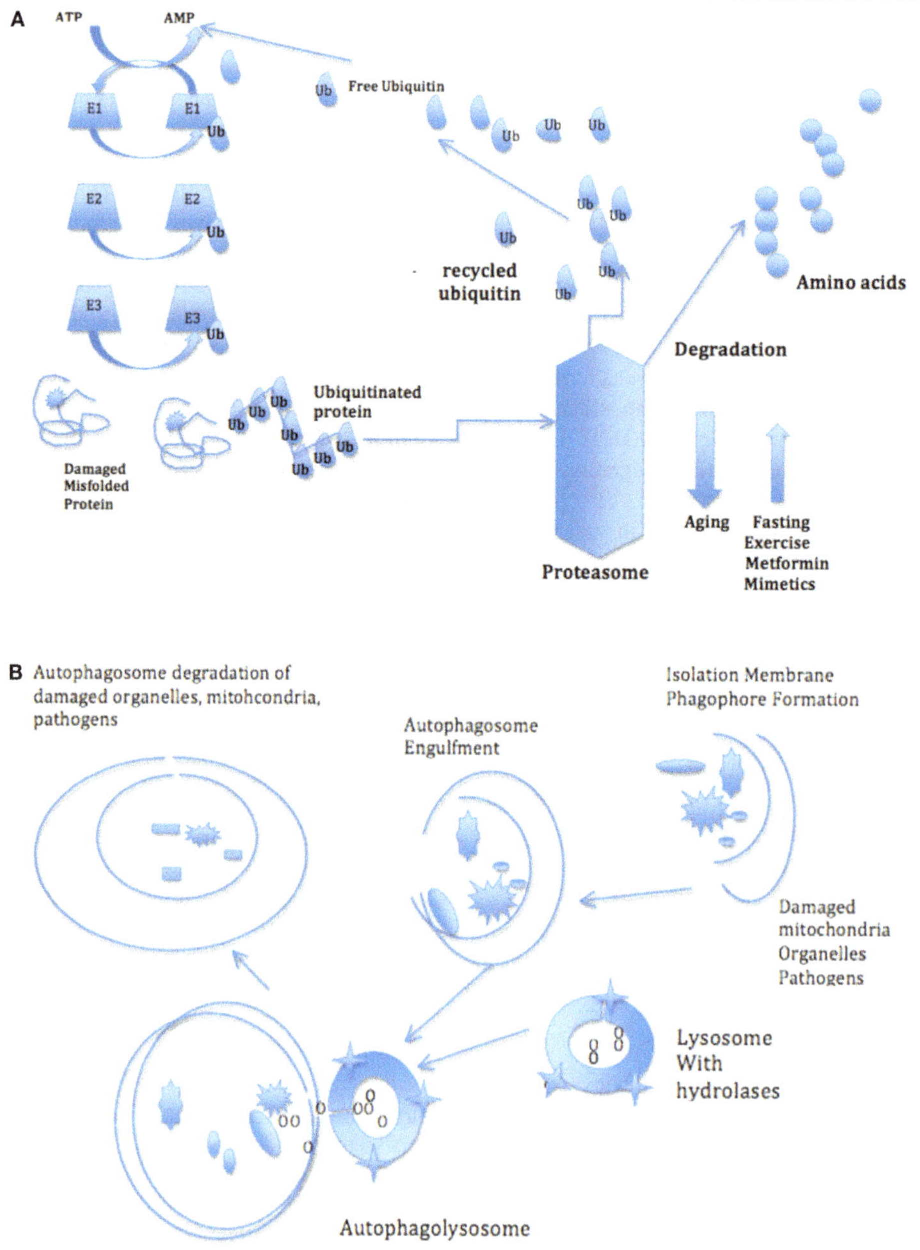

FIGURE 3 | (A) The ubiquitin–proteasome pathway of protein degradation. Three different sets of enzymes—E1, E2, and E3, identify and categorize proteins in order to link ubiquitin or ubiquitin complexes to the damaged proteins. The ubiquitin-protein complexes pass through the proteasome where they are degraded and discharged as free amino acids into the cytoplasm. **(B)** The autophagy pathway of degradation of damaged organelles and pathogens. The autophagy system degrades larger aggregated proteins and cellular organelles, such as mitochondria, peroxisomes, and infectious organisms. The process involves membrane formation, fusion, and degradation. A small separate membrane called a phagophore forms and then forms the autophagosome that fuses with the lysosome. The autophagosome contents are degraded by lysosomal hydrolases.

attractive molecular pathway to target to improve the quality of aging.

Two groups of drugs, the mammalian target of rapamycin (mTOR) inhibitors and AMP-activated protein kinase (AMPK) activators are promising pharmacological agents which stimulate autophagic degradation (78–80). Other drugs, such as the diabetic drug metformin and the oncology agent 5-aminimidazole-4-carboxamide ribonucleoside are pharmacological activators of AMPK, which are soon planned for clinical studies in relation to aging (81–83). A number of substances, such as curcumin, berberine, and quercetin, regularly available in normal diets, appear able to mimic the action of AMPK and upregulate autophagy. The action of AMPK has important anti-inflammatory and immunosuppressive effects (83). By upregulating autophagic activity, AMPK promotes effective clearing of DAMPs and by preventing the activation of the inflammasome, it reduces the triggering of the inflammatory cascade. Further evidence of the anti-inflammatory role comes from research with the AMPK agonist A-769662 that mimics AMPK activity (84). This AMPK mimetic has been shown to suppress inflammatory arthritis in mice and reduce IL-6 expression in serum and arthritic joints, suggesting that targeted AMPK activation could be an effective therapeutic strategy for IL-6-dependent inflammatory arthritis (85).

Non-pharmacological life-style changes also upregulate autophagy. One of the best researched is the effect of exercise which improves mitochondrial mitogenesis and stimulates mitogeny, so improving the quality of muscle function and exercise performance, with improvement in the quality of aging (86, 87). Furthermore in animal model studies, both modulated caloric restriction and exercise increase autophagy, downregulate endotoxin-induced IL-1β production, improve the aging-related pro-inflammatory profile, and reduce disease symptoms (78, 88).

Further understanding of molecular pathways of the signaling networks underpinning autophagy should help to identify other novel drug targets. Important research areas include those that could improve the sensitivity of degradation inhibitors useful to improve anticancer treatment, or new drugs to upregulate autophagy to maintain good cellular housekeeping, with the potential for improving the quality of aging and the management of age-related degenerative diseases.

Senescent Cells

Senescent cells increase with age and are considered important contributors to the pro-inflammatory phenotype (89). The two major hallmarks of cellular senescence are an irreversible arrest of cell proliferation and production of the pro-inflammatory secretome, called the SASP. When replicative senescence was first identified in serial cell passage studies (90), telomere attrition was considered to cause the cellular growth arrest that acted as a mechanism to stop damaged or transformed cells from proliferation and transiting to tumor initiation. Today senescence is considered to have much broader role as both a contributor to damage protection and in the control of cellular growth, or as both a "friend and foe" depending on the cellular context. Senescence together with apoptosis is recognized to play an important physiological role in normal embryonic development, in ongoing tissue homeostasis throughout life (91, 92), but is increasingly considered to have a role in causing or exacerbating aging and age-related diseases (91, 93–95).

Senescence is a stress response triggered not only by telomere attrition as originally described (90, 96), but also by stress insults, such as genomic instability, DNA damage, protein misfolding and/or aggregation, and ROS. There is also an association between senescent cells and the dysregulated mitochondrial network and associated metabolic dysfunction that is seen with increasing age (97). Through the SASP, the senescent cell has an important influence on the extrinsic microenvironment, which suggests a link between senescence and alterations in intracellular and intercellular communications (93).

Cells that express senescence markers accumulate with age in some tissues in studies in mice and man (98–100). Senescent cells are found in association with age-related diseases, such as atherosclerosis, RA, neurodegenerative diseases, and cancer (101–104). In RA patients T-cells are described as showing a pre-aged phenotype with apparent loss of CD28 expression that reduces T-cell activation and this in association with reduced RA-related NK surveillance, could allow senescent cells and the associated SASP to persist. In cancer, SASP factors promote angiogenesis, cell proliferation, and cancer invasiveness. Cells attracted by SASP influence the local microenvironment with the potential to promote tumor invasion and cancer progression (105). Senescent cells have been seen in atherosclerotic plaques (101). Recent data from several laboratories has suggested that both aging and age-related neurodegenerative diseases show an increase in SASP-expressing senescent cells of non-neuronal origin in the brain, which correlated with changes in neurodegeneration (103).

The SASP consists of a complex combination of growth factors, proteases, chemokines, matrix metalloproteinases, and is particularly enriched in pro-inflammatory cytokines, especially IL-6 (106–108). The SASP-secreting cells respond by switching on a self-perpetuating intracellular pro-inflammatory signaling loop, centered around the NF-κB, TGF-β, IL-1α, IL-6 pathway (109–111), with suggested mechanisms related to higher basal phosphorylation and altered threshold signaling (112) or alternative splicing (113). Senescent cells influence other cells by paracrine and bye-stander effects (114). There appears to be multi-level control of senescence and the SASP secretome, which includes the tumor suppressor pathways involved in the cell cycle arrest and the NF-κB and persistent damage response (DAMP) pathway, involved in triggering transcription of the SASP-related factors (115). Several pathways of investigation suggest that senescent primary human CD8+ T cells use anaerobic glycolysis to generate energy for effector functions and that p38 mitogen-activated protein kinase (p38 MAPK) blockade may reverse senescence *via* the mTOR-independent pathway (116). Low doses of glucocorticoid suppress elements of the SASP in patients with RA and improve clinical symptoms (117). Senescent cells effectively recruit the immune system to organize their removal, but with increasing age, removal becomes sluggish or otherwise impaired (118, 119).

It can be argued that the increase in senescent cells with aging reflects either an increase in their rate of generation or a decrease in their rate of clearance because the immune response is attenuated or weakened with aging and less capable of clearing senescent cells (120–122). Senescent cells express ligands for cytotoxic immune cells, such as natural killer (NK) cells, and have been shown to be able to be specifically eliminated by the immune system (123, 124). Through a proteomics analysis of senescent cell chromatin, the NF-κB pathway appeared to act as a master regulator of the SASP, with NF-κB suppression causing escape from immune recognition by NK cells (125). Other studies show that processes which eliminate senescent cells with p16(Ink4a)-positive markers, delay age-related pathologies in the mouse model of aging though side-effects can be problematical (126, 127). Therapies that specifically recognize and trigger the elimination of senescent cells would seem important to enhance the immune system in older people. New methods are in the process of being developed to enhance the immune clearance and autophagy of the increased senescent cell burden in aging and age-related disease (128).

Inflammasome NLRP3

The inflammasomes, intra-cellular multiprotein sensors that recognize danger signals, are likely key players in initiating and maintaining the pro-inflammatory phenotype found associated with aging. The NLRP3 is a major inflammasome sensor for intracellular stress molecules called DAMPs, which together with damaged aggregated proteins that are released from destabilized lysosomes and damaged mitochondria contribute to the cellular stress (ROS) and trigger NLRP3 activation (129). Once activated, the NLRP3 inflammasome initiates the inflammatory response cascade by stimulating caspase-1 (casp-1) that acts to induce the active precursors of pro-inflammatory cytokines, such as IL-1β, IL-1α, and IL-18, and on-going interaction with NF-κB (130, 131) (**Figure 4**). Although the baseline activity of NLRP3 is low, the initiation process of the inflammatory cascade requires a complex oligomerization-priming phase that includes association with NF-κB and so contributes several layers of regulatory control.

Nod-like receptor 3 has been shown to be able to activate NF-κB and induce cytokines in response to sterile signals, such as monosodium urate crystals and aluminum adjuvant, suggesting that NLRP3 could initiate NF-κB activation to both pathogen-induced and sterile inflammation (132). Conversely NF-κB, which primes the NLPR3 inflammasome for activation also prevents excessive inflammation and restrains NLRP3 activation by enhancing the NF-κB-p62 mitophagy pathway. By self-limiting the host response, the NF-κB-p62 mitophagy pathway maintains homeostasis which under normal conditions leads to tissue repair (75). It is, however, unclear if this layer of control of NF-κB function remains as tightly controlled in aging and age-related disease.

The NLRP3 inflammasome is a key component of the innate inflammatory response to pathogenic infection and tissue damage. It responds to a wide range of cellular stress and is considered to contribute to the aging process and to age-related diseases (133). Zhou and colleagues identified that mitochondrial ROS was involved in the activation of NLRP3 (58). This study emphasized the important role of mitochondria in maintaining a correct balance between cellular energy production and ROS production and that effective clearance of damaged mitochondria through autophagy was an important regulatory activity. Damaged mitochondria increase with aging and age-related diseases (134). Mitochondrial dysfunction drives mitochondrial mutagenesis, affecting respiratory chain genes, and compromising the efficiency of oxidative phosphorylation, which may lead to further mt-DNA mutations and more cell damage. The subsequent mitochondrial impairment leads to more ROS that further reduce ATP generation and increases the chance of cell death. Mitochondria have been identified as a key source of DAMPs, the so-called mito-DAMPs, which have been considered to play a role in DAMPS-modulated inflammation in diseases, such as RA, cancer, and heart disease (135–138) as well as in the aging process (139). Degraded mt-DNA has also been reported in neuroinflammation (140). Dysfunctional mitochondria seem to be able to initiate an auto-feedback loop to increase autophagy, so that damaged mitochondria or misfolded proteins are degraded which reduces inflammasome activation and risk of further tissue injury, though this system is less efficient in aging (141).

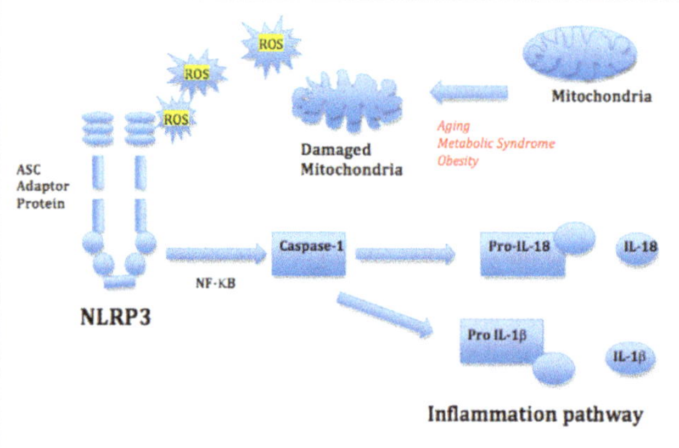

FIGURE 4 | Mitochondrial reactive oxygen species (ROS) and nod-like receptor 3 (NLRP3) activation of inflammation pathway. Mitochondrial ROS from damaged mitochondria triggers the inflammasome NLRP3, stimulating NF-κB and the IL-1β and IL-18-mediated inflammatory cascade. The adapter protein ASC mediates innate signaling by bridging the interaction between the damage recognition receptor and the NF-κB caspase-1 inflammasome complex.

Lysosomal destabilization is also associated with NLRP3 activation and can be induced by a number of molecules, including cholesterol crystals in macrophages linking atherosclerosis progression with inflammation (142). There is deposition of other harmful intra- and extracellular material in several age-related diseases. The aggregates compromise cellular homeostasis and can provoke the activation of the NLRP3 inflammasome. Research has shown that amyloid fibrils and Alzheimer's amyloid-β can trigger NLRP3 inflammasomes and in that way stimulate inflammation and enhance pathogenesis and association between type 2 diabetes and Alzheimer's disease, respectively (143). Palmitate, a saturated fatty acid has been shown to activate NLPR3, whereas oleic acid did not initiate the same inflammatory response (144). The inflammasome has been implicated in the development of the metabolic syndrome through impairment of adipose tissue sensitivity. Evidence showed that obesity triggered NLRP3 activation, and that the secreted IL-1β impaired insulin signaling which promoted insulin resistance in mice (145). Other research has shown that obesity was associated with the activation of the NLRP3 in adipose tissues (146, 147).

A number of intracellular processes seem likely to work together to stimulate and augment the inflammasome pathway and contribute to pro-inflammatory cytokine upregulation associated with increased age and age-related diseases. Both the redox-sensitive inflammatory pathway and the senescent cell-related SASP activate the inflammasome through the NF-κB and IL-α cascade, causing persistence of the inflammatory response that delays resolution and healing (125, 138). Similarly, reduced autophagy processes allow the accumulation of damaged intracellular proteins and senescent cells that further perpetuate and amplify the pro-inflammatory milieu that is found with increased age and is associated with age-related diseases.

PRO-INFLAMMATORY AND ANTI-INFLAMMATORY CYTOKINE DYSREGULATION

Pro-Inflammatory Cytokines in Aging and Age-Related Disease

Various biomarkers and biochemical indices are used in medicine and age-related diseases as a way of improving diagnosis, beyond the well-recognized clinical signs. Modest increases in concentration of C-reactive protein, a circulating marker of inflammation, have been widely reported to be associated with a large number of age-related conditions and lifestyles felt to be associated with poor health; these conditions represent or reflect minor metabolic stresses. Alongside C-reactive proteins, cytokines have come under investigation as the molecular processes and pathways underpinning inflammation have become better identified. A common finding in aging and age-related diseases is "inflamm-aging," a dysregulation of the cytokine network and its homeostasis. Downstream from NF-κB signaling, the pro-inflammatory cytokines play a central role in the remodeling of the immune system with age (**Figure 5**).

The major pro-inflammatory cytokines, such as IL-6, TNF-α, and IL-1α contribute significantly to the phenomenon of inflamm-aging in healthy elderly individuals (8), while also playing a major role in many age-related diseases (11, 27, 148–151). The key to healthy aging must lie in the ability to maintain a balanced response to these immune messengers and a prompt and integrated return to inflammation resolution and immune homeostasis (17). A summary of the changes that have been described in pro-inflammatory and anti-inflammatory cytokines in aging and some age-related diseases are outlined in this section.

Interleukin-1 (IL-1) Family

IL-1α and IL-1β, known as IL-1, and IL-18 are important cytokine initiators of the stress-induced inflammatory cascade (152). IL-1β and IL-18 are cleaved to active forms by Casp-1, whereas IL-1α is activated by calpain protease. All bind to and activate the IL-1R that is downregulated by the receptor anatagonist IL-1Rα, which blocks IL-1-mediated signal transduction.

Studies in elderly people, including centenarians have reported an age-related rise in the IL-1R antagonist, (IL-1Rα), whereas IL-1β showed no detectable age-related trend. The age-related rise is associated with increased co-morbidity, age-related disease, and mortality (153–156).

Certain IL-1 haplotype-carriers produce increased IL-1β, and IL-1 gene variations associate with earlier onset or more severe progression of cardiovascular and Alzheimer's disease, but not with osteoporosis (157–161). In centenarians, no single IL-1 gene polymorphism showed a survival advantage, but in Swedish elderly males an IL-1 gene polymorphism shortened life expectancy (153, 162, 163). IL-1 gene variants appear to increase the risk of age-related diseases and recombinant drugs, such as IL-1Rα-blockers may have a role in the clinical control of inflammation (164).

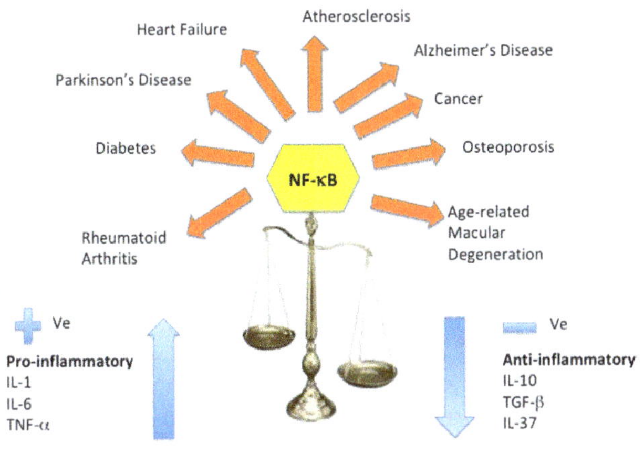

FIGURE 5 | Cytokine dysregulation and NF-κB inflammation pathway. This reshaping of cytokine expression pattern with a progressive tendency toward a pro-inflammatory phenotype has been called "inflamm-aging" and is found associated with age-related diseases. Several molecular pathways have been identified that trigger the inflammasome and stimulate the NF-κB and the IL-1β-mediated inflammatory cascade of cytokines.

Interleukin-18 (IL-18)

Interleukin-18, a linked IL-1 pro-inflammatory cytokine, signals in a complex with IL-18 receptors α (Rα) and β (Rβ) chains and induces IFN-γ that is essential for defense against infections (165). IL-18's multiple pro-inflammatory effects are modulated through IL-18 binding protein (166).

Higher levels of IL-18 have been found in centenarians, associated with heart failure, ischemic heart disease, and type 1 diabetes in patients, and in the Alzheimer's disease brain (167–172). IL-18 levels associate with physical functioning and with a frailty index in the English longitudinal study of aging, where carriers of IL-18 gene polymorphism that reduced IL-18 levels, showed improved walking speed (173–175). Evidence consistently shows that IL-1 and IL-18 are mediators of inflammation and associated with the aging process (168). Drugs blocking binding between IL-18 and the receptors are currently in development and may provide benefit in the treatment in diabetes, macular degeneration, and autoimmune disease (176).

Interleukin-6 (IL-6)

Interleukin-6 has been long recognized as important in aging and age-related disease and has been called the "gerontologist's cytokine" (177, 178). IL-6 plays a key role in the acute phase response, in the transition from innate to acquired immunity, in metabolic control, and in the pathogenesis many chronic diseases (11, 148–151, 179). It has both pro- and anti-inflammatory activities, and modulates the acute inflammatory response by producing IL-1 Rα and soluble tumor necrosis factor receptor p55 (sTNF-R55), which suppresses TNF-α and IL-1.

Interleukin-6 is normally present in low levels in the blood, but is increased in aging and in subjects with markers of frailty and chronic disease, where it tracks with mortality (180–183). IL-6 is a risk factor associated with cardiovascular disease and is associated with sarcopenia and muscle loss (184, 185).

The G allele of IL-6-174C/G polymorphism shows higher IL-6 levels and associates with cognitive decline and mortality in age-related vascular disease, whereas CC allele carriers show decreased

Alzheimer's risk (186–191). In a meta-analysis of longevity in a large cohort of European nonagenarians and centenarians there was longevity benefit for carriers of the lower cytokine producing IL-6 allele, with similar supporting findings for this IL-6 allele in a case control study (192, 193). IL-6 or IL-6 receptor blockers are already used successfully in the treatment of RA, and are proof of concept that damping down IL-6, a product of the NF-κB pro-inflammatory cascade, can improve clinical symptoms. Studies are either in progress or planned to assess the outcome of blocking IL-6-related inflammation in other age-related diseases with the potential for contributing to more successful aging (194, 195).

Tumor Necrosis Factor Alpha

Another major player in the immune response is the pro-inflammatory cytokine TNF-α, which increases with age and is associated with age-related disease (196). It is a pro-inflammatory mediator that can be beneficial when it acts locally in the tissues, but can be highly harmful when released systemically.

Tumor necrosis factor-α has been reported to be increased in intracellular aging studies in elderly people, in centenarians and octogenarians with atherosclerosis, and associated with mortality (197–202). In post-MI patients, a rise in TNF-α increased risk of recurrent cardiac events and in renal patients TNF-α receptors predicted cardiovascular disease (203–205). In genetic studies, the A allele of TNF-α 308 G/A gene associated with risk for MI, whereas TNF-α polymorphisms and TNF-α itself, have been variably associated with increased Alzheimer's disease risk (206–210). TNF-α mediates metabolic changes and increased TNF-α was found in type 2 diabetes mellitus and was associated with lower muscle mass and strength in older groups (211).

In studies in nonagenarian/centenarian groups from three European countries, there was no attrition of the TNF-α-308 A/G polymorphism in centenarians (162, 212, 213). With increasing evidence of an association between increases in TNF-α and age-related diseases, research re-purposing anti-inflammatory drugs are under development. Research has demonstrated that TNF-α inhibitors may have possible prophylactic or ameliorating roles in cardiovascular and Alzheimer's disease in animal models (214, 215).

Other Pro-Inflammatory Cytokines

Other pro-inflammatory cytokines are increasingly being recognized as dysregulated in association with aging and age-related disease.

Interleukin-2

Interleukin-2 plays a pivotal role in the immune response. It is a growth factor that promotes NK cell activity and the differentiation of naïve T cells into Th1 and Th2 cells (216). Conversely, IL-2, acting *via* STAT5 pathway negatively regulates interleukin 17 (IL-17) production (217). Most studies show that lymphocytes in elderly people produce significantly less IL-2, compared to young people (218–220). Intracellular cytokine studies have shown variable results for IL-2, whereas mitogen-induced stimulation of mononuclear cells from elderly subjects showed significant decreases in IL-2 and IFNγ production (197, 221).

The IL-7/IL-7R

The IL-7/IL-7R network is essential at various stages in T-cell development and survival (222). It has an important role in the maintenance of a vigorous health span and higher IL7R gene expression is associated with long life (223–225). Serum IL-7 is increased in some age-related diseases, including osteoarthritis and genetic variation in the IL7RA/IL7 pathway increased susceptibility to multiple sclerosis (226, 227). Research has suggested that silencing of the IL-7R gene may be an important mechanism underpinning an aging-related loss of binding to NK-κB (228), linking IL-7R gene to the NF-κB pathway and inflammation control.

Interleukin-12

Interleukin-12, a pro-inflammatory member of the IL-6 family has an active role in the development of cardiovascular diseases, such as atherosclerosis, MI, and stroke (229). Patients with cardiovascular disease show increased levels of IL-12, 23, and 27 with higher IL-12 predicting poorer long-term outcome after acute MI (230). Other research shows variable results for IL-12 and its receptor antagonist, with increased IL-12 (total) and IL-12p40 in apparently healthy nonagenarians, lower IL-12p70 and IL-23 production in association with frailty and IL-12/23p40 ameliorating Alzheimer's disease in animal models (231–233).

Interleukin 17

Interleukin 17 is a key pro-inflammatory cytokine that belongs to a family of six cytokine members (A–F). IL-17A (referred to as IL-17) plays a central role in host defense against invading pathogens and is produced by a subset of CD4+ cells (234, 235). Elderly people (age ≥65) have shown a decreased frequency of IL-17-producing cells in memory subset of CD4+ T cells compared to healthy younger people (236). IL-17 enhances production of IL-6, TNF-α, the acute phase reactants, C-reactive protein, and serum amyloid A and activates the induction of IL-6, IL-8, and G-CSF in non-immune cells, such as fibroblasts and epithelial cells, in part through activation of the NF-κB transcription factor (237). IL-17 promotes inflammation and is overexpressed in many autoimmune diseases, such as RA, systemic lupus erythematosus, inflammatory bowel disease, and psoriasis and its effects are stabilized by IL-23 (238–241). An IL-17 expressing CD8+ T subset of cells has also been reported to be involved in psoriatic arthritis and some other autoimmune diseases (242, 243).

Interleukin-8

Interleukin-8 (or CXCL8) is a chemokine secreted by monocyte/macrophages whose key role in the inflammation process is the recruitment and activation of neutrophils. IL-8 has been implicated in a number of inflammatory conditions, such as cystic fibrosis, asthma, chronic pulmonary disease, inflammatory bowel disease, and some autoimmune diseases, including RA and psoriasis.

Increased levels of IL-8 have been detected after LPS-stimulation of leukocytes from elderly individuals (244). In one small study of centenarians, IL-8 was proposed as a possible longevity factor (245). A single study of IL-8 polymorphisms found no significant difference in IL-8 -251 A/T polymorphisms in nonagenarians compared to young controls (212). IL-8 signaling occurs *via* the MAPK and PI3K pathways, by binding to the IL-8 receptors-CXCR1/2. Several agents that block IL-8-CXCR1/2 signaling have been developed in an attempt to target inflammatory pathways in cancer, asthma, chronic obstructive pulmonary disease, psoriasis, and RA (246).

Anti-Inflammatory Cytokines in Aging and Age-Related Disease

The anti-inflammatory cytokines play a key role in balancing the immune response, and in preventing the tipping of the steady state of immune homeostasis across into inflamm-aging and a disease-inducing state. Anti-inflammatory cytokines are an important arm of inflammation resolution. They block or modulate the synthesis of IL-1α, TNF, and other major pro-inflammatory cytokines and damp down the inflammatory response, so that inflammation resolution can begin. Specific cytokine receptors for IL-1, TNF-α, and IL-18, together with soluble receptor antagonists, chemokines, microRNA, siRNAs, also function as inhibitors for pro-inflammatory cytokines. The anti-inflammatory cytokines and families of soluble receptor antagonists work within a complex network of control of immune regulation. They are critical for balancing the inflammatory outcome and together with pro-resolving lipoxins are critical to resolving inflammation in an integrated and organized manner.

As age increases and in age-related diseases, a chronic inflammatory state predominates, which is not properly contained or resolved and the anti-inflammatory side of the immune system seems to be similarly dysregulated, and unable to damp down the inflammatory episode in a timely effective manner. The following cytokines are the major players in the anti-inflammatory pathway of the control of inflammation and changes in their production and expression have been quite widely reported in aging and age-related disease. Where increases in anti-inflammatory cytokines have been reported, one interpretation would be that increases might reflect the immune system's attempt to suppress the persistent pro-inflammatory response and support a return to immune homeostasis.

IL-10 Family

Interleukin 10 is one of the key anti-inflammatory cytokines, which suppresses the actions of IL-6, TNF-α, and IL-8 (247, 248). Higher IL-10 serum levels and production by both lymphocytes and monocytes have been reported in elderly people (155, 244, 249). Conversely an age and gender-related decline in cellular stimulation studies has been reported (250).

In age-related disease, IL-10 has been reported to be associated with vascular protection in atherosclerosis and improved endothelial dysfunction (251–253). However, at variance, the authors from the ERA (254) and PROSPER (255) studies, concluded that elevated IL-10 increased cardiovascular risk among elderly groups, and suggested that IL-10 blockers merited investigation. In male Sicilian centenarians, male carriers of the high producing GG 1,082 allele of the IL-10 promoter polymorphism showed a survival advantage, suggesting that IL-10 anti-inflammatory activities might be a marker for male longevity (213). This result was not replicated in Sardinian, Irish, or Finnish nonagenarian/centenarians (162, 212, 256). It has been argued that an enhanced anti-inflammatory phenotype could be beneficial and contribute to longevity by controlling the pro-inflammatory milieu that predominates in later life and contributes to increased morbidity and mortality (9, 11, 257).

TGF-β

TGF-β, another important anti-inflammatory cytokine limits both the acute phase response, and is involved in tissue repair post-damage or infection (258). Several authors have reported that TGF-β was increased in octogenarians and centenarians (148, 259). It is also involved in aging-related disease, such as in obesity, in vascular wall integrity, in muscle loss and sarcopenia, in osteoarthritis, and with frailty in the Newcastle longitudinal study (260–264). In stroke, TGF-β signaling was increased in microglia and macrophages suggesting that increased TGF-β likely regulated glial scar formation (265). Reports have linked TGF-β or its polymorphisms with atherosclerosis and Alzheimer's disease (266–268). Other research found TGF-β genotypes associated with longevity in Italian centenarians, a finding not replicated in BELFAST nonagenarians (212, 269). Context-specific environmental factors, epigenetic regulation, and non-coding RNAs are suggested to play a role in TGF-β's paradoxical pro-and anti-inflammatory functions (7, 270, 271), but important uses have been found for TGF-β in fibrosis management and oncology (272).

Interleukin-37

Interleukin-37, formerly an IL-1 cytokine, limits innate inflammation *via* suppression of pro-inflammatory cytokine production (273). Carriage of an IL-37 haplotype that decreases IL-37 levels contributes to increased inflammation. Research demonstrates that IL-37 reduces TNF-α and IL-1β cytokine production from human macrophages, is increased in chronic heart failure patients and attenuated the production of inflammatory cytokines in serum or synovial joints in RA, suggesting IL-37 may have a role in clinical disease (274–276).

AGE-RELATED DISEASES

Cancer

Cancer increases with aging, with one in two people likely to develop malignant tumors in their lifetime. Probable reasons for this age-related increase include exposure to environmental toxins, declining immune surveillance, and increasingly ineffective DNA repair mechanisms. Inflammation is involved at different stages of tumor development, at initiation, promotion, malignant conversion, invasion, and metastasis, has a paracrine bystander role and is an essential part of the tumor micro-environment. Inflammation also affects immune surveillance and responses to therapy (277). Thus, malignancy is a major threat to successful aging.

While inflammatory pathways are vital to promote immune homeostasis, over-activation or dysregulation can be pathological and lead to malignant progression. Prolonged inflammation, either as a result of chronic infections, or reduced homeostasis in the inflammatory response, plays a role through the production of pro-inflammatory cytokines that may be directly or indirectly implicated in the oncogenesis (278, 279). More recent investigations have focused on the role of the inflammasone pathway, whose biochemical function is to activate casp-1, which leads to the activation of the IL-1β and IL-18 pathways and induction of pyroptosis, a form of cell death. Although inflammasomes have an important role in inhibiting cancer, through the triggering of the programmed-death pathway, they both initiate and maintain carcinogenesis, dependent on tumor type and the tumor environment (280, 281).

Bacterial and viral infections are associated with malignancies. For example, *Helicobacter pylori* (*H. pylori*) infection of the gut is associated with both gastric cancer and mucosa-associated lymphoid tissue (MALT) lymphoma (282). Epstein–Barr virus (EBV) is a causative agent in Hodgkin's disease (HD), where chronic inflammation is considered a major contributory factor (283), human papilloma virus is implicated in most cases of cervical cancer (284), while human T-lymphotrophic virus 1 (HTLV-1) is a causative agent in adult T-cell leukemia lymphoma (285). A common factor is the association of infection with oncogenesis, with chronic inflammation a contributory factor.

In *H. pylori* chronic infection, elevated levels of IL-1β are detected and recognized as important in the development of gastric carcinoma. Normally gastric acid in the stomach does not permit bacterial survival, but in circumstances of low stomach acidity, *H. pylori* grow vigorously in the mucosa and induces caspase-mediated cleavage of pro-IL-1β and pro-IL-18 in association with the NLRP3 inflammasome. The overexpression of IL-1β induces NF-κB activation and the transcription and expression of IL-6, TNF-α, and IL-10. The proinflammatory cytokine milieu increases the risk for developing both gastric carcinoma and MALT lymphoma (286). Persistently high levels of IL-1β and IL-18 suppress acid secretion, allow hypoacidity in the stomach, loss of parietal cells, gastric atrophy, metaplasia, and eventually gastric cancer. In addition, IL-1β inhibits gastric acid secretion and carriers of IL-1β polymorphisms producing higher IL-1β carry increased gastric cancer risk (287, 288). *H. pylori* infection of gastric mucosa can cause a monoclonal B cell proliferation, with a histological diagnosis of MALT lymphoma. This tumor-like proliferation of gastric mucosal cells and clonal B cells can regress after eradication of the *H. pylori* infection with combined antibiotic therapy and proton pump inhibitor treatment (289).

Viral infections strongly stimulate inflammatory responses and may lead to malignant transformation of the host cell (290). Although the activation of the inflammasome benefits the clearance of viruses and the regression of cancer, there are several examples of viruses, such as EBV and HTLV-1 developing strategies to evade detection, triggering the inflammasome, and high-jacking the inflammatory cascade to induce, and amplify the cancer spread. For example, when EBV infects B-lymphocytes and nasopharyngeal cells through its receptor CD21 (291), this leads to a proliferation of infected B cells, followed by an increase in CD8+ T cells, that controls the infected cells by lysis. However, where the normal infection-limiting response is "exhausted" or dysregulated, B cell proliferation continues unabated leading to chromosomal damage, which drives cell proliferation outside normal control mechanisms and may result in an aggressive non-Hodgkin's or Burkitt's lymphoma (292). NLRP3 activation has been demonstrated in EBV-associated cancerous tissues (293). Furthermore, EBV has been shown to be able to overcome the immune response by means of EBV miRNA binding to the 3′-untranslated region of NLRP3 (294), so preventing effective immune activation and control mechanisms.

Retro-viruses stimulate inflammatory responses and are associated with malignant transformation of host cells. They reverse transcribe their RNA into the host cell's DNA, leading to dysregulation of cellular proliferation and programmed cell death responses, and elicit a pro-inflammatory response. HTLV-1 causes adult T-cell leukemia by targeting CD4+ T cells that express CD25 (IL-2Rα) and FoxP3, similar to Tregs (295, 296). The persistent activation of the NF-κB pathway in HTLV-1-infected T cells and the associated NF-κB oncoprotein Tax contribute to the oncogenic transformation (297). The resulting hijacking of the NF-κB pathway, allows uncontrolled upregulation of cellular genes that govern growth-signal transduction, amplify the pro-inflammatory cytokines (IL-2, IL-6, IL-15, TNF), together with increasing expression of proto-oncogenes (c-Myc), and antiapoptotic proteins (bcl-xl) Hiscott Rayet (298, 299). Inter-individual susceptibility to HTLV-1 infection has been associated with allele carrier status of the NLRP3 gene (300).

In summary, the interaction of infective agents, host cells, adaptive immune cells, cytokine production, and the inflammasome response is complex and incompletely understood. Many cancers arise from sites of infection, chronic irritation, and inflammation, which although sometimes reversible in the pre-malignant phase by eradicating the causative virus or bacterium, often treatments are too delayed to prevent the cancer development. There needs to be improved understanding about the roles of inflammation, the inflammatory cells, and the paracrine effects that allow tumor cell proliferation, survival, and migration. Does the pro-inflammatory environment found in aging enhance and facilitate cancer cell proliferation or does it alternatively represent an upregulated immune surveillance mechanism to deal with increased damaged and dangerous cancer cells? Improved understanding of the pathways involved should begin to provide insights that could contribute to new anticancer and anti-inflammatory therapeutic approaches through manipulation of autophagy for cancer treatment regimes or conversely tagging cancer cells for destruction through proteasome or autophagy upregulation (301).

Rheumatoid Arthritis

Chronic tissue inflammation has an important role in the etiology and immunopathogenesis of RA (302), with genetic and environmental factors contributing to a predilection to develop the disease. In the *pre-clinical* asymptomatic phase of RA disease, the immune system is characterized by reduced self-tolerance and production of autoantibodies, whereas in the *clinical* phase (303) innate and adaptive immune cells infiltrate the synovial joints and produce symptoms of joint pain and stiffness (304, 305). As RA progresses, immune cells and synovial fibroblasts produce a pro-inflammatory environment in the joint (306, 307) leading to joint destruction (302). Cell-specific cytokines, include TNF-α, IL-1, and IL-6 from macrophages, IL-6, IL-7, and IL-15 from memory T-cells, IL-1 and IL-17 from helper T-cells, and IL-1, IL-6, IL-18, GM-CSF, and TGF-β from synovial fibroblasts (303, 308). This complex cytokine milieu attracts further immune cells, promotes abnormal angiogenesis and osteoclastogenesis, poorly formed leaky vasculature and leads to systemic effects (309).

There is evidence to suggest that activation of the NLRP3-inflammasome contributes to the inflammatory processes in RA. Active RA subjects have increased expression of NLRP3 and NLRP3-mediated IL-18 secretion in whole blood upon stimulation *via* TLR3 and TLR4, but not TLR2 receptors (310, 311). Functional polymorphisms in the genes coding for NLRP3 and its component parts, including CARD8 has been shown to contribute to higher disease activity at diagnosis and for response in the early months of treatment (312, 313).

Patients with RA show premature immune aging and accumulation of $CD28^-$ pre-aged effector T cells that associate with disease activation and prognosis (314, 315). A novel T-cell subset $CD28^-$ Treg-like cell has been described that produce pro-inflammatory cytokines, mirroring the SASP associated with senescent cells (316). RA patients who show $CD28^-$ senescent Treg-like cells in blood seem to demonstrate earlier and more severe osteoporosis (317).

Limiting inflammation before damage occurs is central to successful RA management and the use of specific monoclonal antibodies has been a key therapeutic strategy. The central roles of TNF and IL-6 in RA have been corroborated by clinical trials of biologic drugs, which can specifically target and neutralize these cytokines. Evidence from RA clinical subgroups stratified by responses to specific biologic drugs strongly suggest that for a particular individual, inflammation is coordinated by a predominant cytokine pathway, such as TNF or IL-6 (318).

Anti-TNF biologics, such as adalimumab, etanercept, and infliximab reduce inflammation, pain, neovascularization, lymphocyte infiltration, and increase macrophage apoptosis (318–321). Anti-IL-6R biologics, such as tociluzimab and anti-IL-6, such as sirukumab, strongly reduce disease activity and erosive progression (322, 323). Evidence suggests that the predominant cell cytokines seen in synovial histopathology may act as prognostic biomarkers for stratification of RA patients (324–326).

Studies of TNF and IL-6 gene polymorphisms further support their role in RA risk and severity. SNPs in IL-6 and IL-6R genes associate with increased RA risk and joint damage (327–329), and the TNF 308 G gene polymorphism with RA disease severity and poor response to anti-TNF treatment (330–334). In the elderly person with RA, there is difficulty in distinguishing whether chronic inflammation or genetic "predisposition" initiates disease or if late-onset RA is hastened by the pro-inflammatory phenotype associated with aging. TNF-α inhibitors used as disease-modifying agents in RA improve not only the clinical symptoms of RA, but also decrease the associated vascular risk (335), suggesting that a stratified biologic approach may be of use to therapeutically dampen chronic systemic inflammation related to aging and other age-related diseases.

Like other age-related diseases and aging itself, there is evidence for dysregulation in both the autophagy–lysosomal and the ubiquitin–proteasomal systems in RA (102). Autophagy seems to be activated in RA in a TNFα-dependent manner and regulates osteoclast differentiation and bone resorption, emphasizing a central role for autophagy in joint destruction (336). Gene and allele frequency population differences seem also to contribute to how effectively cellular autophagy processes work within the cell in removing damaged proteins and other necrotic cellular debris. Polymorphisms of the ubiquitn E3 ligase gene that directly influence autophagy have also been identified and have been associated with the etiology and response to drug treatment in RA (337, 338). Both are likely important contributors to the action and effectiveness of disease modifying and monoclonal biological drugs used in RA treatment. The role of the NLPR3 inflammasome may give opportunities for developing other disease-modifying drugs by targeting upstream triggers of the NLPR3 pathway.

Atherosclerosis

Atherosclerosis is recognized as a chronic inflammatory condition (339) and atherosclerotic plaques show cellular senescence (340, 341). Cytokines are involved in all stages of the pathogenesis of atherosclerosis, having both pro- or anti-atherogenic effects (342, 343). In response to increased low-density lipoprotein (LDL), hypertension, and subsequent shear stress, cytokines modulate endothelial cell permeability and recruit monocytes and T-lymphocytes (344, 345). The continuous monocyte recruitment, foam cell and fatty steak formation eventually result in unstable plaque development, thrombosis, and a cardiac event (345, 346).

Chronic unresolved inflammation is a key feature in atherosclerosis and the levels of SPMs, particularly resolvin D1, and the ratio of SPMs to pro-inflammatory leukotriene B_4 (LTB_4), are significantly decreased in the vulnerable plaque regions (27). Vulnerable atherosclerotic plaques are recognized as having distinct features; increased inflammation; oxidative stress; areas of necrosis overlain by a thin protective layer of collagen (fibrous cap). In advanced atherosclerotic plaques, macrophages have more abundant nuclear 5-LOX, which is suggested to lead to conversion of AA to proinflammatory LTs, with the potential to contribute to plaque rupture (27).

The NLRP3 inflammasome, a central regulator of inflammation (58), is activated by cholesterol crystals and oxidized LDL (347, 348) that drives the IL-1β inflammation pathway. Recent research targeting IL-1β inflammation in atherosclerosis using cannakinumab, a therapeutic monoclonal antibody, has shown up to 15% lower rates of recurrent cardiovascular events, which was independent of lipid lowering (349). As well as playing a major role in chronic inflammation, NLRP3 is also upregulated during endothelial cell senescence (350) *via* ROS, and is negatively regulated by autophagy (351, 352). The NLRP3 inflammasome, therefore, appears to warrant further investigation as a potential target for inflamm-aging related to atherosclerosis given that such mechanisms are now of well known importance in atherosclerosis (353).

The gut microbiome has been implicated in age-related inflammation (354) with numerous studies reporting bacterial organisms in arterial plaque (355–357). Emerging research reports bacterial DNA in blood associated with a personal microbiota fingerprint as a predictor of cardiovascular events and stool microbiome as a signature of cardiovascular disease (358, 359). Similarly, bacterial DNA has been noted in cell-free plasma in cardiovascular and chronic renal disease patients (360, 361). Altered gut microbiota composition or dysbiosis is also seen in elderly people, and is associated with inflammatory markers (354). Aging leads to changes in intestinal permeability in gut bacterial milieu (362), and the increased circulatory bacterial DNA observed associated with atherosclerosis support further investigation of the microbiome as a contributory factor to age-related inflammation and atherosclerosis.

Neuroinflammation and Neurodegenerative Disease

Inflammation has been well established as a major component of neurodegenerative disorders, but it has never been clear if this was a direct cause of the disease or a consequence of the progressive degenerative process that was occurring (363, 364). The central role of cytokines in regulating the immune response has been implicated in neurodegeneration, but over the past decade, there has been a revolution in our understanding of how cytokines contribute to the etiology of the leading neurodegenerative disorders, including Alzheimer's (AD) and Parkinson's disease (PD).

In AD, central events seem to include the inflammasome, the NF-κB pathway, and the activation of microglia by a variety of factors, including beta amyloid and pro-inflammatory cytokines (172). Microglia, the primary components of the CNS innate immune system (365), produce cytokines and monitor the integrity of CNS. Together with astrocytes, microglia are the primary effectors of neuroinflammation and express PPRs that allow early recognition of PAMPs and DAMPs. When the NLRP3 inflammasome is activated, the inflammation cascade begins with casp-1 that facilitates the processing of IL-1β and IL18. These proinflammatory cytokines drive the inflammatory cascade through downstream signaling pathways and lead to neuronal damage and death (366). The activated microglia release proinflammatory cytokines, such as IL-1β, IL-6, TNF-α, and IL-18, that contributes to neuronal death and dysfunction.

There is interest in the role of sphingolipid metabolites, such as ceramide and sphingosine-1-phosphate, which regulate a diverse range of cellular processes that are important in immunity, inflammation, and inflammatory diseases (367). Growing evidence suggests that ceramide may play a critical role in NLRP3 inflammasome assembly in neuroinflammation. Research has shown that microglia treated with sodium palmitate (PA) induce *de novo* ceramide synthesis, triggering the expression of NLRP3 inflammasome assembly and resulting in release of IL-1β (368), linking neuroinflammation with dietary lipids. Recent insights into the molecular mechanisms of action of sphingolipid metabolites suggest roles in altering membrane composition, with effects on cellular interactions and signaling pathways with potential causal relationships to neuroinflammatory disease.

Dysregulated autophagy has been considered to play a role in neurodegenerative diseases, particularly AD, and is felt to be a key regulator of Aβ abnormal protein generation and clearance (369). In AD the maturation of autophagolysosomes (i.e., autophagosomes that have undergone fusion with lysosomes) and their clearance are hindered. Evidence suggests that Aβ peptides are released from neurons in an autophagy-dependent manner and that the accumulation of intracellular Aβ plaques is toxic to brain cells leading to AD pathology (370). Furthermore, lysosomal and autophagocytic dysfunction has been associated with both Alzheimer's and Parkinson's diseases (71, 72). Senescent cells too, accumulate abnormal protein aggregates in the cytoplasm that contribute to neurodegenerative disease (72). Cellular senescence has been reported in the aging brain with an increase in SASP-expressing senescent cells of non-neurological origin that are likely to contribute to the pro-inflammatory background (103, 371).

In AD and PD, the application of genome-wide association studies (GWAS) has demonstrated a number of key genes, relating to immunity, including the human leukocyte antigen (HLA) complex on chromosome six that regulates the immune and inflammatory response (372, 373). In the most recent Parkinson's disease GWAS a locus containing the IL-1R2 gene was identified as significantly associated with disease risk and awaits further investigation (372). There is some evidence that carriage of certain pro-inflammatory cytokine gene alleles may confer increased Alzheimer's disease risk. Single studies have reported that carriers of the A allele of the TNF-α 308 G/A gene were variably associated with increased risk of Alzheimer's disease (207–210) and that carriage the higher IL-6 producing allele of IL-6 (174 G/C) may confer increased risk (186, 190, 191). Animal studies have provided some clearer understanding of the role of TNF-α in Alzheimer's disease with evidence of disease modulation with the use of anti-TNF agents (215). Three studies, published in 2013, confirmed a role for the immune response in AD identifying the microglia-related gene TREM2 as harboring an intermediate effect size variant in risk of AD that has also been implicated in other related neurodegenerative diseases (374–376). A recent study of rare variants has also implicated a role for microglial-mediated innate immunity in AD (377).

A better understanding of the molecular pathways involved in the use of established drugs, such as non-steroidal anti-inflammatory or statin drugs in risk and progression of neurological disorders may provide further opportunities to treat earlier or prevent disease onset (378–380). It has been considered that downregulation of the type and magnitude of the pro-inflammatory immune response in neurodegeneration might be a key to earlier and more successful targeting of these pathways. However results, to date, have been disappointing and anti-TNF-α therapies and targeted treatment of TNF-α levels that are elevated in cerebrospinal fluid and in patients' serum, have produced, at best, modest results (381). Multiple sclerosis patients have benefited from treatment with fingolimod (FTY720) that has been reported to attenuate neuroinflammation, by regulating the activation and neuroprotective effects of microglia, by modulating the sphingosine-1-phosphate receptor (S1P receptor) (382). Given the success of FTY720 for treatment of multiple sclerosis, it is hoped that next-generation

S1PR1 modulators will find wider therapeutic uses in other inflammatory disorders. Fingolimod is now under a phase 2 clinical trials for acute stroke and phase 4 for neurodegeneration (383).

FUTURE CONSIDERATIONS

Aging is heterogeneous among people and highly variable between different organs and tissues. Our genes, our lifestyles, and our response to stress are infinitely individual and variable, so that the immunobiography of each life tells a different story of how each will respond to the internal and external environmental stressors (1–3, 384). But evidence is accumulating that the aging process may be malleable.

Because aging is the major risk factor for age-related diseases, understanding age better and maintaining the health of older people and societies is highly important personally and for societies and governments. Knowledge about the underlying molecular pathways and the genetic and life-style processes associated with age-related disease and aging itself is increasing. Evidence from centenarian and nonagenarian studies suggests that these oldest members of populations have had the ability to delay aging and age-related disease (385, 386). Other studies suggest that centenarians may demonstrate optimized cardiovascular risk factors (387, 388), or have either intuitively or through social example, adopted lifestyles which have interacted with their genes to facilitate a successful aging phenotype (3, 389, 390).

Population studies across the world show that the age-specific incidence of cardiovascular disease, stroke, and dementia is decreasing (391–395). This suggests that better blood pressure and diabetic control and statin use may directly or indirectly link into and downregulate molecular pathways associated with inflammation (396–399). Research into how carriage of certain gene alleles, such as TCF7L2 or IL-6 can increase inflammation or stroke risk, respectively, and can be ameliorated by following a Mediterranean-type diet (42, 400, 401), or how gene splicing and features of senescence may be modulated by resveratrol in food (402), herald research into how gene, diet, and lifestyles can interact, with positive or negative effects on the immune system and health. Increased knowledge is emerging as to how epigenetic modulation can affect cytokine genes with reports linking cytokine epigenetic change to neuroinflammation (403–405). Obesity, smoking, and malnutrition have been shown to have next generational epigenetic effects, and seem likely to contribute to the predilection of offspring developing age-related disease or conversely the longevity phenotype (406–409).

Other strategies should be adopted which link with public health messages and encourage people to adopt behavioral changes in lifestyles. Modifications should include: changes in diets to include more omega-3 containing foods or fruits and vegetables as in the Mediterranean diet (410–413); engagement in regular moderated exercise routines (414–417); continued engagement with social connections and intellectual activities in daily lives (418–420); or best of all a combination of life-style factors (3, 421, 422), all of which have been shown to reduce the inflammatory profile and improve the quality of aging. Although the role of diet on human health and connections through nutrition, inflammation, and cancer are not as linear as those between tobacco, smoking, and lung cancer, obesity is linked to chronic inflammation through several mechanisms, including the dysregulation of autophagy, whereas fasting has anti-inflammatory effects, similar to the effect of exercise (423–426), and may downregulate inflammatory biomarkers (427–429). There is, therefore, considerable interest in the role of the intestinal microbiota and health and the so-called immune-relevant microbiome (324, 354), with important correlations between inflammation and neurodegenerative disease (430), bacterial β-hydroxybutyrate metabolites (431), and the role of vagal stimulation (432).

Increasing evidence shows that many signaling pathways are activated in a stress-type-dependent fashion, and all appear to converge with nuclear factor (NF)-κB signaling, which is a central controller of the immune response, and inflammatory cascade (110, 433–436). With increasing age, immune homeostasis loosens, NF-κB signaling becomes less tightly controlled or is more readily triggered, cytokine dysregulation occurs, and a pro-inflammatory phenotype predominates that underpins most major age-related diseases from atherosclerosis to cancer, and aging itself (**Figure 5**). Understanding how different factors trigger the NF-κB cascade is an important pathway of research (434). In animal models, miRNA-based regulatory networks involving miR-155 and miR-146a, finely regulate NF-κB activity, with miR-146a downregulating and miR-155 upregulating NF-κB expression (435). There is an important temporal separation of miR-155 and miR-146a cellular expression that allows finely controlled NK-κB signaling and enables a precise macrophage inflammatory response, which merits further research.

Therapeutic opportunities may arise through better understanding of the molecular mechanisms that induce senescent cells and SASP in the cellular environments of chronic disease or whether senescent cells can be removed by upregulating autophagy and using sophisticated tagging mechanisms (110). There will be increased opportunities to use the knowledge gained from clinical studies in autoimmune disease, about the roles and actions of monoclonal antibodies in modulating inflammation, which may be able to be utilized in treatments for other age-related diseases involving inflammation (436). The formulations of new and more specific drugs are likely to become available as the modes of action of kinases, such a AMPK and mTOR which control the senescence and inflammation pathways, become better understood (81, 84, 437). Old drugs, such as metformin, still used in diabetes control, are being repurposed and have been shown to have exciting new uses through their ability to modify epigenetic gene expression. Clinical studies are underway to assess any modulating effect of metformin in aging and age-related diseases (81). The use of histone deacetylating drugs is likely to increase as the clinical use of deacetylation and methylation agents is evaluated in cancer with improved knowledge of their effects and safety criteria (438). The current interest in diet and modified diets will encourage further studies assessing how nutrachemicals modify gene expression, for example, through the regulation of intracellular receptors that bind the promoters of certain genes, and may help to design more specific drugs to modify metabolism and benefit health (439).

Turning research to focus on improved understanding of the mechanisms of inflammation resolution in aging and age-related disease, should also be prioritized, since it is an under researched area. Developing synthetic resolvins for use in inflammation resolution may have advantages over the use of single biological anti-inflammatory blockers in autoimmune disease clinical management, since cytokine networks are highly interactive and complex (440), with many auto-regulatory feedback loops. All these molecular pathways are, or have the potential for being developed as drug targets toward clinical interventions useful in damping down and modulating inflammation (441, 442) and may have a role in delaying the onset or treatment of age-related diseases.

Evidence from on-going global studies of the oldest members of our societies, such as centenarians and nonagenarians (443–454) suggests that it may be possible to delay age-related diseases and that aging may be a potentially modifiable risk factor (455). Further investigation has shown that centenarians and super-centenarians also have an enhanced pro-inflammatory background (9, 456, 457), which at first seems surprising, given their long lives. However, studies have demonstrated that the pro-inflammatory background is accompanied and perhaps modulated, by an enhanced anti-inflammatory status in some centenarians. Some have argued that an enhanced anti-inflammatory phenotype could be beneficial as a contributor to longevity by effectively controlling the pro-inflammatory background (9, 11, 257). Others suggest that some inflammation is good, in the same way as hormetic stress triggers systems, and upgrades them but does not overwhelm them (458). Regular exposure to pro-inflammatory stressors could train the immune system to upregulate and fine-tune its cellular processes, so that it responds better and provides better outcomes, when faced with real life-threatening pathogenic threats.

Genome-wide association studies have proved a powerful methodology to assess the influence of common variation in AD and PD disease susceptibility, but by their nature have reflected low effect size variants that likely have a cumulative effect on risk (459). As next-generation sequencing technology becomes more cost-effective, the ability to identify variants that are less common (<1% minor allele frequency) will become more achievable. These unbiased approaches should aid the identification of key players in the inflamm-aging pathway and will play a critical role in the development of therapeutic intervention strategies in neurodegenerative and age-related diseases.

There is the increasing opportunity to link large global datasets with the technologies of genomics, transcriptomics, and proteomics through bioinformatics and artificial intelligence methods to unlock the physiological, genetic, and molecular pathways that underpin the pro-inflammatory aging-phenotype. Using systems biology methods has the potential to lead to the generation of novel therapeutic approaches for old diseases and modern health challenges. Improving knowledge about how to delay or modify the pro-inflammatory aging-phenotype, the hallmark of aging and age-related disease, will give hope of a better quality aging and the longevity dividend for all.

AUTHOR CONTRIBUTIONS

IR conceived and designed the outline of the manuscript. All authors IR, DG, VM, SM, DA, and OR contributed to the manuscript draft. All authors contributed to the drafting and revising of the manuscript and approved the manuscript prior to submission.

ACKNOWLEDGMENTS

VM, DG, and DA were supported by £11.5M grant awarded to Professor Tony Bjourson from European Union Regional Development Fund EU Sustainable Competitiveness Programme for N. Ireland; Northern Ireland Public Health Agency (HSC R&D) & Ulster University and a project supported by the European Union's INTERREG VA Programme, managed by the Special EU Programmes Body. Interreg grant number is IVA 5306. OR receives support from the Mayo Clinic Center of Individualized Medicine. IMR was funded in part by EU Socrates Erasmus Programme for Thematic Network, Interfacing Science, Literature and Humanities ACUME2 (227942-CP-1-2006-1-IT-ERASMUS-TN2006-2371/001 SO2-23RETH), LSH-2002-2.1.4-1—Genetic factors of longevity and healthy ageing, Atlantic Philanthropies, Changing Ageing Partnership Grant, Queens Foundation Trust (R9158PHM) (IMR), Wellcome Trust Project Grant (045519/Z/95/Z) (IMR), Eastern Health and Social Care Board Research Fellowship Grant (IMR) and Belfast Trust Fund (Research and Education into Ageing (0-132) (IMR). IR thanks the nonagenarians from the BELFAST study who enthusiastically engaged in the Super Vivere and Beyond 90 Together projects.

REFERENCES

1. Ter Horst R, Jaeger M, Smeekens SP, Oosting M, Swertz MA, Li Y, et al. Host and environmental factors influencing individual human cytokine responses. *Cell* (2016) 167(4):1111e-24e. doi:10.1016/j.cell.2016.10.018
2. Govindaraju D, Atzmon G, Barzilai N. Genetics, lifestyle and longevity: lessons from centenarians. *Appl Transl Genom* (2015) 4:23–32. doi:10.1016/j.atg.2015.01.001
3. Rea JNM, Carvalho A, McNerlan SE, Alexander HD, Rea IM. Genes and life-style factors in BELFAST nonagenarians: nature, nurture and narrative. *Biogerontology* (2015) 16(5):587–97. doi:10.1007/s10522-015-9567-y
4. Liu Y-Z, Wang Y-X, Jiang C-L. Inflammation: the common pathway of stress-related diseases. *Front Hum Neurosci* (2017) 11:316. doi:10.3389/fnhum.2017.00316
5. Abe K, Hashimoto Y, Yatsushiro S, Yamamura S, Bando M, Hiroshima Y, et al. Simultaneous immunoassay analysis of plasma IL-6 and TNF-α on a microchip. *PLoS One* (2013) 8(1):e53620. doi:10.1371/journal.pone.0053620
6. Battle A, Khan Z, Wang SH, Mitrano A, Ford MJ, Pritchard JK, et al. Genomic variation. Impact of regulatory variation from RNA to protein. *Science* (2015) 347(6222):664–647. doi:10.1126/science.1260793
7. Kubiczkova L, Sedlarikova L, Hajek R, Sevcikova S. TGF-beta – an excellent servant but a bad master. *J Transl Med* (2012) 10:183. doi:10.1186/1479-5876-10-183
8. Franceschi C, Bonafè M, Valensin S, Olivieri F, De Luca M, Ottaviani E, et al. Inflamm-aging. An evolutionary perspective on immunosenescence. *Ann N Y Acad Sci* (2000) 908:244–54. doi:10.1111/j.1749-6632.2000.tb06651.x
9. Franceschi C, Capri M, Monti D, Giunta S, Olivieri F, Sevini F, et al. Inflammaging and antiinflammaging: a systemic perspective on aging and longevity emerged from studies in humans. *Mech Ageing Dev* (2007) 128:92–105. doi:10.1016/j.mad.2006.11.016
10. Medzhitov R. Origin and physiological role of inflammation. *Nature* (2008) 454:428–35. doi:10.1038/nature07201
11. Franceschi C, Campisi J. Chronic inflammation (inflammaging) and its potential contribution to age-associated diseases. *J Gerontol A Biol Sci Med Sci* (2014) 69(Suppl 1):S4–9. doi:10.1093/gerona/glu057
12. Chung HY, Cesari M, Anton S, Marzetti E, Giovannini S, Seo AY, et al. Molecular inflammation: underpinnings of aging and age-related diseases. *Ageing Res Rev* (2009) 8(1):18–30. doi:10.1016/j.arr.2008.07.002
13. Martin SJ. Cell death and inflammation: the case for IL-1 family cytokines as the canonical DAMPs of the immune system. *FEBS J* (2016) 283(14):2599–615. doi:10.1111/febs.13775

14. Kumar V, Abbas A, Aster J. *Robbins & Cotran Pathologic Basis of Disease.* IX ed. Amsterdam: Elsevier (2014).
15. Nathan C. Points of control in inflammation. *Nature* (2002) 420(6917): 846–52. doi:10.1038/nature01320
16. Chiurchiù V, Leuti A, Maccarrone M. Bioactive lipids and chronic inflammation: managing the fire within. *Front Immunol* (2018) 9:38. doi:10.3389/fimmu.2018.00038
17. Serhan CN, Chiang N, Dalli J, Levy BD. Lipid mediators in the resolution of inflammation. *Cold Spring Harb Perspect Biol* (2015) 7(2):a016311. doi:10.1101/cshperspect.a016311
18. Serhan CN, Chiang N, Dalli J. New pro-resolving n-3 mediators bridge resolution of infectious inflammation to tissue regeneration. *Mol Aspects Med* (2017). doi:10.1016/j.mam.2017.08.002
19. Serhan CN. Pro-resolving lipid mediators are leads for resolution physiology. *Nature* (2014) 510(7503):92–101. doi:10.1038/nature134
20. Awad F, Assrawi E, Jumeau C, Georgin-Lavialle S, Cobret L, Duquesnoy P, et al. Impact of human monocyte and macrophage polarization on NLR expression and NLRP3 inflammasome activation. *PLoS One* (2017) 12(4): e0175336. doi:10.1371/journal.pone.0175336
21. Mantovani A, Biswas SK, Galdiero MR, Sica A, Locati M. Macrophage plasticity and polarization in tissue repair and remodelling. *J Pathol* (2013) 229:176–85. doi:10.1002/path.4133
22. Kittan NA, Allen RM, Dhaliwal A, Cavassani KA, Schaller M, Gallagher KA, et al. Cytokine induced phenotypic and epigenetic signatures are key to establishing specific macrophage phenotypes. *PLoS One* (2013) 8(10):e78045. doi:10.1371/journal.pone.0078045
23. Chiurchiù V, Leuti A, Dalli J, Jacobsson A, Battistini L, Maccarrone M, et al. Proresolving lipid mediators resolvin D1, resolvin D2, and maresin 1 are critical in modulating T cell responses. *Sci Transl Med* (2016) 8:353ra111.1. doi:10.1126/scitranslmed.aaf7483
24. Krishnamoorthy N, Burkett PR, Dalli J, Abdulnour RE, Colas R, Ramon S, et al. Cutting edge: maresin-1 engages regulatory T cells to limit type 2 innate lymphoid cell activation and promote resolution of lung inflammation. *J Immunol* (2015) 194(3):863–7. doi:10.4049/jimmunol.1402534
25. Ramon S, Gao F, Serhan CN, Phipps RP. Specialized proresolving mediators enhance human B cell differentiation to antibody-secreting cells. *J Immunol* (2012) 189:1036–42. doi:10.4049/jimmunol.1103483
26. Recchiuti A, Serhan CN. Pro-resolving lipid mediators (SPMs) and their actions in regulating miRNA in novel resolution circuits in inflammation. *Front Immunol* (2012) 3:298. doi:10.3389/fimmu.2012.00298
27. Fredman G, Hellmann J, Proto JD, Kuriakose G, Colas RA, Dorweiler B, et al. An imbalance between specialized pro-resolving lipid mediators and pro-inflammatory leukotrienes promotes instability of atherosclerotic plaques. *Nat Commun* (2016) 7:2859. doi:10.1038/ncomms1285
28. Spite M, Norling LV, Summers L, Spite M, Norling LV, Summers L, et al. Resolvin D2 is a potent regulator of leukocytes and controls microbial sepsis. *Nature* (2009) 461(7268):1287–91. doi:10.1038/nature08541
29. Buckley CD, Gilroy DW, Serhan CN. Pro-Resolving lipid mediators and mechanisms in the resolution of acute inflammation. *Immunity* (2014) 40(3):315–27. doi:10.1016/j.immuni.2014.02.009
30. Arita M, Ohira T, Sun YP, Elangovan S, Chiang N, Serhan CN. Resolvin E1 selectively interacts with leukotriene B4 receptor BLT1 and ChemR23 to regulate inflammation. *J Immunol* (2007) 178:3912–7. doi:10.4049/jimmunol.178.6.3912
31. Liao Z, Dong J, Wu W, Yang T, Wang T, Guo L, et al. Resolvin D1 attenuates inflammation in lipopolysaccharide-induced acute lung injury through a process involving the PPARgamma/NF-kappaB pathway. *Respir Res* (2012) 13:110. doi:10.1186/1465-9921-13-110
32. Chatterjee A, Sharma A, Chen M, Toy R, Mottola G, Conte MS. The pro-resolving lipid mediator maresin 1 (MaR1) attenuates inflammatory signaling pathways in vascular smooth muscle and endothelial cells. *PLoS One* (2014) 9(11):e113480. doi:10.1371/journal.pone.0113480
33. Marcon R, Bento AF, Dutra RC, Bicca MA, Leite DF, Calixto JB. Maresin 1, a proresolving lipid mediator derived from omega-3 polyunsaturated fatty acids, exerts protective actions in murine models of colitis. *J Immunol* (2013) 191:4288–98. doi:10.4049/jimmunol.1202743
34. Perretti M, Norling LV. Actions of SPM in regulating host responses in arthritis. *Mol Aspects Med* (2017) 58:57–64.1. doi:10.1016/j.mam.2017.04.005
35. Sulciner ML, Serhan CN, Gilligan MM, Mudge DK, Chang J, Gartung A, et al. Resolvins suppress tumor growth and enhance cancer therapy. *J Exp Med* (2018) 215(1):115–40. doi:10.1084/jem.20170681
36. Fiala M, Terrando N, Dalli J. Specialized pro-resolving mediators from omega-3 fatty acids improve amyloid-β phagocytosis and regulate inflammation in patients with minor cognitive impairment. *J Alzheimers Dis* (2015) 48:293–301.1. doi:10.3233/JAD-150367
37. Zhu M, Wang X, Hjorth E, Colas RA, Schroeder L, Granholm A-C, et al. Pro-resolving lipid mediators improve neuronal survival and increase Aβ42 phagocytosis. *Mol Neurobiol* (2016) 53:2733–49. doi:10.1007/s12035-015-9544-0
38. Skoldstam L, Hagfors L, Johansson G. An experimental study of a Mediterranean diet intervention for patients with rheumatoid arthritis. *Ann Rheum Dis* (2003) 62(3):208–14. doi:10.1136/ard.62.3.208
39. Fung TT, Rexrode KM, Mantzoros CS, Manson JE, Willett WC, Hu FB. Mediterranean diet and incidence of and mortality from coronary heart disease and stroke in women. *Circulation* (2009) 119(8):1093–100. doi:10.1161/CIRCULATIONAHA.108.816736
40. Esposito K, Maiorino MI, Bellastella G, Chiodini P, Panagiotakos D, Giugliano D. A journey into a Mediterranean diet and type 2 diabetes: a systematic review with meta-analyses. *BMJ Open* (2015) 5:e008222. doi:10.1136/bmjopen-2015-008222
41. Demarin V, Lisak M, Morović S. Mediterranean diet in healthy lifestyle and prevention of stroke. *Acta Clin Croat* (2011) 50(1):67–77.
42. Corella D, Carrasco P, Sorlí JV, Estruch R, Rico-Sanz J, Martínez-González MÁ, et al. Mediterranean diet reduces the adverse effect of the TCF7L2-rs7903146 polymorphism on cardiovascular risk factors and stroke incidence: a randomized controlled trial in a high-cardiovascular-risk population. *Diabetes Care* (2013) 36:3803–11. doi:10.2337/dc13-0955
43. Harman D. Aging: a theory based on free radical and radiation chemistry. *J Gerontol* (1956) 11:298–300. doi:10.1093/geronj/11.3.298
44. Bedard K, Krause KH. The NOX family of ROS-generating NADPH oxidases: physiology and pathophysiology. *Physiol Rev* (2007) 87:245–313. doi:10.1152/physrev.00044.2005
45. Daiber A. Redox signaling (cross-talk) from and to mitochondria involves mitochondrial pores and reactive oxygen species. *Biochim Biophys Acta* (2010) 1797(6–7):897–906. doi:10.1016/j.bbabio.2010.01.032
46. Marcus RL, Addison O, Kidde JP, Dibble LE, Lastayo PC. Skeletal muscle fat infiltration: impact of age, inactivity, and exercise. *J Nut Health Aging* (2010) 14:362–6. doi:10.1007/s12603-010-0081-2
47. Rea IM. Towards ageing well: use it or lose it: exercise, epigenetics and cognition. *Biogerontology* (2017) 18(4):679–91. doi:10.1007/s10522-017-9719-3
48. Diot A, Morten K, Poulton J. Mitophagy plays a central role in mitochondrial ageing. *Mamm Genome* (2016) 27:381–95. doi:10.1007/s00335-016-9651-x
49. Sohal RS, Orr WC. The redox stress hypothesis of aging. *Free Radic Biol Med* (2012) 52(3):539–55. doi:10.1016/j.freeradbiomed.2011.10.445
50. Takac I, Schroder K, Brandes RP. The Nox family of NADPH oxidases: friend or foe of the vascular system? *Curr Hypertens Rep* (2012) 14:70–8. doi:10.1007/s11906-011-0238-3
51. Babior BM, Lambeth JD, Nauseef W. The neutrophil NADPH oxidase. *Arch Biochem Biophys* (2002) 397(2):342–324. doi:10.1006/abbi.2001.2642
52. Nguyen GT, Green ER, Mecsas J. Neutrophils to the ROScue: mechanisms of NADPH oxidase activation and bacterial resistance. *Front Cell Infect Microbiol* (2017) 7:373. doi:10.3389/fcimb.2017.00373
53. Drummond GR, Sobey CG. Endothelial NADPH oxidases: which NOX to target in vascular disease? *Trends Endocrinol Metab* (2014) 25(9):452–63. doi:10.1016/j.tem.2014.06.012
54. Youn J-Y, Zhang J, Zhang Y, Chen H, Liu D, Ping P, et al. Oxidative stress in atrial fibrillation: an emerging role of NADPH oxidase. *J Mol Cell Cardiol* (2013) 62:72–9. doi:10.1016/j.yjmcc.2013.04.019
55. Marnett LJ, Rowlinson SW, Goodwin DC, Kalgutkar AS, Lanzo CA. Arachidonic acid oxygenation by COX-1 and COX-2. Mechanisms of catalysis and inhibition. *J Biol Chem* (1999) 274:22903–6. doi:10.1074/jbc.274.33.22903
56. Cho K-J, Seo J-M, Kim J-H. Bioactive lipoxygenase metabolites stimulation of NADPH oxidases and reactive oxygen species. *Mol Cells* (2011) 32(1):1–5. doi:10.1007/s10059-011-1021-7
57. Kienhofer J, Haussler DJF, Ruckelshausen F, Muessig E, Weber K, Pimentel D, et al. Association of mitochondrial antioxidant enzymes with mitochondrial

DNA as integral nucleoid constituents. *FASEB J* (2009) 23(7):2034–44. doi:10.1096/fj.08-113571
58. Zhou R, Yazdi AS, Menu P, Tschopp J. A role for mitochondria in NLRP3 inflammasome activation. *Nature* (2011) 469:221–5. doi:10.1038/nature09663
59. Tschopp J. Mitochondria: sovereign of inflammation? *Eur J Immunol* (2011) 41:1196–202. doi:10.1002/eji.201141436
60. Abais JM, Xia M, Zhang Y, Boini KM, Li P-L. Redox regulation of NLRP3 inflammasomes: ROS as trigger or effector? *Antioxid Redox Signal* (2015) 22(13):1111–29. doi:10.1089/ars.2014.5994
61. Ciechanover A. Intracellular protein degradation: from a vague idea thru the lysosome and the ubiquitin-proteasome system and onto human diseases and drug targeting. *Biochim Biophys Acta* (2012) 1824:3–13. doi:10.1038/sj.cdd.4401692
62. Tanida I. Autophagosome formation and molecular mechanism of autophagy. *Antioxid Redox Signal* (2011) 14(11):2201–14. doi:10.1089/ars.2010.3482
63. Gelino S, Hansen M. Autophagy – an emerging anti-aging mechanism. *J Clin Exp Pathol* (2012) Suppl 4:006.
64. Brunk UT, Terman A. The mitochondrial-lysosomal axis theory of aging. Accumulation of damaged mitochondria as a result of imperfect autophagocytosis. *Eur J Biochem* (2002) 269:1996–2002. doi:10.1046/j.1432-1033.2002.02869.x
65. Carrard G, Bulteau A-L, Petropoulos I, Friguet B. Impairment of proteasome structure and function in aging. *Int J Biochem Cell Biol* (2002) 34:1461–74. doi:10.1016/S1357-2725(02)00085-7
66. Rubinsztein DC, Marino G, Kroemer G. Autophagy and aging. *Cell* (2011) 146:682–95. doi:10.1016/j.cell.2011.07.030
67. de Duve C. The lysosome turns fifty. *Nat Cell Biol* (2005) 7:847–9. doi:10.1038/ncb0905-847
68. Orenstein SJ, Cuervo AM. Chaperone-mediated autophagy: molecular mechanisms and physiological relevance. *Semin Cell Dev Biol* (2010) 21(7):719–26. doi:10.1016/j.semcdb.2010.02.005
69. Green DR, Galluzzi L, Kroemer G. Mitochondria and the autophagy-inflammation-cell death axis in organismal aging. *Science* (2011) 333: 1109–12. doi:10.1126/science.1201940
70. Jiang P, Mizushima N. Autophagy and human diseases. *Cell Res* (2014) 24:69–79. doi:10.1038/cr.2013.161
71. Wolfe DM, Lee J-H, Kumar A, Lee S, Orenstein SJ, Nixon RA. Autophagy failure in Alzheimer's disease and the role of defective lysosomal acidification. *Eur J Neurosci* (2013) 37:1949–61. doi:10.1111/ejn.12169
72. Nah J, Yuan J, Jung Y-K. Autophagy in neurodegenerative diseases: from mechanism to therapeutic approach. *Mol Cells* (2015) 38(5):381–9. doi:10.14348/molcells.2015.0034
73. Cuervo AM, Macian F. Autophagy and the immune function in aging. *Curr Opin Immunol* (2014) 29:97–104. doi:10.1016/j.coi.2014.05.006
74. Shi C-S, Shenderov K, Huang N-N, Kabat J, Abu-Asab M, Fitzgerald KA, et al. Activation of autophagy by inflammatory signals limits IL-1a production by targeting ubiquitinated inflammasomes for destruction. *Nat Immunol* (2012) 13(3):255–63. doi:10.1038/ni.2215
75. Zhong Z, Umemura A, Sanchez-Lopez E, Liang S, Shalapour S, Wong J, et al. NF-κB restricts inflammasome activation via elimination of damaged mitochondria. *Cell* (2016) 164(5):896–910. doi:10.1016/j.cell.2015.12.057
76. Nam T, Han JH, Sushil Devkota S, Lee H-W. Emerging paradigm of crosstalk between autophagy and the ubiquitin-proteasome system. *Mol Cells* (2017) 40(12):897–905. doi:10.14348/molcells.2017.0226
77. Mizushima N, Levine B, Cuervo AM, Klionsky DJ. Autophagy fights disease through cellular self-digestion. *Nature* (2008) 451:1069–75. doi:10.1038/nature06639
78. Blagosklonny MV. Linking calorie restriction to longevity through sirtuins and autophagy: any role for TOR. *Cell Death Dis* (2010) 1:e12. doi:10.1038/cddis.2009.17
79. Blagosklonny MV. Rapamycin extends life- and health span because it slows aging. *Aging (Albany NY)* (2013) 5(8):592–8. doi:10.18632/aging.100591
80. Zoncu R, Efeyan A, Sabatini DM. mTOR: from growth signal integration to cancer, diabetes and ageing. *Nat Rev Mol Cell Biol* (2011) 12:21–35. doi:10.1038/nrm3025
81. Barzilai NR. Targeting aging with metformin (TAME). *Innov Aging* (2017) doi:10.1093/geroni/igx004.2682
82. Vaiserman AM, Marotta F. Longevity-promoting pharmaceuticals: is it a time for implementation? *Trends Pharmacol Sci* (2016) 37(5):331–3. doi:10.1016/j.tips.2016.02.003
83. Fogarty S, Hardie DG. Development of protein kinase activators: AMPK as a target in metabolic disorders and cancer. *Biochim Biophys Acta* (2010) 1804:581–91. doi:10.1016/j.bbapap.2009.09.012
84. O'Neill LA, Hardie DG. Metabolism of inflammation limited by AMPK and pseudo-starvation. *Nature* (2013) 493:346–55. doi:10.1038/nature11862
85. Guma M, Wang Y, Viollet B, Liu-Bryan R. AMPK Activation by A-769662 controls IL-6 expression in inflammatory arthritis. *PLoS One* (2015) 10(10):e0140452. doi:10.1371/journal.pone.0140452
86. Grumati P, Coletto L, Schiavinato A, Castagnaro S, Bertaggia E, Sandri M, et al. Physical exercise stimulates autophagy in normal skeletal muscles but is detrimental for collagen VI-deficient muscles. *Autophagy* (2011) 7:1415–23. doi:10.4161/auto.7.12.17877
87. Yan Z, Lira VA, Greene NP. Exercise training-induced regulation of mitochondrial quality. *Exerc Sport Sci Rev* (2012) 40(3):159–64. doi:10.1097/JES.0b013e3182575599
88. Ferreira-Marques M, Aveleira CA, Carmo-Silva S, Botelho M, de Almeida LP, Cavadas C. Caloric restriction stimulates autophagy in rat cortical neurons through neuropeptide Y and ghrelin receptors activation. *Aging (Albany NY)* (2016) 8(7):1470–84. doi:10.18632/aging.100996
89. Campisi J. Aging, cellular senescence, and cancer. *Annu Rev Physiol* (2013) 75:685–705. doi:10.1146/annurev-physiol-030212-183653
90. Hayflick L, Moorhead PS. The serial cultivation of human diploid cell strains. *Exp Cell Res* (1961) 25:585–621. doi:10.1016/0014-4827(61)90192-6
91. Muñoz-Espín D, Cañamero M, Maraver A, Gómez-López G, Contreras J, Murillo-Cuesta S, et al. Programmed cell senescence during mammalian embryonic development. *Cell* (2013) 155:1104–11. doi:10.1016/j.cell.2013.10.019
92. Storer M, Mas A, Robert-Moreno A, Pecoraro M, Ortells MC, Di Giacomo V, et al. Senescence is a developmental mechanism that contributes to embryonic growth and patterning. *Cell* (2013) 155(5):1119–30. doi:10.1016/j.cell.2013.10.041
93. McHugh D, Gil J. Senescence and aging: causes, consequences, and therapeutic avenues. *J Cell Biol* (2018) 217(1):65–77. doi:10.1083/jcb.201708092
94. Wiley CD, Campisi J. From ancient pathways to aging cells—connecting metabolism and cellular senescence. *Cell Metab* (2016) 23(6):1013–21. doi:10.1016/j.cmet.2016.05.010
95. Serrano M. Senescence helps regeneration. *Dev Cell* (2014) 31(6):671–2. doi:10.1016/j.devcel.2014.12.007
96. Bodnar AG, Ouellette M, Frolkis M, Holt SE, Chiu CP, Morin GB, et al. Extension of life-span by introduction of telomerase into normal human cells. *Science* (1998) 279(5349):349–52. doi:10.1126/science.279.5349.349
97. Sun N, Youle RJ, Finkel T. The mitochondrial basis of aging. *Mol Cell* (2016) 61(5):654–66. doi:10.1016/j.molcel.2016.01.028
98. Dimri GP, Lee X, Basile G, Acosta M, Scott G, Roskelley C, et al. A biomarker that identifies senescent human cells in culture and in aging skin in vivo. *Proc Natl Acad Sci U S A* (1995) 92(20):9363–7. doi:10.1073/pnas.92.20.9363
99. Jeyapalan JC, Sedivy JM. Cellular senescence and organismal aging. *Mech Ageing Dev* (2008) 129(7–8):467–74. doi:10.1016/j.mad.2008.04.001
100. Krizhanovsky V, Yon M, Dickins RA, Hearn S, Simon J, Miething C, et al. Senescence of activated stellate cells limits liver fibrosis. *Cell* (2008) 134(4):657–67. doi:10.1016/j.cell.2008.06.049
101. Erusalimsky JD, Kurz DJ. Cellular senescence in vivo: its relevance in ageing and cardiovascular disease. *Exp Gerontol* (2005) 40(8–9):634–42. doi:10.1016/j.exger.2005.04.010
102. Chalan P, van den Berg A, Kroesen B-J, Brouwer L, Boots A. Rheumatoid arthritis, immunosenescence and the hallmarks of aging. *Curr Aging Sci* (2015) 8(2):131–46. doi:10.2174/1874609808666150727110744
103. Chinta SJ, Woods G, Rane A, Demaria M, Campisi J, Andersen JK. Cellular senescence and the aging brain. *Exp Gerontol* (2015) 68:3–7. doi:10.1016/j.exger.2014.09.018
104. Campisi J, Andersen J, Kapahi P, Melov S. Cellular senescence: a link between cancer and age-related degenerative disease? *Semin Cancer Biol* (2011) 21(6):354–9. doi:10.1016/j.semcancer.2011.09.001
105. Ghosh K, Capell BC. The senescence-associated secretory phenotype: critical effector in skin cancer and aging. *J Invest Dermatol* (2016) 136(11):2133–9. doi:10.1016/j.jid.2016.06.621

106. Coppé JP, Desprez PY, Krtolica A, Campisi J. The senescence-associated secretory phenotype: the dark side of tumor suppression. *Annu Rev Pathol* (2010) 5:99–118. doi:10.1146/annurev-pathol-121808-102144
107. Kuilman T, Michaloglo C, Mooi WJ, Peeper DS. The essence of senescence. *Genes Dev* (2010) 24:2463–79. doi:10.1101/gad.1971610
108. Rodier F, Campisi J. Four faces of cellular senescence. *J Cell Biol* (2011) 192(4):547–56. doi:10.1083/jcb.201009094
109. Ovadya Y, Krizhanovsky V. Senescent cells: SASPected drivers of age-related pathologies. *Biogerontology* (2014) 15:627–42. doi:10.1007/s10522-014-9529-9
110. Freund A, Orjalo AV, Desprez PY, Campisi J. Inflammatory networks during cellular senescence: causes and consequences. *Trends Mol Med* (2010) 16(5):238–46. doi:10.1016/j.molmed.2010.03.003
111. Salminen A, Kauppinen A, Kaarniranta K. Emerging role of NF-κB signaling in the induction of senescence-associated secretory phenotype (SASP). *Cell Signal* (2012) 24(4):835–45. doi:10.1016/j.cellsig.2011.12.006
112. Fulop T, Witkowski JM, Le Page A, Fortin C, Pawelec G, Larbi A. Intracellular signalling pathways: targets to reverse immunosenescence. *Clin Exp Immunol* (2017) 187:35–43. doi:10.1111/cei.12836
113. Deschênes M, Chabot B. The emerging role of alternative splicing in senescence and aging. *Aging Cell* (2017) 16:918–33. doi:10.1111/acel.12646
114. Nelson G, Wordsworth J, Wang C, Jurk D, Lawless C, Martin-Ruiz C, et al. A senescent cell bystander effect: senescence-induced senescence. *Aging Cell* (2012) 11:345–9. doi:10.1111/j.1474-9726.2012.00795.x
115. Watanabe S, Kawamoto S, Ohtani N, Hara E. Impact of senescence-associated secretory phenotype and its potential as a therapeutic target for senescence-associated diseases. *Cancer Sci* (2017) 108(4):563–9. doi:10.1111/cas.13184
116. Hongo A, Okumura N, Nakahara M, Kay EP, Koizumi N. The Effect of a p38 mitogen-activated protein kinase inhibitor on cellular senescence of cultivated human corneal endothelial cells. *Invest Ophthalmol Vis Sci* (2017) 58(9):3325–34. doi:10.1167/iovs.16-21170
117. Laberge RM, Zhou L, Sarantos MR, Rodier F, Freund A, de Keizer PL, et al. Glucocorticoids suppress selected components of the senescence-associated secretory phenotype. *Aging Cell* (2012) 11:569–78. doi:10.1111/j.1474-9726.2012.00818.x
118. Akbar AN. The convergence of senescence and nutrient sensing during lymphocyte ageing. *Clin Exp Immunol* (2016) 187:4–5. doi:10.1111/cei.12876
119. Henson SM, Lanna A, Riddell NE, Franzese O, Macaulay R, Griffiths SJ, et al. p38 signaling inhibits mTORC1-independent autophagy in senescent human CD8? T cells. *J Clin Invest* (2014) 124(9):4004–16. doi:10.1172/JCI75051
120. Hoenicke L, Zender L. Immune surveillance of senescent cells – biological significance in cancer- and non-cancer pathologies. *Carcinogenesis* (2012) 33(6):1123–6. doi:10.1093/carcin/bgs124
121. Kang TW, Yevsa T, Woller N, Hoenicke L, Wuestefeld T, Dauch D, et al. Senescence surveillance of pre-malignant hepatocytes limits liver cancer development. *Nature* (2011) 479(7374):547–51. doi:10.1038/nature10599
122. McElhaney JE, Effros RB. Immunosenescence: what does it mean to health outcomes in older adults? *Curr Opin Immunol* (2009) 21:418–24. doi:10.1016/j.coi.2009.05.023
123. Krishnamurthy J, Torrice C, Ramsey MR, Kovalev GI, Al-Regaiey K, Su L, et al. Ink4a/Arf expression is a biomarker of aging. *J Clin Invest* (2004) 114(9):1299–307. doi:10.1172/JCI22475
124. Xue W, Zender L, Miething C, Dickins RA, Hernando E, Krizhanovsky V, et al. Senescence and tumour clearance is triggered by p53 restoration in murine liver carcinomas. *Nature* (2007) 445(7128):656–60. doi:10.1038/nature05529
125. Chien Y, Scuoppo C, Wang X, Fang X, Baigley B, Bolden JE, et al. Control of the senescence-associated secretory phenotype by NF-κB promotes senescence and enhances chemosensitivity. *Genes Dev* (2011) 25:2125–36. doi:10.1101/gad.17276711
126. Baker DJ, Wijshake T, Tchkonia T, LeBrasseur NK, Childs BG, van de Sluis B, et al. Clearance of p16Ink4a-positive senescent cells delays ageing-associated disorders. *Nature* (2011) 479(7372):232–6. doi:10.1038/nature10600
127. Baker DJ, Childs BG, Durik M, Wijers ME, Sieben CJ, Zhong J, et al. Naturally occurring p16Ink4a-positive cells shorten healthy lifespan. *Nature* (2016) 530(7589):184–9. doi:10.1038/nature16932
128. Velarde MC, Demaria M, Campisi J. Senescent cells and their secretory phenotype as targets for cancer therapy. *Interdiscip Top Gerontol* (2013) 38:17–27. doi:10.1159/000343572
129. Cruz CM, Rinna A, Forman HF, Ventura ALM, Persechini PM, Ojcius DM. ATP activates a reactive oxygen species-dependent oxidative stress response and secretion of proinflammatory cytokines in macrophages. *J Biol Chem* (2007) 282:2871–9. doi:10.1074/jbc.M608083200
130. Chen G, Shaw MH, Kim YG, Nunez G. NOD-like receptors; role in innate immunity and inflammatory disease. *Annu Rev Pathol* (2009) 4:365–98. doi:10.1146/annurev.pathol.4.110807.092239
131. Schroder K, Tschopp J. The inflammasomes. *Cell* (2010) 140:821–32. doi:10.1016/j.cell.2010.01.040
132. Kinoshita T, Imamura R, Kushiyama H, Suda T. NLRP3 mediates NF-κB activation and cytokine induction in microbially induced and sterile inflammation. *PLoS One* (2015) 10(3):e0119179. doi:10.1371/journal.pone.0119179
133. Youm YH, Grant RW, McCabe LR, Albarado DC, Nguyen KY, Ravussin A, et al. Canonical Nlrp3 inflammasome links systemic low-grade inflammation to functional decline in aging. *Cell Metab* (2013) 18:519–32. doi:10.1016/j.cmet.2013.09.015
134. Payne BAI, Chinnery PF. Mitochondrial dysfunction in aging: much progress but many unresolved questions. *Biochim Biophys Acta* (2015) 1847(11): 1347–53. doi:10.1016/j.bbabio.2015.05.022
135. Fang C, Wei X, Wei Y. Mitochondrial DNA in the regulation of innate immune responses. *Protein Cell* (2016) 7(1):11–6. doi:10.1007/s13238-015-0222-9
136. Collins LV, Hajizadeh S, Holme E, Jonsson IM, Tarkowski A. Endogenously oxidized mitochondrial DNA induces in vivo and in vitro inflammatory responses. *J Leukoc Biol* (2004) 7(5):995–1000. doi:10.1189/jlb.0703328
137. Ding Z, Liu S, Wang X, Khaidakov M, Dai Y, Mehta JL. Oxidant stress in mitochondrial DNA damage, autophagy and inflammation in atherosclerosis. *Sci Rep* (2013) 3:1077. doi:10.1038/srep01077
138. Escames G, López LC, Garcıa JA, Garcıa-Corzo L, Ortiz F, Acun ~a-Castroviejo D. Mitochondrial DNA and inflammatory diseases. *Hum Genet* (2012) 131:161–73. doi:10.1007/s00439-011-1057-y
139. Salminen A, Ojala J, Kaarniranta K, Kauppinen A. Mitochondrial dysfunction and oxidative stress activate inflammasomes: impact on the aging process and age-related diseases. *Cell Mol Life Sci* (2012) 69(18):2999–3013. doi:10.1007/s00018-012-0962-0
140. Mathew A, Lindsley TA, Sheridan A, Bhoiwala DL, Hushmendy SF, Yager EJ, et al. Degraded mitochondrial DNA is a newly identified subtype of the damage associated molecular pattern (DAMP) family and possible trigger of neurodegeneration. *J Alzheimers Dis* (2012) 30:617–27. doi:10.3233/JAD-2012-120145
141. Scherz-Shouval R, Elazar Z. Regulation of autophagy by ROS: physiology and pathology. *Trends Biochem Sci* (2011) 36:30–8. doi:10.1016/j.tibs.2010.07.007
142. Rajamaki L, Lappalainen J, Oorni K, Vallimaki E, Matikanien S, Kovanen PT, et al. Cholesterol crystals activate the NLRP3 inflammasome in human macrophages: a novel link between cholesterol metabolism and inflammation. *PLoS One* (2010) 5:e11765. doi:10.1371/journal.pone.0011765
143. Masters SL, O'Nelll LA. Disease-associated amyloid and misfolded protein aggregrates activate the inflammasome. *Trends Mol Med* (2011) 17:276–82. doi:10.1016/j.molmed.2011.01.005
144. Wen H, Fris D, Lei Y, Jha S, Zhang L, Huang MTH, et al. Fatty acid induced NLRP-3AS inflammasome activation interferes with insulin signaling. *Nat Immunol* (2011) 12:408–15. doi:10.1038/ni.2022
145. Mori MA, Bezy O, Kahn CR. Metabolic Syndrome: is Nlrp3 inflammasome a trigger or a target of insulin resistance? *Circ Res* (2011) 108(10):1160–2. doi:10.1161/RES.0b013e318220b57b
146. Vandanmagsar B, Youm YH, Ravussin A, Galgani JE, Stadler K, Mynatt RL, et al. The NLRP3 inflammasome instigates obesity-induced inflammation and insulin resistance. *Nat Med* (2011) 17(2):179–88. doi:10.1038/nm.2279
147. Schroder K, Zhou R, Tschopp J. The NLRP3 inflammasome: a sensor for metabolic danger? *Science* (2010) 327:296–300. doi:10.1126/science.1184003
148. Forsey RJ, Thompson JM, Ernerudh J, Hurst TL, Strindhall J, Johnsson B, et al. Plasma cytokine profiles in elderly humans. *Mech Ageing Devel* (2003) 124:487–93. doi:10.1016/S0047-6374(03)00025-3

149. Ferrucci L, Harris TB, Guralnik JM, Tracy RP, Corti MC, Cohen HJ, et al. Serum IL-6 level and the development of disability in older persons. *J Am Geriatr Soc* (1999) 47(6):639–46. doi:10.1111/j.1532-5415.1999.tb01583.x
150. Harris TB, Ferrucci L, Tracy RP, Corti MR, Wacholder S, Ettinger WH Jr, et al. Associations of elevated interleukin-6 and C-reactive protein levels with mortality in the elderly. *Am J Med* (1999) 106(5):506–12. doi:10.1016/S0002-9343(99)00066-2
151. Wei J, Xu H, Davies JL, Hemmings JP. Increase of plasma IL-6 concentration with age in healthy subjects. *Life Sci* (1992) 51(25):1953–6. doi:10.1016/0024-3205(92)90112-3
152. Sims JE, Smith DE. The IL-1 family: regulators of immunity. *Nat Rev Immunol* (2010) 10:89–102. doi:10.1038/nri2691
153. Cavallone L, Bonafe M, Olivieri F, Cardelli M, Marchegiani F, Giovagnetti S, et al. The role of IL-1 gene cluster in longevity: a study in Italian population. *Mech Ageing Dev* (2003) 124:533–8. doi:10.1016/S0047-6374(03)00033-2
154. Di Iorio A, Ferrucci L, Sparvieri E, Cherubini A, Volpato S, Corsi A, et al. Serum IL-1beta levels in health and disease: a population based study. "The InCHIANTI Study". *Cytokine* (2003) 22:198–205. doi:10.1016/S1043-4666(03)00152-2
155. Sansoni P, Vescovini R, Fagnoni F, Biasini C, Zanni F, Zanlari L, et al. The immune system in extreme longevity. *Exp Gerontol* (2008) 43(2):61–5. doi:10.1016/j.exger.2007.06.008128-
156. Jylha M, Paavilainen P, Lehtimäki T, Goebeler S, Karhunen PJ, Hervonen A, et al. Interleukin-1 receptor antagonist, interleukin-6, and C-reactive protein as predictors of mortality in nonagenarians: the vitality 90+ study. *J Gerontol A Biol Sci Med Sci* (2007) 62(9):1016–21. doi:10.1093/gerona/62.9.1016
157. Zhou L, Cai J, Liu G, Wei Y, Tang H. Associations between interleukin-1 gene polymorphisms and coronary heart disease risk: a meta-analysis. *PLoS One* (2012) 7(9):e45641. doi:10.1371/journal.pone.0045641
158. Mun M-J, Kim J-H, Choi J-Y, Jang W-C. Genetic polymorphisms of interleukin genes and the risk of Alzheimer's disease: an update meta-analysis. *Meta Gene* (2016) 8:1–10. doi:10.1016/j.mgene.2016.01.001
159. Trompet S, de Craen AJ, Slagboom P, Shepherd J, Blauw GJ, Murphy MB, et al. Genetic variation in the interleukin-1 beta-converting enzyme associates with cognitive function. The PROSPER study. *Brain* (2008) 131(4):1069–77. doi:10.1093/brain/awn023
160. Mrak RE, Griffin WS. Interleukin-1 and the immunogenetics of Alzheimer disease. *J Neuropathol Exp Neurol* (2000) 59(6):471–6. doi:10.1093/jnen/59.6.471
161. Langdahl BL, Lokke E, Carstens M, Stenkjaer LL, Eriksen EF. Osteoporotic fractures are associated with an 86-base pair repeat polymorphism in the interleukin-1 receptor antagonist gene but not with polymorphisms in the interleukin-1beta gene. *J Bone Miner Res* (2000) 15(3):402–14. doi:10.1359/jbmr.2000.15.3.402
162. Wang XY, Hurme M, Jylha M, Hervonen A. Lack of association between human longevity and polymorphisms of IL-1 cluster, IL-6, IL-10 and TNF-alpha genes in Finnish nonagenarians. *Mech Ageing Dev* (2001) 123:29–38. doi:10.1016/S0047-6374(01)00338-4
163. Cederholm T, Persson M, Andersson P, Stenvinkel P, Nordfors L, Madden J, et al. Polymorphisms in cytokine genes influence long-term survival differently in elderly male and female patients. *J Intern Med* (2007) 262:215–23. doi:10.1111/j.1365-2796.2007.01803.x
164. Dinarello CA, Simon A, van der Meer JWM. Treating inflammation by blocking interleukin-1 in a broad spectrum of diseases. *Nat Rev Drug Discov* (2012) 11:633–52. doi:10.1038/nrd3800
165. Smith DE. The biological paths of IL-1 family members IL-18 and IL-33. *J Leukoc Biol* (2011) 89(3):383–92. doi:10.1189/jlb.0810470
166. Dinarello CA, Novick D, Kim S, Kaplanski G. Interleukin-18 and IL-18 binding protein. *Front Immunol* (2013) 4:289. doi:10.3389/fimmu.2013.00289
167. Gangemi S, Basile G, Merendino RA, Minciullo PL, Novick D, Rubinstein M, et al. Increased circulating interleukin-18 levels in centenarians with no signs of vascular disease: another paradox of longevity? *Exp Gerontol* (2003) 38:669–72. doi:10.1016/S0531-5565(03)00061-5
168. Dinarello CA. Interleukin 1 and interleukin 18 as mediators of inflammation and the aging process. *Am J Clin Nutr* (2006) 83(2):447S–55S. doi:10.1093/ajcn/83.2.447S
169. Mallat Z, Heymes C, Corbaz A, Logeart D, Alouani S, Cohen-Solal A, et al. Evidence of altered interleukin (IL)-18 pathway in human heart failure. *FASET J* (2004) 18(14):1752–4. doi:10.1096/fj.04-2426fje
170. Jefferis BJ, Papacosta O, Owen CG, Wannamethee SG, Humphries SE, Woodward M, et al. Interleukin 18 and coronary heart disease: prospective study and systematic review. *Atherosclerosis* (2011) 217(1):227–33. doi:10.1016/j.atherosclerosis.2011.03.015
171. Harms RZ, Yarde DN, Guinn Z, Lorenzo-Arteaga KM, Corley KP, Cabrera MS, et al. Increased expression of IL-18 in the serum and islets of type 1 diabetics. *Mol Immunol* (2015) 64(2):306–12. doi:10.1016/j.molimm.2014.12.012
172. Liu L, Chan C. The role of inflammasome in Alzheimer's disease. *Ageing Res Rev* (2014) 15:6–15. doi:10.1016/j.arr.2013.12.007
173. Thomas K, Radiq S, Frayling T, Ebrahim S, Kumari M, Gallacher J, et al. Interleukin-18 polymorphism and physical functioning in older people: a replication study and meta-analysis. *J Gerontol A Biol Sci Med Sci* (2009) 64(11):1177–82. doi:10.1093/gerona/glp092
174. Mekli K, Marshall A, Nazroon J, Vanhoutte B, Pendleton N. Genetic variant of Interleukin-18 gene is associated with the frailty index in the English longitudinal study of ageing. *Age Ageing* (2015) 44(6):938–42. doi:10.1093/ageing/afv122
175. Frayling TM, Rafiq S, Murray A, Hurst AJ, Weedon MN, Henley W, et al. Aninterleukin-18 polymorphism is associated with reduced serum concentrations and better functioning in older people. *J Gerontol A Biol Sci Med Sci* (2007) 62:73–8. doi:10.1093/gerona/62.1.73
176. Doyle SL, Ozaki E, Brennan K, Humphries MM, Mulfaul K, Keaney J, et al. IL-18 attenuates experimental choroidal neovascularization as a potential therapy for wet age-related macular degeneration. *Sci Transl Med* (2014) 6(230):230ra44. doi:10.1126/scitranslmed.3007616
177. Ershler WB. Interleukin-6: a cytokine for gerontologists. *J Am Geriatr Soc* (1993) 41:176–81. doi:10.1111/j.1532-5415.1993.tb02054.x
178. Ershler WB, Keller ET. Age-associated increased interleukin-6 gene expression, late-life diseases, and frailty. *Annu Rev Med* (2000) 51:245–70. doi:10.1146/annurev.med.51.1.245
179. Weiss TW, Arnesen H, Seljeflot I. Components of the interleukin-6 trans-signalling system are associated with the metabolic syndrome, endothelial dysfunction and arterial stiffness. *Metabolism* (2013) 62(7):1008–13. doi:10.1016/j.metabol.2013.01.019
180. Puzianowska-Kuźnicka M, Owczarz M, Wieczorowska-Tobis K, Nadrowski P, Chudek J, Slusarczyk P, et al. Interleukin-6 and C-reactive protein, successful aging, and mortality: the PolSenior study. *Immun Ageing* (2016) 13:21. doi:10.1186/s12979-016-0076-x
181. Van Epps P, Oswald D, Higgins PA, Hornick TR, Aung H, Banks RE, et al. Frailty has a stronger association with inflammation than age in older veterans. *Immun Ageing* (2016) 13:27. doi:10.1186/s12979-016-0082-z
182. Varadhan R, Yao W, Matteini A, Beamer BA, Xue QL, Yang H, et al. Simple biologically informed inflammatory index of two serum cytokines predicts 10 year all-cause mortality in older adults. *J Gerontol A Biol Sci Med Sci* (2014) 69:165–73. doi:10.1093/gerona/glt023
183. Hubbard RE, O'Mahony MS, Savva GM, Calver BL, Woodhouse KW. Inflammation and frailty measures in older people. *J Cell Mol Med* (2009) 13:3103–9. doi:10.1111/j.1582-4934.2009.00733
184. Alemán H, Esparza J, Ramirez FA, Astiazaran H, Payette H. Longitudinal evidence on the association between interleukin-6 and C-reactive protein with the loss of total appendicular skeletal muscle in free-living older men and women. *Age Ageing* (2011) 40(4):469–75. doi:10.1093/ageing/afr040
185. Ridker PM, Rifai N, Stampfer MJ, Hennekens CH. Plasma concentration of interleukin-6 and the risk of future myocardial infarction among apparently healthy men. *Circulation* (2000) 101:1767–72. doi:10.1161/01.CIR.101.15.1767
186. Fishman D, Faulds G, Jeffery R, Mohamed-Ali V, Yudkin JS, Humphries S, et al. The effect of novel polymorphisms in the interleukin-6 (IL- 6) gene on IL-6 transcription and plasma IL-6 levels, and an association with systemic-onset juvenile chronic arthritis. *J Clin Invest* (1998) 102:1369–76. doi:10.1172/JCI2629
187. Mooijaart SP, Sattar N, Trompet S, Lucke J, Stott DJ, Ford I, et al. Circulating interleukin-6 concentration and cognitive decline in old age: the PROSPER study. *J Intern Med* (2013) 274:77–85. doi:10.1111/joim.12052
188. Miwa K, Okazaki S, Sakaguchi M, Mochizuki H, Kitagawa K. Interleukin-6, interleukin-6 receptor gene variant, small-vessel disease and incident dementia. *Eur J Neurol* (2016) 23(3):656–63. doi:10.1111/ene.12921
189. Spoto B, Mattace-Raso F, Sijbrands E, Leonardis D, Testa A, Pisano A, et al. Association of IL-6 and a functional polymorphism in the IL-6 Gene with

cardiovascular events in patients with CKD. *Clin J Am Soc Nephrol* (2014) 10:232–40. doi:10.2215/CJN.07000714

190. Dai L, Liu D, Guo H, Wang Y, Bai Y. Association between polymorphism in the promoter region of Interleukin 6 (174 G/C) and risk of Alzheimers disease: a meta-analysis. *J Neurol* (2012) 259(3):414–9. doi:10.1007/s00415-011-6164-0
191. Qi H-P, Qu Z-Y, Duan S-R, Wei S-Q, Wen S-R, Bi S. IL-6-174 G/C and 572 C/G polymorphisms and risk of Alzheimer's disease. *PLoS One* (2012) 7(6):e37858. doi:10.1371/journal.pone.0037858
192. Di Bona D, Vasto S, Capurso C, Christiansen L, Deiana L, Franceschi C, et al. Effect of interleukin-6 polymorphisms on human longevity: a systematic review and meta-analysis. *Ageing Res Rev* (2009) 8:36–42. doi:10.1016/j.arr.2008.09.001
193. Soerensen M, Dato S, Tan Q, Thinggaard M, Kleindorp R, Beekman M, et al. Evidence from case-control and longitudinal studies supports associations of genetic variation in APOE, CETP, and IL6 with human longevity. *Age* (2013) 35(2):487–500. doi:10.1007/s11357-011-9373-7
194. Interleukin-6 Receptor Mendelian Randomisation Analysis (IL6R MR) Consortium, Swerdlow DI, Holmes MV, Kuchenbaecker KB, Engmann JEL, Shah T, et al. The interleukin-6 receptor as a target for prevention of coronary heart disease: a Mendelian randomisation analysis. *Lancet* (2012) 379:1214–24. doi:10.1016/S0140-6736(12)60110-X
195. Davies R, Choy E. Clinical experience of IL-6 blockade in rheumatic diseases—implications on IL-6 biology and disease pathogenesis. *Semin Immunol* (2014) 26:97–104. doi:10.1016/j.smim.2013.12.002
196. Ferruci L, Corsi A, Lauretani F, Bandinelli S, Bartali B, Taub DD, et al. The origins of age-related proinflammatory state. *Blood* (2005) 105(6):2294–9. doi:10.1182/blood-2004-07-2599
197. McNerlan SE, Rea IM, Alexander HD. A whole blood method for measurement of intracellular TNFα, IFNγ an IL-2 expression in stimulated CD3+ lymphocytes: differences between young and elderly subjects. *Exp Gerontol* (2002) 37:227–37. doi:10.1016/S0531-5565(01)00188-7
198. O'Mahoney L, Holland J, Jackson J, Feighery C, Hennessy TP, Mealy K. Quantitative intracellular cytokine measurement: age-related changes in proinflammatory cytokine production. *Clin Exp Immunol* (1998) 113(2):213–9. doi:10.1046/j.1365-2249.1998.00641.x
199. Armstrong ME, Alexander HD, Ritchie JL, McMillan SA, Rea IM. Age-related alterations in basal expression and in vitro, tumour necrosis factor alpha mediated, upregulation of CD11b. *Gerontology* (2001) 47:180–5. doi:10.1159/000052795
200. Bruunsgaard H, Pedersen AN, Schroll M, Skinhoj P, Pedersen BK. Ageing, TNF-α and atherosclerosis. *Clin Exp Immunol* (2000) 121:255–60. doi:10.1046/j.1365-2249.2000.01281.x
201. Bruunsgaard H, Ladelund S, Pedersen AN, Schroll M, Jørgensen T, Pedersen BK. Predicting death from tumour necrosis factor-alpha and interleukin-6 in 80 year old people. *Clin Exp Immunol* (2003) 132:24–31. doi:10.1046/j.1365-2249.2003.02137.x
202. Bruunsgaard H, Andersen-Ranberg K, Hjelmborg JV, Pedersen BK, Jeune B. Elevated levels of tumour necrosis factor alpha and mortality in centenarians. *Am J Med* (2003) 115:278–83. doi:10.1016/S0002-9343(03)00329-2
203. Ridker PM, Rifai N, Pfeffer M, Sacks F, Lepage S, Braunwald E. Elevation of tumor necrosis factor-alpha and increased risk of recurrent coronary events after myocardial infarction. *Circulation* (2000) 101(18):2149–53. doi:10.1161/01.CIR.101.18.2149
204. Nilsson L, Szymanowski A, Swahn E, Jonasson L. Soluble TNF receptors are associated with infarct size and ventricular dysfunction in ST-elevation myocardial infarction. *PLoS One* (2013) 8:e55477. doi:10.1371/journal.pone.0055477
205. Bae E, Cha R-H, Kim YC, An JN, Kim DK, Yoo KD, et al. Circulating TNF receptors predict cardiovascular disease in patients with chronic kidney disease. *Medicine* (2017) 96(19):e6666. doi:10.1097/MD.0000000000006666
206. Zhang P, Wu X, Li G, He Q, Dai H, Ai C, et al. Tumor necrosis factor-alpha gene polymorphisms and susceptibility to ischemic heart disease: a systematic review and meta-analysis. *Medicine* (2017) 96(14):e6569. doi:10.1097/MD.0000000000006569
207. Wang T. TNF-alpha G308A polymorphism and the susceptibility to Alzheimer's disease: an updated meta-analysis. *Arch Med Res* (2015) 46(1):24.e–30.e. doi:10.1016/j.arcmed.2014.12.006
208. McCusker SM, Curran MD, Dynan KB, McCullagh CD, Urquhart DD, Middleton D, et al. Association between polymorphism in regulatory region of gene encoding tumour necrosis factor alpha and risk of Alzheimer's disease and vascular dementia: a case-control study. *Lancet* (2001) 357:436–9. doi:10.1016/S0140-6736(00)04008-3
209. Collins JS, Perry RT, Watson B Jr, Harrell LE, Acton RT, Blacker D, et al. Association of a haplotype for tumour necrosis factor in siblings with late-onset Alzheimer disease. The NIMH Alzheimer disease genetics initiative. *Am J Med Genet* (2000) 96:823–30. doi:10.1002/1096-8628(20001204)96:6<823::AID-AJMG26>3.0.CO;2-I
210. Zheng C, Zhou Z-W, Wang J-Z. The dual roles of cytokines in Alzheimer's disease: update on interleukins, TNF-α, TGF-β and IFN-γ. *Transl Neurodegener* (2016) 5(1):7. doi:10.1186/s40035-016-0054-4
211. Nilsson J, Jovinge S, Niemann A, Reneland R, Lithell H. Relation between plasma tumour necrosis factor-α and insulin sensitivity in elderly men with non-insulin-dependent diabetes mellitus. *Arterioscler Thromb Vasc Biol* (1998) 18(8):1199. doi:10.1161/01.ATV.18.8.1199
212. Ross OA, Curran MD, Meenagh A, Williams F, Barnett YA, Middleton D, et al. Study of age-association with cytokine gene polymorphisms in an aged Irish population. *Mech Ageing Dev* (2003) 124(2):199–206. doi:10.1016/S0047-6374(02)00132-X
213. Lio D, Scola L, Crivello A, Colonna-Romano G, Candore G, Bonafè M, et al. Inflammation, genetics and longevity: further studies on the prospective effects in men of IL-10-1082 promoter SNP and its interaction with TNF-alpha-308 promoter SNP. *J Med Genet* (2003) 40:296–9. doi:10.1136/jmg.40.4.296
214. Ruparelia N, Chai JT, Fisher EA, Choudhury RP. Inflammatory processes in cardiovascular disease: a route to targeted therapies. *Nat Rev Cardiol* (2017) 14:133–44. doi:10.1038/nrcardio.2017.33
215. Shamim D, Laskowski M. Inhibition of inflammation mediated through the tumor necrosis factor α biochemical pathway can lead to favorable outcomes in Alzheimer disease. *J Cent Nerv Syst Dis* (2017) 9:1179573517722512. doi:10.1177/1179573517722512
216. Mosmann TR, Sad S. The expanding universe of T cell subsets: Th1, Th2 and more. *Immunol Today* (1996) 17:138–46. doi:10.1016/0167-5699(96)80606-2
217. Laurence A, Tato CM, Davidson S, Kano Y, Chen Z, Yao Z, et al. Interleukin-2 signaling via STAT5 constrains T helper 17 cell generation. *Immunity* (2009) 26(3):371–81. doi:10.1016/j.immuni.2007.02.009
218. Gillis S, Watson J. Interleukin-2 dependent culture of cytolytic T cells. *Immunol Rev* (1981) 54:81–109. doi:10.1111/j.1600-065X.1981.tb00435.x
219. Caruso C, Candore G, Cigna D, DiLorenzo G, Sireci G, Dieli F, et al. Cytokine production pathway in the elderly. *Immunol Res* (1996) 15:84–90. doi:10.1007/BF02918286
220. Rea IM, Stewart M, Campbell P, Alexander HD, Crockard AD, Morris TCM. Changes in lymphocyte subsets, interleukin 2 and soluble interleukin 2 receptor in old and very old age. *Gerontology* (1996) 42:69–78. doi:10.1159/000213775
221. Pietschmann P, Gollob E, Brosch S, Hahn P, Kudlacek S, Willheim M, et al. The effect of age and gender on cytokine production by human peripheral blood mononuclear cells and markers of bone metabolism. *Exp Gerontol* (2003) 38:1119–27. doi:10.1016/S0531-5565(03)00189-X
222. Aspinall R. T cell development, ageing and interleukin-7. *Mech Ageing Dev* (2006) 127:572–8. doi:10.1016/j.mad.2006.01.016
223. Nguyen V, Mendelsohn A, LarricK JW. Interleukin-7 and Immunosenescence. *J Immunol Res* (2017) 2017:4807853. doi:10.1155/2017/4807853
224. Passtoors WM, Boer JM, Goeman JJ, van den Akker EB, Deelen J, Zwaan BJ. Transcriptional prefiling of human familial longevity indicates a role for ASF1A and IL-7R. *PLoS One* (2012) 7(1):e27759. doi:10.1371/journal.pone.0027759
225. Passtoors WM, van den Akker EB, Deelen J, Maier AB, van der Breggen R, Jansen R, et al. IL7R gene expression network associates with human healthy ageing. *Immun Ageing* (2015) 12:21. doi:10.1186/s12979-015-0048-6
226. Rübenhagen R, Schüttrumpf JP, Stürmer KM, Frosch KH. Interleukin-7 levels in synovial fluid increase with age and MMP-1 levels decrease with progression of osteoarthritis. *Acta Orthop* (2012) 83(1):59–64. doi:10.3109/17453674.2011.645195
227. Zuvich RL, McCauley JL, Oksenberg JR, Sawcer SJ, De Jager PL. Consortium international multiple sclerosis genetics, haines JL. genetic variation in the

IL7RA/IL7 pathway increases multiple sclerosis susceptibility. *Hum Genet* (2010) 127(5):525–35. doi:10.1007/s00439-010-0789-4
228. Ucar D, Márquez EJ, Chung C-H, Marches R, Rossi RJ, Uyar A, et al. The chromatin accessibility signature of human immune aging stems from CD8+ T cells. *J Exp Med* (2017) 214(10):3123–44. doi:10.1084/jem.20170416
229. van der Heijden T, Bot I, Kuiper J. IL-12 cytokine family in cardiovascular disease. *Cytokine* (2017) 816:1–2. doi:10.1016/j.cyto.2017.10.010
230. Zykov MV, Barbarash OL, Kashtalap W, Kutikhin AG, Barbarash LS. Interleukin 12 serum level has prognostic value in patients with ST-segment elevation myocardial infarction. *Heart Lung* (2016) 45:336–40. doi:10.1016/j.hrtlng.2016.03.007
231. Rea IM, McNerlan SE, Alexander HD. Serum IL-12 and IL12p40 but not IL-12p70 are increased in the serum of older subjects: relationship to CD3+ and NK subsets. *Cytokine* (2000) 12(2):156–9. doi:10.1006/cyto.1999.0537
232. Compte N, Zouaoui Boudjeltia K, Vanhaeverbeek M, De Bruecker S, Tassignon J, Trelcat A, et al. Frailty in old age is associated with decreased interleukin 12/23 production in response to toll-like receptor ligation. *PLoS One* (2013) 8:e65325. doi:10.1371/journal.pone.0065325
233. Tan MS, Yu JT, Jiang T, Zhu XC, Guan HS, Tan L. Il-12/23 p40 inhibition ameliorates alzheimers disease-associated neuropathology and spatial memory in SAMP8 mice. *J Alzheimers Dis* (2014) 38(3):633–46. doi:10.1371/journal.pone.0176760
234. O'Quinn D, Palmer M, Lee Y, Weaver C. Emergence of the Th17 pathway and its role in host defense. *Adv Immunol* (2008) 99:115–63. doi:10.1016/S0065-2776(08)00605-6
235. Korn T, Bettelli E, Oukka M, Kuchroo VK. IL-17 and Th17 cells. *Annu Rev Immunol* (2009) 27:485–517. doi:10.1146/annurev.immunol.021908.132710
236. Lee JS, Lee WW, Kim SH, Kang Y, Lee N, Shin MS, et al. Age-associated alteration in naive and memory Th17 cell response in humans. *Clin Immunol* (2011) 140(1):84–91. doi:10.1016/j.clim.2011.03.018
237. Gaffen SL. The role of interleukin-17 in the pathogenesis of rheumatoid arthritis. *Curr Rhematol Rep* (2009) 11:365–70. doi:10.1007/s11926-009-0052-y
238. Zambrano-Zaragoza JF, Romo-Martínez EJ, Durán-Avelar Mde J, García-Magallanes N, Vibanco-Pérez N. Th17 cells in autoimmune and infectious diseases. *Int J Inflam* (2014) 2014:651503. doi:10.1155/2014/651503
239. McKensie BS, Kastelein RA, Cua DJ. Understanding the IL-23-IL-17 immune pathway. *Trends Immunol* (2006) 27:17–23. doi:10.1016/j.it.2005.10.003
240. Garrett-Sinha LA, John S, Gaffen SL. IL-17 and the Th17 lineage in systemic lupus erythematosus. *Curr Opin Rheumatol* (2008) 20:519–25. doi:10.1007/s10067-014-2656-5
241. Dong C. Regulation and pre-inflammatory function of interleukin-17 family cytokines. *Immunol Rev* (2008) 226:80–6. doi:10.1111/j.1600-065X.2008.00709.x
242. Srenathan U, Steel K, Taams LS. IL-17+ CD8+ T cells: differentiation, phenotype and role in inflammatory disease. *Immunol Lett* (2016) 178:20–6. doi:10.1016/j.imlet.2016.05.001
243. Menon B, Gullick NJ, Walter GJ, Rajasekhar M, Garrood T, Evans HG, et al. IL-17+ CD8+ T cells are enriched in the joints of patients with psoriatic arthritis and correlate with disease activity and joint damage progression. *Arthritis Rheum* (2014) 66:1272–81. doi:10.1002/art.38376
244. Rink L, Cakman I, Kirchner H. Altered cytokine production in the elderly. *Mech Ageing Dev* (1998) 102:199–209. doi:10.1016/S0047-6374(97)00153-X
245. Wieczorowska-Tobis K, Niemir ZI, Podkówka R, Korybalska K, Mossakowska M, Bręborowicz A. Can an increased level of circulating IL-8 be a predictor of human longevity? *Med Sci Monit* (2006) 12:CR118–21.
246. Campbell LM, Maxwell PJ, Waugh DJ. Rationale and means to target pro-inflammatory interleukin-8 (CXCL8) signaling in cancer. *Pharmaceuticals (Basel)* (2013) 6(8):929–59. doi:10.3390/ph6080929
247. Ouyang W, Rutz S, Crellin NK, Valdez PA, Hymowitz SG. Regulation and functions of the IL-10 family of cytokines in inflammation and disease. *Annu Rev Immunol* (2011) 29:71–109. doi:10.1146/annurev-immunol-031210-101312
248. Commins S, Steinke JW, Borish L. The extended IL-10 superfamily: IL-10, IL-19, IL-20, IL-22, IL-24, IL-26, IL-28, and IL-29. *J Allergy Clin Immunol* (2008) 121(5):1108–11. doi:10.1016/j.jaci.2008.02.026
249. Rea IM. IL-10 production from monocyte monolayers in very old age. *Immunology* (1996) 89(Suppl 1):68.
250. Hirokawa K, Utsuyama M, Hayashi Y, Kitagawa M, Makinodan T, Fulop T. Slower immune system aging in women versus men in the Japanese population. *Immun Ageing* (2013) 10:19. doi:10.1186/1742-4933-10-19
251. Didion SP, Kinzenbaw DA, Schrader LI, Chu Y, Faraci FM. Endogenous interleukin-10 inhibits angiotensin II-induced vascular dysfunction. *Hypertension* (2009) 54(3):619–24. doi:10.1161/HYPERTENSIONAHA.109.137158
252. Kinzenbaw DA, Chu Y, Peña Silva RA, Didion SP, Faraci FM. Interleukin-10 protects against aging-induced endothelial dysfunction. *Physiol Rep* (2013) 1(6):e00149. doi:10.1002/phy2.149
253. Fichtlscherer S, Breuer S, Heeschen C, Dimmeler S, Zeiher AM. Interleukin-10 serum levels and systemic endothelial vasoreactivity in patients with coronary artery disease. *J Am Coll Cardiol* (2004) 44(1):44–9. doi:10.1016/j.jacc.2004.02.054
254. Lakoski SG, Liu Y, Brosnihan KB, Herrington DM. Interleukin-10 concentration and coronary heart disease (CHD) event risk in the estrogen replacement and atherosclerosis (ERA) study. *Atherosclerosis* (2008) 197(1):443–7. doi:10.1016/j.atherosclerosis.2007.06.033
255. Welsh P, Murray HM, Ford I, Trompet S, de Craen AJ, Jukema JW, et al. Circulating interleukin-10 and risk of cardiovascular events a prospective study in the elderly at risk. *Arterioscler Thromb Vasc Biol* (2011) 31(10):2338–44. doi:10.1161/ATVBAHA.111.231795
256. Pes GM, Lio D, Carru C, Deiana L, Baggio G, Franceschi C, et al. Association between longevity and cytokine gene polymorphisms. A study in Sardinian centenarians. *Aging Clin Exp Res* (2004) 16(3):244–8. doi:10.1007/BF03327391
257. Westendorp RG, Langermans JAM, Huizinga TWJ, Elouali AH, Verweij CL, Boomsma DI, et al. Genetic influence on cytokine production in meningococcal disease. *Lancet* (1997) 349:170–3. doi:10.1016/S0140-6736(96)06413-6
258. Yoshimura A, Wakabayashi Y, Mori T. Cellular and molecular basis for the regulation of inflammation by TGF-beta. *J Biochem* (2010) 147(6):781–92. doi:10.1093/jb/mvq043
259. Rea IM, Maxwell LD, McNerlan SE, Alexander HD, Curran MD, Middleton D, et al. Killer immunoglobulin-like receptors (KIR) haplogroups A and B track with natural killer cells and cytokine profile in aged subjects: observations from octo/nonagenarians in the belfast elderly longitudinal free-living aging study (BELFAST). *Immun Ageing* (2013) 10(1):35. doi:10.1186/1742-4933-10-35
260. Krieglstein K, Miyazono K, Ten Dijke P, Unsicker K. TGF-beta in aging and disease. *Cell Tissue Res* (2012) 347:5–9. doi:10.1007/s00441-011-1278-1273
261. Pastrana JL, Sha X, Virtue A, Mai J, Cueto R, Lee IA, et al. Regulatory T cells and atherosclerosis. *J Clin Exp Cardiolog* (2012) (Suppl 12):002. doi:10.4172/2155-9880.S12-002
262. Burks TN, Cohn RD. Role of TGF-β signaling in inherited and acquired myopathies. *Skelet Muscle* (2011) 1:19. doi:10.1186/2044-5040-1-19
263. Baugé C, Girard N, Lhuissier E, Bazille C, Boumediene K. Regulation and role of TGFβ signaling pathway in aging and osteoarthritis joints. *Aging Disease* (2014) 5(6):394–405. doi:10.14336/AD.2014.0500394
264. Mitnitski A, Collerton J, Martin-Ruiz C, Jagger C, von Zglinicki T, Rockwood K, et al. Age-related frailty and its association with biological markers of ageing. *BMC Med* (2015) 13:161. doi:10.1186/s12916-015-0400-x
265. Doyle KP, Cekanaviciute E, Mamer LE, Buckwalter MS. TGFβ signaling in the brain increases with aging and signals to astrocytes and innate immune cells in the weeks after stroke. *J Neuroinflammation* (2010) 7:62. doi:10.1186/1742-2094-7-62
266. Yang Q, Wang E-Y, Jia H-W, Wang Y-P. Association between polymorphisms in transforming growth factor-β1 and sporadic Alzheimer's disease in a Chinese population. *Int J Neurosci* (2016) 126:979–84. doi:10.3109/00207454.2015.1088849
267. Bosco P, Ferri R, Salluzzo MG, Castellano S, Signorelli M, Nicoletti F, et al. Role of the transforming-growth-factor-β1 gene in late-onset Alzheimer's disease: implications for the treatment. *Curr Genomics* (2013) 14(2):147–56. doi:10.2174/1389202911314020007
268. Mallat Z, Gojova A, Marchiol-Fournigault C, Esposito B, Kamate C, Merval R, et al. Inhibition of transforming growth factor-beta signaling accelerates atherosclerosis and induces an unstable plaque phenotype in mice. *Circ Res* (2001) 89(10):930–4. doi:10.1161/hh2201.099415
269. Carrieri G, Marzi E, Olivieri F, Marchegiani F, Cavallone L, Cardelli M, et al. The G/C 915 polymorphism of transforming growth factor β1 is associated with human longevity: a study in Italian centenarians. *Aging Cell* (2004) 3:443–8. doi:10.1111/j.1474-9728.2004.00129.x

270. Tran Dat Q. TGF-β: the sword, the wand, and the shield of FOXP3+ regulatory T cells. *J Mol Cell Biol* (2012) 4(1):29–37. doi:10.1093/jmcb/mjr033
271. Han G, Li F, Singh TP, Wolf P, Wan X-J. The Pro-inflammatory Role of TGFβ1: a Paradox? *Int J Biol Sci* (2012) 8(2):228–35. doi:10.7150/ijbs.8.228
272. Akhurst RJ, Hata A. Targeting the TGFb signaling pathway in disease. *Nat Rev Drug Discov* (2012) 11:790–811. doi:10.1038/nrd3810
273. Nold MF, Nold-Petry CA, Zepp JA, Palmer BE, Bufler P, Dinarello CA. IL-37 is a fundamental inhibitor of innate immunity. *Nat Immunol* (2010) 11(11):1014–22. doi:10.1038/ni.1944
274. Shou X, Lin J, Xie C, Wang Y, Sun C. Plasma IL-37 elevated in patients with chronic heart failure and predicted major adverse cardiac events: a 1-year follow-up study. *Dis Markers* (2017) 2017:9134079. doi:10.1155/2017/913407
275. Dinarello CA, Nold-Petry C, Nold M, Fujita M, Li S, Kim S, et al. Suppression of innate inflammation and immunity by interleukin-37. *Eur J Immunol* (2016) 46(5):1067–81. doi:10.1002/eji.20154582854
276. Xu WD, Zhao Y, Liu Y. Insights into IL-37, the role in autoimmune diseases. *Autoimmun Rev* (2015) 14(12):1170–5. doi:10.1016/j.autrev.2015.08.006
277. Balkwill F, Charles KA, Mantovani A. Smoldering and polarized inflammation in the initiation and promotion of malignant disease. *Cancer Cell* (2005) 7:211–7. doi:10.1016/j.ccr.2005.02.013
278. Coussens LM, Werb Z. Inflammation and cancer. *Nature* (2002) 420(6917):860–7. doi:10.1038/nature01322
279. Grivennikov SI, Greten FR, Karin M. Immunity, inflammation, and cancer. *Cell* (2010) 140(6):883–99. doi:10.1016/j.cell.2010.01.025
280. Kantono M, Guo B. Inflammasomes and cancer: the dynamic role of the inflammasome in tumor development. *Front Immunol* (2017) 8:1132. doi:10.3389/fimmu.2017.01132
281. Lin C, Zhang J. Inflammasomes in inflammation- induced cancer. *Front Immunol* (2017) 8:271. doi:10.3389/fimmu.2017.00271
282. Venerito M, Vasapolli R, Rokkas T, Delchier JC, Malfertheiner P. Helicobacter pylori, gastric cancer and other gastrointestinal malignancies. *Helicobacter* (2017) 22(Suppl):1. doi:10.1111/hel.12413
283. Vockerodt M, Cader FZ, Shannon-Lowe C, Murray P. Epstein-Barr virus and the origin of Hodgkin lymphoma. *Chin J Cancer* (2014) 33(12):591–7. doi:10.5732/cjc.014.10193
284. de Sanjosé S, Brotons M, Pavón MA. The natural history of human papillomavirus infection. *Best Pract Res Clin Obstet Gynaecol* (2017). doi:10.1016/j.bpobgyn.2017.08.015
285. Greaves MF, Verbi W, Tilley R, Lister TA, Habeshaw J, Guo HG, et al. Human T-cell leukemia virus (HTLV) in the United Kingdom. *Int J Cancer* (1984) 33(6):795–806. doi:10.1002/ijc.2910330614
286. Diaconu S, Predescu A, Moldoveanu A, Pop CS, Fierbinteanu-Braticevici C. *Helicobacter pylori* infection: old and new. *J Med Life* (2017) 10(2):112–7.
287. El-Omar EM, Rabkin CS, Gammon MD, Vaughan TL, Risch HA, Schoenberg JB, et al. Increased risk of noncardia gastric cancer associated with proinflammatory cytokine gene polymorphisms. *Gastroenterology* (2003) 124: 1193–201.
288. El-Omar EM, Carrington M, Chow WH, McColl KE, Bream JH, Young HA, et al. Interleukin-1 polymorphisms associated with increased risk of gastric cancer. *Nature* (2000) 404:398–402. doi:10.1038/35006081
289. Iwamuro M, Takenaka R, Nakagawa M, Moritou Y, Saito S, Hori S, et al. Management of gastric mucosa-associated lymphoid tissue lymphoma in patients with extra copies of the MALT1 gene. *World J Gastroenterol* (2017) 23(33):6155–63. doi:10.3748/wjg.v23.i33.6155
290. Lupfer C, Malik A, Kanneganti TD. Inflammasome control of viral infection. *Curr Opin Virol* (2015) 12:38–46. doi:10.1016/j.coviro.2015.02.007
291. Fingeroth JD, Clabby ML, Strominger JD. Characterization of a T-lymphocyte Epstein-Barr virus/C3d receptor (CD21). *J Virol* (1988) 62(4):1442–7.
292. Bernheim A, Berger R, Lenoir G. Cytogenetic studies on African Burkitt's lymphoma cell lines: t(8;14), t(2;8) and t(8;22) translocations. *Cancer Genet Cytogenet* (1981) 3(4):307–15. doi:10.1016/0165-4608(81)90039-X
293. Chen LC, Wang LJ, Tsang NM, Ojcius DM, Chen CC, Ouyang CN, et al. Tumour inflammasome-derived IL-1beta recruits neutrophils and improves local recurrence-free survival in EBV-induced nasopharyngeal carcinoma. *EMBO Mol Med* (2012) 4(12):1276–93. doi:10.1002/emmm.201201569
294. Haneklaus M, Gerlic M, Kurowska-Stolarska M, Rainey AA, Pich D, McInnes IB, et al. Cutting edge: miR-223 and EBV miR-BART15 regulate the NLRP3 inflammasome and IL-1beta production. *J Immunol* (2012) 189(8):3795–9. doi:10.4049/jimmunol.1200312
295. Longo DL, Gelmann EP, Cossman J, Young RA, Gallo RC, O'Brien SJ, et al. Isolation of HTLV-transformed B-lymphocyte clone from a patient with HTLV-associated adult T-cell leukaemia. *Nature* (1984) 310(5977):505–6. doi:10.1038/310505a0
296. Bangham CR, Toulza F. Adult T cell leukemia/lymphoma: FoxP3(+) cells and the cell-mediated immune response to HTLV-1. *Adv Cancer Res* (2011) 111:163–82. doi:10.1016/B978-0-12-385524-4.00004-0
297. Oliere S, Douville R, Sze A, Belgnaoui SM, Hiscott J. Modulation of innate immune responses during human T-cell leukemia virus (HTLV-1) pathogenesis. *Cytokine Growth Factor Rev* (2011) 22(4):197–210. doi:10.1016/j.cytogfr.2011.08.002
298. Rayet B, Gélinas C. Aberrant rel/nfkb genes and activity in human cancer. *Oncogene* (1999) 18(49):6938–47. doi:10.1038/sj.onc.1203221
299. Hiscott J, Kwon H, Génin P. Hostile takeovers: viral appropriation of the NF-kB pathway. *J Clin Invest* (2001) 107(2):143–51. doi:10.1172/JCI11918
300. Kamada AJ, Pontillo A, Guimarães RL, Loureiro P, Crovella S, Brandão LAC. NLRP3 polymorphism is associated with protection against human T-lymphotropicvirus 1 infection. *Mem Inst Oswaldo Cruz* (2014) 109(7): 960–3. doi:10.1590/0074-0276140154
301. Wang D, DuBois RN. The role of COX-2 in intestinal inflammation and colorectal cancer. *Oncogene* (2010) 29(6):781–8. doi:10.1038/onc.2009.421
302. Smolen JS, Aletaha D, McInnes IB. Rheumatoid arthritis. *Lancet* (2016) 388:2023–38. doi:10.1016/S0140-6736(16)30173-8
303. Firestein GS, McInnes IB. Immunopathogenesis of rheumatoid arthritis. *Immunity* (2017) 46:183–96. doi:10.1016/j.immuni.2017.02.006
304. van de Sande MG, de Hair MJ, Schuller Y, van de Sande GP, Wijbrandts CA, Dinant HJ, et al. The features of the synovium in early rheumatoid arthritis according to the 2010 ACR/EULAR classification criteria. *PLoS One* (2012) 7:e36668. doi:10.1371/journal.pone.0036668
305. van der Ven M, van der Veer-Meerkerk M, Ten Cate DF, Rasappu N, Kok MR, Csakvari D, et al. Absence of ultrasound inflammation in patients presenting with arthralgia rules out the development of arthritis. *Arthritis Res Ther* (2017) 19:202. doi:10.1186/s13075-017-1405-y
306. Noack M, Miossec P. Selected cytokine pathways in rheumatoid arthritis. *Semin Immunopathol* (2017) 39:365–83. doi:10.1007/s00281-017-0619-z
307. van de Sande MG, Baeten DL. Immunopathology of synovitis: from histology to molecular pathways. *Rheumatology (Oxford)* (2016) 55:599–606. doi:10.1093/rheumatology/kev330
308. Bottini N, Firestein GS. Duality of fibroblast-like synoviocytes in RA: passive responders and imprinted aggressors. *Nat Rev Rheumatol* (2013) 9:24–33. doi:10.1038/nrrheum.2012.190
309. McInnes IB, Schett G. The pathogenesis of rheumatoid arthritis. *N Engl J Med* (2011) 365:2205–19. doi:10.1056/NEJMra1004965
310. Ruscitti P, Cipriani P, Di Benedetto P, Liakouli V, Berardicurti O, Carubbi F, et al. Monocytes from patients with rheumatoid arthritis and type 2 diabetes mellitus display an increased production of interleukin (IL)-1β via the nucleotide-binding domain and leucine-rich repeat containing family pyrin 3(NLRP3)-inflammasome activation: a possible implication for therapeutic decision in these patients. *Clin Exp Immunol* (2015) 182:35–44. doi:10.1111/cei.12667
311. Choulaki C, Papadaki G, Repa A, Kampouraki E, Kambas K, Ritis K, et al. Enhanced activity of NLRP3 inflammasome in peripheral blood cells of patients with active rheumatoid arthritis. *Arthritis Res Ther* (2015) 17:257. doi:10.1186/s13075-015-0775-2
312. Mathews RJ, Robinson JI, Battellino M, Wong C, Taylor JC; Biologics in Rheumatoid Arthritis Genetics and Genomics Study Syndicate (BRAGGSS), et al. Evidence of NLRP3-inflammasome activation in rheumatoid arthritis (RA); genetic variants within the NLRP3-inflammasome complex in relation to susceptibility to RA and response to anti-TNF treatment. *Ann Rheum Dis* (2014) 73(6):1202–10. doi:10.1136/annrheumdis-2013-203276
313. Jenko B, Praprotnik S, Tomšic M, Dolžan V. NLRP3 and CARD8 polymorphisms influence higher disease activity in rheumatoid arthritis. *J Med Biochem* (2016) 35:319–23. doi:10.1515/jomb-2016-0008
314. Weyand CM, Yang Z, Goronzy JJ. T cell aging in rheumatoid arthritis. *Curr Opin Rheumatol* (2014) 26(1):93–100. doi:10.1097/BOR.0000000000000011
315. Boots AM, Maier AB, Stinissen P, Masson P, Lories RJ, De Keyser F. The influence of ageing on the development and management of rheumatoid arthritis. *Nat Rev Rheumatol* (2013) 9(10):604–13. doi:10.1038/nrrheum.2013.92

316. Fessler J, Raicht A, Husic R, Ficjan A, Schwarz C, Duftner C, et al. Novel senescent regulatory T-cell subset with impaired suppressive function in rheumatoid arthritis. *Front Immunol* (2017) 20(8):300. doi:10.3389/fimmu.2017.00300
317. Fessler J, Husic R, Schwetz V, Lerchbaum E, Aberer F, Fasching P, et al. Senescent T-cells promote bone loss in rheumatoid arthritis. *Front Immunol* (2018) 1(9):95. doi:10.3389/fimmu.2018.00095
318. Catrina AI, Trollmo C, af Klint E, Engstrom M, Lampa J, Hermansson Y, et al. Evidence that anti-tumor necrosis factor therapy with both etanercept and infliximab induces apoptosis in macrophages, but not lymphocytes, in rheumatoid arthritis joints: extended report. *Arthritis Rheum* (2005) 52:61–72. doi:10.1002/art.20764
319. Hess A, Axmann R, Rech J, Finzel S, Heindl C, Kreitz S, et al. Blockade of TNF-alpha rapidly inhibits pain responses in the central nervous system. *Proc Natl Acad Sci U S A* (2011) 108:3731–6. doi:10.1073/pnas.1011774108
320. Izquierdo E, Canete JD, Celis R, Santiago B, Usategui A, Sanmarti R, et al. Immature blood vessels in rheumatoid synovium are selectively depleted in response to anti-TNF therapy. *PLoS One* (2009) 4:e8131. doi:10.1371/journal.pone.0008131
321. Nadkarni S, Mauri C, Ehrenstein MR. Anti-TNF-alpha therapy induces a distinct regulatory T cell population in patients with rheumatoid arthritis via TGF-beta. *J Exp Med* (2007) 204:33–9. doi:10.1084/jem.20061531
322. Smolen JS, Weinblatt ME, Sheng S, Zhuang Y, Hsu B. Sirukumab, a human anti-interleukin-6 monoclonal antibody: a randomised, 2-part (proof-of-concept and dose-finding), phase II study in patients with active rheumatoid arthritis despite methotrexate therapy. *Ann Rheum Dis* (2014) 73:1616–25. doi:10.1136/annrheumdis-2013-205137
323. Nishimoto N, Hashimoto J, Miyasaka N, Yamamoto K, Kawai S, Takeuchi T, et al. Study of active controlled monotherapy used for rheumatoid arthritis, an IL-6 inhibitor (SAMURAI): evidence of clinical and radiographic benefit from an x ray reader-blinded randomised controlled trial of tocilizumab. *Ann Rheum Dis* (2007) 66:1162–7. doi:10.1136/ard.2006.068064
324. Astorri E, Nerviani A, Bombardieri M, Pitzalis C. Towards a stratified targeted approach with biologic treatments in rheumatoid arthritis: role of synovial pathobiology. *Curr Pharm Des* (2015) 21:2216–24. doi:10.2174/1381612821666150310145758
325. Dennis G Jr, Holweg CT, Kummerfeld SK, Choy DF, Setiadi AF, Hackney JA, et al. Synovial phenotypes in rheumatoid arthritis correlate with response to biologic therapeutics. *Arthritis Res Ther* (2014) 16:R90. doi:10.1186/ar4555
326. Robinson WH, Lindstrom TM, Cheung RK, Sokolove J. Mechanistic biomarkers for clinical decision making in rheumatic diseases. *Nat Rev Rheumatol* (2013) 9:267–76. doi:10.1038/nrrheum.2013.14
327. Dar SA, Haque S, Mandal RK, Singh T, Wahid M, Jawed A, et al. Interleukin-6-174G > C (rs1800795) polymorphism distribution and its association with rheumatoid arthritis: a case-control study and meta-analysis. *Autoimmunity* (2017) 50:158–69. doi:10.1080/08916934.2016.1261833
328. Ferreira RC, Freitag DF, Cutler AJ, Howson JM, Rainbow DB, Smyth DJ, et al. Functional IL6R 358Ala allele impairs classical IL-6 receptor signaling and influences risk of diverse inflammatory diseases. *PLoS Genet* (2013) 9:e1003444. doi:10.1371/journal.pgen.1003444
329. Lopez-Lasanta M, Julia A, Maymo J, Fernandez-Gutierrez B, Urena-Garnica I, Blanco FJ, et al. Variation at interleukin-6 receptor gene is associated to joint damage in rheumatoid arthritis. *Arthritis Res Ther* (2015) 17:242–215. doi:10.1186/s13075-015-0737-8
330. Hussein YM, Mohamed RH, Pasha HF, El-Shahawy EE, Alzahrani SS. Association of tumor necrosis factor alpha and its receptor polymorphisms with rheumatoid arthritis in female patients. *Cell Immunol* (2011) 271:192–6. doi:10.1016/j.cellimm.2011.06.023
331. O'Rielly DD, Roslin NM, Beyene J, Pope A, Rahman P. TNF-alpha-308 G/A polymorphism and responsiveness to TNF-alpha blockade therapy in moderate to severe rheumatoid arthritis: a systematic review and meta-analysis. *Pharmacogenomics J* (2009) 9:161–7. doi:10.1038/tpj.2009.7
332. Stojanovic S, Bojana S, Stoimenov TJ, Nedovic J, Zivkovic V, Despotovic M, et al. Association of tumor necrosis factor-alpha (G-308A) genetic variant with matrix metalloproteinase-9 activity and joint destruction in early rheumatoid arthritis. *Clin Rheumatol* (2017) 36:1479–85. doi:10.1007/s10067-017-3699-1
333. Suarez-Gestal M, Perez-Pampin E, Calaza M, Gomez-Reino JJ, Gonzalez A. Lack of replication of genetic predictors for the rheumatoid arthritis response to anti-TNF treatments: a prospective case-only study. *Arthritis Res Ther* (2010) 12:R72. doi:10.1186/ar2990
334. Zeng Z, Duan Z, Zhang T, Wang S, Li G, Gao J, et al. Association between tumor necrosis factor-alpha (TNF-alpha) promoter -308 G/A and response to TNF-alpha blockers in rheumatoid arthritis: a meta-analysis. *Mod Rheumatol* (2013) 23:489–95. doi:10.1007/s10165-012-0699-5
335. Barnabe C, Martin BJ, Ghali WA. Systematic review and meta-analysis: anti-tumor necrosis factor α therapy and cardiovascular events in rheumatoid arthritis. *Arthritis Care Res* (2011) 63:522–9. doi:10.1002/acr.20371
336. Lin NY, Beyer C, Giessl A, Kireva T, Scholtysek C, Uderhardt S, et al. Autophagy regulates TNFα-mediated joint destruction in experimental arthritis. *Ann Rheum Dis* (2013) 72(5):761–8. doi:10.1136/annrheumdis-2012-201671
337. Kawaida R, Yamada R, Kobayashi K, Tokuhiro S, Suzuki A, Kochi Y, et al. CUL1, a component of E3 ubiquitin ligase, alters lymphocyte signal transduction with possible effect on rheumatoid arthritis. *Genes Immun* (2005) 6(3):194–202. doi:10.1038/sj.gene.6364177
338. Negi S, Kumar A, Thelma BK, Juyal RC. Association of cullin1 haplotype variants with rheumatoid arthritis and response to methotrexate. *Pharmacogenet Genomics* (2011) 21(9):590–3. doi:10.1097/FPC.0b013e3283492af7
339. Kannel WB, Vasan RS. Is age really a non-modifiable cardiovascular risk factor? *Am J Cardiol* (2009) 104(9):1307–10. doi:10.1016/j.amjcard.2009.06.051
340. Bolton E, Rajkumar C. The ageing cardiovascular system. *Rev Clin Gerontol* (2011) 21:99–109. doi:10.1017/S0959259810000389
341. Lv L, Ye M, Duan R, Yuan K, Chen J, Liang W, et al. Downregulation of Pin1 in human atherosclerosis and its association with vascular smooth muscle cell senescence. *J Vasc Surg* (2017). doi:10.1016/j.jvs.2017.09.006
342. Ramji DP, Davies TS. Cytokines in atherosclerosis: key players in all stages of disease and promising therapeutic targets. *Cytokine Growth Factor Rev* (2015) 26(6):673–85. doi:10.1016/j.cytogfr.2015.04.003
343. Moss JW, Ramji DP. Cytokines: roles in atherosclerosis disease progression and potential therapeutic targets. *Future Med Chem* (2016) 8(11):1317–30. doi:10.4155/fmc-2016-0072
344. McLaren JE, Michael DR, Ashlin TG, Ramji DP. Cytokines, macrophage lipid metabolism and foam cells: implications for cardiovascular disease therapy. *Prog Lipid Res* (2011) 50:331–47. doi:10.1016/j.plipres.2011.04.002
345. Ait-Oufella H, Taleb S, Mallat Z, Tedgui A. Recent advances on the role of cytokines in atherosclerosis. *Arterioscler Thromb Vasc Biol* (2011) 31:969–79. doi:10.1161/ATVBAHA.110.207415
346. Moore KJ, Sheedy FJ, Fisher EA. Macrophages in atherosclerosis: a dynamic balance. *Nat Rev Immunol* (2013) 13:709–21. doi:10.1038/nri3520
347. Karasawa T, Takahashi M. The crystal-induced activation of NLRP3 inflammasomes in atherosclerosis. *Inflamm Regen* (2017) 37:18. doi:10.1186/s41232-017-0050-9
348. Sheedy FJ, Grebe A, Rayner KJ, Kalantari P, Ramkhelawon B, Carpenter SB, et al. CD36 coordinates NLRP3 inflammasome activation by facilitating intracellular nucleation of soluble ligands into particulate ligands in sterile inflammation. *Nat Immunol* (2013) 14:812–20. doi:10.1038/ni.2639
349. Ridker PM, Everett BM, Thuren T, MacFadyen JG, Chang WH, Ballantyne C, et al. Anti inflammatory therapy with canakinumab for atherosclerotic disease. *N Engl J Med* (2017) 377(12):1119–31. doi:10.1056/NEJMoa1707914
350. Yin Y, Zhou Z, Liu W, Chang Q, Sun G, Dai Y. Vascular endothelial cells senescence is associated with NOD-like receptor family pyrin domain-containing 3 (NLRP3) inflammasome activation via reactive oxygen species (ROS)/thioredoxin-interacting protein (TXNIP) pathway. *Int J Biochem Cell Biol* (2017) 84:22–34. doi:10.1016/j.biocel.2017.01.001
351. Karasawa T, Takahashi M. Role of NLRP3 inflammasomes in atherosclerosis. *J Atheroscler Thromb* (2017) 24(5):443–51. doi:10.5551/jat.RV17001
352. Qian S, Fan J, Billiar TR, Scott MJ. Inflammasome and autophagy regulation: a two-way street. *Mol Med* (2017) 23:188–95. doi:10.2119/molmed.2017.00077
353. Sergin I, Evans TD, Zhang X, Bhattacharya S, Stokes CJ, Song E, et al. Exploiting macrophage autophagy-lysosomal biogenesis as a therapy for atherosclerosis. *Nat Commun* (2017) 8:15750. doi:10.1038/ncomms15750
354. Buford TW. (Dis)Trust your gut: the gut microbiome in age-related inflammation, health, and disease. *Microbiome* (2017) 5:80. doi:10.1186/s40168-017-0296-0
355. Håheim LL. The infection hypothesis revisited: oral infection and cardiovascular disease. *Epidemiol Res Int* (2014) 2014:735378. doi:10.1155/2014/735378
356. Tang WH, Hazen SL. The contributory role of gut microbiota in cardiovascular disease. *J Clin Invest* (2014) 124(10):4204–11. doi:10.1172/JCI72331

357. Renko J, Koskela KA, Lepp PW, Oksala N, Levula M, Lehtimäki T, et al. Bacterial DNA signatures in carotid atherosclerosis represent both commensals and pathogens of skin origin. *Eur J Dermatol* (2013) 23:53–8. doi:10.1684/ejd.2012.1908
358. Amar J, Lange C, Payros G, Garret C, Chabo C, Lantieri O, et al. Blood microbiota dysbiosis is associated with the onset of cardiovascular events in a large general population: the D.E.S.I.R. study. *PLoS One* (2013) 8(1):e54461. doi:10.1371/journal.pone.0054461
359. Jie Z, Xia H, Zhong S, Feng Q, Li S, Liang S, et al. The gut microbiome in atherosclerotic cardiovascular disease. *Nat Commun* (2017) 8(1):845. doi:10.1038/s41467-017-00900-1
360. Szeto C-C, Kwan BC-H, Chow K-M, Kwok JS-S, Lai K-B, Cheng PM-S, et al. Circulating bacterial-derived DNA fragment level is a strong predictor of cardiovascular disease in peritoneal dialysis patients. *PLoS One* (2015) 10(5):e0125162. doi:10.1371/journal.pone.0125162
361. Dinakaran V, Rathinavel A, Pushpanathan M, Sivakumar R, Gunasekaran P, Rajendhran J. Elevated levels of circulating dna in cardiovascular disease patients: metagenomic profiling of microbiome in the circulation. *PLoS One* (2014) 9(8):e105221. doi:10.1371/journal.pone.0105221
362. Thevaranjan N, Puchta A, Schulz C, Naidoo A, Szamosi JC, Verschoor CP, et al. Age-associated microbial dysbiosis promotes intestinal permeability, systemic inflammation, and macrophage dysfunction. *Cell Host Microbe* (2017) 21(4):455.e–66.e. doi:10.1016/j.chom.2017.03.002
363. McGeer PL, Rogers J, McGeer EG. Inflammation, antiinflammatory agents, and Alzheimer's disease: the last 22 years. *J Alzheimers Dis* (2016) 54(3):853–7. doi:10.3233/JAD-160488
364. McGeer PL, McGeer EG. Inflammation and neurodegeneration in Parkinson's disease. *Parkinsonism Relat Disord* (2004) 10(Suppl 1):S3–7. doi:10.1016/j.parkreldis.2004.01.005
365. Sousa C, Biber K, Michelucci A. Cellular and molecular characterization of microglia: a unique immune cell population. *Front Immunol* (2017) 8:198. doi:10.3389/fimmu.2017.00198
366. Song L, Pei L, Yao S, Wu Y, Shang Y. NLRP3 inflammasome in neurological diseases, from functions to therapies. *Front Cell Neurosci* (2017) 11:63. doi:10.3389/fncel.2017.00063
367. Maceyka M, Spiegel S. Sphingolipid metabolites in inflammatory disease. *Nature* (2014) 510(7503):58–67. doi:10.1038/nature13475
368. Scheiblich H, Schlütter A, Golenbock DT, Latz E, Martinez-Martinez P, Heneka MT. Activation of the NLRP3 inflammasome in microglia: the role of ceramide. *J Neurochem* (2017) 143(5):534–50. doi:10.1111/jnc.14225
369. Nilsson P, Saido TC. Dual roles for autophagy: degradation and secretion of Alzheimer's disease abeta peptide. *Bioessays* (2014) 36:570–8. doi:10.1002/bies.201400002
370. Nilsson P, Loganathan K, Sekiguchi M, Matsuba Y, Hui K, Tsubuki S, et al. A beta secretion and plaque formation depend on autophagy. *Cell Rep* (2013) 5:61–9. doi:10.1016/j.celrep.2013.08.042
371. Boccardi V, Pelini L, Ercolani S, Ruggiero C, Mecocci P. From cellular senescence to Alzheimer's disease: the role of telomere shortening. *Ageing Res Rev* (2015) 22:1–8. doi:10.1016/j.arr.2015.04.003
372. Chang D, Nalls MA, Hallgrímsdóttir IB, Hunkapiller J, van der Brug M, Cai F, et al. A meta-analysis of genome-wide association studies identifies 17 new Parkinson's disease risk loci. *Nat Genet* (2017) 49(10):1511–6. doi:10.1038/ng.3955
373. Lambert JC, Ibrahim-Verbaas CA, Harold D, Naj AC, Sims R, Bellenguez C, et al. Meta-analysis of 74,046 individuals identifies 11 new susceptibility loci for Alzheimer's disease. *Nat Genet* (2013) 45(12):1452–8. doi:10.1038/ng.2802
374. Rayaprolu S, Mullen B, Baker M, Lynch T, Finger E, Seeley WW, et al. TREM2 in neurodegeneration: evidence for association of the p.R47H variant with frontotemporal dementia and Parkinson's disease. *Mol Neurodegener* (2013) 8:19. doi:10.1186/1750-1326-8-19
375. Jonsson T, Stefansson H, Steinberg S, Jonsdottir I, Jonsson PV, Snaedal J, et al. Variant of TREM2 associated with the risk of Alzheimer's disease. *N Engl J Med* (2013) 368(2):107–16. doi:10.1056/NEJMoa1211103
376. Guerreiro R, Wojtas A, Bras J, Carrasquillo M, Rogaeva E, Majounie E, et al. TREM2 variants in Alzheimer's disease. *N Engl J Med* (2013) 368(2):117–27. doi:10.1056/NEJMoa1211851
377. Sims R, van der Lee SJ, Naj AC, Bellenguez C, Badarinarayan N, Jakobsdottir J, et al. Rare coding variants in PLCG2, ABI3, and TREM2 implicate microglial-mediated innate immunity in Alzheimer's disease. *Nat Genet* (2017) 49(9):1373–84. doi:10.1038/ng.3916
378. Carroll CB, Wyse RHK. Simvastatin as a potential disease-modifying therapy for patients with Parkinson's disease: rationale for clinical trial, and current progress. *J Parkinsons Dis* (2017) 7(4):545–68. doi:10.3233/JPD-171203
379. Klegeris A, McGeer EG, McGeer PL. Therapeutic approaches to inflammation in neurodegenerative disease. *Curr Opin Neurol* (2007) 20(3):351–7. doi:10.1097/WCO.0b013e3280adc943
380. McGeer PL, Guo JP, Lee M, Kennedy K, McGeer EG. Alzheimer's disease can be spared by non steroidal anti-inflammatory drugs. *J Alzheimers Dis* (2017) 30:1–4. doi:10.3233/JAD-170706
381. Decourt B, Lahiri DK, Sabbagh MN. Targeting tumor necrosis factor alpha for Alzheimer's disease. *Curr Alzheimer Res* (2017) 4(4):412–25. doi:10.2174/1567205013666160930110551
382. Kolahdooz Z, Nasoohi S, Asle-Rousta M, Ahmadiani A, Dargahi L. Sphingosin-1-phosphate receptor 1: a potential target to inhibit neuroinflammation and restore the sphingosin-1-phosphate metabolism. *Can J Neurol Sci* (2015) 42(3):195–202. doi:10.1017/cjn.2015.19
383. Park S-J, Im D-S. Sphingosine 1-phosphate receptor modulators and drug discovery. *Biomol Ther (seoul)* (2017) 25(1):80–90. doi:10.4062/biomolther.2016.160
384. Franceschi C, Salvioli S, Garagnani P, de Equileor M, Monti D, Capri M. Immunobiography and the heterogeneity of immune responses in the elderly: a focus on inflammaging and trained immunity. *Front Immunol* (2017) 8:982. doi:10.3389/fimmu.2017.00982
385. Garagnani P, Giuliani C, Pirazzini C, Olivieri F, Bacalini MG, Ostan R, et al. Centenarians as super-controls to assess the biological relevance of genetic risk factors for common age-related diseases: a proof of principle on type 2 diabetes. *Aging (Albany NY)* (2013) 5:373–85. doi:10.18632/aging.100562
386. Evert J, Lawler E, Bogan H, Perls T. Morbidity Profiles of centenarians: survivors, delayers and escapers. *J Gerontol A Biol Sci Med Sci* (2003) 58:232–7. doi:10.1093/gerona/58.3.M232
387. Bennati E, Murphy A, Cambien F, Whitehead AS, Archbold GPR, Young IS, et al. BELFAST centenarians: a case of optimised cardiovascular risk? *Curr Pharm Des* (2010) 16:789–95. doi:10.2174/138161210790883697
388. Terry DF, Wilcox M, McCormick MA, Lawler E, Perls TT. Cardiovascular advantages among the offspring of centenarians. *J Gerontol A Biol Sci Med Sci* (2004) 59:M385–9. doi:10.1093/gerona/59.4.M385
389. Rea M. Living long and ageing well: insights from nonagenarians. In: Davidson S, Goodwin J, Rossall P editors. *Improving Later Life: Understanding The Oldest Old Age*. London (2013). p. 74–8.
390. Laland KN, Odling-Smee J, Myles S. How culture shaped the human genome: bridging genetics and the human sciences together. *Nat Rev Gen* (2010) 11:137–48. doi:10.1038/nrg2734
391. Herrington W, Lacey B, Sherliker P, Armitage J, Lewington S. Epidemiology of atherosclerosis and the potential to reduce the global burden of atherothrombotic disease. *Circ Res* (2016) 118(4):535–46. doi:10.1161/CIRCRESAHA.115.307611
392. Roth GA, Forouzanfar MH, Moran AE, Barber R, Nguyen G, Feigin VL, et al. Demographic and epidemiologic drivers of global cardiovascular mortality. *N Engl J Med* (2015) 372:1333–41. doi:10.1056/NEJMoa1406656
393. Koton S, Schneider AL, Rosamond WD, Shahar E, Sang Y, Gottesman RF, et al. Stroke incidence and mortality trends in US communities, 1987 to 2011. *JAMA* (2014) 312(3):259–68. doi:10.1001/jama.2014.7692
394. Prince M. The global prevalence of dementia: a systemic review and meta-analysis. *Alzheimers Dement* (2013) 9(1):63–75. doi:10.1016/j.jalz.2012.11.007
395. Lee S, Shafe ACE, Cowie MR. UK stroke incidence, mortality and cardiovascular risk management 1999e2008: time-trend analysis from the general practice research database. *BMJ Open* (2011) 1:e000269. doi:10.1136/bmjopen-2011-000269
396. Xie X, Atkins E, Lv J, Bennett A, Neal B, Ninomiya T, et al. Effects of intensive blood pressure lowering on cardiovascular and renal outcomes: updated systematic review and meta-analysis. *Lancet* (2016) 387(10017):435–43. doi:10.1016/S0140-6736(15)00805-3
397. Ali MK, Bullard KM, Saaddine JB, Cowie CC, Imperatore G, Gregg EW. Achievement of goals in U.S. diabetes care, 1999-2010. *N Engl J Med* (2013) 368:1613–24. doi:10.1056/NEJMsa1213829

398. Satoh M, Tabuchi T, Itoh T, Nakamura M. NLRP3 inflammasome activation in coronary artery disease: results from prospective and randomized study of treatment with atorvastatin or rosuvastatin. *Clin Sci (Lond)* (2014) 126:233–41. doi:10.1042/CS20130043
399. Baigent C, Blackwell L, Emberson J, Holland LE, Reith C, Bhala N, et al. Efficacy and safety of more intensive lowering of LDL cholesterol: a meta-analysis of data from 170,000 participants in 26 randomised trials. *Lancet* (2010) 376:1670–81. doi:10.1016/S0140-6736(10)61350-5
400. Razquin C, Martinez JA, Martinez-Gonzalez MA, Fernández-Crehuet J, Santos JM, Marti A. A Mediterranean diet rich in virgin olive oil may reverse the effects of the -174G/C IL6 gene variant on 3-year body weight change. *Mol Nutr Food Res* (2010) 54(Suppl 1):S75–82. doi:10.1002/mnfr.200900257
401. Corella D, González JI, Bulló M, Carrasco P, Portolés O, Díez-Espino J, et al. The IL6 Gene Promoter SNP and Plasma IL-6 in Response to Diet Intervention. *J Nutr* (2009) 139(1):128–34. doi:10.3945/jn.108.093054
402. Latorre E, Birar VC, Sheerin AN, Jeynes CC, Hooper A, Dawe HR, et al. Small molecule modulation of splicing factor expression is associated with rescue from cellular senescence. *BMC Cell Biol* (2017) 18:31. doi:10.1186/s12860-017-0147-7
403. Falvo JV, Jasenosky LD, Kruidenier L, Goldfeld AE. Epigenetic control of cytokine gene expression: regulation of the TNF/LT Locus and T helper cell differentiation. *Adv Immunol* (2013) 118:37–128. doi:10.1016/B978-0-12-407708-9.00002-9
404. Freytag V, Carrillo-Roa T, Milnik A, Samann PG, Vukojevic V, Coynek D, et al. A peripheral epigenetic signature of immune system genes is linked to neocortical thickness and memory. *Nat Commun* (2017) 8:15193. doi:10.1038/ncomms15193
405. Kaminska B, Mot M, Pizzi M. Signal transduction and epigenetic mechanisms in the control of microglia activation during neuroinflammation. *Biochim Biophys Acta* (2016) 1862(3):339–51. doi:10.1016/j.bbadis.2015.10.026
406. Bauer M, Fink B, Thürmann L, Eszlinger M, Herberth G, Lehmann I. Tobacco smoking differently influences cell types of the innate and adaptive immune system—indications from CpG site methylation. *Clin Epigenet* (2016) 8:83. doi:10.1186/s13148-016-0249-7
407. Bell JT, Tsai PC, Yang TP, Pidsley R, Nisbet J, Glass D, et al. Epigenome-wide scans identify differentially methylated regions for age and age-related phenotypes in a healthy ageing population. *PLoS Genet* (2012) 8:e1002629. doi:10.1371/journal.pgen.1002629
408. Moskalev AA, Aliper AM, Smit-McBride Z, Buzdin A, Zhavoronkov A. Genetics and epigenetics of aging and longevity. *Cell Cycle* (2014) 13(7):1063–77. doi:10.4161/cc.28433
409. Rea IM, Dellet M, Mills KI; ACUME2 Project. Living long and ageing well: is epigenomics the missing link between nature and nurture? *Biogerontology* (2016) 17(1):33–54. doi:10.1007/s10522-015-9589-5
410. Martínez-González MA, Salas-Salvadó J, Estruch R, Corella D, Fitó M, Ros E, et al. Benefits of the Mediterranean diet: insights from the PREDIMED study. *Prog Cardiovasc Dis* (2015) 58(1):50–60. doi:10.1016/j.pcad.2015.04.003
411. Estruch R, Ros E, Salas-Salvadó J, Covas MI, Corella D, Martínez-González MA, et al. Primary prevention of cardiovascular disease with a Mediterranean diet. *N Engl J Med* (2013) 369:676–7. doi:10.1056/NEJMoa1200303
412. Camargo A, Delgado-Lista J, Garcia-Rios A, Cruz-Teno C, Yubero-Serrano EM, Perez-Martinez P, et al. Expression of pro-in- flammatory, pro-atherogenic genes is reduced by the Mediterranean diet in elderly people. *Br J Nutr* (2012) 108(3):500–8. doi:10.1017/S0007114511005812
413. de Lorgeril M, Salen P. The mediterranean-style diet for the prevention of cardiovascular diseases. *Public Health Nutr* (2006) 9(1):118–23. doi:10.1079/PHN2005933
414. Almeida OP, Khan KM, Hankey GJ, Yeap BB, Golledge J, Flicker L. 150 minutes of vigorous physical activity per week predicts survival and successful ageing: a population-based 11-year longitudinal study of 12,201 older Australian men. *Br J Sports Med* (2014) 48(3):220–5. doi:10.1136/bjsports-2013-092814
415. Carvalho A, Rea IM, Parimon T, Cusack BJ. Physical activity and cognitive function in individuals over 60 years of age: a systematic review. *Clin Interv Aging* (2014) 9:661–82. doi:10.2147/CIA.S55520
416. Hamer M, Lavoie KL, Bacon SL. Taking up physical activity in later life and healthy ageing: the English longitudinal study of ageing. *Br J Sports Med* (2014) 48(3):239–43. doi:10.1136/bjsports-2013-092993
417. Elosua R, Bartali B, Ordovas JM, Corsi AM, Lauretani F, Ferrucci L, et al. Association between physical activity, physical performance, and inflammatory biomarkers in an elderly population: the InCHIANTI study. *J Gerontol A Biol Sci Med Sci* (2005) 60(6):760–7. doi:10.1093/gerona/60.6.760
418. Yang YC, Boen C, Gerken K, Li T, Schorrp K, Harris KM. Social relationships and physiological determinants of longevity across the human life span. *Proc Natl Acad Sci U S A* (2016) 113(3):578–83. doi:10.1073/pnas.1511085112
419. Vemuri P, Lesnick TG, Przybelsk SA, Machulda M, Knopman DS, Mielke MM, et al. Association of lifetime intellectual enrichment with cognitive decline in the older population. *JAMA Neurol* (2014) 71(8):1017–24. doi:10.1001/jamaneurol.2014.963
420. Rea M, Rea S. *Super Vivere: Reflections on Long Life and Ageing Well.* Belfast: Blackstaff Press (2011). 187 p.
421. Yates LB, Djousse L, Kurth T, Buring JE, Gaziano M. Exceptional longevity in men: modificable factors associated with survival and function to age 90 years. *Arch Intern Med* (2008) 168:284–90. doi:10.1001/archinternmed.2007.77
422. Knoops KT, de Groot LC, Kromhout D, Perrin AE, Moreiras-Varela O, Menotti A, et al. Mediterranean diet, lifestyle factors, and 10-year mortality in elderly European men and women: the HALE project. *JAMA* (2004) 292(12):1433–9. doi:10.1001/jama.292.12.1433
423. Tam CS, Redman LM. Adipose tissue inflammation and metabolic dysfunction: a clinical perspective. *Horm Mol Biol Clin Investig* (2013) 15(1):19–24. doi:10.1515/hmbci-2013-0032
424. Holloszy JO, Fontana L. Caloric restriction in humans. *Exp Gerontol* (2007) 42(8):709–12. doi:10.1016/j.exger.2007.03.009
425. Jung SH, Park HS, Kim KS, Choi WH, Ahn CW, Kim BT, et al. Effect of weight loss on some serum cytokines in human obesity: increase in IL-10 after weight loss. *J Nutr Biochem* (2008) 19:371–5. doi:10.1016/j.jnutbio.2007.05.007
426. Picca A, Pesce V, Lezza AM. Does eating less make you live longer and better? An update on calorie restriction. *Clin Interv Aging* (2017) 12:1887–902. doi:10.2147/CIA.S126458
427. Jung KJ, Lee EK, Kim JY, Zou Y, Sung B, Heo HS, et al. Effect of short term calorie restriction on pro-inflammatory NF-kB and AP-1 in aged rat kidney. *Inflamm Res* (2009) 58:143–50. doi:10.1007/s00011-008-7227-2
428. Cronin O, Keohane DM, Molloy MG, Shanahan F. The effects of exercise interventions on inflammatory biomarkers in healthy, physically inactive subjects: a systemati review. *QJM Int J Med* (2017) 110:629–37. doi:10.1093/qjmed/hcx091
429. Wohlgemuth SE, Seo AY, Marzetti E, Lees HA, Leeuwenburgh C. Skeletal muscle autophagy and apoptosis during aging: effects of calorie restriction and life-long exercise. *Exp Gerontol* (2010) 45:138–48. doi:10.1016/j.exger.2009.11.002
430. Sampson TR, Debelius JW, Thron T, Janssen S, Shastri GG, Ilhan ZE, et al. Gut microbiota regulate motor deficits and neuroinflammation in a model of Parkinson's disease. *Cell* (2016) 167(6):1469.e–80.e. doi:10.1016/j.cell.2016.11.018
431. Youm Y-H, Nguyen KY, Grant RW, Goldberg EL, Bodogai M, Kim D, et al. The ketone metabolite β-hydroxybutyrate blocks NLRP3 inflammasome-mediated inflammatory disease. *Nat Med* (2015) 21:263–9. doi:10.1038/nm.3804
432. Forsythe P, Bienenstock J, Kunze WA. Vagal pathways for microbiome-brain-gut axis communication. *Adv Exp Med Biol* (2014) 817:115–33. doi:10.1007/978-1-4939-0897-4_5
433. Salminen A, Huuskonen K, Ojala J, Kauppinen A, Kaarniranta K, Suuronen T. Activation of innate immunity system during ageing.: NF-kB signaling is the molecular culprit of inflamm-aging. *Ageing Res Rev* (2008) 7(2):83–105. doi:10.1016/j.arr.2007.09.002
434. Goldberg EL, Dixit VD. Drivers of age-related inflammation and strategies for healthspan extension. *Immunol Rev* (2015) 265(1):63–74. doi:10.1111/imr.12295
435. Mann M, Mehta A, Zhao JL, Lee K, Mariov GK, Garcia-Flores Y, et al. An NF-κB-microRNA regulatory network tunes macrophage inflammatory responses. *Nat Commun* (2017) 8:851. doi:10.1038/s41467-017-00972-z
436. Xu X, Ning Y-C, Wang W, Liu J, Bai X, Sun X, et al. Anti-inflamm-aging effects of long-term caloric restriction via overexpression of SIGIRR to inhibit NF-κB signaling pathway. *Cell Physiol Biochem* (2015) 37:1257–70. doi:10.1159/000430248

437. Dinarello CA. Anti-inflammatory agents: present and future. *Cell* (2010) 140(6):935–50. doi:10.1016/j.cell.2010.02.043
438. Falantes J, Pleyer L, Thépot S, Almeida AM, Maurillo L, Martínez-Robles V, et al. European ALMA + investigators. Real life experience with frontline azacitidine in a large series of older adults with acute myeloid leukemia stratified by MRC/LRF score: results from the expanded international E-ALMA series (E-ALMA+). *Leuk Lymphoma* (2018) 59(5):1113–20. doi:10.1080/10428194.2017.1365854
439. Joven J, Micol V, Segura-Carretero A, Alonso-Villaverde C, Menéndez JA, Bioactive Food Components Platform. Polyphenols and the modulation of gene expression pathways: can we eat our way out of the danger of chronic disease? *Crit Rev Food Sci Nutr* (2014) 54(8):985–1001. doi:10.1080/10408398.2011.621772
440. Uguccioni M, Teixeira MM, Locati M, Mantovani A. Editorial: regulation of inflammation, its resolution and therapeutic targeting. *Front Immunol* (2017) 8:415. doi:10.3389/fimmu.2017.00415
441. Figueira I, Fernandes A, Miadenovi DA, Lopez-Contreras A, Henriques CM, Selman C, et al. Interventions for age-related diseases: shifting the paradigm. *Mech Ageing Develop* (2016) 160:69–92. doi:10.1016/j.mad.2016.09.009
442. De Cabo R, Carmona-Gutierrez D, Bernier M, Hall MN, Madeo F. The search for antiaging interventions: from elixirs to fasting regimens. *Cell* (2014) 157:1515–26. doi:10.1016/j.cell.2014.05.031
443. Broer L, Buchman AS, Deelen J, Evans DS, Faul JD, Lunetta KL, et al. GWAS of longevity in CHARGE consortium confirms APOE and FOXO3 candidacy. *J Gerontol A Biol Sci Med Sci* (2015) 70(1):110–8. doi:10.1093/gerona/glu166
444. Deelen J, Beekman M, Uh H-W, Broer L, Ayers KL, Tan Q, et al. Genome-wide association meta-analysis of human longevity identifies a novel locus conferring survival beyond 90 years of age. *Hum Mol Genet* (2014) 23:4420–32. doi:10.1093/hmg/ddu139
445. Lu F, Guan H, Gong B, Liu X, Zhu R, Wang Y, et al. Genetic variants in PVRL2-TOMM40-APOE region are associated with human longevity in a Han Chinese population. *PLoS One* (2014) 9(6):e99580. doi:10.1371/journal.pone.0099580
446. Beekman M, Blanché H, Perola M, Hervonen A, Bezrukov V, Sikora E, et al. Genome-wide linkage analysis for human longevity: genetics of healthy ageing study. *Aging Cell* (2013) 12(2):184–93. doi:10.1111/acel.12039
447. Brooks-Wilson A. Genetics of healthy aging and longevity. *Hum Genet* (2013) 132:1323–38. doi:10.1007/s00439-013-1342-z
448. Murabito JM, Yuan R, Lunetta KL. The search for longevity and healthy aging genes: insights from epidemiological studies and samples of long-lived individuals. *J Gerontol A Biol Sci Med Sci* (2012) 67(5):470–9. doi:10.1093/gerona/gls089
449. Sebastiani P, Solovieff N, DeWan AT, Walsh KM, Puca A, Hartley SW, et al. Genetic signatures of exceptional longevity in humans. *PLoS One* (2012) 7(1):e29848. doi:10.1371/journal.pone.0029848
450. Deelan J, Beekman M, Hae-Won UH, Helmer Q, Kuningas M, Christiansen L, et al. Genome-wide association study identifies a single major locus contributing to survival into old age: the APOE locus revisited. *Aging Cell* (2011) 10:686–98. doi:10.1111/j.1474-9726.2011.00705.x
451. Soerensen M, Dato S, Christensen K, McGue M, Stevnsner T, Bohr VA, et al. Replication of an association of variation in the FOXO3A gene with human longevity using both case-control and longitudinal data. *Aging Cell* (2010) 9:1010–7. doi:10.1111/j.1474-9726.2010.00627.x
452. Willcox DC, Willcox BJ, Poon LW. Centenarian studies: important contributors to our understanding of the aging process and longevity. *Curr Gerontol Geriatr Res* (2010) 2010:6. doi:10.1155/2010/484529
453. Willcox BJ, Willcox DC, Ferrucci L. Secrets of healthy aging and longevity from exceptional survivors around the globe: lessons from octogenarians to supercentenarians. *J Gerontol A Biol Sci Med Sci* (2008) 63(11):1181–5. doi:10.1093/gerona/63.11.1181
454. Franceschi C, Bezrukov V, Blanche H, Bolund L, Christensen K, De Benedictis G, et al. Genetics of healthy aging in Europe: the EU-integrated project GEHA (GEnetics of healthy aging). *Ann N Y Acad Sci* (2007) 1100:21–45. doi:10.1196/annals.1395.003
455. Franceschi C. Inflammaging as a major characteristic of old people: can it be prevented or cured? *Nutr Rev* (2007) 65(12):S173–6. doi:10.1111/j.1753-4887.2007.tb00358.x
456. Arai Y, Martin-Ruiz C, Takayama M, Abe Y, Takbayashi T, Koyasu S, et al. Inflammation, but not telomere length, predicts successful ageing at extreme old age: a longitudinal study of semi-supercentenarians. *EBioMedicine* (2015) 2(10):1316–7. doi:10.1016/j.ebiom.2015.07.029
457. Baggio G, Donazzan S, Monti D, Mari D, Martini S, Gabelli C, et al. Lipoprotein(a) and lipoprotein profile in healthy centenarians: a reappraisal of vascular risk factors. *FASEB J* (1998) 12(6):433–7. doi:10.1096/fasebj.12.6.433
458. Calabrese EJ. Hormetic dose-response relationships in immunology: occurrence, quantitative features of the dose response, mechanistic foundations, and clinical implications. *Crit Rev Toxicol* (2005) 35(2–3):89–295. doi:10.1080/10408440590917044
459. Holmans P, Moskvina V, Jones L, Sharma M; International Parkinson's Disease Genomics Consortium, Vedernikov A, et al. A pathway-based analysis provides additional support for an immune-related genetic susceptibility to Parkinson's disease. *Hum Mol Genet* (2013) 22(5):1039–49. doi:10.1093/hmg/dds492

9

Immunosenescence and Inflamm-Aging as Two Sides of the Same Coin: Friends or Foes?

Tamas Fulop[1], Anis Larbi[2], Gilles Dupuis[3], Aurélie Le Page[1], Eric H. Frost[4], Alan A. Cohen[5], Jacek M. Witkowski[6] and Claudio Franceschi[7]*

*[1] Research Center on Aging, Graduate Program in Immunology, Faculty of Medicine and Health Sciences, University of Sherbrooke, Sherbrooke, QC, Canada, [2] Singapore Immunology Network (SIgN), Biopolis, Agency for Science Technology and Research (A*STAR), Singapore, Singapore, [3] Department of Biochemistry, Graduate Program in Immunology, Faculty of Medicine and Health Sciences, University of Sherbrooke, Sherbrooke, QC, Canada, [4] Department of Infectious Diseases and Microbiology, Faculty of Medicine and Health Sciences, University of Sherbrooke, Sherbrooke, QC, Canada, [5] Department of Family Medicine, Faculty of Medicine and Health Sciences, University of Sherbrooke, Sherbrooke, QC, Canada, [6] Department of Pathophysiology, Medical University of Gdańsk, Gdańsk, Poland, [7] Italian National Research Center on Aging, Department of Experimental Pathology, University of Bologna, Bologna, Italy*

Correspondence:
Tamas Fulop
tamas.fulop@usherbrooke.ca

The immune system is the most important protective physiological system of the organism. It has many connections with other systems and is, in fact, often considered as part of the larger neuro–endocrine–immune axis. Most experimental data on immune changes with aging show a decline in many immune parameters when compared to young healthy subjects. The bulk of these changes is termed immunosenescence. Immunosenescence has been considered for some time as detrimental because it often leads to subclinical accumulation of pro-inflammatory factors and inflamm-aging. Together, immunosenescence and inflamm-aging are suggested to stand at the origin of most of the diseases of the elderly, such as infections, cancer, autoimmune disorders, and chronic inflammatory diseases. However, an increasing number of immune-gerontologists have challenged this negative interpretation of immunosenescence with respect to its significance in aging-related alterations of the immune system. If one considers these changes from an evolutionary perspective, they can be viewed preferably as adaptive or remodeling rather than solely detrimental. Whereas it is conceivable that global immune changes may lead to various diseases, it is also obvious that these changes may be needed for extended survival/longevity. Recent cumulative data suggest that, without the existence of the immunosenescence/inflamm-aging duo (representing two sides of the same phenomenon), human longevity would be greatly shortened. This review summarizes recent data on the dynamic reassessment of immune changes with aging. Accordingly, attempts to intervene on the aging immune system by targeting its rejuvenation, it may be more suitable to aim to maintain general homeostasis and function by appropriately improving immune-inflammatory-functions.

Keywords: inflamm-aging, immunosenescence, immunometabolism, immune-adaptation, immunoremodeling, longevity, healthspan

INTRODUCTION

Aging is one of the most intricate and complex biological phenomenon. A comprehensive understanding of aging requires an integrated approach of all physiological systems (1–3). This has captured human imagination from immemorial centuries and the search for a "Fountain of Youth" is still ongoing. Aging is often termed "senescence," which literally means to grow old. Despite this clear and simple definition, the common interpretation of senescence and related senescent states is shadowed with a negative connotation associated with growing old, that is the only aspect which is inescapably considered is death instead of the process *per se*.

One physiological system that shows marked changes during aging is the immune system (4–7). The interest of the immune system in aging is related to the fact that this is an interacting master regulatory system that keeps the organism free of invaders, either internal or external. Since the introduction of the notion of immunosenescence, many scientists have questioned the justification for unidirectional implication of the immune system and its decreased efficiency associated with aging (8). Whereas some functions are indeed decreased, others are increased. Therefore; changes are not as uniform as the designation would suggest. In this review, we will describe recent advances in the domain of changes in the immune system with aging and outline our vision on how these changes can be dynamically reconsidered from immunosenescence to immunoadaptation/immunoremodeling.

IMMUNE CHANGES WITH AGING: IMMUNOSENESCENCE AND INFLAMM-AGING, AS THE TWO SIDES OF THE SAME COIN

The prevailing current opinion is that the most marked changes that occur with aging in the adaptive immune system determine the state of immunosenescence (9–11). It is of note that since the 1980s it has been recognized that the innate system is influenced by aging but perhaps not always in the same direction (12–14). At the turn of the century, a new concept has been put forward by Claudio Franceschi. This concept suggested that aging was associated with a chronic, sterile, low-grade inflammation called inflamm-aging (15). The first related question that arises is what are the characteristic aging-associated changes in the various compartments of the immune system? Furthermore, are these changes faithful indicators of senescence (and progressive incapacitation of the system) or an adaptation, as well as ultimately whether they have any clinical significance. The second question is what the relationship between immunosenescence and inflamm-aging is and how it can be integrated into the broader mechanism of the aging process? Finally, the third question is whether we should attempt to intervene to modulate it.

Innate Immune Changes

The innate immune response is the most phylogenetically conserved protection in the animal kingdom that allows the organism to efficiently defend against an impressive number of aggressive pathogens (16). This compartment is meant to recognize and react to the conserved pathogen-associated molecular patterns (external threats) and danger-associated molecular patterns (internal threats) by way of specific receptors that play a key role in elimination of the aggressors (17, 18). There are three classes of pattern-recognition receptors (PRRs), each one having distinct roles although all of them elicit some form of inflammation. The first class of PRR comprises the Toll-like receptors which, using various intracellular signaling pathways, results in NF-κB activation and production of various mediators such as cytokines and chemokines (19). The second class comprises the NOD-like receptors, which are able to stimulate the inflammasome complex and that results in the production of IL-1, IL-18, and IL-33 (20). The third class includes the Rig-like receptors that act through the interferon response elements (21). There are also other receptors which are crucial for the functionality of innate immune cells, such as various Fcγ receptors, chemokine receptors such as fMLP receptors, and complement receptors (14). One of the most important observations of these last years, besides the discovery of PRR, is the fact that the innate immune system possesses some sort of memory which has been termed trained innate immune memory (22, 23). As described by Franceschi et al., the innate immune system may be viewed as possessing the "bow tie" architecture where many signals converge to a few sensors but result in many effectors (24). These coordinated events help to elicit a precise and efficient response.

Whereas many immune changes have been described with aging, we will not describe in details all the aging-associated changes for each immune cell type, as this topic has been comprehensively reviewed recently (25, 26). Collectively, the main characteristics of aging with respect to the innate system are immune stimulation at the basal level on the one hand and, immune paralysis when specific functions such as free radical production are needed, on the other hand (8). This dichotomy was initially proposed to be at the basis of the inflamm-aging concept, which stated that the relatively maintained innate response overrode the more altered adaptive immune response, resulting in higher production of pro-inflammatory mediators. Since that original observation, it became obvious that other processes may contribute to inflamm-aging, such as cell senescence, mitochondrial dysfunction, and microbiota changes (dysbiosis) (27, 28). Furthermore, under some circumstances the effects of oxidative stress were included as part of the process (oxy-inflamm-aging), emphasizing the role of the oxidative stress in the complex mechanisms of aging (29). Whatever the nature and the involvement of the components of inflamm-aging are, it is a fact that the phenomenon results in subclinical low-grade inflammation. For instance, life-long antigenic stimulation by pathogens would maintain this quiescent state of innate immune system activation. The innate immune system can also be stimulated by the so-called internal GARBage system (30). Thus, a heightened inflamm-aging state is produced as a consequence of (1) dysfunctional mitochondria, (2) defective autophagy/mitophagy (disposal of dysfunctional organelles), (3) endoplasmic reticulum stress, (4) activation of inflammasome by cell debris and misplaced self molecules, (5) defective ubiquitin/proteasome system (misfolded/oxidized proteins), (6) activation of DNA damage response, (7) senescent T cells and their senescence-associated secretory phenotype (SASP), and (8) age-related changes in the composition of gut microbiota (dysbiosis) (27–29).

The demonstration of trained immune memory may explain, at least partially, some of the immune aspects of aging (22, 23). Following their response, innate immune cells return to a quiescent state due to epigenetic changes and modulation of cell metabolism alternating between (aerobic) oxidative phosphorylation (OX-PHOS) and anaerobic glycolysis (Warburg effect) (31). A subsequent stimulation (e.g., by the same or different type of pathogen) elicits a faster and higher response than the first one due to trained innate memory (32).

The hypothesis of trained innate memory may, at least in part, explain why aging innate immune cells are in a state of sustained activation (14). This concept is relatively novel and was first observed after a specific stimulation, such as the Calmette–Guérin bacillus (BCG). Even after 3 months following challenge, innate cells (monocyte/macrophages) were still able to sustain a certain "memory" of the initial infection and to react in the absence of BCG to any other stimulation (22). This observation has led to the concept that the innate immune system has a certain "memory," which was not foreseen from the previous paradigm of the immune system function.

Within the context of the aging innate immune system, it can also be suggested that the sustained trained immune memory is (or may be) leading to a sustained state of activation even in the absence of a specific challenge (6). This memory is likely due to a shift in the epigenetic landscape (epigenome) of the innate cells and fueled by an energetic shift of these cells. As yet, there is no formal proof for the contribution of these phenomena to the basic activation of innate immune cells, but this seems strongly probable. If this was the case, the epigenome and pathways involved in energy production, use, and conservation by immune cells could be targets of choice for immune modulation in the elderly. This possibility may explain the suggestions that macrophages are at center stage of inflamm-aging (15). Macrophages are able to modify their phenotype, produce pro- and anti-inflammatory mediators, and orchestrate many vital functions. Moreover, this phenomenon may to some extent resemble hormesis, providing a possibility to better react after each repeated stimulation (33, 34). Finally, it has recently been reported that not only does a high low-grade controlled inflammation was present in aged individuals (centenarians) but also that inflammation showed a better correlation with longevity than any other parameters, according to two longitudinal studies (35, 36).

The epigenetic clock notion in aging whole-organism has been proposed recently (37). ELOVL2 (elongase of omega 3 and 6 fatty acids) was found to be the most powerful single epigenetic biomarker of aging (38). Furthermore, Franceschi's group has shown that centenarians and their offsprings are epigenetically younger than one could deduct from their chronological age. According to this study (39), semi-supercentenarians are on average 8.7 years younger than expected based on chronological age, and offsprings of aged greater than 105 years are 5.2 years younger than age-matched controls where DNA methylation age and chronological age overlap. These findings reinforce the idea that epigenome control of the innate trained memory and its possible dysregulation with aging lead to DAMAge by inflamm-aging. Can this be reconciled with the heightened inflamm-aging in centenarians? Perhaps trained immune memory is the key regulated by epigenetic changes. The methylation age observed in centenarians suggests that the heightened inflamm-aging is either not connected to it or, paradoxically, methylation age should be younger. These observations may represent a trade-off between a potentially harmful process which, when under tight control, may remain beneficial. It is tempting to suggest that inflamm-aging may be considered the essence of life and the real "Fountain of Youth." In this context, centenarians may be considered as the standard and not the exception and may serve as model for the better understanding the role of inflammation and epigenetics in aging.

Chronic challenges during aging are paralleled by intracellular changes such as mitochondrial dysfunction, altered autophagy and changes in DNA repair mechanisms. However; immune cells are constantly maintained in an alert state due to chronic low-grade inflammation. However, this state may be counterbalanced by anti-inflammatory molecules as shown in the case of centenarians (40–42). Chronic low-grade inflammation (inflamm-aging) is a physiological response to the life-long antigenic stress and represents an efficient defense mechanism as long as it is under control. Without the essential counter-regulation by anti-inflammatory molecules as seen in aging, it is now clear how damaging this physiological state may be to the whole organism (43). Centenarians seem to represent an exception to the inflamm-aging effects on physiological aging or, perhaps, they present the physiological dynamics of aging. Thus, we may suggest that the norm (successful) aging is exemplified by centenarians whereas individuals that do not reach this age are the biological exceptions that lack the individual epigenetic history and machinery to reach that pinnacle.

The corollary of chronic low-grade inflammation is the down-regulation of the innate immune functions or immune paralysis or eventually a sort of innate immune tolerance (8). This physiological condition protects the organism against further self-induced damage even if it is at the expense of the defense from pathogens or from GARBAge. However, it is a reductionist view to assume that this immune paralysis is equal to a non-functional state. Although there are functional alterations in elderly individuals when compared to young subjects, a straightforward assumption that immune cells of elderly humans lose their protective functions. For instance, most elderly humans are able to defend against many types of infections even if the adaptive immune response is somewhat less functional. However, there are relatively few longitudinal studies concerning innate immune function changes with age. Therefore, we do not know whether this is a continuous phenomenon or whether they remain stable during aging. We can speculate that incongruent results of cross-sectional studies suggest that there is not a uniform decrease either related to cell type or to immune cell functions.

Could there be any advantage associated with innate immune paralysis? It can easily be conceptualized that maintenance of identical intensities in the innate cell functions in elderly subjects to the level of young individuals would be energetically very difficult. For instance, this is illustrated by the situation of the large amounts of energy needed for maintaining a M1 (pro-inflammatory and anti-cancer) phenotype in the case of macrophages (44). On the other hand, the M2 phenotype (healing, promoting angiogenesis and cancer growth) consumes much less energy and, therefore, is not as much affected. A decreased production of free radicals can be considered harmful for the eradication of pathogens. However, low free radical production may protect the whole body against further age- and oxidative stress-related damages. Decreased chemotactic activity may also be suggested to be harmful for pathogen destruction, although a sterile inflammatory process may protect against excessive tissue damage. Thus, the question is within the context of evolution, what is most rewarding for the body in an aged organism? On the one hand, is it to destroy pathogens at any cost? On the other hand, is it to maintain physiological integrity by way of chronic inflammation? This dichotomy can mirror recent findings on mitochondria where a certain degree of dysfunction was linked to successful aging and longevity, in contrast to normal or excessively altered functioning in unsuccessful aging (45). This mild impairment may work as a hormetic signal (46). Although there is at present no definitive answer to this question, it illustrates the fact that a broader perspective is needed to understand changes in the innate immune system with aging.

The innate immune system influences the adaptive immune response in many ways. One of these cases is antigen presentation by dendritic cells (DCs). There are conflicting results in this domain and it seems that DCs are less able to prime CD4^{+} T cells in the elderly (47). It is not clear whether the problem is related to antigen presentation or to reaction to antigen presentation. In likelihood; both aspects may be affected by aging. The processing of antigenic peptides by the immune proteasome may not be so efficient and perhaps either the T cell receptor (TCR) itself or TCR-dependent-signaling could be altered (48, 49). The interaction may also occur through an interplay with the cytokines that are secreted by the innate immune system cells. Increased levels of pro-inflammatory cytokine production by the innate cells during aging may also influence the reactivity of the CD4^{+} T cells; e.g., the increased amounts of TNFα may downregulate the expression of CD28 which will negatively affect clonal expansion (50). Moreover, these cytokines may elicit increased free radical production in T cells, which will paralyze their function by increasing inhibitory events of signaling (51). In sum, alterations in the innate immune system may also impact adaptive immune changes with aging.

Adaptive Immune System

The adaptive immune system is composed of the cellular and the humoral immune response. T cells are orchestrating the cellular immune responses. These cells are basically divided into CD4^{+} and CD8^{+} T cell populations, which possess very clearly defined functions. CD4^{+} T cells are helper cells that regulate the functions of all the other immune cells. They also possess effector functions (52). CD8^{+} T cells are effector and memory T cells responsible for clearing the aggressors (53). The CD4^{+} compartment may be subdivided, taking into account functionalities, in Th1, Th2, Th17, and regulatory T cell (Treg) subpopulations (54). Phenotypically, CD4^{+} and CD8^{+} T cell compartments are subdivided into four functionally distinct subpopulations, which are naïve, central memory, effector memory, and T effector memory cells re-expressing CD45RA (TEMRA) (55).

Many alterations in the adaptive immune system have been described in aging (11, 56, 57). With respect to T cell subpopulations, aging is characterized by two main changes: a decrease in naïve T cells that leads to the shrinking of the TCR repertoire and an increase in memory T cells that is primed by different aggressors. Recent thymic emigrants of new naïve cells are vanishingly rare in the elderly because of thymic involution at puberty and acute and chronic antigenic stress over the lifetime and, age-associated hematopoietic stem cell insufficiency (9, 10), This phenomenon is considered as one of the most basic changes in the adaptive immune system with aging. How does this situation happen? This seems to be the main explanation for the increased incidence of infections, cancers and the failure of vaccination in elderly (58–60). These observations mean that elderly individuals are less able to respond to neo-antigens than young individuals. However, this idea has been seriously challenged in recent years, mainly on the basis that there may not be a dramatic shrinkage of the TCR repertoire involving the remaining and slowly produced new emigrants, as supposed for decades (60). Moreover, the newly reconsidered homeostatic proliferation of naïve T cells under IL-7 stimulation may replace the failing thymus, at least partially. The recently discovered Stem Cell-like Memory T cells may also participate in incomplete replenishment of the naïve T cell compartment (61). Overall, the alterations may not be so dramatic and even the T cell repertoire may be relatively sufficient to supply the demand. Indeed, centenarians do not present more cancer, as its prevalence plateaus after the age of 90. Furthermore, there is no tendency for these individuals to suffer from unknown new pathogen-induced infections. Findings of two longitudinal studies led to the conclusion that having more CD8^{+} naïve T cells was not considered a survival advantage (62, 63). These new data shed serious doubts on the present concept of "immunosenescence," at least in the adaptive compartment. However, the debate between immunologists and gerontologists is far from being settled.

There could be some evolutionary reasons for thymic involution. First, the maintenance of an organ so metabolically active may be very resource-demanding in the situation where the whole organism tends to reduce energy consumption during aging. This phenomenon can parallel the other two very energy-demanding organ shrinkage situations seen in aging, namely those of muscles and bone marrow. Second, during life, the organism has already encountered most of the pathogens typically active in the temporal and spatial region of its dwelling. Thus, resources must be allocated preferentially to combat these "usual," cognate pathogens by the memory part of the immune system rather than spend energy for a useless fight, which may be terminated in any event by destruction of the invading organism.

Thymic involution is a double-edged sword. On the one hand, it may indirectly be responsible for the death of the organism which would then lack the right TCR to mount an effective response against neo-antigen(s). On the other hand, it results in lower energy consumption which becomes available for other survival-supportive functions and activities of the organism. Given the relative rarity of direct infectious causes of death in the elderly, it would appear that downregulation of capacity to respond to novel pathogens during aging does not come at an excessive cost.

The increase in the number of memory T cells may be very rewarding for the aging organism as this will continuously assure survival against attacks by cognate pathogens that may threaten the survival of the organism. T cells are all directed against specific internal and external aggressors. The body hosts many latent infections which can re-activate from time to time under specific conditions (55). One well characterized pathogen of this type is the cytomegalovirus (CMV) (62). CMV was once considered the main cause of age-related immune changes in the elderly. Although accumulating data are still quite contradictory, the current belief is that the presence of CMV infection does not seem to be only detrimental (63–66). On the contrary, CMV infection may be considered a recurrent stimulation that maintains a sustained immunological alertness that favors a better immune response, e.g., to vaccination (67). The global response to the many various CMV antigens has even been linked to better survival (68). Thus, the increased number of committed memory T cells may not be considered unequivocally as detrimental or related only to aging.

One of the most important features of aging is the notion of senescent cells (69). This idea has re-gained popularity in recent years as a way to explain the decreased functionality of the immune system with aging (70). Senescent cells conform to the model of Hayflick replicative senescence as they are not proliferating but remain metabolically active and secrete several pro-inflammatory substances (SASP) (71, 72). Formerly, accumulated memory T cells were considered "senescent" (70). However, experimental evidence suggests that these cells are still able to function when pathogens such as CMV are re-activated (64, 65). Furthermore, there are no universally accepted markers of cell senescence (7). Finally, cell senescence is also a double-edged sword as these cells are needed in the case of some physiological functions, for instance repair and fight against cancerous transformation, whereas they are detrimental—to other cell functions (73, 74).

There is also a large confusion in the field of aging with respect to the number and distinction between senescent and exhausted cells (75–77). Senescent and exhausted immune cells are to be distinguished as the former may be functionally inert, whereas the latter may be functionally "dormant." This distinction is crucial when considering immune functions in relationship to aging. Exhausted T cells can be awakened by modulation of some surface receptors called the immune checkpoint inhibitors and, they can then resume function (78, 79). The most important of these receptors are PD-1, CTLA-4, LAG-3, TIM-3, and TIMIN. This distinction has gained considerable importance since it has been reported that a number of cancers in some elderly subjects could be successfully modulated and T cells engineered to be immunotoxic toward such cancers, namely melanoma and NSCLC (80–82).

One additional aspect where the literature has not, in our view, paid enough attention is the age-associated impairment of metabolic regulation of immune cell functions which is of vital importance for an adequate immune response. Quiescent cells compared to activated cells require different metabolic responses (83–87). Whereas quiescent cells use the OX-PHOS pathway for their functions that generates 36 ATP per metabolized glucose, activated cells use anaerobic glycolysis, which generate two ATP. Why is it so? When cells are activated, they need energy very quickly which cannot be provided by the OX-PHOS pathway, but only by aerobic glycolysis (Warburg effect). This is another example where the body is trading efficiency for rapidity, as in many circumstances in the aging immune system. Not only do the quiescent and activated states have different metabolic requirements but also the differentiation of the various subtypes of T cells is dependent on the specific metabolic pathways used (88). The master of cellular metabolism is the mTOR pathway that regulates clonal expansion, whereas its inhibition drives (*via* autophagy) the reconstruction of damaged cells (89). Very few studies in aging have addressed the metabolic changes that occur in immune cells with aging (90). However, one of these studies has emphasized the metabolic differences in T cells of young and elderly subjects (91). T cells of elderly individuals suffer from insufficient substrate to feed mitochondrial respiration and, consequently, are energy deprived. Instead of breaking down glucose, they shunt it into the pentose phosphate pathway, promoting an anabolic state. One of the metabolic consequences is the accumulation of reductive elements, particularly NADPH and reduced glutathione, and the scavenging of reactive oxygen species (91). Energy-deprived T cells upregulate activation of the energy sensor 5′-AMP-activated protein kinase (AMPK). A downstream target of inappropriately activated AMPK in aging T cells is the dual-specificity protein phosphatase 4 (DUSP4) (92), which negatively regulates members of the MAPK superfamily, in particular ERK1, ERK2, and JNK. ERK is also subject to increased negative regulation by another dual-specificity protein phosphatase, DUSP6 (93). ERK is a key regulator of the T-cell receptor signaling cascade, and its dephosphorylation by DUSP4 and DUSP6 functions as a suppressive mechanism, weakening the TCR-induced signal and dampening T-cell function. Thus, it may be very important to take into account age-related changes to determine how the extrinsic nutritional availability of glucose, amino-acids, and lipids will modulate age-related changes in immune system functioning.

Once immune cells are stimulated as a result of recognition of cognate antigen presentation, they initiate signaling pathways that result in the transcription of the appropriate molecules required for the expected functions (94–96). In elderly subjects, this cascade of events has been found to be altered, from impaired immune synapse formation to defects associated with translocation of transcription factors (49). Interestingly, detailed investigations of these alterations have revealed that they were mostly related to factors which could be considered modulable. One of the key factors that are involved in these changes are the composition and the organization of components of the plasma membrane, which orchestrates assembly of signaling molecules in cholesterol/ganglioside-containing nanoclusters (97). Thus, changes that were once considered a part of the aging process could be viewed as only the manifestation of some environmental interference and modulated by lifestyle factors such as exercise and nutrition (98).

WHAT IS THE RELATIONSHIP BETWEEN IMMUNOSENESCENCE AND INFLAMM-AGING?

According to the original concept of inflamm-aging, a consequence of immunosenescence, the relatively conserved innate immune system overtakes the more altered adaptive immune system in aging. However, recent data are more in line with the interpretation that this is not a unidirectional relationship, but a mutually maintained state where immunosenescence is induced by inflamm-aging and *vice versa*. The main changes in the aging adaptive immune system occur in the T cell compartment (57, 91). There is an increase in the number of memory $CD8^+$ T cells, which were originally considered relatively non-functional (99). These cells are characterized by the loss of naïve T cell surface markers, such as CD28, CD27, and the emergence of new senescent markers such as KLRG1. It has been found that the increase in the number of memory T cells and, later on, that of B cells may be due to a continuous chronic antigenic stimulation similar to the phenomenon of inflamm-aging. Infection by CMV emerged above all the large variety of potential stimulating agents (62). However, some data indicate that CMV infection could not be differentiated from inflamm-aging between seropositive and seronegative individuals (100). It is conceivable that the body devotes a huge part of its immune resources to contain this specific infection throughout life. Consequently, the immune space becomes filled with CMV-specific memory $CD8^+$ T cells. These cells have been previously considered to be inactive but recent data have shown that they are metabolically active and their senescent phenotype (SASP) can participate in the development of inflamm-aging (76). Thus, chronic antigenic stimulation leads both to the phenomenon of inflamm-aging and the increase of the number of senescent T cells. One additional consequence of chronic stimulation is the phenomenon of exhaustion, characterized by the emergence of inhibitory receptors, such as PD-1, CTLA-4, and many others (75). Other cell types of the adaptive immune system are also affected by aging but to various extents. For instance, the $CD4^+$ T cell population also undergoes similar changes to $CD8^+$ T cells but to a different extent (55). The Treg population also increases with aging as well as the pro-inflammatory Th17 subpopulation (101). Finally, the B cell compartment is also altered with aging (102). The functional consequences of these overall changes result collectively in the decreased ability to fight new challenges. Thus, clonal expansion, cytokine production, and specific antibody production are compromised. This situation leads to increased infections, cancer, and chronic diseases in the elderly (43). It appears that inflamm-aging and immunosenescence progress in parallel and form a vicious cycle. Increased production of inflammatory mediators characteristic of inflamm-aging contributes to the decrease of the adaptive immune response and, eventually, to immunosenescence. In contrast, the decrease of the adaptive immune response reinforces the stimulation of the innate immune response (as the means to protect organism from infections in the circumstances when adaptive immunity fails) leading to inflamm-aging. Both processes are important not only as causes of immune changes in the elderly but also (or even mainly) because of their consequences in the aging organism.

IMMUNOSENESCENCE/INFLAMM-AGING; WHY DOES IT MATTER?

One can ask why all these changes in the immune system with aging do matter. The paradigm for many years has been that immunosenescence and inflamm-aging are the fertile soil for the development of diseases mostly considered as age-related, either acute such as infections, or chronic such as cancer, frailty, Alzheimer's disease (AD), and cardiovascular diseases (CVD) (43). The bulk of these observations has led to the field of geroscience (103–105). The consequence of this new field leads to a novel approach that consists in targeting the aging process as the single most important risk factor instead of treating each disease separately. This notion should be nuanced by individual aging, suggesting that all individuals do not age in the same way and perhaps the underlying mechanisms may be different (6).

Alterations in T cell functions, more precisely the decrease in the number of naïve T cells and the increase in number of memory T cells, has been considered the main explanation for increased incidence of infections and cancers in the elderly (43). However, there is still no direct evidence from experimental observations or longitudinal studies, which could really support this hypothesis. It is of note to mention that the overall incidence of malignancies decreases after the age of 90 (106). However, would the incidence of infections, which is claimed to increase; still be true if one would only take into account elderly individuals with healthy aging? It is also of note that relatively few elderly subjects die of infections, even if severe and requiring hospital treatment. For example, in Canada in 2013, only 4.1% of deaths in individuals aged more than 65 years could be directly attributable to infectious causes (International Classification of Diseases A00-A99, B00-B99, G00-G03, J09-J21) (Statistics Canada: http://www5.statcan.gc.ca/cansim/pick-choisir?lang=eng&searchTypeByValue=1&id=1020561, accessed Oct 23, 2017).

It has also been commonly believed for decades that elderly individuals responded poorly to vaccination, which sometimes led to generalized doubts about the efficacy of vaccination in old age in general. Among the many vaccines which were considered less efficient (107), influenza vaccination was generally cited as the gold standard (108, 109). It is now established that there are many factors besides immunosenescence, which influence effectiveness of this vaccine and others. In fact, knowledge and better understanding of these factors has already led to enormous enhancement of efficacy of vaccination (e.g., against herpesviruses) (110).

Inflamm-aging could play a role in the late manifestation of diseases such as AD, frailty syndrome (FS), and CVD. It is of note that, besides FS, the onset of these diseases start in young or middle age when the immune system is still efficient, that is before signs of immunosenescence or inflamm-aging are detectable. Frailty can be considered a manifestation of (unsuccessful) aging and may represent the clinical sign of biological age, in contrast to chronological age (111). Furthermore, in a longitudinal study, inflammation was found to be the most important factor to account for longevity, especially in semi-super centenarians (36). In conclusion, there is no doubt that immunosenescence and inflamm-aging contribute to the increased incidence of age-related diseases. However, their exact role is not yet well defined, and in some case, it may be even doubtful. There has been little exploration of the possibility that there are optimum levels of immunosenescence and inflamm-aging and that too much or too little could exacerbate the risks of various diseases in the elderly.

HOW CAN SUCCESSES IN VACCINATION AND IMMUNOTHERAPY BE INTERPRETED IN LIGHT OF IMMUNOSENESCENCE?

There has been recent reports of therapeutic successes in domains which were strongly considered to have the potential to overcome immunosenescence, namely the decreased immune response of the elderly to vaccination and the failures in treatment of some cancers. For example, in one study a new vaccine was tested for herpes zoster (shingles) prevention. This study showed that the administration of the antigen in combination with an adjuvant induced a strong immune response even in subjects older than 80 years of age (110). Furthermore, protection by this vaccine was high even after the 3.2 years of follow-up. This report should serve as a lead to question whether reported lack of vaccine efficacy in the elderly is due to immunosenescence or to improperly designed vaccines. Alternatively, even if a decrease in the immune response occurs it may be overcome by a well targeted vaccine (110). Recently, there has been a rise of immune checkpoint inhibitors as effective therapeutics in cancer treatment. While still sparse, the observations of effectiveness in elderly subjects are very encouraging. For example, in the case of metastatic melanoma, the use of Nivolumab® and Ipilimumab® either alone or in combination had survival effects in elderly subjects similar to young patients (80–82). This is a remarkable result that suggests that the exhausted T cells of the elderly are still able to respond to inhibition of their inhibitory receptors with a recovery of cytotoxic activity. It is to be mentioned that immunotherapy often works well in the elderly, but the treatment has to be adapted to the patients and be different than for young people (112). What works for one does not necessarily work for the other, but this does not mean that the elderly will not respond. The longevity advantage in some cases of CMV infection may also militate against the exclusively detrimental effect of the immunosenescence and inflamm-aging (68).

HOW SHOULD WE INTERPRET IMMUNOSENESCENCE AND INFLAMM-AGING?

We suggest that there is a need for a complete reconsideration of immune changes with aging to gain access to a better understanding of their mechanisms and to ensure that eventual interventions do more good than harm. The question does follow: which immune changes in the elderly may be beneficial? The answer to this question would require careful reinterpretation of current data, but it could also be highly useful to cope with an extended perspective of aging. There are several potential changes in the adaptive immune system with aging. First, increased proportions of adaptive memory cells may be beneficial to fight cognate pathogens more efficiently. Thymic involution may be considered as needed for reduction of energy consumption by an organ which is not absolutely necessary for survival and the maintenance of which is energy-costly. Finally, the increased proportions of Tregs observed in the elderly may prevent autoimmune onslaught.

There are some alterations that may not be solely detrimental in the innate immune system. For instance, increased proportions of innate ("trained") memory cells may help to efficiently fight cognate—and some not so cognate—pathogens. Increased asymptomatic pro-inflammatory state (conceptualized as increased "readiness" of innate immunity to pathogen challenge) may have some evolutionary advantages and could even be considered necessary if it is well regulated, i.e., not excessive. However, too much of a good thing could ultimately lead to disastrous consequences at any age, e.g., free radicals.

Accordingly, we can propose a new paradigm for dynamic immune changes with aging (**Figure 1**). We suggest that aging leads to modified/modulated responses of the immune system, making it more adapted to cope with challenges (pathogens) in a given (local) environment, and not just to an eventually terminal deterioration of the immune system. From an evolutionary perspective, this is a simple optimization of the resources of the aging body, even if it ultimately leads to pathologies and death. From this perspective, many or most age-related changes in the immune system may be desirable adaptations to the aging process, and thus no need for rejuvenation seems to be necessary.

TWO IMPORTANT RECENT APPROACHES TO BETTER UNDERSTAND IMMUNE CHANGES WITH AGING, SUPPORTING THE NEED FOR A CHANGE OF THE CURRENT PARADIGM

There are two new approaches which can be adopted to re-conceptualize immune changes with aging. These integrate almost all aspects mentioned above. Immune systems of the elderly are remodeled with fewer naive cells and dysfunctional (exhausted vs. senescent) memory cells, due to chronic antigenic stimulation (including, but not limited to, CMV and neo-antigens from emerging malignant cells) and thymic involution, with altered innate immune response resulting in inflamm-aging eventually contributing to some age-related disease development (**Table 1**).

How do Inflamm-Aging and Immunosenescence Stand from an Evolutionary Perspective?

Considering all the alterations in the immune system with aging, the question arises whether and how inflamm-aging and immunosenescence can be the cause of these numerous age-related alterations and pathologies attributed to them. Recent

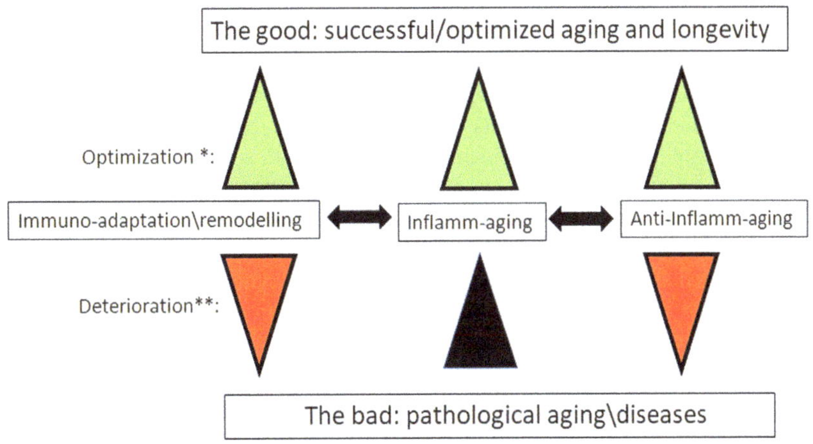

FIGURE 1 | The new paradigm for the role of inflamm-aging and immunoadaptation/remodeling in the aging process. *Optimization: all three processes increase in concert, balancing each other. **Deterioration: inflamm-aging increases, and is not balanced by opposite processes of anti-inflamm-aging and immune-adaptation/remodeling, which are decreasing. We mean by anti-inflamm-aging all compensatory mechanisms which emerged to compensate the chronic inflamm-aging. The most important diseases that could have an inflamm-aging component are cancers, cardiovascular diseases, and neurodegenerative diseases.

TABLE 1 | Summary of some immune changes associated with aging in innate and adaptive immune systems.

Features	Increase	Decrease	No change
Innate immunity			
Phagocytosis	–	√	√
Free radical production	√	√	–
Chemotaxis	–	√	–
Cytokine production	√	–	–
Myeloid cell number	√	–	–
Adaptive immunity			
Naïve cell number	–	√	–
Memory cell number	√	–	–
T regulatory cell number	√	–	–
T regulatory cell function	–	√	–
Proliferation	–	√	–
IL-2 production	–	√	–
B regulatory cell number/function	–	√	–
B cell immunoglobulin production	–	√	–
B cell autoantibody production	√	–	–

Changes are indicated with a checkmark (√) and, absence of changes with a horizontal bar (—).

observations tend to challenge the established view of the role of immune changes with aging. The publication of Lal et al. cited above that reported a positive response to a new herpes zoster vaccine even in the very old raises the question of the role of immunosenescence and inflamm-aging in the decreased response to vaccination (110). An additional recent report has further suggested that inflammation is a driving force for longevity in super semi-centenarians (36). In another study (113), Franceschi's group determined HCMV prevalence in 132 centenarians, 245 centenarian offspring, and 101 offspring of non-long-lived parents. These authors found that infection did not impact on the longevity of these elderly individuals. Finally, the studies concerning the diversity of the microbiota in centenarians may also support this changing paradigm as dysbiosis is not always the equivalent of dysregulated inflamm-aging, particularly in centenarians and semi-super centenarians. The changes in the composition of the gut microbiota with age in subjects ranging from 22 to 109 years can be mentioned as one of the best example of remodeling, with possible large influence on inflamm-aging and immunosenescence, taking into account how important is the gut microbiota for the immune system. An increase in sub-dominant species and among them, species which are considered very "good," was observed in Italian, Japanese, and Chinese centenarians despite the differences of diet and genetics in aged subjects, particularly in semi-supercentenarians (114, 115).

This situation did not involve a chronic uncontrolled inflammation, but the well-balanced inflammatory and anti-inflammatory equilibrium. Immune changes observed during aging may thus only represent an adaptation to a challenging environment (containing mostly the cognate pathogens, with the exception of cancer cells generated by semi-random mutations) that results in maintenance of homeostasis *via* hormesis. However, under conditions of not previously encountered pressure (i.e., contact with a novel, previously unknown pathogen), the aging immune system either can adapt by using the available reserves. Conversely, if it is unable to do so, that leads to a maladaptation manifested by age-related diseases or a lethal outcome.

From this perspective, it is interesting to consider the putative role of inflamm-aging in frailty. The definition of frailty is already controversial as two main designations exist, namely the phenotypic definition (116) and the multiple composite burden (deficit accumulation) (117). Frailty in fact can be conceptualized from an evolutionary point of view as the decrease of the physiological/biological/molecular reserves of the aging organs/organism, leading to less efficient responses to stresses and, therefore, producing deleterious effects, even death (4, 111). This could be considered normal (usual) aging, in contrast to successful aging on the one hand or pathological aging on the other hand. Independently of its definition, one of the most accepted causes of frailty is inflamm-aging (4, 118) that represents the biological threshold between successful and pathological aging. This event suggests a dynamic process that could still be reversed if the underlying causes such as inflamm-aging were contained. However, this situation may also progress to death through diseases when it becomes uncontrolled and hyperinflammatory, as would be predicted by the trained innate memory process (8). From this perspective, the extent of symptoms included in the clinical picture of frailty may be considered as a surrogate measure for biological age independently of chronological age, indicating whether inflamm-aging tends toward health or disease/vulnerability. Then an "optimal inflamm-aging" may be defined for longevity and health (optimal aging). Eventually, as is the case with all biological processes, an equilibrium is needed with functional checkpoint gatekeepers. If, for any reason, this equilibrium is perturbed the pathological pathway may prevail. The aim of optimization efforts and approaches would be to help maintain this very complex equilibrium to achieve an adequate functional longevity for optimal aging.

A Dysregulatory Approach Integrating the Immune System and Other Systems

Clearly, the immune system does not exist in isolation but is influenced by and, in turn, influences many other systems such as the central and the peripheral nervous system, the endocrine system and others (3, 4, 119). This fact fits perfectly with the new approach of the study of aging which states that aging is the sum of results of the dysregulation of different system(s) from a normal regulatory level (i.e., a homeostatic state). This state is not necessarily identical between young and old subjects and may well reflect adaptations to intrinsic (GARBAge) and extrinsic changes (mainly pathogens and adverse environmental influences) related to aging. Thus, dysregulations are neither obligatorily detrimental nor beneficial but indicate a state of dyshomeostasis. This statement leads to the important insight that the pro-inflammatory state cannot be considered separately from the anti-inflammatory state (41). In this respect, this possibility will likely be expanded and nuanced by inclusion of other systems and cellular subsystems, e.g., mitochondrial metabolism. More broadly, this approach suggests that there are clear limits to the relatively linear, pathway-based, reductionist approaches to understanding physiology in general and immunology in particular. "Optimal" levels of various cell types, surface markers, and cytokines are unlikely to be very high or very low, but often intermediate, suggesting non-linear associations with risk. These optimal levels are also likely to vary depending on many other factors, such that it will be quite tricky to identify generally healthy or unhealthy states. Because of the possibility that changes with age or health state represent adaptations rather than aspects of pathology, substantial care must be exercised when interpreting changes in the system.

This way of thinking is a completely innovative approach which can be studied by various statistical analyses using smaller or larger databases obtained in the studies of elderly subjects. This approach can also lead to the discovery of new biomarkers and their use in clinical settings. Such a broad approach would allow the integration of the omics, single cell assessment and systems biology. Different statistical approaches may be warranted both in cases when the dysregulation(s) follow a single unidirectional pathway (as appears to be the case for inflamm-aging and likely metabolic syndrome) (119, 120), as well as in cases where dysregulation can produce a wide array of phenotypes sharing little beyond their departure from a homeostatic state (121–123). An appealing hypothesis is that canalized dysregulations occur as a result of adaptations to the aging process and thus reflect an optimized response to an imperfect situation. In contrast, non-canalized dysregulations reflect a true loss of homeostatic control and may themselves be the imperfect situation causing the canalized responses.

Identification of cell types in both the innate and adaptive immune systems that are affected by age-related changes would be an additional application of these kinds of integrative statistical approaches. Immunology has generally considered individual cells to belong to discrete types that can be distinguished based on their surface markers. Certainly, this is a valid paradigm for many of the major classes of immune cells (T-cells vs., B-cells, $CD4^+$ vs. $CD8^+$, etc.), but many examples of less distinct, partially overlapping classes are starting to emerge: classes based on the levels of surface receptors rather than just their presence or absence, or classes confounded by some subpopulations that are simultaneously expressing two markers that were supposed to distinguish populations (e.g., $CD45RA^+$ vs. $CD45RO^+$). It would thus appear that variation in cell surface receptors can happen in different ways. Discrete variation produces populations of cells with distinct functions and properties ("classes" or "types"), whereas continuous variation produces cells with functions and properties that vary along a gradient. This distinction is important because if one wrongly considers cells varying along a gradient as being from discrete classes, one is likely to (a) misidentify many cells with intermediate phenotypes and (b) to fail to understand the true biological processes driving cell diversity, thus wrongly interpreting the functional consequences of this diversity. For example, one can suppose that a population of cells varies along a gradient that determines their affinity for two types of pathogens (say, A and B). The cells with high affinity for A would have low affinity for B and *vice versa*. If there were a true gradient, a reasonable strategy would be to have a large population of cells with an intermediate affinity for both, maximizing the flexibility of the response. This may be a particularly good strategy during aging when the total cell population declines and the ability to maintain large numbers of cells at both extremes of the gradient is compromised. If one wrongly divides cells into A-affinitive and B-affinitive types, one may obtain uninterpretable or confusing results, depending on where along the gradient the threshold is set. It would then be not possible to understand any strategies that involve the use of intermediate values along the gradient.

Should We Intervene and How?

If we consider immune changes related to aging as an adaptation/remodeling, interventions are presently very difficult to foresee. In particular, a single, generalized immune intervention does not appear to be likely. Anti-inflammatory interventions may depend on the state (level) of inflammation and its duration and, on interactions of the innate immune system with other systems, as well as on the appropriate inflammatory state of the individual given age and disease status. If one assumes that the immune/inflammatory system in the elderly/aged organism is adapted/remodeled in order to provide the best possible anti-pathogen protection when the adaptive immune system fails, the rejuvenation approach as currently proposed (e.g., IL-7/IL-15) seems likely to cause potential long-term harm in the aged organism.

Perhaps, more general, however, purposeful interventions may be necessary, such as lifestyle interventions with personalized exercise and nutrition. Specific epigenetic diets may have their role in this modulation (124, 125). Some drugs with global action have been suggested to decrease the (over)activation of the immune/inflammatory system. One such drug is metformin, suspected for a long time to be a powerful modulator of aging (126). Still, its effects in aging immune/inflammatory system are not yet clear. In any case, any interventions will need to be personalized and the immune history (immunobiography) of the individual will have to be taken into account.

CONCLUSION AND FUTURE PERSPECTIVES

Aging is a highly complex process but an increased understanding of the process should lead to the efficient treatment of the many age-related diseases. The immune system interacts with many other systems in the organism (mainly the neural, metabolic, and the endocrine systems) and is, therefore, one of the most ubiquitous master systems of the organism. As such, it orchestrates health when it functions well but, when maladapted, it leads to diseases in the aging organism. Many changes in the immune system with age have been described and most of them have been considered deleterious and causes of many age-related diseases. Changes occur in both the innate and the adaptive immune arms of the immune system, but perhaps not to the same extent or with the same consequences. There is an intricate interrelationship between inflamm-aging and immunosenescence, which are nearly identical in some ways but very different in other aspects and, occurring in concert, mutually influencing each other. Future studies are obviously necessary to elucidate these interactions and raise targets for new interventions to decrease the deleterious effects of aging and use the beneficial effects for a better health and functionspan in the elderly.

Therefore, the phenomenon traditionally termed "immunosenescence" may be considered an immunoremodeling/adaptation as a result of chronic aggressions and time. Immunosenescence may be necessary for an adequate response to known antigens, but detrimental for responses to new antigens in most circumstances. The discovery of new processes, new immune cell subtypes, and the integration of genetic/epigenetic/metabolic and environmental factors (nutrition) will nuance our «evil» and apparently mistaken perception that aging-associated immune changes are only detrimental. Immunosenescence/inflamm-aging may contribute to diseases such as cancer but its role during aging is still controversial. Elderly in clinical settings are doing much better than predicted from experiments thus, human studies in particular are badly needed.

In view of the successes of cancer immunotherapy and vaccination in the elderly, no such intervention should be refused to an elderly subject based on a dogmatic assumption that aging-related immune changes are detrimental. Thus, time is of the essence; and the future is already now for the elderly.

AUTHOR CONTRIBUTIONS

TF has written and conceptualized the article; AL, GD, AP, EF, AC, JW, and CF have contributed to the writing and critically read it.

FUNDING

This work was partly supported by grants from the Canadian Institutes of Health Research (No. 106634 and No. 106701) to TF, the Université de Sherbrooke, and its Research Center on Aging; the Polish Ministry of Science and Higher Education (statutory grant 02-0058/07/262) to JW, the Agency for Science Technology and Research (A*STAR) to AL. AC is supported by a New Investigator Salary Award from the Canadian Institutes of Health Research and is a member of the Fonds de Recherche du Québec-Santé (FRQS)-supported Centre de Recherche sur le Vieillissement and Centre de Recherche Clinique du Centre Hospitalier Universitaire de Sherbrooke (CHUS). CF is supported by progetto CARIPLO rif. 2015-0564.

REFERENCES

1. Zierer J, Menni C, Kastenmüller G, Spector TD. Integration of 'omics' data in aging research: from biomarkers to systems biology. *Aging Cell* (2015) 14(6):933–44. doi:10.1111/acel.12386
2. Jazwinski SM, Yashin AI. Aging and health – a systems biology perspective. introduction. *Interdiscip Top Gerontol* (2015) 40:VII–XII.
3. Cohen AA. Complex systems dynamics in aging: new evidence, continuing questions. *Biogerontology* (2016) 17(1):205–20. doi:10.1007/s10522-015-9584-x
4. Fulop T, McElhaney J, Pawelec G, Cohen AA, Morais JA, Dupuis G, et al. Frailty, inflammation and immunosenescence. *Interdiscip Top Gerontol Geriatr* (2015) 41:26–40. doi:10.1159/000381134
5. Pawelec G. Does the human immune system ever really become "senescent"? *F1000Res* (2017) 6(F1000 Faculty Rev):1323. doi:10.12688/f1000research.11297.1
6. Franceschi C, Salvioli S, Garagnani P, de Eguileor M, Monti D, Capri M. Immunobiography and the heterogeneity of immune responses in the elderly: a focus on inflammaging and trained immunity. *Front Immunol* (2017) 8:982. doi:10.3389/fimmu.2017.00982
7. Xu W, Larbi A. Markers of T cell senescence in humans. *Int J Mol Sci* (2017) 18(8):E1742. doi:10.3390/ijms18081742
8. Fulop T, Dupuis G, Baehl S, Le Page A, Bourgade K, Frost E, et al. From inflamm-aging to immune-paralysis: a slippery slope during aging for immune-adaptation. *Biogerontology* (2016) 17(1):147–57. doi:10.1007/s10522-015-9615-7

9. Goronzy JJ, Fang F, Cavanagh MM, Qi Q, Weyand CM. Naïve T cell maintenance and function in human ageing. *J Immunol* (2015) 194:4073–80. doi:10.4049/jimmunol.1500046
10. Pawelec G. Hallmarks of human "immunosenescence": adaptation or dysregulation? *Immun Ageing* (2012) 9:15. doi:10.1186/1742-4933-9-15
11. Yanes RE, Gustafson CE, Weyand CM, Goronzy JJ. Lymphocyte generation and population homeostasis throughout life. *Semin Hematol* (2017) 54:33–8. doi:10.1053/j.seminhematol.2016.10.003
12. Solana R, Tarazona R, Gayoso I, Lesur O, Dupuis G, Fulop T. Innate immunosenescence: effect of aging on cells and receptors of the innate immune system in humans. *Semin Immunol* (2012) 24:331–41. doi:10.1016/j.smim.2012.04.008
13. Montgomery RR, Shaw AC. Paradoxical changes in innate immunity in aging: recent progress and new directions. *J Leukoc Biol* (2015) 98(6):937–43. doi:10.1189/jlb.5MR0315-104R
14. Fülöp T Jr, Fóris G, Wórum I, Leövey A. Age-dependent alterations of Fc gamma receptor-mediated effector functions of human polymorphonuclear leucocytes. *Clin Exp Immunol* (1985) 61(2):425–32.
15. Franceschi C, Bonafè M, Valensin S, Olivieri F, De Luca M, Ottaviani E, et al. Inflamm-aging. An evolutionary perspective on immunosenescence. *Ann N Y Acad Sci* (2000) 908:244–54. doi:10.1111/j.1749-6632.2000.tb06651.x
16. Müller L, Fülöp T, Pawelec G. Immunosenescence in vertebrates and invertebrates. *Immun Ageing* (2013) 10(1):12. doi:10.1186/1742-4933-10-12
17. Rivera A, Siracusa MC, Yap GS, Gause WC. Innate cell communication kick-starts pathogen-specific immunity. *Nat Immunol* (2016) 17(4):356–63. doi:10.1038/ni.3375
18. Kaufmann SH, Dorhoi A. Molecular determinants in phagocyte-bacteria interactions. *Immunity* (2016) 44(3):476–91. doi:10.1016/j.immuni.2016.02.014
19. Vidya MK, Kumar VG, Sejian V, Bagath M, Krishnan G, Bhatta R. Toll-like receptors: significance, ligands, signaling pathways, and functions in mammals. *Int Rev Immunol* (2017) 13:1–17. doi:10.1080/08830185.2017.1380200
20. Kufer TA, Nigro G, Sansonetti PJ. Multifaceted functions of NOD-like receptor proteins in myeloid cells at the intersection of innate and adaptive immunity. *Microbiol Spectr* (2016) 4(4):429–36. doi:10.1128/microbiolspec.MCHD-0021-2015
21. Barik S. What really rigs up RIG-I? *J Innate Immun* (2016) 8(5):429–36. doi:10.1159/000447947
22. Kleinnijenhuis J, Quintin J, Preijers F, Joosten LA, Ifrim DC, Saeed S, et al. Bacille Calmette-Guerin induces NOD2-dependent nonspecific protection from reinfection via epigenetic reprogramming of monocytes. *Proc Natl Acad Sci U S A* (2012) 109:17537–42. doi:10.1073/pnas.1202870109
23. Netea MG, van der Meer JW. Trained immunity: an ancient way of remembering. *Cell Host Microbe* (2017) 21(3):297–300. doi:10.1016/j.chom.2017.02.003
24. Tieri P, Grignolio A, Zaikin A, Mishto M, Remondini D, Castellani GC, et al. Network, degeneracy and bow tie. Integrating paradigms and architectures to grasp the complexity of the immune system. *Theor Biol Med Model* (2010) 11(7):32. doi:10.1186/1742-4682-7-32
25. Bektas A, Schurman SH, Sen R, Ferrucci L. Human T cell immunosenescence and inflammation in aging. *J Leukoc Biol* (2017) 102(4):977–88. doi:10.1189/jlb.3RI0716-335R
26. Molony RD, Malawista A, Montgomery RR. Reduced dynamic range of antiviral innate immune responses in aging. *Exp Gerontol* (2017) S0531-5565(17):30483-7. doi:10.1016/j.exger.2017.08.019
27. Byun HO, Lee YK, Kim JM, Yoon G. From cell senescence to age-related diseases: differential mechanisms of action of senescence-associated secretory phenotypes. *BMB Rep* (2015) 48(10):549–58. doi:10.5483/BMBRep.2015.48.10.122
28. Biagi E, Candela M, Fairweather-Tait S, Franceschi C, Brigidi P. Aging of the human metaorganism: the microbial counterpart. *Age (Dordr)* (2012) 34(1):247–67. doi:10.1007/s11357-011-9217-5
29. Bauer ME, Fuente Mde L. The role of oxidative and inflammatory stress and persistent viral infections in immunosenescence. *Mech Ageing Dev* (2016) 158:27–37. doi:10.1016/j.mad.2016.01.001
30. Franceschi C, Garagnani P, Vitale G, Capri M, Salvioli S. Inflammaging and 'Garb-aging'. *Trends Endocrinol Metab* (2017) 28(3):199–212. doi:10.1016/j.tem.2016.09.005
31. van der Heijden CD, Noz MP, Joosten LAB, Netea MG, Riksen NP, Keating ST. Epigenetics and trained immunity. *Antioxid Redox Signal* (2017). doi:10.1089/ars.2017.7310
32. Bekkering S, Blok BA, Joosten LA, Riksen NP, van Crevel R, Netea MG. In vitro experimental model of trained innate immunity in human primary monocytes. *Clin Vaccine Immunol* (2016) 23(12):926–33. doi:10.1128/CVI.00349-16
33. Calabrese EJ, Dhawan G, Kapoor R, Iavicoli I, Calabrese V. What is hormesis and its relevance to healthy aging and longevity? *Biogerontology* (2015) 16(6):693–707. doi:10.1007/s10522-015-9601-0
34. Martucci M, Ostan R, Biondi F, Bellavista E, Fabbri C, Bertarelli C, et al. Mediterranean diet and inflammaging within the hormesis paradigm. *Nutr Rev* (2017) 75(6):442–55. doi:10.1093/nutrit/nux013
35. Ostan R, Bucci L, Capri M, Salvioli S, Scurti M, Pini E, et al. Immunosenescence and immunogenetics of human longevity. *Neuroimmunomodulation* (2008) 15(4–6):224–40. doi:10.1159/000156466
36. Arai Y, Martin-Ruiz CM, Takayama M, Abe Y, Takebayashi T, Koyasu S, et al. Inflammation, but not telomere length, predicts successful ageing at extreme old age: a longitudinal study of semi-supercentenarians. *EBioMedicine* (2015) 2(10):1549–58. doi:10.1016/j.ebiom.2015.07.029
37. Lowe D, Horvath S, Raj K. Epigenetic clock analyses of cellular senescence and ageing. *Oncotarget* (2016) 7(8):8524–31. doi:10.18632/oncotarget.7383
38. Garagnani P, Bacalini MG, Pirazzini C, Gori D, Giuliani C, Mari D, et al. Methylation of ELOVL2 gene as a new epigenetic marker of age. *Aging Cell* (2012) 11(6):1132–4. doi:10.1111/acel.12005
39. Horvath S, Pirazzini C, Bacalini MG, Gentilini D, Di Blasio AM, Delledonne M, et al. Decreased epigenetic age of PBMCs from Italian semi-supercentenarians and their offspring. *Aging (Albany NY).* (2015) 7(12):1159–70. doi:10.18632/aging.100861
40. Franceschi C, Capri M, Monti D, Giunta S, Olivieri F, Sevini F, et al. Inflammaging and anti-inflammaging: a systemic perspective on aging and longevity emerged from studies in humans. *Mech Ageing Dev* (2007) 128(1):92–105. doi:10.1016/j.mad.2006.11.016
41. Morrisette-Thomas V, Cohen AA, Fülöp T, Riesco É, Legault V, Li Q, et al. Inflamm-aging does not simply reflect increases in pro-inflammatory markers. *Mech Ageing Dev* (2014) 139:49–57. doi:10.1016/j.mad.2014.06.005
42. Monti D, Ostan R, Borelli V, Castellani G, Franceschi C. Inflammaging and human longevity in the omics era. *Mech Ageing Dev* (2017) 165(Pt B):129–38. doi:10.1016/j.mad.2016.12.008
43. Fülöp T, Dupuis G, Witkowski JM, Larbi A. The role of immunosenescence in the development of age-related diseases. *Rev Invest Clin* (2016) 68(2):84–91.
44. Geeraerts X, Bolli E, Fendt SM, Van Ginderachter JA. Macrophage metabolism as therapeutic target for cancer, atherosclerosis, and obesity. *Front Immunol* (2017) 15(8):289. doi:10.3389/fimmu.2017.00289
45. Rose G, Santoro A, Salvioli S. Mitochondria and mitochondria-induced signalling molecules as longevity determinants. *Mech Ageing Dev* (2017) 165(Pt B):115–28. doi:10.1016/j.mad.2016.12.002
46. Calabrese V, Santoro A, Monti D, Crupi R, Paola RD, Latteri S, et al. Aging and Parkinson's disease: inflammaging, neuroinflammation and biological remodeling as key factors in pathogenesis. *Free Radic Biol Med* (2017) 115:80–91. doi:10.1016/j.freeradbiomed.2017.10.379
47. Agrawal A, Agrawal S, Gupta S. Role of dendritic cells in inflammation and loss of tolerance in the elderly. *Front Immunol* (2017) 8:896. doi:10.3389/fimmu.2017.00896
48. Johnston-Carey HK, Pomatto LC, Davies KJ. The immunoproteasome in oxidative stress, aging, and disease. *Crit Rev Biochem Mol Biol* (2015) 51(4):268–81. doi:10.3109/10409238.2016.1172554
49. Fulop T, Le Page A, Fortin C, Witkowski JM, Dupuis G, Larbi A. Cellular signaling in the aging immune system. *Curr Opin Immunol* (2014) 29:105–11. doi:10.1016/j.coi.2014.05.007
50. Bryl E, Witkowski JM. Decreased proliferative capability of $CD4^+$ cells of elderly people is associated with faster loss of activation-related antigens and accumulation of regulatory T cells. *Exp Gerontol* (2004) 39(4):587–95. doi:10.1016/j.exger.2003.10.029
51. Rider DA, Sinclair AJ, Young SP. Oxidative inactivation of CD45 protein tyrosine phosphatase may contribute to T lymphocyte dysfunction in the elderly. *Mech Ageing Dev* (2003) 124(2):191–8. doi:10.1016/S0047-6374(02)00120-3

52. Das A, Ranganathan V, Umar D, Thukral S, George A, Rath S, et al. Effector/memory CD4 T cells making either Th1 or Th2 cytokines commonly co-express T-bet and GATA-3. *PLoS One* (2017) 12(10):e0185932. doi:10.1371/journal.pone.0185932
53. Mittrücker HW, Visekruna A, Huber M. Heterogeneity in the differentiation and function of CD8? T cells. *Arch Immunol Ther Exp (Warsz)* (2014) 62(6):449–58. doi:10.1007/s00005-014-0293-y
54. Golubovskaya V, Wu L. Different subsets of T cells, memory, effector functions, and CAR-T Immunotherapy. *Cancers (Basel)* (2016) 8(3):E36. doi:10.3390/cancers8030036
55. Larbi A, Fulop T. From "truly naïve" to "exhausted senescent" T cells: when markers predict functionality. *Cytometry A* (2014) 85(1):25–35. doi:10.1002/cyto.a.22351
56. Kim C, Fang F, Weyand CM, Goronzy JJ. The life cycle of a T cell after vaccination – where does immune ageing strike? *Clin Exp Immunol* (2017) 187(1):71–81. doi:10.1111/cei.12829
57. Tu W, Rao S. Mechanisms underlying T cell immunosenescence: aging and Cytomegalovirus infection. *Front Microbiol* (2016) 7:2111. doi:10.3389/fmicb.2016.02111
58. Appay V, Sauce D. Naive T cells: the crux of cellular immune aging? *Exp Gerontol* (2014) 54:90–3. doi:10.1016/j.exger.2014.01.003
59. Nguyen THO, Sant S, Bird NL, Grant EJ, Clemens EB, Koutsakos M, et al. Perturbed CD8+ T cell immunity across universal influenza epitopes in the elderly. *J Leukoc Biol* (2017). doi:10.1189/jlb.5MA0517-207R
60. Pawelec G. Immunosenescence and cancer. *Biogerontology* (2017) 18:717–21. doi:10.1007/s10522-017-9682-z
61. Gattinoni L, Speiser DE, Lichterfeld M, Bonini C. T memory stem cells in health and disease. *Nat Med* (2017) 23(1):18–27. doi:10.1038/nm.4241
62. Pawelec G. Immunosenenescence: role of cytomegalovirus. *Exp Gerontol* (2014) 54:1–5. doi:10.1016/j.exger.2013.11.010
63. Derhovanessian E, Maier AB, Hähnel K, Zelba H, de Craen AJ, Roelofs H, et al. Lower proportion of naïve peripheral CD8+ T cells and an unopposed pro-inflammatory response to human Cytomegalovirus proteins in vitro are associated with longer survival in very elderly people. *Age (Dordr)* (2013) 35(4):1387–99. doi:10.1007/s11357-012-9425-7
64. Solana R, Tarazona R, Aiello AE, Akbar AN, Appay V, Beswick M, et al. CMV and immunosenescence: from basics to clinics. *Immun Ageing* (2012) 9(1):23. doi:10.1186/1742-4933-9-23
65. Pawelec G, McElhaney JE, Aiello AE, Derhovanessian E. The impact of CMV infection on survival in older humans. *Curr Opin Immunol* (2012) 24:507–11. doi:10.1016/j.coi.2012.04.002
66. Söderberg-Nauclér C, Fornara O, Rahbar A. Cytomegalovirus driven immunosenescence-an immune phenotype with or without clinical impact? *Mech Ageing Dev* (2016) 158:3–13. doi:10.1016/j.mad.2016.06.005
67. McElhaney JE, Garneau H, Camous X, Dupuis G, Pawelec G, Baehl S, et al. Predictors of the antibody response to influenza vaccination in older adults with type 2 diabetes. *BMJ Open Diabetes Res Care* (2015) 3(1):e000140. doi:10.1136/bmjdrc-2015-000140
68. Bajwa M, Vita S, Vescovini R, Larsen M, Sansoni P, Terrazzini N, et al. CMV-specific T-cell responses at older ages: broad responses with a large central memory component may be key to long-term survival. *J Infect Dis* (2017) 215(8):1212–20. doi:10.1093/infdis/jix080
69. Campisi J, Robert L. Cell senescence: role in aging and age-related diseases. *Interdiscip Top Gerontol* (2014) 39:45–61. doi:10.1159/000358899
70. Effros RB. Replicative senescence: the final stage of memory T cell differentiation? *Curr HIV Res* (2003) 1:153–65. doi:10.2174/1570162033485348
71. Coppé JP, Patil CK, Rodier F, Sun Y, Muñoz DP, Goldstein J, et al. Senescence-associated secretory phenotypes reveal cell-nonautonomous functions of oncogenic RAS and the p53 tumor suppressor. *PLoS Biol* (2008) 6(12):2853–68. doi:10.1371/journal.pbio.0060301
72. Rao SG, Jackson JG. SASP: tumor suppressor or promoter? Yes! *Trends Cancer* (2016) 2:676–87. doi:10.1016/j.trecan.2016.10.001
73. Capece D, Verzella D, Tessitore A, Alesse E, Capalbo C, Zazzeroni F. Cancer secretome and inflammation: the bright and the dark sides of NF-κB. *Semin Cell Dev Biol* (2017). doi:10.1016/j.semcdb.2017.08.004
74. Campisi J. Cellular senescence and lung function during aging. Yin and Yang. *Ann Am Thorac Soc* (2016) 13(Suppl_5):S402–6. doi:10.1513/AnnalsATS.201609-703AW
75. Wherry EJ, Kurachi M. Molecular and cellular insights into T cell exhaustion. *Nat Rev Immunol* (2015) 15(8):486–99. doi:10.1038/nri3862
76. Akbar AN, Henson SM, Lanna A. Senescence of T lymphocytes: implications for enhancing human immunity. *Trends Immunol* (2016) 37(12):866–76. doi:10.1016/j.it.2016.09.002
77. Henson SM, Macaulay R, Riddell NE, Nunn CJ, Akbar AN. Blockade of PD-1 or p38 MAP kinase signaling enhances senescent human $CD8^+$ T-cell proliferation by distinct pathways. *Eur J Immunol* (2015) 45:1441–51. doi:10.1002/eji.201445312
78. Zou W, Wolchok JD, Chen L. PD-L1 (B7-H1) and PD-1 pathway blockade for cancer therapy: mechanisms, response biomarkers, and combinations. *Sci Transl Med* (2016) 8:328rv324. doi:10.1126/scitranslmed.aad7118
79. Zarour HM. Reversing T-cell dysfunction and exhaustion in cancer. *Clin Cancer Res* (2016) 22:1856–64. doi:10.1158/1078-0432.CCR-15-1849
80. Elias R, Karantanos T, Sira E, Hartshorn KL. Immunotherapy comes of age: immune aging & checkpoint inhibitors. *J Geriatr Oncol* (2017) 8:229–35. doi:10.1016/j.jgo.2017.02.001
81. Daste A, Domblides C, Gross-Goupil M, Chakiba C, Quivy A, Cochin V, et al. Immune checkpoint inhibitors and elderly people: a review. *Eur J Cancer* (2017) 82:155–66. doi:10.1016/j.ejca.2017.05.044
82. Hurez V, Padrón ÁS, Svatek RS, Curiel TJ. Considerations for successful cancer immunotherapy in aged hosts. *Clin Exp Immunol* (2017) 187:53–63. doi:10.1111/cei.12875
83. MacIver NJ, Michalek RD, Rathmell JC. Metabolic regulation of T lymphocytes. *Annu Rev Immunol* (2013) 31:259–83. doi:10.1146/annurev-immunol-032712-095956
84. Michalek RD, Rathmell JC. The metabolic life and times of a T-cell. *Immunol Rev* (2010) 236:190–202. doi:10.1111/j.1600-065X.2010.00911.x
85. Kouidhi S, Elgaaied AB, Chouaib S. Impact of metabolism on T-cell differentiation and function and cross talk with tumor microenvironment. *Front Immunol* (2017) 8:270. doi:10.3389/fimmu.2017.00270
86. Liu H, Yang H, Chen X, Lu Y, Zhang Z, Wang J, et al. Cellular metabolism modulation in T lymphocyte immunity. *Immunology* (2014). doi:10.1111/imm.12321
87. Peng M, Yin N, Chhangawala S, Xu K, Leslie CS, Li MO. Aerobic glycolysis promotes T helper 1 cell differentiation through an epigenetic mechanism. *Science* (2016) 354:481–4. doi:10.1126/science.aaf6284
88. Buck MD, Sowell RT, Kaech SM, Pearce EL. Metabolic instruction of immunity. *Cell* (2017) 169(4):570–86. doi:10.1016/j.cell.2017.04.004
89. Henson SM, Lanna A, Riddell NE, Franzese O, Macaulay R, Griffiths SJ, et al. p38 signaling inhibits mTORC1-independent autophagy in senescent human $CD8^+$T cells. *J Clin Invest* (2014) 124(9):4004–16. doi:10.1172/JCI75051
90. Akbar AN. The convergence of senescence and nutrient sensing during lymphocyte ageing. *Clin Exp Immunol* (2017) 187(1):4–5. doi:10.1111/cei.12876
91. Weyand CM, Goronzy JJ. Aging of the immune system. Mechanisms and therapeutic targets. *Ann Am Thorac Soc* (2016) 13(Suppl_5):S422–8. doi:10.1513/AnnalsATS.201602-095AW
92. Yu M, Li G, Lee WW, Yuan M, Cui D, Weyand CM, et al. Signal inhibition by the dual-specific phosphatase 4 impairs T cell-dependent B-cell responses with age. *Proc Natl Acad Sci U S A* (2012) 109(15):E879–88. doi:10.1073/pnas.1109797109
93. Li G, Yu M, Lee WW, Tsang M, Krishnan E, Weyand CM, et al. Decline in miR-181a expression with age impairs T cell receptor sensitivity by increasing DUSP6 activity. *Nat Med* (2012) 18:1518–24. doi:10.1038/nm.2963
94. Chakraborty AK, Weiss A. Insights into the initiation of TCR signaling. *Nat Immunol* (2014) 15:798–807. doi:10.1038/ni.2940
95. Porciello N, Tuosto L. CD28 costimulatory signals in T lymphocyte activation: emerging functions beyond a qualitative and quantitative support to TCR signalling. *Cytokine Growth Factor Rev* (2016) 28:11–9. doi:10.1016/j.cytogfr.2016.02.004
96. Dustin ML, Depoil D. New insights into the T cell synapse from single molecule techniques. *Nat Rev Immunol* (2011) 11:672–84. doi:10.1038/nri3066
97. Larbi A, Dupuis G, Khalil A, Douziech N, Fortin C, Fülöp T Jr. Differential role of lipid rafts in the functions of CD4+ and CD8+ human T lymphocytes with aging. *Cell Signal* (2006) 18(7):1017–30. doi:10.1016/j.cellsig.2005.08.016

98. Turner JE, Brum PC. Does regular exercise counter T cell immunosenescence reducing the risk of developing cancer and promoting successful treatment of malignancies? *Oxid Med Cell Longev* (2017)2017:4234765. doi:10.1155/2017/4234765
99. Weltevrede M, Eilers R, de Melker HE, van Baarle D. Cytomegalovirus persistence and T-cell immunosenescence in people aged fifty and older: a systematic review. *Exp Gerontol* (2016) 77:87–95. doi:10.1016/j.exger.2016.02.005
100. Bartlett DB, Firth CM, Phillips AC, Moss P, Baylis D, Syddall H, et al. The age-related increase in low-grade systemic inflammation (inflammaging) is not driven by cytomegalovirus infection. *Aging Cell* (2012) 11(5):912–5. doi:10.1111/j.1474-9726.2012.00849.x
101. van der Geest KS, Abdulahad WH, Tete SM, Lorencetti PG, Horst G, Bos NA, et al. Aging disturbs the balance between effector and regulatory CD4+ T cells. *Exp Gerontol* (2014) 60:190–6. doi:10.1016/j.exger.2014.11.005
102. Frasca D, Diaz A, Romero M, Blomberg BB. The generation of memory B cells is maintained, but the antibody response is not, in the elderly after repeated influenza immunizations. *Vaccine* (2016) 34(25):2834–40. doi:10.1016/j.vaccine.2016.04.023
103. Sonntag WE, Ungvari Z. GeroScience: understanding the interaction of processes of aging and chronic diseases. *Age (Dordr)* (2016) 38(5–6):377–8. doi:10.1007/s11357-016-9953-7
104. Franceschi C, Garagnani P. Suggestions from geroscience for the genetics of age-related diseases. *PLoS Genet* (2016) 12(11):e1006399. doi:10.1371/journal.pgen.1006399
105. Sierra F. The emergence of geroscience as an interdisciplinary approach to the enhancement of health span and life span. *Cold Spring Harb Perspect Med* (2016) 6(4):a025163. doi:10.1101/cshperspect.a025163
106. Yang Y, Li T, Nielsen ME. Aging and cancer mortality: dynamics of change and sex differences. *Exp Gerontol* (2012) 47:695–705. doi:10.1016/j.exger.2012.06.009
107. Weinberger B, Schirmer M, Matteucci Gothe R, Siebert U, Fuchs D, Grubeck-Loebenstein B. Recall responses to tetanus and diphtheria vaccination are frequently insufficient in elderly persons. *PLoS One* (2013) 8(12):e82967. doi:10.1371/journal.pone.0082967
108. Merani S, Pawelec G, Kuchel GA, McElhaney JE. Impact of aging and Cytomegalovirus on immunological response to influenza vaccination and infection. *Front Immunol* (2017) 8:784. doi:10.3389/fimmu.2017.00784
109. Haq K, McElhaney JE. Immunosenescence: influenza vaccination and the elderly. *Curr Opin Immunol* (2014) 29:38–42. doi:10.1016/j.coi.2014.03.008
110. Lal H, Cunningham AL, Godeaux O, Chlibek R, Diez-Domingo J, Hwang SJ, et al. Efficacy of an adjuvanted herpes zoster subunit vaccine in older adults. *N Engl J Med* (2015) 372(22):2087–96. doi:10.1056/NEJMoa1501184
111. Fulop T, Larbi A, Witkowski JM, McElhaney J, Loeb M, Mitnitski A, et al. Aging, frailty and age-related diseases. *Biogerontology* (2010) 11(5):547–63. doi:10.1007/s10522-010-9287-2
112. Hurez V, Padrón Á, Svatek RS, Curiel TJ. Considerations for successful cancer immunotherapy in aged hosts. *Exp Gerontol* (2017). doi:10.1016/j.exger.2017.10.002
113. Sansoni P, Vescovini R, Fagnoni FF, Akbar A, Arens R, Chiu YL, et al. New advances in CMV and immunosenescence. *Exp Gerontol* (2014) 55:54–62. doi:10.1016/j.exger.2014.03.020
114. Santoro A, Ostan R, Candela M, Biagi E, Brigidi P, Capri M, et al. Gut microbiota changes in the extreme decades of human life: a focus on centenarians. *Cell Mol Life Sci* (2017). doi:10.1007/s00018-017-2674-y
115. Biagi E, Franceschi C, Rampelli S, Severgnini M, Ostan R, Turroni S, et al. Gut microbiota and extreme longevity. *Curr Biol* (2016) 26(11):1480–5. doi:10.1016/j.cub.2016.04.016
116. Fried LP, Tangen CM, Walston J, Newman AB, Hirsch C, Gottdiener J, et al. Frailty in older adults evidence for a phenotype. *J Gerontol A Biol Sci Med Sci* (2001) 56:M146–57. doi:10.1093/gerona/56.3.M146
117. Rockwood K, Andrew M, Mitnitski A. A comparison of two approaches to measuring frailty in elderly people. *J Gerontol A Biol Sci Med Sci* (2007) 62:738–43. doi:10.1093/gerona/62.7.738
118. Wu IC, Lin CC, Hsiung CA. Emerging roles of frailty and inflammaging in risk assessment of age-related chronic diseases in older adults: the intersection between aging biology and personalized medicine. *Biomedicine (Taipei)* (2015) 5(1):1. doi:10.7603/s40681-015-0001-1
119. Cohen AA, Milot E, Li Q, Bergeron P, Poirier R, Dusseault-Bélanger F, et al. Detection of a novel, integrative aging process suggests complex physiological integration. *PLoS One* (2015) 10(3):e0116489. doi:10.1371/journal.pone.0116489
120. Dusseault-Belanger F, Cohen AA, Hivert MF, Courteau J, Vanasse A. Validating metabolic syndrome through principal component analysis in a medically diverse, realistic cohort. *Metab Syndr Relat Disord* (2013) 11(1):21–8. doi:10.1089/met.2012.0094
121. Li Q, Wang S, Milot E, Bergeron P, Ferrucci L, Fried LP, et al. Homeostatic dysregulation proceeds in parallel in multiple physiological systems. *Aging Cell* (2015) 14(6):1103–12. doi:10.1111/acel.12402
122. Milot E, Morissette-Thomas V, Li Q, Fried LP, Ferrucci L, Cohen AA. Trajectories of physiological dysregulation predicts mortality and health outcomes in a consistent manner across three populations. *Mech Ageing Dev* (2014) 14(1–142):56–63. doi:10.1016/j.mad.2014.10.001
123. Arbeev KG, Cohen AA, Arbeeva LS, Milot E, Stallard E, Kulminski AM, et al. Optimal versus realized trajectories of physiological dysregulation in aging and their relation to sex-specific mortality risk. *Front Public Health* (2016) 4:3. doi:10.3389/fpubh.2016.00003
124. Szarc vel Szic K, Declerck K, Vidaković M, Vanden Berghe W. From inflammaging to healthy aging by dietary lifestyle choices: is epigenetics the key to personalized nutrition? *Clin Epigenetics* (2015) 7:33. doi:10.1186/s13148-015-0068-2
125. Quach A, Levine ME, Tanaka T, Lu AT, Chen BH, Ferrucci L, et al. Epigenetic clock analysis of diet, exercise, education, and lifestyle factors. *Aging (Albany NY)* (2017) 9(2):419–46. doi:10.18632/aging.101168
126. Campbell JM, Bellman SM, Stephenson MD, Lisy K. Metformin reduces all-cause mortality and diseases of ageing independent of its effect on diabetes control: a systematic review and meta-analysis. *Ageing Res Rev* (2017) 40:31–44. doi:10.1016/j.arr.2017.08.003

10

Aging, Obesity and Inflammatory Age-Related Diseases

Daniela Frasca[1], Bonnie B. Blomberg[1] and Roberto Paganelli[2]*

[1] *Department of Microbiology and Immunology, University of Miami Miller School of Medicine, Miami, FL, United States,*
[2] *Dipartimento di Medicina e Scienze dell'Invecchiamento, Università degli Studi 'G. d'Annunzio' Chieti-Pescara, Chieti, Italy*

Correspondence:
Daniela Frasca
dfrasca@med.miami.edu

The increase in the prevalence of obesity represents a worldwide phenomenon in all age groups and is pathologically and genetically correlated with several metabolic and cardiovascular diseases, representing the most frequent age-related diseases. Obesity superimposed on aging drastically increases chronic low-grade inflammation (inflammaging), which is an important link between obesity, insulin resistance, and age-associated diseases. Immune cells of both the innate and the adaptive immune systems infiltrate the adipose tissue (AT) and during obesity induce inflammatory responses associated with metabolic switches and changes in phenotypes and function of immune cell subsets. Obesity poses new health problems especially when it occurs in the context of other diseases, many of them frequently affect elderly subjects. An emerging problem is the decreased proportion of patients with obesity achieving clinical response to therapy. In this review, we will discuss the reciprocal influences of immune cell and AT inflammation in aging and age-associated diseases and the complex relationship of nutrient and energy-sensing homeostatic checkpoints, which contribute to shape the phenotype of the AT. We will specifically examine type-2 diabetes, rheumatoid arthritis, osteoarthritis, cognitive impairment, and dementia, where obesity plays a significant role, also in shaping some clinical aspects.

Keywords: aging, obesity, inflammation, type-2 diabetes, rheumatoid arthritis

INTRODUCTION

The increase in prevalence of overweight and obesity represents a worldwide phenomenon, which is associated with several chronic diseases such as type-2 diabetes (T2D), cancer, rheumatoid arthritis and osteoarthritis (OA), cognitive impairment and dementia, and those affecting the cardiovascular (CV) system.

The global obesity pandemic affects all age groups. Recent studies examining body mass index (BMI) data in 68 million people in 195 countries showed both increased prevalence and disease burden of high BMI subjects globally over the past 20 years (1). Although the prevalence of obesity among children is lower than in adults, its rate of increase exceeds that of adults (2). The global burden of disease related to high BMI is calculated in individuals without underlying conditions, and it increases at a slower pace in adults mainly because of the reduction of other risk factors for CV diseases and for effective clinical intervention. However, increased BMI has been shown to be pathogenetically related to several diseases. Among these, insulin resistance (IR) and T2D have a strong link to obesity, and the metabolic syndrome represents a cluster of risk factors for severe CV events (coronary artery disease, stroke). Obesity superimposed on aging represents an additional risk factor for older age groups in which the prevalence of chronic disease as well as the occurrence of complications increases (3–5). The disease burden of high BMI in children (≤18 years of age) has not been addressed in the same detail.

The aging process is characterized by a state of chronic inflammation, known as inflammaging. Several factors contribute to inflammaging, including polymorphisms in the promoter regions of pro-inflammatory genes, chronic stimulation of immune cells with viruses such as cytomegalovirus, changes in the gut microbiome, and increased permeability from the intestine [reviewed in Ref. (6)]. It has been recently proposed that continuous engagement of innate receptors by endogeneous signals such as damage-associated molecular patterns drives a chronic state of background inflammation, which needs to be counterbalanced by anti-inflammatory mechanisms. Cellular senescence and the acquisition of the senescence-associated secretory phenotype (SASP) by fibroblasts (7) and endothelial (8) and immune cells (9–11) has also been pinpointed as a significant contributor to inflammaging. Cell senescence induces the accumulation of terminally differentiated B, T, and NK cells with dysregulated function through the activation of pathways integrating senescence and energy-sensing signals.

Inflammaging is an important link among obesity, IR, aging, and age-associated diseases such as cognitive impairment, atherosclerosis, cancer, and autoimmunity. Elevated pro-inflammatory cytokines are associated with decreased insulin sensitivity. Chronic low-grade (sterile) inflammation causes IR, which leads to the transition from metabolically normal obesity to metabolic syndrome. This occurs through both systemic inflammation and metaflammation (12), a process whereby excess nutrients promote chronic low-grade inflammation, and whose metabolic hallmarks are high levels of lipids, free fatty acids (FFAs), glucose, and reactive oxygen species (ROS).

Immune cells of the innate and adaptive immune systems infiltrate insulin responsive tissues, such as the visceral adipose tissue (VAT) and with obesity incite inflammatory responses. Immune cells (macrophages, T, B, NK, NKT cells, and neutrophils) have been implicated in adipose tissue (AT) inflammation and IR (13–17). Inflammation leads to local and systemic increases in pro-inflammatory molecules, such as tumor necrosis factor (TNF)-α, interleukin (IL)-1β, IL-6, interferon (IFN)-γ, inflammatory adipokines, chemokines, and FFAs [reviewed in Ref. (16)].

LINKS OF OBESITY TO INSULIN RESISTANCE (IR) AND T2D

IR is the lack of appropriate response to circulating insulin in several tissues, including liver, muscle, and AT (18). It frequently associates with obesity, hypertension (integrating features of the metabolic syndrome), and CV disease and typically precedes the onset of T2D. In the pancreas, β-cells adapt to hyperglycemia with an expansion of the total β-cell mass and with increased secretion of insulin (hyperinsulinemia), which is able not only to control normal levels of glycemia but also can induce β-cell stress, causing β-cell failure, and then T2D (19). Poor glycemic control in individuals with T2D results in severe complications, such as renal failure, blindness, neuropathy, and CV disorders (20).

It is not completely clear how obesity causes the development of IR. Although many molecular mechanisms have been proposed, including ER stress, oxidative stress, dysregulation of lipid homeostasis, mitochondrial dysfunction, hypoxia, and impairment of the insulin signaling pathway in insulin-responsive cells, there is evidence that obesity-induced inflammation may be a key factor for IR (21). **Figure 1** summarizes the main pathways leading to inflammation in the obese AT.

Production of Pro-inflammatory Mediators in the Obese AT

High levels of TNF-α in the AT are associated with chronically elevated basal lipolysis, the process of hydrolysis of tryglycerides to release FFAs and lipids (22). These provide chronic stimulation to macrophages leading to FFA-induced TNF-α production, causing IR. It has been proposed that adipocyte-derived TNF-α contributes to elevated levels of FFAs in the blood of obese individuals (22), and neutralization of TNF-α *in vivo* in obese mice decreases circulating levels of FFAs (23). TNF-α has also been shown to reduce the expression of proteins stabilizing lipid droplet (perilipins) (24), leading to ectopic lipid deposition in insulin-sensitive tissues. Lipids and lipid-derived molecules have direct effects on insulin-sensitive tissues and induce IR (25).

Other major pro-inflammatory cytokines released by the obese AT are IFN-γ secreted by $CD8^+$ T cells (26) and NK cells (27) and IL-17 secreted by $CD4^+$ T cells (28).

Hypoxia and Release of "Self" Antigens in the Obese AT

During the development of obesity, the supply of oxygen to the expanding AT becomes inadequate, resulting in areas of hypoxia (29, 30). This phenomenon of poorly oxygenated AT not only activates the transcription factor hypoxia-inducible factor-1α (HIF-1α) and further release of pro-inflammatory cytokines (31) but also induces cell death and release of "self" antigens, which stimulate class switch and the production of IgG pathogenic antibodies. Hypoxia in the AT has been the only mechanism suggested so far for the release of "self" antigens in the obese AT.

Immune Cell Infiltration in the Obese AT

Data from obese mice and humans have indicated that the hypertrophied AT becomes heavily infiltrated by a variety of immune cells displaying a pro-inflammatory phenotype, characterized by secretion of SASP markers (32), and their numbers inversely correlate with insulin sensitivity. Cells with an anti-inflammatory phenotype have also been reported in the obese AT, but these cells are present at low frequencies. These are B1 B cells producing IL-10 (15, 33) and innate lymphoid cells type 2, which produce large amounts of Th2 cytokines such as IL-4, IL-5, and IL-13 (34). Tregs have also been reported but only in the lean AT (35).

Macrophage infiltration within the AT has been considered a major driver of inflammation, due to the secretion of pro-inflammatory cytokines and chemokines involved in the

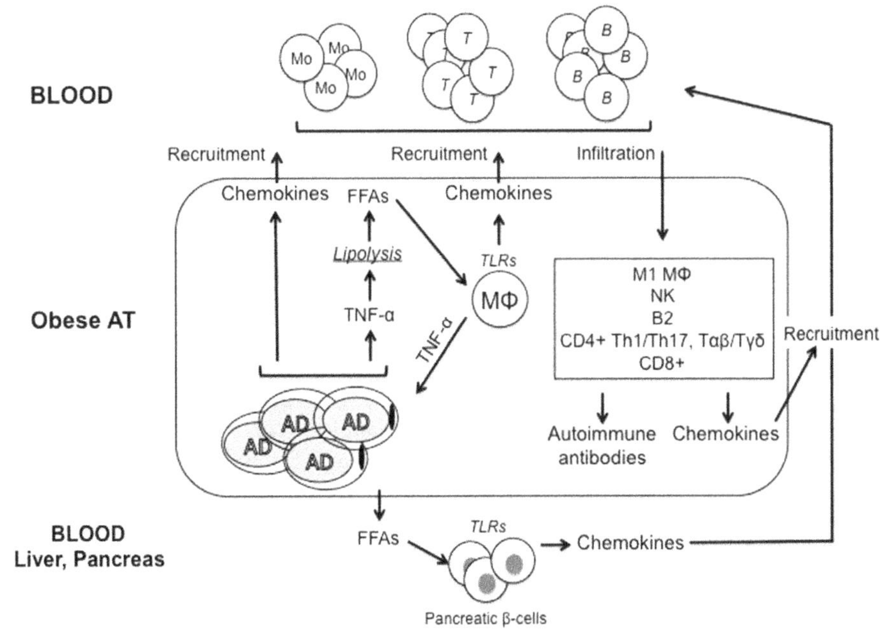

FIGURE 1 | Model for regulation of inflammatory pathways in the obese adipose tissue (AT). Adipocytes (AD) in the obese AT are highly inflammatory and secrete several pro-inflammatory cytokines and chemokines, which recruit immune cells, thus contributing to the establishment and maintenance of local and systemic inflammation. Among these inflammatory mediators, tumor necrosis factor (TNF)-α released by both AD and immune cells induces lipolysis and release of free fatty acids (FFAs), which activate tissue-resident macrophages (MΦ) to release cytokines and chemokines. FFAs are also released in blood and cause both insulin resistance and inflammation in major insulin target tissues. Immune cells recruited to the obese AT differentiate into inflammatory subsets and secrete additional pro-inflammatory mediators. We hypothesize that these cells would generate suboptimal immune responses in obese individuals by circulating to peripheral lymphoid organs. Pathogenic antibodies may be secreted by B cells in the AT. These antibodies may form immune complexes with "self"-antigens, which in turn activate complement and Fc receptors on immune cells, leading to enhanced local inflammation, remodeling of the AT, impairment of adipocyte function and nutrient metabolism, and exacerbation of obesity-associated conditions. These antibodies can also exert additional detrimental effects both locally and systemically targeting distinct clusters of self proteins. One mechanisms for the release of "self"-antigens in the obese AT is the decreased supply of oxygen, resulting in areas of hypoxia, which leads to further release of pro-inflammatory cytokines, as well as to the release of "self"-antigens, such as intracellular proteins, cell-free DNA, and lipids.

recruitment of immune cells to the AT. However, adipocytes also secrete pro-inflammatory mediators (cytokines, chemokines, and adipokines) and in larger amounts compared with immune cells (36). Therefore, with obesity, a crosstalk between adipocytes and the immune cells infiltrating the AT contributes to the establishment of chronic inflammation, a prerequisite for IR. Macrophages in the AT are almost exclusively M1, they depend on glycolysis for their inflammatory function, and their stimulation in the AT induces glucose transporter expression and glucose intake and utilization (37). Hypoxia (via HIF-1α) potentiates glycolysis and stabilizes the inflammatory phenotype (38). In M1 macrophages, the inflammasome NLRP3 activates caspase 1 and the secretion of IL-1β (39), which is directly toxic to pancreatic β-cells and induces IR (40). Increased inflammasome activity has been reported in monocyte-derived macrophages from T2D patients (41).

T cells in the AT are Th1 $CD4^+$ and IFN-γ-producing $CD8^+$ T cells (26). These promote secretion of pro-inflammatory cytokines from M1 macrophages leading to both local and systemic IR (42). Similar to macrophages, T cell subset skewing in the AT occurs through modulation of substrate metabolism regulated by hormones (leptin) and intracellular nutrient sensing kinases, such as AMPK/mTOR (43). Th1 $CD4^+$ T cells express high levels of membrane glucose transporters and are highly glycolytic (44), a trait supporting inflammatory responses.

Interferon-γ, the signature Th1 cytokine, induces macrophages and T cells to secrete chemokines, which recruit immune cells to the obese AT (45, 46). Moreover, IFN-γ facilitates the M2 to M1 polarization (47) and decreases insulin receptor signaling by reducing the expression of insulin receptors and glucose transporters (48). IFN-γ production is regulated by T-bet, a T-box family transcription factor first identified as a transcriptional inducer of IFN-γ in $CD4^+$ T cells (49). T-bet plays a critical role in the development of IR in animal models of obesity, and T-bet-deficient mice fed a high-fat diet are refractory to the induction of IR (50). These mice show improved insulin sensitivity and glucose tolerance, reduced numbers of immune cells in the AT ($CD4^+/CD8^+$ T cells, NK cells, and macrophages), and reduced production of pro-inflammatory cytokines per gram of fat (IFN-γ, TNF-α, IL-1β, and IL-6).

Obese and T2D patients have alterations in the composition of their microbiome, with reduced proportions of Bacteroidetes (beneficial bacteria) in obese versus lean individuals (51). Moreover, it has been reported that the gut microflora regulates the development of obesity in animal models (52). T-bet regulates mucosal T cell activation (53), and T-bet deficiency alters the composition of microflora (54). T-bet deficiency may also alter the microbiome in individuals with obesity leading to the inflammatory and metabolic processes that regulate T2D.

B cells also accumulate in the obese AT (15, 55, 56). B cell recruitment can initiate T cell-induced M1 polarization and IR. Obesity and hyperglycemia have direct influence on antibody production, and IgG secretion from inflamed VAT modulate the function of resident macrophages. It has been reported that B cells in AT are induced to produce pathogenic IgG autoantibodies, due to the dysregulated expression of autoantigens by hypoxic adipocytes. B cells also support the activation of inflammatory T cells, which are the main pathogenic drivers in systemic inflammation and IR.

Recently, a new lymphoid tissue called fat-associated lymphoid clusters (FALCs) has been identified in the mesenteric AT of mice and humans. FALCs are rapidly induced after inflammatory stimuli and support B cell proliferation and differentiation regulating antibody production within the AT (57).

OBESITY AND RHEUMATOID ARTHRITIS (RA): EVIDENCES AND MECHANISTIC LINKS

RA is a debilitating chronic autoimmune disease that causes synovial inflammation and destruction of joints including the cartilage and the adjacent bone. It generally occurs between the fourth and sixth decades of life and affects more women than men. It is characterized by joint stiffness, pain, and swelling and is accompanied by extraarticular manifestations and systemic inflammation. RA has been associated with muscle wasting and cachexia due to uncontrolled inflammation driven by TNF-α, which fuels hypercatabolism (58). However, BMI rarely falls below normal because loss of lean tissue is compensated by increased AT, and this characterizes rheumatoid cachexia, also called "cachectic obesity" (59, 60). It has been observed that in RA patients, despite adequate nutrient intake, but inflammatory cytokine dominance and reduced activity due to pain, joint deformity, and decreased muscle strength (61), cachexia appears to be similar to that occurring in aged subjects with disability. Abnormal body composition in RA can be defined as a sarcopenic obesity (62) with characteristic changes that in the elderly contribute to frailty (63, 64). Moreover, the percentage of obese RA patients has increased (65), and the impact of obesity on RA has become a relevant issue not much for the negligible risk of developing RA (66), but for its negative effects on disease activity, response to therapy, and CV risk. Obese RA patients are indeed less likely to achieve sustained remission in response to therapy with conventional chemical (4) or biologic (TNF-α inhibitors) agents (67). Despite opposite results with some treatments (68), obesity decreases the rate of remission in RA and negatively affects disease activity (69) and patient-reported outcomes during therapy (70).

The "Obesity Paradox" in RA

Obesity represents an important link with comorbidities such as metabolic syndrome (71) and CV diseases (72); however, in some studies, increased BMI had the opposite effect of reduced mortality (70, 73), which has been described as the "obesity paradox" (74). Moreover, in overweight RA patients, progression of bone destruction was reduced (75, 76), the number of swollen joints is not increased, and better quality of life has been reported (77). Weight loss and cachexia represent major determinants for a greater risk of death (78) and worse quality of life (77), thus strengthening the paradoxical observation of lower mortality in obese patients. However, follow-up studies have demonstrated that in RA patients with a history of obesity reduced BMI is strongly associated with death. Therefore, the "obesity paradox" does not entail a biologically protective role of obesity (73), raising the question whether the use of BMI is a valid tool for assessing obesity in RA (65).

High BMI contributes to disease activity in RA by affecting both biomechanics and the metabolic status, and obese RA patients show worse subjective assessment of symptoms (79). Hyperglycemia, as a part of the metabolic syndrome, is more common in early RA (80), whereas active RA shows decreased lipid levels (81) despite an increased risk of CV events, due to the lipid-lowering effect of systemic inflammation (82). An increase in VAT, e.g., the epicardial fat (83), and the more abundant macrophage infiltrate are associated with systemic inflammation, metabolic syndrome, and IR (84). Anti-TNF-α therapy improves insulin sensitivity in RA patients who are resistant, but despite controlling inflammation, it does not achieve the same extent of improvement in obese RA patients (85). In addition, even when therapy succeeds in the control of disease activity, it fails to restore the altered body composition and improve physical function (86). Adipokines (leptin, adiponectin, visfatin, resistin, and chemerin) have been postulated to be the mediators linking AT and RA activity (87). Adipokine imbalance may underlie the higher degree of inflammation (88), the levels of autoantibodies (leptin and adiponectin differentially regulate the generation of Treg cells, which are abundant in normal VAT), and also the lower amount of bone resorption observed in obese patients (89). On another level, the association of RA with both the metabolic syndrome and atherosclerosis is probably also mediated by VAT through altered secretion of adipokines. Therefore, adipokines contribute decisively to the systemic inflammation underlying RA, which represents an independent risk factor for CV diseases.

Since weight reduction may have possible contraindications (lower BMI being associated with accelerated mortality in RA), and the assessment of the inflammatory milieu of VAT in RA patients is still incomplete, much research has been devoted to uncovering the metabolic changes occurring in the development and chronicization of RA. This field has been recently reviewed (90) and can be summarized in the two distinct stages of early and chronic RA. In the first stage, there is a high metabolic demand in all cell types involved, due to proliferative signaling, angiogenesis, cellular de-differentiation, and unbalanced bone turnover. However, in RA T cells, at variance with other types of inflammatory metabolic changes, the glycolytic pathway is reduced in favor of the pentose phosphate shunt (91), reduced ROS generation, and decreased AMPK function. In early stages, AMPK activation (e.g., by Metformin) may be an attractive target because its activity is decreased in several tissues of obese or IR patients. In the late (erosive) stage of RA, the inflamed joint is a hypermetabolic lesion (90), T cells undergo a metabolic switch to aerobic glycolysis due to hypoxic conditions, and mitochondrial dysfunction with increased lactate production causes acidification of the synovia. The reprogramming of T cells accounts for pro-inflammatory Th1/Th17 phenotypes and premature T cell aging (92). Several aspects of immunosenescence have been found to be relevant in RA pathogenesis (93–96), and rejuvenation of the immune system has been proposed as therapy, including mTOR inhibitors (97, 98).

Role of B Cells in RA Pathogenesis

The key role played by autoreactive B cells is highlighted by the presence of diagnostic autoantibodies, and rheumatoid factor (RF) (99) and anticyclic-citrullinated peptide antibodies (ACPAs) (100) are well-established indicators of disease and disease severity and may precede the onset of disease. The role of B cells in RA pathogenesis in the context of overweight/obesity has not been addressed yet and deserves thorough attention. A primary defect in early B cell tolerance has been detected since the majority of naive B lymphocytes express polyreactive autoantibodies, including RF and ACPA. These B cells are resistant to Fas-induced apoptosis and therefore not suppressed by Treg (101). However, B cells are involved in RA by other mechanisms, in a bidirectional support of helper T lymphocytes, as self-antigen-presenting cells, with the release of inflammatory mediators, and with the promotion of lymphoid neogenesis (which is prominent in RA synovitis). RF^+ B cells are able to take up IgG-containing immune complexes and present antigen to T cells, thus activating a reciprocally reinforced response (102).

The phenotype of B lymphocytes in RA has been extensively studied in peripheral blood and in synovial tissue, with some discordant data owing to examination of different stages of the disease. The general consensus is the increased presence of memory ($CD27^+$) B cells with an activated ($CD95^+$, $CD21^{low}$) phenotype both in peripheral blood and in the synovial compartment (103). These cells increased even more significantly after B cell depletion therapy (BCDT) with rituximab. There is also agreement on the fact that response to BCDT relies on elimination of memory B cells, and their repopulation, along with transitional B lymphocytes, may predict relapse (103). The role of homeostatic lymphoproliferation of both memory B cells and the extent of BCDT in bone marrow and synovial tissue represent critical points still to be elucidated. Since it has been observed that $CD4^+$ T cell activation decrease after BCDT (104), changes in not only B cell subsets but also T cell subsets may underlie the response of RA patients to therapy. The Treg compartment is less affected by RA treatments (105), but the presence of Breg lymphocytes (decreased in untreated RA) seem to play a role in balancing immune abnormalities and predict the treatment outcome (106). Cytokine production by B cell subsets is also relevant to RA pathogenesis and disease activity [reviewed in Ref. (107)], with inflammatory cytokines predominating in untreated severe RA, as activated memory B cells preferentially secrete TNF-α, whereas BCDT induced a shift to subpopulations producing IL-10. The recent identification of a subset of B cells able to produce large amounts of RANKL (108) provides a mechanistic link between activated memory B cells and bone resorption through induction of osteoclastogenesis. It is relevant to mention that ACPAs are associated with more joint and bone damage and that therapy does not eliminate ACPA-producing autoreactive B cells in the synovial tissue. The central role of B lymphocytes in RA pathogenesis and in tissue damage makes these cells and their products attractive targets for treatment; however, there is still uncertainty about the beneficial or even protective effects of B cell subsets.

OSTEOARTHRITIS (OA), AGING, AND OBESITY

In the elderly, arthritis is frequently associated with other diseases with multiple aging or degenerative features (109). OA and RA share common features in elderly patients and significantly contribute to disability (110). OA is usually differentiated from RA by age at diagnosis, duration of morning stiffness, pattern of joint involvement, and radiographic findings. Distinguishing between the diseases can be challenging, but in the >60 years of age group, OA is by far more common. Despite the fact that OA directly correlates with age, the real cause of this association is not clear, and OA development can be separated into aging-dependent and aging-independent processes (111–114). Both increased production of matrix metalloproteinases and cytokines, reduced levels of collagen type II synthesis, and increased production of ROS induce age-related changes in chondrocytes (114). These changes alter cartilage function, and sarcopenia further leads to decreased joint stability (115). Cellular senescence, impaired regeneration, and repair are recognized factors contributing to cartilage damage with aging (115, 116).

In patients younger than 60 years of age with symptomatic OA, joint pain and disabilities are less recognized as inevitable consequences of growing old, compared to OA patients older than 70 years (117). Several factors contribute to the development of OA: acute injury (including fracture), excessive mechanical overloading (113, 118), diabetes, and chronic tobacco smoking, all playing a role in the amplification of senescence-inducing stresses (118–121). These factors develop before symptoms appearance and may cause early onset of OA; multimorbidity including OA and obesity can be seen at an adult age (122). The prevalence of arthritis is increasing, with 29.3% ever reported doctor-diagnosed arthritis in individuals aged 45–64 years versus 49.6% in individuals aged 65 or older in the United States (123). However, obesity prevalence did not change significantly over time among middle-aged and younger adults with doctor-diagnosed arthritis (124) despite increasing significantly over time among older adults with RA and remaining also higher when compared with adults without RA. Obesity impacts progression of OA and has a negative influence on outcomes (125). Exercise and loss of at least 10% of body weight can effectively lead to improvement in symptoms, pain relief, and physical function. Physical activity may reactivate a regenerative process by mobilizing stem cells and increase proteoglycan production, restoring the cartilage structure (113, 115, 126).

COGNITIVE IMPAIRMENT, DEMENTIA, AND RELATIONSHIP TO AGE-ASSOCIATED DISEASES AND OBESITY

Our summary of conditions where inflammation, obesity, and aging converge in defining particular features and outcomes of disease must also briefly mention the dementias, whose prevalence has been reported to be declining among older US adults between 2000 and 2012 (127). However, dementia rates are growing at an alarming proportion in most regions of the world and are related to population aging (128). Prevalence varies in countries with different mean population ages. However, differences persist after adjusting for age (129). The decline in the United States occurred in those older than 65 years and was related to increased number of years in education despite the age- and sex-adjusted increase in the prevalence of hypertension, diabetes, and obesity in the same years. There is a long unresolved debate on the prodromal phase of the neurodegenerative disorders with inflammatory features, such as Alzheimer's dementia, but it is undisputed that prevalence of dementias of all types increase with old age, from about 2–3% among those aged 70–75 years to 20–25% among those aged 85 years or more (130). The known risk factors include obesity, depression, diabetes, decreased physical activity, hypertension, smoking, hypercholesterolemia, coronary heart disease, and alcohol use; and assessment of these provide an estimate of the risk of developing dementia (131) despite the fact that in the oldest-old (80–97 years old), these factors did not increase the risk for dementia, so that age plays a major role.

Taken together for the two most frequent types of dementia (Alzheimer's and Vascular) (129), vascular risk factors such as dietary fat intake, high cholesterol, obesity, T2D, and hypertension have emerged as the most important determinants (132). Vascular risk is seldom isolated and is accompanied by alterations in hormonal metabolism. Overweight/obesity, due to excess AT, increase the CV risk and also for late-onset dementia. This is exemplified in the prodromal phases of dementia, as vascular and metabolic parameters decline in direct relation to cognitive impairment and in a way which seems to differ from that occurring in "normal" aging. With regard to obesity, its presence at midlife is associated with an increased risk of dementia and Alzheimer's later in life (133), and in particular central obesity in midlife increases the risk of dementia independent of diabetes and CV comorbidities (134). The risk is reversed when late-life BMI is considered: underweight persons had an increased risk of dementia, whereas being overweight was not associated and being obese reduced the risk of dementia compared with normal BMI. This has been dubbed as an "obesity paradox" also in this case (135). A recent systematic review and meta-analysis suggests a positive association between obesity in mid-life and later dementia but the opposite in late life (136). A successive study confirmed the association of mid-life obesity and dementia, but that of being underweight and dementia remained controversial (137). It is difficult to draw a clear distinction between visceral adiposity and total body fat in most studies, and this is reflected on the paucity of mechanistic hypotheses supported by experimental data. The attention has been focused on the role of several adipokines and mainly the two major hormones produced by the AT, leptin and adiponectin, that interact directly with the brain (138). They have the capability to cross the blood–brain barrier and influence dementia processes within the brain (139), but evidence for a direct role is missing. Another postulated link is through altered gut microbial flora, which may participate in the development of obesity, T2D, and subsequent initiation of AD (140). Also lacking is the evidence that weight reduction in mid-life may produce beneficial effects on dementia development. However, in older adults, regular exercise provides numerous health benefits that include improvements in blood pressure, coronary artery disease, diabetes, lipid profile, OA, osteoporosis, mood, neurocognitive function, and overall morbidity so that studies in this area should be encouraged.

CONCLUDING REMARKS

Immunity and metabolism are highly integrated factors in aging and age-related diseases. This is an expanding field of investigation. Obesity and related complications are a major global epidemic. Scientific research must be a crucial part of the solution to understand all implications of obesity, but this research is still in its initial phase. The investigation of the mechanisms whereby inflammation and immune activation disrupt a functional immune response adds novel insights to the understanding of the relationship between inflammation and long-term metabolic disease outcome and opens new ways for effective therapeutic interventions.

AUTHOR CONTRIBUTIONS

All authors were involved in writing the article and had final approval of the submitted version.

FUNDING

This study was supported by NIH AG-32576 (BBB), AI096446, AG042826, and AG032576 (BBB and DF).

REFERENCES

1. Collaborators GBD, Afshin A, Forouzanfar MH, Reitsma MB, Sur P, Estep K, et al. Health effects of overweight and obesity in 195 countries over 25 years. *N Engl J Med* (2017) 377(1):13–27. doi:10.1056/NEJMoa1614362
2. Hruby A, Hu FB. The epidemiology of obesity: a big picture. *Pharmacoeconomics* (2015) 33(7):673–89. doi:10.1007/s40273-014-0243-x
3. Ottaviani S, Allanore Y, Tubach F, Forien M, Gardette A, Pasquet B, et al. Body mass index influences the response to infliximab in ankylosing spondylitis. *Arthritis Res Ther* (2012) 14(3):R115. doi:10.1186/ar3841
4. Sandberg ME, Bengtsson C, Kallberg H, Wesley A, Klareskog L, Alfredsson L, et al. Overweight decreases the chance of achieving good response and low disease activity in early rheumatoid arthritis. *Ann Rheum Dis* (2014) 73(11):2029–33. doi:10.1136/annrheumdis-2013-205094

5. George MD, Baker JF. The obesity epidemic and consequences for rheumatoid arthritis care. *Curr Rheumatol Rep* (2016) 18(1):6. doi:10.1007/s11926-015-0550-z
6. Frasca D, Blomberg BB. Inflammaging decreases adaptive and innate immune responses in mice and humans. *Biogerontology* (2016) 17(1):7–19. doi:10.1007/s10522-015-9578-8
7. Freund A, Orjalo AV, Desprez PY, Campisi J. Inflammatory networks during cellular senescence: causes and consequences. *Trends Mol Med* (2010) 16(5):238–46. doi:10.1016/j.molmed.2010.03.003
8. Olivieri F, Lazzarini R, Recchioni R, Marcheselli F, Rippo MR, Di Nuzzo S, et al. MiR-146a as marker of senescence-associated pro-inflammatory status in cells involved in vascular remodelling. *Age (Dordr)* (2013) 35(4):1157–72. doi:10.1007/s11357-012-9440-8
9. Lanna A, Henson SM, Escors D, Akbar AN. The kinase p38 activated by the metabolic regulator AMPK and scaffold TAB 1 drives the senescence of human T cells. *Nat Immunol* (2014) 15(10):965–72. doi:10.1038/ni.2981
10. Muller-Durovic B, Lanna A, Covre LP, Mills RS, Henson SM, Akbar AN. Killer cell lectin-like receptor G1 inhibits NK cell function through activation of adenosine 5'-monophosphate-activated protein kinase. *J Immunol* (2016) 197(7):2891–9. doi:10.4049/jimmunol.1600590
11. Frasca D, Diaz A, Romero M, Blomberg BB. Human peripheral late/exhausted memory B cells express a senescent-associated secretory phenotype and preferentially utilize metabolic signaling pathways. *Exp Gerontol* (2017) 87(Pt A):113–20. doi:10.1016/j.exger.2016.12.001
12. Hotamisligil GS. Inflammation, metaflammation and immunometabolic disorders. *Nature* (2017) 542(7640):177–85. doi:10.1038/nature21363
13. Weisberg SP, McCann D, Desai M, Rosenbaum M, Leibel RL, Ferrante AW Jr. Obesity is associated with macrophage accumulation in adipose tissue. *J Clin Invest* (2003) 112(12):1796–808. doi:10.1172/JCI19246
14. Winer S, Chan Y, Paltser G, Truong D, Tsui H, Bahrami J, et al. Normalization of obesity-associated insulin resistance through immunotherapy. *Nat Med* (2009) 15(8):921–9. doi:10.1038/nm.2001
15. Winer DA, Winer S, Shen L, Wadia PP, Yantha J, Paltser G, et al. B cells promote insulin resistance through modulation of T cells and production of pathogenic IgG antibodies. *Nat Med* (2011) 17(5):610–7. doi:10.1038/nm.2353
16. Grant RW, Dixit VD. Adipose tissue as an immunological organ. *Obesity (Silver Spring)* (2015) 23(3):512–8. doi:10.1002/oby.21003
17. Boulenouar S, Michelet X, Duquette D, Alvarez D, Hogan AE, Dold C, et al. Adipose type one innate lymphoid cells regulate macrophage homeostasis through targeted cytotoxicity. *Immunity* (2017) 46(2):273–86. doi:10.1016/j.immuni.2017.01.008
18. Schenk S, Saberi M, Olefsky JM. Insulin sensitivity: modulation by nutrients and inflammation. *J Clin Invest* (2008) 118(9):2992–3002. doi:10.1172/JCI34260
19. Weir GC, Bonner-Weir S. Five stages of evolving beta-cell dysfunction during progression to diabetes. *Diabetes* (2004) 53(Suppl 3):S16–21. doi:10.2337/diabetes.53.suppl_3.S16
20. Brownlee M. Biochemistry and molecular cell biology of diabetic complications. *Nature* (2001) 414(6865):813–20. doi:10.1038/414813a
21. Shoelson SE, Lee J, Goldfine AB. Inflammation and insulin resistance. *J Clin Invest* (2006) 116(7):1793–801. doi:10.1172/JCI29069
22. Langin D, Arner P. Importance of TNFalpha and neutral lipases in human adipose tissue lipolysis. *Trends Endocrinol Metab* (2006) 17(8):314–20. doi:10.1016/j.tem.2006.08.003
23. Hotamisligil GS, Murray DL, Choy LN, Spiegelman BM. Tumor necrosis factor alpha inhibits signaling from the insulin receptor. *Proc Natl Acad Sci U S A* (1994) 91(11):4854–8. doi:10.1073/pnas.91.11.4854
24. Bezaire V, Mairal A, Anesia R, Lefort C, Langin D. Chronic TNFalpha and cAMP pre-treatment of human adipocytes alter HSL, ATGL and perilipin to regulate basal and stimulated lipolysis. *FEBS Lett* (2009) 583(18):3045–9. doi:10.1016/j.febslet.2009.08.019
25. Chavez JA, Summers SA. A ceramide-centric view of insulin resistance. *Cell Metab* (2012) 15(5):585–94. doi:10.1016/j.cmet.2012.04.002
26. Nishimura S, Manabe I, Nagasaki M, Eto K, Yamashita H, Ohsugi M, et al. CD8+ effector T cells contribute to macrophage recruitment and adipose tissue inflammation in obesity. *Nat Med* (2009) 15(8):914–20. doi:10.1038/nm.1964
27. O'Rourke RW, Metcalf MD, White AE, Madala A, Winters BR, Maizlin II, et al. Depot-specific differences in inflammatory mediators and a role for NK cells and IFN-gamma in inflammation in human adipose tissue. *Int J Obes (Lond)* (2009) 33(9):978–90. doi:10.1038/ijo.2009.133
28. Chen Y, Tian J, Tian X, Tang X, Rui K, Tong J, et al. Adipose tissue dendritic cells enhances inflammation by prompting the generation of Th17 cells. *PLoS One* (2014) 9(3):e92450. doi:10.1371/journal.pone.0092450
29. Pasarica M, Sereda OR, Redman LM, Albarado DC, Hymel DT, Roan LE, et al. Reduced adipose tissue oxygenation in human obesity: evidence for rarefaction, macrophage chemotaxis, and inflammation without an angiogenic response. *Diabetes* (2009) 58(3):718–25. doi:10.2337/db08-1098
30. Lawler HM, Underkofler CM, Kern PA, Erickson C, Bredbeck B, Rasouli N. Adipose tissue hypoxia, inflammation, and fibrosis in obese insulin-sensitive and obese insulin-resistant subjects. *J Clin Endocrinol Metab* (2016) 101(4):1422–8. doi:10.1210/jc.2015-4125
31. Imtiyaz HZ, Simon MC. Hypoxia-inducible factors as essential regulators of inflammation. *Curr Top Microbiol Immunol* (2010) 345:105–20. doi:10.1007/82_2010_74
32. Franceschi C. Healthy ageing in 2016: obesity in geroscience – is cellular senescence the culprit? *Nat Rev Endocrinol* (2017) 13(2):76–8. doi:10.1038/nrendo.2016.213
33. Wu L, Parekh VV, Hsiao J, Kitamura D, Van Kaer L. Spleen supports a pool of innate-like B cells in white adipose tissue that protects against obesity-associated insulin resistance. *Proc Natl Acad Sci U S A* (2014) 111(43):E4638–47. doi:10.1073/pnas.1324052111
34. Brestoff JR, Kim BS, Saenz SA, Stine RR, Monticelli LA, Sonnenberg GF, et al. Group 2 innate lymphoid cells promote beiging of white adipose tissue and limit obesity. *Nature* (2015) 519(7542):242–6. doi:10.1038/nature14115
35. Kolodin D, van Panhuys N, Li C, Magnuson AM, Cipolletta D, Miller CM, et al. Antigen- and cytokine-driven accumulation of regulatory T cells in visceral adipose tissue of lean mice. *Cell Metab* (2015) 21(4):543–57. doi:10.1016/j.cmet.2015.03.005
36. Kern PA, Saghizadeh M, Ong JM, Bosch RJ, Deem R, Simsolo RB. The expression of tumor necrosis factor in human adipose tissue. Regulation by obesity, weight loss, and relationship to lipoprotein lipase. *J Clin Invest* (1995) 95(5):2111–9. doi:10.1172/JCI117899
37. Freemerman AJ, Johnson AR, Sacks GN, Milner JJ, Kirk EL, Troester MA, et al. Metabolic reprogramming of macrophages: glucose transporter 1 (GLUT1)-mediated glucose metabolism drives a proinflammatory phenotype. *J Biol Chem* (2014) 289(11):7884–96. doi:10.1074/jbc.M113.522037
38. Taylor CT, Colgan SP. Regulation of immunity and inflammation by hypoxia in immunological niches. *Nat Rev Immunol* (2017) 17(12):774–85. doi:10.1038/nri.2017.103
39. Wen H, Ting JP, O'Neill LA. A role for the NLRP3 inflammasome in metabolic diseases – did Warburg miss inflammation? *Nat Immunol* (2012) 13(4):352–7. doi:10.1038/ni.2228
40. Wen H, Gris D, Lei Y, Jha S, Zhang L, Huang MT, et al. Fatty acid-induced NLRP3-ASC inflammasome activation interferes with insulin signaling. *Nat Immunol* (2011) 12(5):408–15. doi:10.1038/ni.2022
41. Lee HM, Kim JJ, Kim HJ, Shong M, Ku BJ, Jo EK. Upregulated NLRP3 inflammasome activation in patients with type 2 diabetes. *Diabetes* (2013) 62(1):194–204. doi:10.2337/db12-0420
42. Lumeng CN, Bodzin JL, Saltiel AR. Obesity induces a phenotypic switch in adipose tissue macrophage polarization. *J Clin Invest* (2007) 117(1):175–84. doi:10.1172/JCI29881
43. Galic S, Fullerton MD, Schertzer JD, Sikkema S, Marcinko K, Walkley CR, et al. Hematopoietic AMPK beta1 reduces mouse adipose tissue macrophage inflammation and insulin resistance in obesity. *J Clin Invest* (2011) 121(12):4903–15. doi:10.1172/JCI58577
44. Michalek RD, Gerriets VA, Jacobs SR, Macintyre AN, MacIver NJ, Mason EF, et al. Cutting edge: distinct glycolytic and lipid oxidative metabolic programs are essential for effector and regulatory CD4+ T cell subsets. *J Immunol* (2011) 186(6):3299–303. doi:10.4049/jimmunol.1003613
45. Neumann B, Emmanuilidis K, Stadler M, Holzmann B. Distinct functions of interferon-gamma for chemokine expression in models of acute lung inflammation. *Immunology* (1998) 95(4):512–21. doi:10.1046/j.1365-2567.1998.00643.x

46. Singh UP, Singh S, Iqbal N, Weaver CT, McGhee JR, Lillard JW Jr. IFN-gamma-inducible chemokines enhance adaptive immunity and colitis. *J Interferon Cytokine Res* (2003) 23(10):591–600. doi:10.1089/107999003322485099
47. O'Rourke RW, White AE, Metcalf MD, Winters BR, Diggs BS, Zhu X, et al. Systemic inflammation and insulin sensitivity in obese IFN-gamma knockout mice. *Metabolism* (2012) 61(8):1152–61. doi:10.1016/j.metabol.2012.01.018
48. McGillicuddy FC, Chiquoine EH, Hinkle CC, Kim RJ, Shah R, Roche HM, et al. Interferon gamma attenuates insulin signaling, lipid storage, and differentiation in human adipocytes via activation of the JAK/STAT pathway. *J Biol Chem* (2009) 284(46):31936–44. doi:10.1074/jbc.M109.061655
49. Szabo SJ, Kim ST, Costa GL, Zhang X, Fathman CG, Glimcher LH. A novel transcription factor, T-bet, directs Th1 lineage commitment. *Cell* (2000) 100(6):655–69. doi:10.1016/S0092-8674(00)80702-3
50. Stolarczyk E, Vong CT, Perucha E, Jackson I, Cawthorne MA, Wargent ET, et al. Improved insulin sensitivity despite increased visceral adiposity in mice deficient for the immune cell transcription factor T-bet. *Cell Metab* (2013) 17(4):520–33. doi:10.1016/j.cmet.2013.02.019
51. Ley RE, Turnbaugh PJ, Klein S, Gordon JI. Microbial ecology: human gut microbes associated with obesity. *Nature* (2006) 444(7122):1022–3. doi:10.1038/4441022a
52. Backhed F, Manchester JK, Semenkovich CF, Gordon JI. Mechanisms underlying the resistance to diet-induced obesity in germ-free mice. *Proc Natl Acad Sci U S A* (2007) 104(3):979–84. doi:10.1073/pnas.0605374104
53. Neurath MF, Weigmann B, Finotto S, Glickman J, Nieuwenhuis E, Iijima H, et al. The transcription factor T-bet regulates mucosal T cell activation in experimental colitis and Crohn's disease. *J Exp Med* (2002) 195(9):1129–43. doi:10.1084/jem.20011956
54. Garrett WS, Lord GM, Punit S, Lugo-Villarino G, Mazmanian SK, Ito S, et al. Communicable ulcerative colitis induced by T-bet deficiency in the innate immune system. *Cell* (2007) 131(1):33–45. doi:10.1016/j.cell.2007.08.017
55. DeFuria J, Belkina AC, Jagannathan-Bogdan M, Snyder-Cappione J, Carr JD, Nersesova YR, et al. B cells promote inflammation in obesity and type 2 diabetes through regulation of T-cell function and an inflammatory cytokine profile. *Proc Natl Acad Sci U S A* (2013) 110(13):5133–8. doi:10.1073/pnas.1215840110
56. Frasca D, Diaz A, Romero M, Vazquez T, Blomberg BB. Obesity induces pro-inflammatory B cells and impairs B cell function in old mice. *Mech Ageing Dev* (2017) 162:91–9. doi:10.1016/j.mad.2017.01.004
57. Benezech C, Luu NT, Walker JA, Kruglov AA, Loo Y, Nakamura K, et al. Inflammation-induced formation of fat-associated lymphoid clusters. *Nat Immunol* (2015) 16(8):819–28. doi:10.1038/ni.3215
58. Roubenoff R, Roubenoff RA, Ward LM, Holland SM, Hellmann DB. Rheumatoid cachexia: depletion of lean body mass in rheumatoid arthritis. Possible association with tumor necrosis factor. *J Rheumatol* (1992) 19(10):1505–10.
59. Summers GD, Deighton CM, Rennie MJ, Booth AH. Rheumatoid cachexia: a clinical perspective. *Rheumatology (Oxford)* (2008) 47(8):1124–31. doi:10.1093/rheumatology/ken146
60. Roubenoff R. Rheumatoid cachexia: a complication of rheumatoid arthritis moves into the 21st century. *Arthritis Res Ther* (2009) 11(2):108. doi:10.1186/ar2658
61. Rall LC, Roubenoff R. Rheumatoid cachexia: metabolic abnormalities, mechanisms and interventions. *Rheumatology (Oxford)* (2004) 43(10):1219–23. doi:10.1093/rheumatology/keh321
62. Giles JT, Ling SM, Ferrucci L, Bartlett SJ, Andersen RE, Towns M, et al. Abnormal body composition phenotypes in older rheumatoid arthritis patients: association with disease characteristics and pharmacotherapies. *Arthritis Rheum* (2008) 59(6):807–15. doi:10.1002/art.23719
63. Roubenoff R. Sarcopenia: a major modifiable cause of frailty in the elderly. *J Nutr Health Aging* (2000) 4(3):140–2.
64. Kalinkovich A, Livshits G. Sarcopenic obesity or obese sarcopenia: a cross talk between age-associated adipose tissue and skeletal muscle inflammation as a main mechanism of the pathogenesis. *Ageing Res Rev* (2017) 35:200–21. doi:10.1016/j.arr.2016.09.008
65. Stavropoulos-Kalinoglou A, Metsios GS, Koutedakis Y, Kitas GD. Obesity in rheumatoid arthritis. *Rheumatology (Oxford)* (2011) 50(3):450–62. doi:10.1093/rheumatology/keq266
66. Iannone F, Lopalco G, Rigante D, Orlando I, Cantarini L, Lapadula G. Impact of obesity on the clinical outcome of rheumatologic patients in biotherapy. *Autoimmun Rev* (2016) 15(5):447–50. doi:10.1016/j.autrev.2016.01.010
67. Gonzalez-Gay MA, Gonzalez-Juanatey C. Rheumatoid arthritis: obesity impairs efficacy of anti-TNF therapy in patients with RA. *Nat Rev Rheumatol* (2012) 8(11):641–2. doi:10.1038/nrrheum.2012.158
68. Iannone F, Courvoisier DS, Gottenberg JE, Hernandez MV, Lie E, Canhao H, et al. Body mass does not impact the clinical response to intravenous abatacept in patients with rheumatoid arthritis. Analysis from the "pan-European registry collaboration for abatacept (PANABA)". *Clin Rheumatol* (2017) 36(4):773–9. doi:10.1007/s10067-016-3505-5
69. Alvarez-Nemegyei J, Buenfil-Rello FA, Pacheco-Pantoja EL. Association between body composition and disease activity in rheumatoid arthritis. A systematic review. *Reumatol Clin* (2016) 12(4):190–5. doi:10.1016/j.reuma.2015.09.001
70. Liu Y, Hazlewood GS, Kaplan GG, Eksteen B, Barnabe C. Impact of obesity on remission and disease activity in rheumatoid arthritis: a systematic review and meta-analysis. *Arthritis Care Res (Hoboken)* (2017) 69(2):157–65. doi:10.1002/acr.22932
71. Hallajzadeh J, Safiri S, Mansournia MA, Khoramdad M, Izadi N, Almasi-Hashiani A, et al. Metabolic syndrome and its components among rheumatoid arthritis patients: a comprehensive updated systematic review and meta-analysis. *PLoS One* (2017) 12(3):e0170361. doi:10.1371/journal.pone.0170361
72. Chung CP, Oeser A, Solus JF, Avalos I, Gebretsadik T, Shintani A, et al. Prevalence of the metabolic syndrome is increased in rheumatoid arthritis and is associated with coronary atherosclerosis. *Atherosclerosis* (2008) 196(2):756–63. doi:10.1016/j.atherosclerosis.2007.01.004
73. Wolfe F, Michaud K. Effect of body mass index on mortality and clinical status in rheumatoid arthritis. *Arthritis Care Res (Hoboken)* (2012) 64(10):1471–9. doi:10.1002/acr.21627
74. Sattar N, McInnes IB. Rheumatoid arthritis: debunking the obesity-mortality paradox in RA. *Nat Rev Rheumatol* (2015) 11(8):445–6. doi:10.1038/nrrheum.2015.93
75. Baker JF, George M, Baker DG, Toedter G, Von Feldt JM, Leonard MB. Associations between body mass, radiographic joint damage, adipokines and risk factors for bone loss in rheumatoid arthritis. *Rheumatology (Oxford)* (2011) 50(11):2100–7. doi:10.1093/rheumatology/ker294
76. Caplan L, Davis LA, Bright CM, Kerr GS, Lazaro DM, Khan NA, et al. Body mass index and the rheumatoid arthritis swollen joint count: an observational study. *Arthritis Care Res (Hoboken)* (2013) 65(1):101–6. doi:10.1002/acr.21734
77. Fukuda W, Omoto A, Ohta T, Majima S, Kimura T, Tanaka T, et al. Low body mass index is associated with impaired quality of life in patients with rheumatoid arthritis. *Int J Rheum Dis* (2013) 16(3):297–302. doi:10.1111/1756-185X.12079
78. Baker JF, Billig E, Michaud K, Ibrahim S, Caplan L, Cannon GW, et al. Weight loss, the obesity paradox, and the risk of death in rheumatoid arthritis. *Arthritis Rheumatol* (2015) 67(7):1711–7. doi:10.1002/art.39136
79. Vidal C, Barnetche T, Morel J, Combe B, Daien C. Association of body mass index categories with disease activity and radiographic joint damage in rheumatoid arthritis: a systematic review and metaanalysis. *J Rheumatol* (2015) 42(12):2261–9. doi:10.3899/jrheum.150224
80. Muller R, Kull M, Polluste K, Aart A, Eglit T, Lember M, et al. The metabolic profile in early rheumatoid arthritis: a high prevalence of metabolic obesity. *Rheumatol Int* (2017) 37(1):21–7. doi:10.1007/s00296-016-3464-9
81. Kerekes G, Nurmohamed MT, Gonzalez-Gay MA, Seres I, Paragh G, Kardos Z, et al. Rheumatoid arthritis and metabolic syndrome. *Nat Rev Rheumatol* (2014) 10(11):691–6. doi:10.1038/nrrheum.2014.121
82. McGrath CM, Young SP. Lipid and metabolic changes in rheumatoid arthritis. *Curr Rheumatol Rep* (2015) 17(9):57. doi:10.1007/s11926-015-0534-z
83. Ormseth MJ, Lipson A, Alexopoulos N, Hartlage GR, Oeser AM, Bian A, et al. Association of epicardial adipose tissue with cardiometabolic risk and metabolic syndrome in patients with rheumatoid arthritis. *Arthritis Care Res (Hoboken)* (2013) 65(9):1410–5. doi:10.1002/acr.22027
84. Giles JT, Ferrante AW, Broderick R, Zartoshti A, Rose J, Downer K, et al. Adipose tissue macrophages in rheumatoid arthritis: prevalence, disease

related indicators, and associations with cardiometabolic risk factors. *Arthritis Care Res (Hoboken)* (2017). doi:10.1002/acr.23253
85. Stavropoulos-Kalinoglou A, Metsios GS, Panoulas VF, Nightingale P, Koutedakis Y, Kitas GD. Anti-tumour necrosis factor alpha therapy improves insulin sensitivity in normal-weight but not in obese patients with rheumatoid arthritis. *Arthritis Res Ther* (2012) 14(4):R160. doi:10.1186/ar3900
86. Lemmey AB, Wilkinson TJ, Clayton RJ, Sheikh F, Whale J, Jones HS, et al. Tight control of disease activity fails to improve body composition or physical function in rheumatoid arthritis patients. *Rheumatology (Oxford)* (2016) 55(10):1736–45. doi:10.1093/rheumatology/kew243
87. Scrivo R, Vasile M, Muller-Ladner U, Neumann E, Valesini G. Rheumatic diseases and obesity: adipocytokines as potential comorbidity biomarkers for cardiovascular diseases. *Mediators Inflamm* (2013) 2013:808125. doi:10.1155/2013/808125
88. Tolusso B, Alivernini S, Gigante MR, Ferraccioli G, Gremese E. Biomolecular features of inflammation in obese rheumatoid arthritis patients: management considerations. *Expert Rev Clin Immunol* (2016) 12(7):751–62. doi:10.1586/1744666X.2016.1159132
89. Gomez R, Conde J, Scotece M, Gomez-Reino JJ, Lago F, Gualillo O. What's new in our understanding of the role of adipokines in rheumatic diseases? *Nat Rev Rheumatol* (2011) 7(9):528–36. doi:10.1038/nrrheum.2011.107
90. Weyand CM, Goronzy JJ. Immunometabolism in early and late stages of rheumatoid arthritis. *Nat Rev Rheumatol* (2017) 13(5):291–301. doi:10.1038/nrrheum.2017.49
91. Yang Z, Shen Y, Oishi H, Matteson EL, Tian L, Goronzy JJ, et al. Restoring oxidant signaling suppresses proarthritogenic T cell effector functions in rheumatoid arthritis. *Sci Transl Med* (2016) 8(331):331ra338. doi:10.1126/scitranslmed.aad7151
92. Weyand CM, Yang Z, Goronzy JJ. T-cell aging in rheumatoid arthritis. *Curr Opin Rheumatol* (2014) 26(1):93–100. doi:10.1097/BOR.0000000000000011
93. Fulop T Jr, Larbi A, Dupuis G, Pawelec G. Ageing, autoimmunity and arthritis: perturbations of TCR signal transduction pathways with ageing – a biochemical paradigm for the ageing immune system. *Arthritis Res Ther* (2003) 5(6):290–302. doi:10.1186/ar1019
94. Weyand CM, Fulbright JW, Goronzy JJ. Immunosenescence, autoimmunity, and rheumatoid arthritis. *Exp Gerontol* (2003) 38(8):833–41. doi:10.1016/S0531-5565(03)00090-1
95. Boots AM, Maier AB, Stinissen P, Masson P, Lories RJ, De Keyser F. The influence of ageing on the development and management of rheumatoid arthritis. *Nat Rev Rheumatol* (2013) 9(10):604–13. doi:10.1038/nrrheum.2013.92
96. van Onna M, Boonen A. The challenging interplay between rheumatoid arthritis, ageing and comorbidities. *BMC Musculoskelet Disord* (2016) 17:184. doi:10.1186/s12891-016-1038-3
97. Weyand CM, Fujii H, Shao L, Goronzy JJ. Rejuvenating the immune system in rheumatoid arthritis. *Nat Rev Rheumatol* (2009) 5(10):583–8. doi:10.1038/nrrheum.2009.180
98. Cejka D, Hayer S, Niederreiter B, Sieghart W, Fuereder T, Zwerina J, et al. Mammalian target of rapamycin signaling is crucial for joint destruction in experimental arthritis and is activated in osteoclasts from patients with rheumatoid arthritis. *Arthritis Rheum* (2010) 62(8):2294–302. doi:10.1002/art.27504
99. Steiner G, Smolen J. Autoantibodies in rheumatoid arthritis and their clinical significance. *Arthritis Res* (2002) 4(Suppl 2):S1–5. doi:10.1186/ar551
100. Abdul Wahab A, Mohammad M, Rahman MM, Mohamed Said MS. Anti-cyclic citrullinated peptide antibody is a good indicator for the diagnosis of rheumatoid arthritis. *Pak J Med Sci* (2013) 29(3):773–7.
101. Rapetti L, Chavele KM, Evans CM, Ehrenstein MR. B cell resistance to Fas-mediated apoptosis contributes to their ineffective control by regulatory T cells in rheumatoid arthritis. *Ann Rheum Dis* (2015) 74(1):294–302. doi:10.1136/annrheumdis-2013-204049
102. Baker K, Rath T, Lencer WI, Fiebiger E, Blumberg RS. Cross-presentation of IgG-containing immune complexes. *Cell Mol Life Sci* (2013) 70(8):1319–34. doi:10.1007/s00018-012-1100-8
103. Adlowitz DG, Barnard J, Biear JN, Cistrone C, Owen T, Wang W, et al. Expansion of activated peripheral blood memory B cells in rheumatoid arthritis, impact of B cell depletion therapy, and biomarkers of response. *PLoS One* (2015) 10(6):e0128269. doi:10.1371/journal.pone.0128269
104. Bouaziz JD, Yanaba K, Venturi GM, Wang Y, Tisch RM, Poe JC, et al. Therapeutic B cell depletion impairs adaptive and autoreactive CD4+ T cell activation in mice. *Proc Natl Acad Sci U S A* (2007) 104(52):20878–83. doi:10.1073/pnas.0709205105
105. Byng-Maddick R, Ehrenstein MR. The impact of biological therapy on regulatory T cells in rheumatoid arthritis. *Rheumatology (Oxford)* (2015) 54(5):768–75. doi:10.1093/rheumatology/keu487
106. Salomon S, Guignant C, Morel P, Flahaut G, Brault C, Gourguechon C, et al. Th17 and CD24hiCD27+ regulatory B lymphocytes are biomarkers of response to biologics in rheumatoid arthritis. *Arthritis Res Ther* (2017) 19(1):33. doi:10.1186/s13075-017-1244-x
107. McInnes IB, Schett G. Cytokines in the pathogenesis of rheumatoid arthritis. *Nat Rev Immunol* (2007) 7(6):429–42. doi:10.1038/nri2094
108. Meednu N, Zhang H, Owen T, Sun W, Wang V, Cistrone C, et al. Production of RANKL by memory B cells: a link between B cells and bone erosion in rheumatoid arthritis. *Arthritis Rheumatol* (2016) 68(4):805–16. doi:10.1002/art.39489
109. Abyad A, Boyer JT. Arthritis and aging. *Curr Opin Rheumatol* (1992) 4(2):153–9. doi:10.1097/00002281-199204000-00004
110. Tutuncu Z, Kavanaugh A. Rheumatic disease in the elderly: rheumatoid arthritis. *Rheum Dis Clin North Am* (2007) 33(1):57–70. doi:10.1016/j.rdc.2006.12.006
111. Hough AJ Jr, Webber RJ. Aging phenomena and osteoarthritis: cause or coincidence? Claude P. Brown memorial lecture. *Ann Clin Lab Sci* (1986) 16(6):502–10.
112. Aigner T, Rose J, Martin J, Buckwalter J. Aging theories of primary osteoarthritis: from epidemiology to molecular biology. *Rejuvenation Res* (2004) 7(2):134–45. doi:10.1089/1549168041552964
113. Jorgensen AEM, Kjaer M, Heinemeier KM. The effect of aging and mechanical loading on the metabolism of articular cartilage. *J Rheumatol* (2017) 44(4):410–7. doi:10.3899/jrheum.160226
114. Li YS, Xiao WF, Luo W. Cellular aging towards osteoarthritis. *Mech Ageing Dev* (2017) 162:80–4. doi:10.1016/j.mad.2016.12.012
115. Hugle T, Geurts J, Nuesch C, Muller-Gerbl M, Valderrabano V. Aging and osteoarthritis: an inevitable encounter? *J Aging Res* (2012) 2012:950192. doi:10.1155/2012/950192
116. Toh WS, Brittberg M, Farr J, Foldager CB, Gomoll AH, Hui JH, et al. Cellular senescence in aging and osteoarthritis. *Acta Orthop* (2016) 87 (Suppl 363):6–14. doi:10.1080/17453674.2016.1235087
117. Appelt CJ, Burant CJ, Siminoff LA, Kwoh CK, Ibrahim SA. Arthritis-specific health beliefs related to aging among older male patients with knee and/or hip osteoarthritis. *J Gerontol A Biol Sci Med Sci* (2007) 62(2):184–90. doi:10.1093/gerona/62.2.184
118. Wang F, Cai F, Shi R, Wang XH, Wu XT. Aging and age related stresses: a senescence mechanism of intervertebral disc degeneration. *Osteoarthritis Cartilage* (2016) 24(3):398–408. doi:10.1016/j.joca.2015.09.019
119. Loeser RF. Aging and osteoarthritis. *Curr Opin Rheumatol* (2011) 23(5):492–6. doi:10.1097/BOR.0b013e3283494005
120. Loeser RF. Aging processes and the development of osteoarthritis. *Curr Opin Rheumatol* (2013) 25(1):108–13. doi:10.1097/BOR.0b013e32835a9428
121. Loeser RF. The role of aging in the development of osteoarthritis. *Trans Am Clin Climatol Assoc* (2017) 128:44–54.
122. de SSMV, Valadares AL, Costa-Paiva LH, Osis MJ, Sousa MH, Pinto-Neto AM. Aging, obesity, and multimorbidity in women 50 years or older: a population-based study. *Menopause* (2013) 20(8):818–24. doi:10.1097/GME.0b013e31827fdd8c
123. Barbour KE, Helmick CG, Boring M, Brady TJ. Vital signs: prevalence of doctor-diagnosed arthritis and arthritis-attributable activity limitation – United States, 2013-2015. *MMWR Morb Mortal Wkly Rep* (2017) 66(9):246–53. doi:10.15585/mmwr.mm6609e1
124. Barbour KE, Helmick CG, Boring M, Qin J, Pan L, Hootman JM. Obesity trends among US adults with doctor-diagnosed arthritis 2009-2014. *Arthritis Care Res (Hoboken)* (2017) 69(3):376–83. doi:10.1002/acr.22958
125. Bliddal H, Leeds AR, Christensen R. Osteoarthritis, obesity and weight loss: evidence, hypotheses and horizons – a scoping review. *Obes Rev* (2014) 15(7):578–86. doi:10.1111/obr.12173
126. Rahmati M, Nalesso G, Mobasheri A, Mozafari M. Aging and osteoarthritis: central role of the extracellular matrix. *Ageing Res Rev* (2017) 40:20–30. doi:10.1016/j.arr.2017.07.004

127. Langa KM, Larson EB, Crimmins EM, Faul JD, Levine DA, Kabeto MU, et al. A comparison of the prevalence of dementia in the United States in 2000 and 2012. *JAMA Intern Med* (2017) 177(1):51–8. doi:10.1001/jamainternmed.2016.6807
128. Kalaria RN, Maestre GE, Arizaga R, Friedland RP, Galasko D, Hall K, et al. Alzheimer's disease and vascular dementia in developing countries: prevalence, management, and risk factors. *Lancet Neurol* (2008) 7(9):812–26. doi:10.1016/S1474-4422(08)70169-8
129. Rizzi L, Rosset I, Roriz-Cruz M. Global epidemiology of dementia: Alzheimer's and vascular types. *Biomed Res Int* (2014) 2014:908915. doi:10.1155/2014/908915
130. Ferri CP, Prince M, Brayne C, Brodaty H, Fratiglioni L, Ganguli M, et al. Global prevalence of dementia: a Delphi consensus study. *Lancet* (2005) 366(9503):2112–7. doi:10.1016/S0140-6736(05)67889-0
131. Vos SJB, van Boxtel MPJ, Schiepers OJG, Deckers K, de Vugt M, Carriere I, et al. Modifiable risk factors for prevention of dementia in midlife, late life and the oldest-old: validation of the libra index. *J Alzheimers Dis* (2017) 58(2):537–47. doi:10.3233/JAD-161208
132. Villringer A. The path from obesity and hypertension to dementia. *Adv Exp Med Biol* (2015) 821:5. doi:10.1007/978-3-319-08939-3_3
133. Kivipelto M, Ngandu T, Fratiglioni L, Viitanen M, Kareholt I, Winblad B, et al. Obesity and vascular risk factors at midlife and the risk of dementia and Alzheimer disease. *Arch Neurol* (2005) 62(10):1556–60. doi:10.1001/archneur.62.10.1556
134. Whitmer RA, Gustafson DR, Barrett-Connor E, Haan MN, Gunderson EP, Yaffe K. Central obesity and increased risk of dementia more than three decades later. *Neurology* (2008) 71(14):1057–64. doi:10.1212/01.wnl.0000306313.89165.ef
135. Fitzpatrick AL, Kuller LH, Lopez OL, Diehr P, O'Meara ES, Longstreth WT Jr, et al. Midlife and late-life obesity and the risk of dementia: cardiovascular health study. *Arch Neurol* (2009) 66(3):336–42. doi:10.1001/archneurol.2008.582
136. Pedditizi E, Peters R, Beckett N. The risk of overweight/obesity in mid-life and late life for the development of dementia: a systematic review and meta-analysis of longitudinal studies. *Age Ageing* (2016) 45(1):14–21. doi:10.1093/ageing/afv151
137. Albanese E, Launer LJ, Egger M, Prince MJ, Giannakopoulos P, Wolters FJ, et al. Body mass index in midlife and dementia: systematic review and meta-regression analysis of 589,649 men and women followed in longitudinal studies. *Alzheimers Dement (Amst)* (2017) 8:165–78. doi:10.1016/j.dadm.2017.05.007
138. Kiliaan AJ, Arnoldussen IA, Gustafson DR. Adipokines: a link between obesity and dementia? *Lancet Neurol* (2014) 13(9):913–23. doi:10.1016/S1474-4422(14)70085-7
139. Arnoldussen IA, Kiliaan AJ, Gustafson DR. Obesity and dementia: adipokines interact with the brain. *Eur Neuropsychopharmacol* (2014) 24(12):1982–99. doi:10.1016/j.euroneuro.2014.03.002
140. Naseer MI, Bibi F, Alqahtani MH, Chaudhary AG, Azhar EI, Kamal MA, et al. Role of gut microbiota in obesity, type 2 diabetes and Alzheimer's disease. *CNS Neurol Disord Drug Targets* (2014) 13(2):305–11. doi:10.2174/1871527313113126660147

11

Negative Effect of Age, but Not of Latent Cytomegalovirus Infection on the Antibody Response to a Novel Influenza Vaccine Strain in Healthy Adults

*Sara P. H. van den Berg[1,2], Albert Wong[3], Marion Hendriks[1], Ronald H. J. Jacobi[1], Debbie van Baarle[1,2] and Josine van Beek[1]**

[1] Centre for Infectious Disease Control, National Institute for Public Health and the Environment, Bilthoven, Netherlands, [2] Laboratory of Translational Immunology, Department of Immunology, University Medical Center Utrecht, Utrecht University, Utrecht, Netherlands, [3] Department of Statistics, Informatics and Mathematical Modelling, National Institute for Public Health and the Environment, Bilthoven, Netherlands

***Correspondence:**
Josine van Beek
josine.van.beek@rivm.nl

Older adults are more vulnerable to influenza virus infection and at higher risk for severe complications and influenza-related death compared to younger adults. Unfortunately, influenza vaccine responses tend to be impaired in older adults due to aging of the immune system (immunosenescence). Latent infection with cytomegalovirus (CMV) is assumed to enhance age-associated deleterious changes of the immune system. Although lower responses to influenza vaccination were reported in CMV-seropositive compared to CMV-seronegative adults and elderly, beneficial effects of CMV infection were observed as well. The lack of consensus in literature on the effect of latent CMV infection on influenza vaccination may be due to the presence of pre-existing immunity to influenza in these studies influencing the subsequent influenza vaccine response. We had the unique opportunity to evaluate the effect of age and latent CMV infection on the antibody response to the novel influenza H1N1pdm vaccine strain during the pandemic of 2009, thereby reducing the effect of pre-existing immunity on the vaccine-induced antibody response. This analysis was performed in a large study population (n = 263) in adults (18–52 years old). As a control, memory responses to the seasonal vaccination, including the same H1N1pdm and an H3N2 strain, were investigated in the subsequent season 2010–2011. With higher age, we found decreased antibody responses to the pandemic vaccination even within this age range, indicating signs of immunosenescence to this novel antigen in the study population. Using a generalized estimation equation regression model, adjusted for age, sex, and previous influenza vaccinations, we observed that CMV infection in contrast did not influence the influenza virus-specific antibody titer after H1N1pdm vaccination. Yet, we found higher residual protection rates (antibody level ≥40 hemagglutinin units (HAU)) in CMV-seropositive individuals than in CMV-seronegative individuals 6 months and 1 year after pandemic vaccination. In the subsequent season, no effect of age or CMV infection on seasonal influenza vaccine response was observed. In conclusion, we observed no evidence for CMV-induced impairment of antibody responses to a novel influenza strain vaccine in adults. If anything, our data suggest that there might be a beneficial effect of latent CMV infection on the protection rate after novel influenza vaccination.

Keywords: cytomegalovirus, influenza vaccine, aging, immunosenescence, pandemic, antibody response, *de novo* immune response

INTRODUCTION

Aging of the population poses an important public health problem. With age, the function of the human immune system declines, a phenomenon also referred to as immunosenescence (1). Profound changes of the immune system include the gradual loss of naïve cells, increase of memory cell numbers, and decreased diversity of the T cell and B cell repertoire (1–3). These changes contribute to reduced protection against infectious diseases and reduced vaccine responses in older adults. Indeed, the incidence of influenza virus infections is increased and accompanied with more complications and higher mortality in older adults (4, 5). Most developed countries recommend yearly influenza vaccination in individuals above 60 or 65 years of age (6), in order to prevent influenza virus infection by the induction of protective antibodies (4, 7). However, the antibody response to influenza vaccination in older adults is impaired, causing a suboptimal protection in this vulnerable group (7–9).

Accumulating evidence indicates that latent cytomegalovirus (CMV) infection is associated with age-related changes of the immune system, and might enhance immunosenescence (2, 10, 11). CMV is a common β-herpesvirus with a prevalence of 45–100% worldwide, which increases with advancing age (12). CMV infection causes morbidity and mortality in severely immunocompromised patients, while the virus rarely causes clinical symptoms in healthy individuals. Despite the ability of the immune system to control primary infection, the virus establishes a latent infection, with episodes of viral reactivation during lifetime (13). The frequent reactivation of CMV causes continuous antigenic stress for the immune system (3). Anti-CMV IgG levels increase with age (14–16) and are thought to increase after viral reactivation episodes, thereby reflecting the amount of experienced CMV antigenic stress during lifetime (12, 14, 17). The profound effect of CMV infection on the immune system is especially shown by the progressive large expansion of oligoclonal CMV-specific CD8 T cells and, to a lesser extent, CD4 T cells. Furthermore, CMV-seropositivity is strongly associated with an inverted CD4/8 ratio (18), bias of the TCR repertoire (19), and an increase of highly differentiated T cells (20).

It has been suggested that CMV-enhanced immunosenescence could impair the immune response to influenza vaccination (21, 22). Indeed, in several studies, CMV-seropositivity or a high anti-CMV IgG titer was associated with lower antibody responses to influenza vaccination in both adults (23–25) and older adults (25–28). However, others did not find an effect of CMV infection (29, 30), or reported even an enhanced antibody response to influenza vaccination in both young (31, 32) and older CMV-seropositive individuals (33).

The overall impact of latent CMV infection on the antibody induction by influenza vaccines remains controversial and depends, among other factors, on pre-existing immunity to influenza virus (34). Most studies investigated the antibody response to seasonal influenza vaccination; a yearly recommended trivalent influenza vaccine that often contains overlapping influenza vaccine strains in consecutive years. Natural exposure to influenza virus and previous vaccination causes pre-existing immunity, which influences the consecutive vaccine response. Higher pre-vaccination antibody titers (pre-titers) indeed were shown to result in lower post-vaccination antibody titers to subsequent vaccination (7, 35). Furthermore, one could expect a larger effect of immunosenescence on *de novo* immune responses (36, 37). A seasonal influenza vaccination is, therefore, a suboptimal study setting to investigate the effect of latent CMV infection on influenza vaccine antibody response.

We hypothesize that the effect of latent CMV infection on the antibody response to influenza vaccination can best be studied when a novel influenza virus strain is introduced into a naïve population. In this study, we had the unique opportunity to investigate the effect of latent CMV infection on the antibody response during the pandemic season of 2009 to the novel H1N1pdm vaccine strain in a large study population and at multiple time points after vaccination. This allowed a sophisticated study design to test the effect of latent CMV infection on a *de novo* influenza vaccine response by minimizing pre-existing immunity due to previous exposure by vaccination or natural infection. As a control, the influence of latent CMV infection on the memory antibody response to the vaccination in the subsequent year was also investigated, which included both the same H1N1pdm vaccine strain and an H3N2 vaccine strain.

MATERIALS AND METHODS

Study Population and Design

The current study is embedded in a trial that evaluated the immune responses to pandemic and seasonal influenza vaccination that was conducted in 2009–2011 (the Pandemic influenza vaccination trial, Netherlands Trial Register NTR2070). This study was carried out in accordance with the recommendations of Good Clinical Practice with written informed consent from all subjects. All subjects gave written informed consent in accordance with the Declaration of Helsinki. The protocol was approved by the Central Committee on Research Involving Human Subjects of the Netherlands. Healthy individuals, between 18 and 52 years of age, were recruited among health care workers in the Utrecht area in the Netherlands. Individuals over 52 years of age were not included because of potential pre-existing immunity due to exposure to the influenza A/H1N1 strain that circulated until 1957 (38). Serum samples and questionnaires were used from the vaccine group of the Pandemic influenza vaccination cohort.

Vaccines

In the pandemic season, individuals received two doses of the monovalent MF59-adjuvanted influenza vaccine containing influenza A/California/7/2009(H1N1pdm09) with a 3-week interval (Focetria, Novartis, Italy). Blood samples were collected before vaccination (T1), 3 weeks after vaccination at which also the second pandemic vaccine dose was given (T2), 6 weeks after the first vaccination (T3), 26 weeks after the first vaccination (T4), and if participants continued with the study during the 2010–2011 season, also 52 weeks after the first vaccination (T5) (**Figure 1**). Self-reported vaccine history (2006–2009) was extracted from the questionnaires. If study subjects received seasonal trivalent vaccination in 2009–2010 (Solvay, the Netherlands), it took place at least 3 weeks prior to the study or at the end of visit at time point 3 of the study. In season 2010–2011, individuals received the seasonal trivalent subunit vaccine Influvac 2010–2011, containing the influenza A vaccine strains A/California/7/2009(H1N1pdm09) and A/Perth/16/2009(H3N2) (Solvay, the Netherlands). Blood was collected before vaccination (T1), 3 weeks after vaccination (T2), and 20 weeks after vaccination (T3).

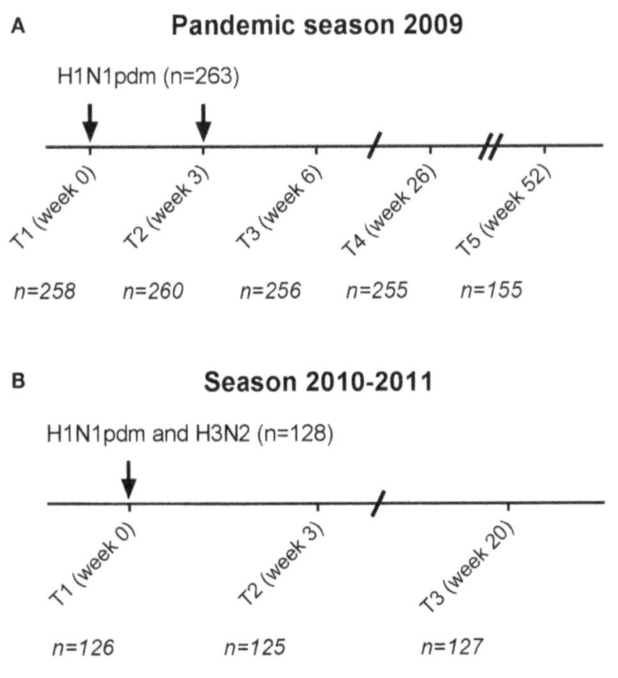

FIGURE 1 | Study schedule. Participants received in the pandemic season two monovalent influenza H1N1pdm vaccinations with a 3-week interval **(A)**. In total, 263 cytomegalovirus (CMV)-seropositive and CMV-seronegative individuals were vaccinated. 155 participants continued for the subsequent year in the study (T5 season 1). In the season 2010–2011, 128 individuals were vaccinated (T1 season 2) with the seasonal trivalent influenza vaccination which contained among others the same H1N1pdm vaccine strain and an H3N2 vaccine strain **(B)**. Arrows (↓) indicate the moment of vaccination. Time points (T) indicate the moment of blood withdrawal. For each time point, the number (*N*) of individuals with data of influenza antibody levels is indicated.

Assessment of Serum Anti-CMV Antibody Titers

Anti-CMV IgG antibody concentrations were measured using a commercial ELISA (IBL international GMBH, Hamburg, Germany) according to manufacturer's instructions. Participants with a CMV antibody level of ≥12 U/ml or higher were considered CMV-seropositive, a level of ≤8 U/ml were considered CMV-seronegative, and a level between 8 and 12 U/ml was considered equivocal and these participants were excluded for further analysis. CMV-seropositive individuals were divided into low anti-CMV levels (≤30 U/ml), medium anti-CMV levels (>30 U/ml, ≤90 U/ml), or high anti-CMV levels (>90 U/ml) according to the standards in the CMV ELISA kit.

Hemagglutination-Inhibition (HI) Assay

Hemagglutination-inhibition assays were performed in the pandemic season for A/California/7/2009(H1N1pdm09) and in season 2010–2011 for A/California/7/2009(H1N1pdm09) and A/Perth/16/2009(H3N2) to determine influenza virus-specific antibody titers before and after vaccination. Briefly, a dilution series of cholera filtrate-treated serum samples was incubated with four hemagglutinin units (HAU) of influenza virus for 20 min, 0.25% turkey erythrocytes for 45 min and scored for agglutination (39). The influenza antibody titer is the inverse of the last dilution of the serum that completely inhibited hemagglutination. A detectable influenza antibody body titer is defined as >5 HAU.

Statistical Analysis

Antibody responses to H1N1pdm influenza vaccination in the pandemic season were expressed in two different ways: (1) influenza antibody titer and (2) protection rate (antibody titer ≥40 HAU). For all statistical analyses, influenza antibody titers were log (base 2) transformed, and presented as geometric mean titer (GMT) with 95% confidence interval (CI) in the figures.

First, a two-tailed Student's *t*-test (for two groups) or one-way ANOVA (for three or more groups) was used to explore group differences in influenza antibody titers (e.g., between low, medium, and high CMV IgG groups). For the two-tailed *T*-test, equality of variances was tested with Levene's test for equality. Group differences in categorical variables were compared with the Fisher exact test.

Second, we investigated the effect of latent CMV infection in a multivariate context; the effect of CMV infection on influenza antibody titers was adjusted for potential confounders using a generalized estimation equation (GEE) regression model (Table S1 in Supplementary Material) (40). This model takes repeated measurements for the same individuals into account. For the continues variable outcome (influenza antibody titer) the normal distribution and for the categorical variable (influenza protection rate) the binomial distribution of the model was used. The effect of CMV infection was investigated in two ways: (a) CMV-serostatus: CMV-seropositive individuals were compared to CMV-seronegative individuals and (b) anti-CMV IgG groups: low, medium, and high anti-CMV IgG levels were compared within CMV-seropositive individuals. Confounders included were age, sex, time, and various variables concerning vaccination history (see Table S1 in Supplementary Material). The model yielded a beta regression coefficient for each variable, which reflects how a category (e.g., highest age group) compares to the reference category (e.g., lowest age group). Regression coefficients of the GEE models are given in Tables S2–S7 in Supplementary Material. The model also yielded adjusted results (i.e., influenza antibody titers or protection rates) for each time point at which comparisons between CMV-serostatus or anti-CMV IgG group were performed, by including an interaction term between time and CMV-serostatus or anti-CMV IgG group in the GEE models. The adjusted outcomes of the models and pairwise comparisons are presented in the figures. These analyses were also performed for the influenza vaccine response in season 2010–2011 for H1N1pdm and H3N2. *P* values of ≤0.10 were considered a trend and of ≤0.05 were considered significant. Data were analyzed using SPSS statistics 22 for Windows (SPSS Inc., Chicago, IL, USA) and R 3.4.0 (https://www.r-project.org/).

RESULTS

Characteristics of the Study Population

In total, 288 individuals were vaccinated with the pandemic influenza vaccine in the pandemic season (**Figure 1**). CMV-serostatus was determined and 25 individuals with an equivocal CMV status were excluded from further analysis. Of the remaining 263 individuals, 171 were CMV-seropositive (65%). Groups of CMV-seropositive and CMV-seronegative individuals were comparable for sex, age, and previous influenza vaccinations (**Table 1**). In season 2010–2011, 128 of the 263 participants were vaccinated with the seasonal vaccination of which 76 (59.4%) were CMV-seropositive. Also, in the subsequent season, no differences in sex, age, and previous influenza vaccinations between CMV-seropositive and CMV-seronegative individuals were observed (**Table 1**).

Negative Effect of Age on Influenza Titers after *De Novo* Pandemic Influenza Vaccination

We investigated if there was an effect of age on the induction of antibodies to the pandemic influenza vaccination in our study population. After pandemic vaccination, H1N1pdm influenza virus-specific antibody titers were negatively correlated with age at all time points post-vaccination except T5 (see Table S8 in Supplementary Material). Representative data are depicted for T2 in **Figure 2A** (T2, $p = 0.0013$, $R = -0.198$). Individuals are divided into three age groups for further analysis by approximately 10-year intervals. Significant differences were also observed between age groups in the H1N1pdm titers (e.g., T2, $p = 0.016$), with lower responses in the oldest age group compared to the youngest two age groups (e.g., T2, 19–30 versus 40–52 year $p = 0.007$) (**Figure 2B**) (see Table S8 in Supplementary Material). Similar results were observed for the different age groups when analyzing the data by protection level, defined by reaching a titer of ≥40 HAU (data not shown). These data indicate that there are already signs of immunosenescence-driven impaired vaccine responses to a novel antigen challenge in middle-aged individuals.

No Effect of CMV-Seropositivity on Antibody Titers after Pandemic Influenza Vaccination

Next, the effect of latent CMV infection on the influenza virus-specific antibody response to the vaccine with the newly introduced H1N1pdm influenza vaccine strain was investigated. CMV-seropositive individuals were compared to CMV-seronegative individuals for influenza titers before and after vaccination. No differences between CMV-seropositive and CMV-seronegative individuals in influenza titer at any time point in both seasons were found (Figure S1A in Supplementary Material). Some individuals did already show a detectable pandemic titer before vaccination, although on average the pre-titer was very low (GMT 9.4 HAU). To correct for this and other potential confounders, influenza titers of CMV-seropositive and CMV-seronegative individuals were analyzed adjusted for pre-titer, sex, age, and previous influenza vaccinations with a GEE model (Table S2 in Supplementary Material). No significant

TABLE 1 | Characteristics of study population for pandemic season and season 2010–2011.

	Pandemic season				Season 2010–2011			
	Total (n = 263)[a]	CMV+ (n = 171)	CMV− (n = 92)	Significance	Total (n = 128)	CMV+ (n = 76)	CMV− (n = 52)	Significance
Age (mean and SD)	39.9 (7.8)	39.3 (8.6)	39.5 (8.5)	$P = 0.88$	41.3 (8.1)	41.7 (7.7)	40.63 (8.6)	$P = 0.43$
Sex (% men)	45.2%	51.1%	42.1%	$P = 0.19$	48.4%	46.1%	51.9%	$P = 0.59$
Previous influenza vaccination before pandemic season	49.0%	49.7%	47.8%	$P = 0.80$	65.6%	63.2%	69.2%	$P = 0.57$
Seasonal vaccination 2009–2010 before study	23.6%	23.4%	23.9%	$P = 1.00$	87.1%[b]	77.6%	78.8%	$P = 1.00$
Seasonal vaccination 2009–2010 during study	37.3%	38.0%	35.9%	$P = 0.79$				

Cytomegalovirus (CMV)-seropositive and CMV-seronegative group are compared with Student's t-test for age and with the Fischer exact test for categorical variables.
[a]Time point 5, 52 weeks after pandemic influenza vaccination, blood was collected of 155 participants who continued in the study for season 2010–2011.
[b]Seasonal vaccination in 2009 before study or during study combined.

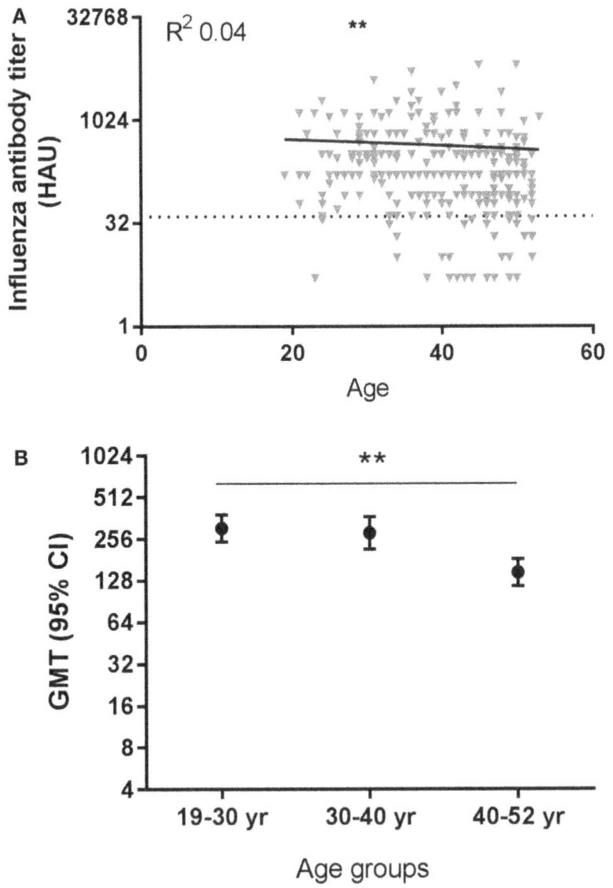

FIGURE 2 | Effect of age on influenza virus-specific antibody titers after influenza vaccination. A representative figure of influenza H1N1pdm antibody titers after pandemic vaccination plotted against age (T2) **(A)**. Dotted horizontal line represents a protective influenza titer of 40 hemagglutinin units (HAU). The geometric mean of the influenza antibody titer **(B)** after vaccination is given for different age groups after vaccination with H1N1pdm for T2 (p = 0.016 ANOVA). Correlations are tested with Pearson correlation. Differences between two age groups are tested with Student's t-test for log-transformed influenza antibody titers. $^{**}p < 0.010$. GMT, geometric mean titers.

differences were found between CMV-seropositive and CMV-seronegative individuals in antibody titers at each individual time point (**Figure 3A**). So although age shows a negative effect on the novel pandemic H1N1pdm antibody response indicative of immunosenescence to *de novo* response (**Figure 2**), no effect of CMV-serostatus on the influenza virus titer is observed after pandemic vaccination in adults (**Figure 3A**).

Higher Residual Protection Rates after Pandemic Influenza Vaccination in CMV-Seropositive Individuals than in CMV-Seronegative Individuals

Subsequently, we investigated whether there was an effect of CMV-serostatus on the protection rate, as defined by antibody titer ≥40 HAU, against influenza virus after influenza vaccination (41). Shortly after vaccination, no effect of CMV-serostatus on the protection rate was observed. However, CMV-seropositivity was associated with enhanced 6 months and 1 year protection rates after pandemic vaccination. The percentage influenza protected individuals is significantly higher for CMV-seropositive individuals than for CMV-seronegative individuals, both 26 weeks ($p = 0.047$) and 52 weeks ($p = 0.044$) after pandemic vaccination (**Figure 3B**) (unadjusted data in Figure S1B in Supplementary Material). Together, this suggests that latent CMV infection did not impair the protection rate after influenza vaccination, but if anything, might be beneficial for persistence of protection after the *de novo* influenza vaccination.

High Anti-CMV IgG Levels As Surrogate Marker of CMV Reactivation Are Not Associated with Impaired Pandemic Influenza Vaccine Response in CMV-Seropositive Individuals

To study in the CMV-seropositive individuals whether the frequency of CMV reactivation has a negative effect on the influenza antibody responses, anti-CMV IgG levels were used as a surrogate marker of CMV reactivation (25, 42) and associated with the influenza antibody response to vaccination. To this end, CMV-seropositive individuals with low anti-CMV IgG levels (≤30 U/ml), medium anti-CMV IgG levels (>30 U/ml, ≤90 U/ml) or high anti-CMV IgG levels (>90 U/ml) were compared for their influenza antibody titer and protection rate both unadjusted (Figures S1C,D in Supplementary Material) and with the GEE model (Table S3 in Supplementary Material). No differences were observed between anti-CMV IgG groups in the H1N1pdm influenza titers or protection rate after the pandemic vaccination (**Figures 3C,D**). This indicates that despite a negative effect of age on the antibody response to the pandemic vaccination (**Figure 2**), no signs of impairment by CMV reactivation were observed. Also this shows that the positive effect of CMV status on long-term protection after pandemic influenza vaccination (**Figure 3B**) could not be explained by differences in anti-CMV IgG groups within CMV-seropositive individuals.

No Effect of Age or CMV-Serostatus on Seasonal Influenza Vaccination with H1N1pdm and H3N2

The same analyses for the effect of age and latent CMV infection on influenza vaccination were performed for the 128 individuals that continued with the study and were vaccinated in season 2010–2011 with the seasonal influenza vaccination containing the same H1N1pdm strain and an H3N2 strain. A trend of a negative effect of age on the H1N1pdm memory response was observed, but no significant differences in antibody titers for H1N1pdm or H3N2 were found between age groups at any time point after vaccination in season 2010–2011 (e.g., T2, respectively, $p = 0.101$ and $p = 0.434$) (**Figure 4A**). Both the influenza antibody titer and the protection rate did not differ between CMV-seropositive and CMV-seronegative individuals (**Figures 4B–D**; Tables S4 and S6 in Supplementary Material). Surprisingly, influenza antibody titers and protection rate after the

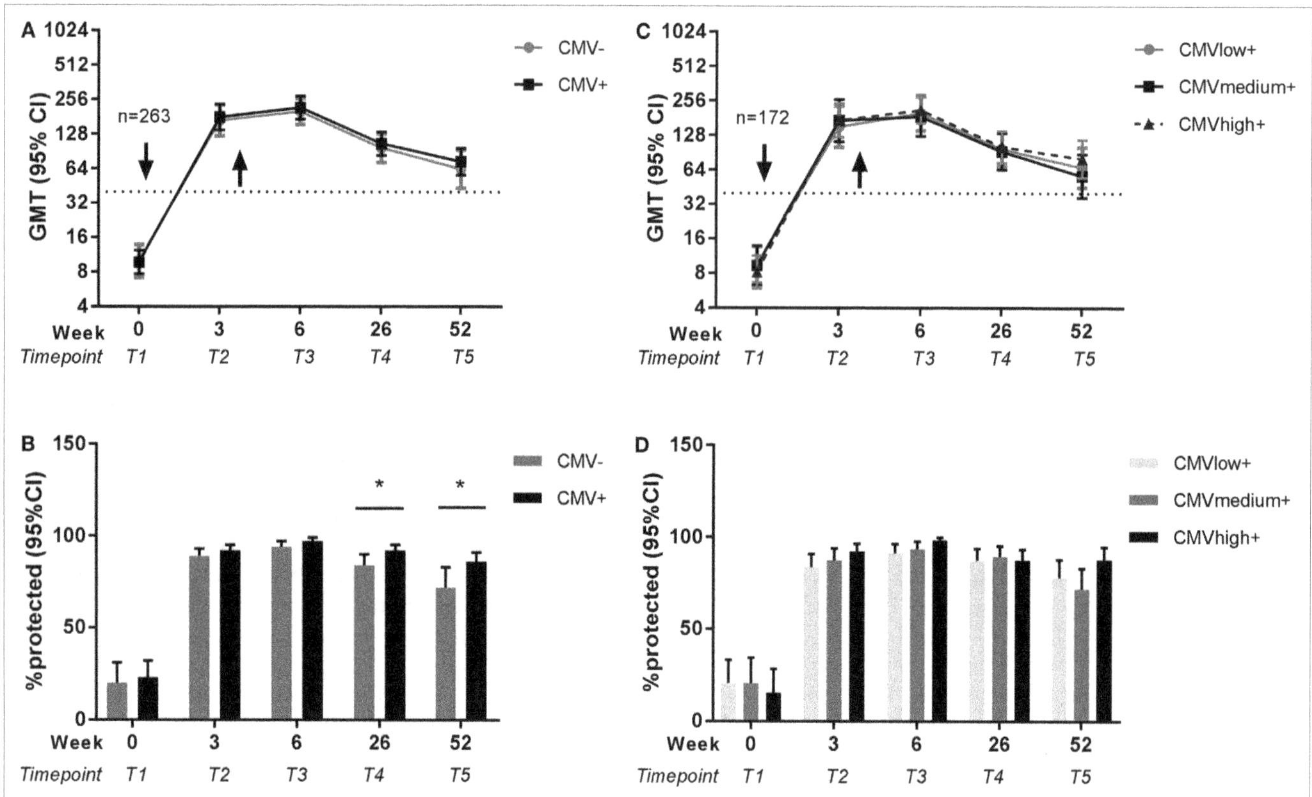

FIGURE 3 | Effect of latent cytomegalovirus (CMV) infection on influenza virus-specific antibody titer and protection rate to pandemic influenza infection. Geometric mean and 95% confidence interval (CI) of influenza antibody titers and the percentage protected (defined as a titer ≥40 HAU) are shown for CMV-seropositive and CMV-seronegative individuals **(A,B)** and for CMV-seropositive individuals with low, medium, and high anti-CMV IgG levels **(C,D)** before and after pandemic vaccination with H1N1pdm in 2009. Arrows (↓) indicate the moment of vaccination. Dotted horizontal line represents a protective influenza titer of 40. Results are adjusted for sex, age group, and previous influenza vaccinations by a generalized estimation equation (GEE) regression model. Significant differences are tested by pairwise comparison between CMV-seropositive and CMV-seronegative individuals or anti-CMV IgG group high and low per separate time point. *$p < 0.05$.

seasonal vaccination were higher for both H1N1pdm and H3N2 in the high anti-CMV IgG levels group compared to low anti-CMV IgG levels group within the CMV-seropositive individuals at most time points after vaccination (**Figures 4E–G**; Tables S5 and S7 in Supplementary Material). In summary, although no clear effect of age or CMV-serostatus, high anti-CMV IgG levels seem to be associated with high influenza antibody titers and protection rate in CMV-seropositive individuals.

DISCUSSION

In this study, we investigated the effect of age and latent CMV infection on the antibody response to a novel influenza vaccine strain in healthy adults. We found evidence of immunosenescence in these adults from the age of 40. However, latent CMV infection did not impair the antibody responses to a *de novo* influenza vaccine response. Interestingly, indications for the contrary were observed: CMV-seropositive individuals even showed a higher long-term influenza protection rate after pandemic influenza vaccination. These results suggest that latent CMV infection does not always further weaken age-related impaired immunity, but if anything, might be beneficial.

Our study showed no negative association between latent CMV infection and the antibody response to influenza vaccination. Other studies did report negative effects in adults (23, 25, 32) and older adults (25, 26, 28, 43). However, most of these studies investigated the effect of latent CMV infection on the influenza vaccine response in the presence of pre-existing immunity. In one study, all subjects were even seroprotected (influenza antibody titer >40 HAU) before influenza vaccination (26). It is known that individuals with high pre-titers show a lower increase in influenza antibody response after influenza vaccination (7, 19, 35, 44). Therefore, high pre-titers are associated with lower seroconversion (antibody titer ≥40 HAU and ≥4-fold increase) and higher protection rate (>40 HAU). Furthermore, in all but two studies (25, 43), vaccine history was not taken into account, while previous vaccination is associated with lower seroconversion independently of pre-titers (7). Not accounting for pre-existing immunity in influenza vaccine responses, therefore, may obscure findings and lead to different findings on the effect of latent CMV infection. Here, we controlled for pre-existing immunity by investigating the effect of latent CMV infection on pandemic vaccination for which pre-existing immunity was low, and by performing analysis adjusted for pre-titers and vaccine history. By doing so, we found that influenza vaccine responses are not

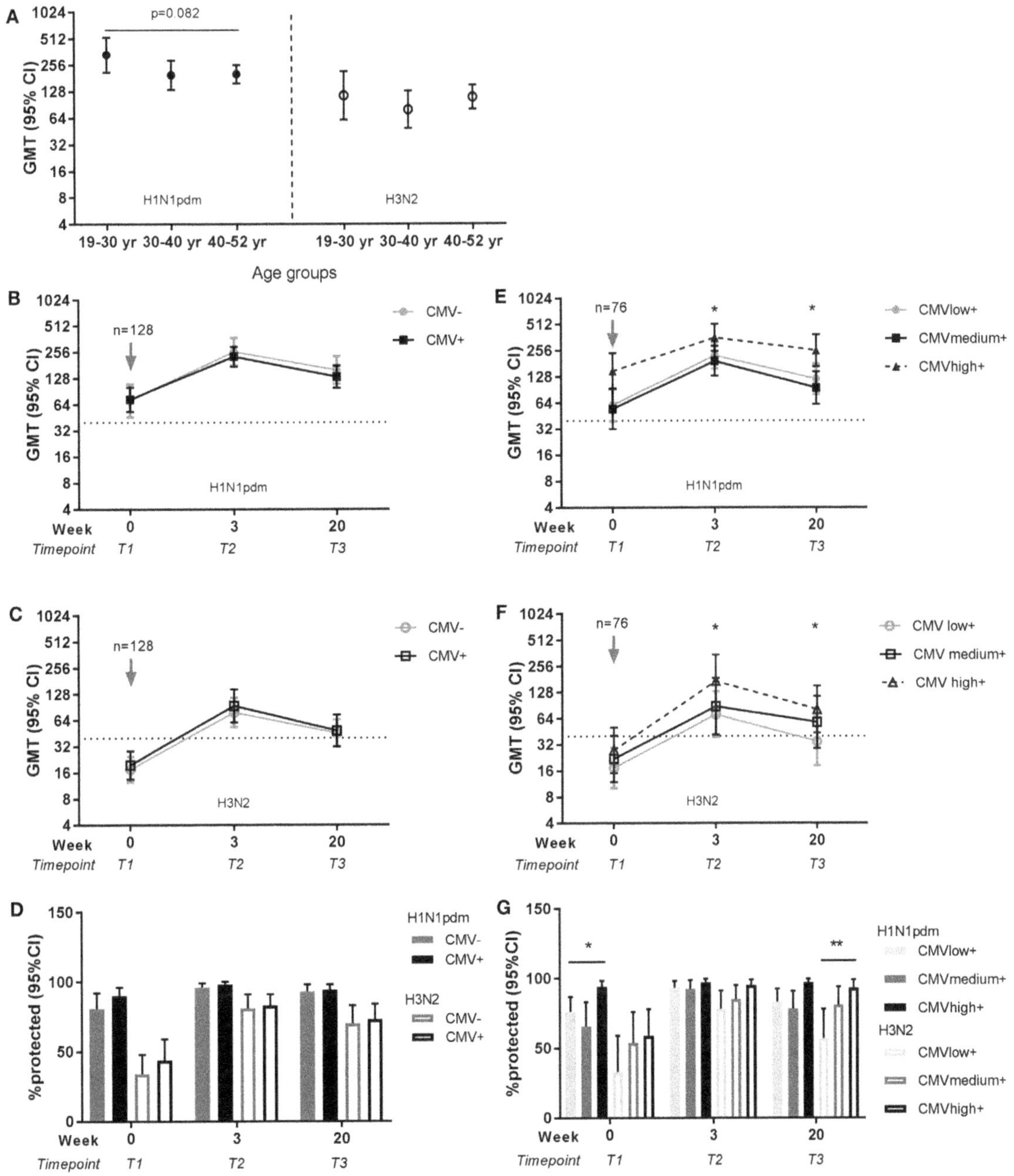

FIGURE 4 | Effect of age and latent cytomegalovirus (CMV) infection on influenza virus-specific antibody titer and protection rate to seasonal influenza infection. Geometric mean and 95% confidence interval (CI) of influenza antibody titers are shown per age group for H1N1pdm (left panel) and H3N2 (right panel) for the representative time point T2 (3 weeks) after seasonal influenza vaccination 2010–2011 **(A)**. Geometric mean and 95% CI of influenza antibody titers **(B,C)** and the percentage protected [defined as a titer ≥40 hemagglutinin units (HAU)] **(D)** are shown for CMV-seropositive and CMV-seronegative individuals for H1N1pdm and H3N2 strain before and after seasonal vaccination 2010–2011. For CMV-seropositive individuals with low, medium, and high anti-CMV IgG levels geometric mean and 95% CI of influenza antibody titers **(E,F)** and the percentage protected (defined as a titer ≥40 HAU) **(G)** are shown for H1N1pdm and H3N2 strain before and after seasonal vaccination 2010–2011. Arrows (↓) indicate the moment of vaccination. Dotted horizontal line represents a protective influenza titer of 40 HAU. Results for the effect of latent CMV infection are adjusted for sex, age group, and previous influenza vaccinations by a generalized estimation equation (GEE) regression model. Significant differences are tested by pairwise comparison between CMV-seropositive and CMV-seronegative individuals or anti-CMV IgG group high and low per separate time point. Significant differences between age groups were tested with ANOVA and differences between two age groups are tested with Student's *t*-test for (log transformed) antibody titers. $^*p < 0.05$.

impaired by latent CMV infection. If anything, signs of enhanced persistence of protection after influenza vaccination were observed in CMV-seropositive individuals. We observed similar results when we analyzed the effect of latent CMV infection on the seroconversion rate. No impairment by CMV-latent infection on the vaccine response was found, but CMV-seropositive individuals showed a higher seroconversion rate 6 months and 1 year after vaccination (T4, $p = 0.044$; T5, $p = 0.02$) (data not shown).

A beneficial effect of latent CMV infection on the immune system has been indicated (10) and is suggested to reflect higher activation status of innate cells after primary CMV infection or reactivation. Accordingly, an increased antibody titer short term after influenza vaccination in young CMV-seropositive compared to young CMV-seronegative individuals was observed (31–33) and suggested to depend on boosting by low-grade inflammation and high levels of circulating IFNγ in CMV-seropositive young individuals (31, 33). A beneficial effect of latent CMV infection on the long-term persistence of protection after vaccination in adults has to our knowledge not been reported. Waning of protection is thought to be most significant in individuals above 65 years of age (45) and accelerated by latent CMV infection (46). Our results might suggest a positive effect of CMV infection in adults on the protection rate. Thereby our data fit in a scenario in which latent CMV infection has a beneficial effect in adults and may become detrimental with aging.

Two studies that reported a short-term negative effect of latent CMV infection in adults did take the factor pre-existing immunity into account by either correcting for antibody titers pre-vaccination (24) or by investigating the effect of latent CMV infection on the novel pandemic vaccine (23). However, these studies differ from our study in terms of vaccine type and analysis of the antibody response. Turner et al. studied the fold increase of influenza antibody titers to seasonal vaccination, corrected for pre-titers before vaccination (24). They reported a negative effect on the influenza antibody fold increase in one strain of the trivalent vaccine in CMV-seropositive adults with high anti-CMV IgG levels compared to CMV-seronegative adults. Wald et al. (23) also reported a negative effect of CMV-seropositivity in adults, by investigating the same pandemic H1N1pdm vaccine response in 2009 as we did. However, they did not adjust for confounders in the analysis (23). These differences in findings of the effect of latent CMV infection on the influenza vaccine response without pre-existing immunity are unexplained. We speculate that the vaccine dose and adjuvant use may be a reason for these differences. In Turner et al., half the recommended dose was used (24). Likewise, an unadjuvanted monovalent vaccine (47) was used in Wald et al., while in our study the vaccine was adjuvanted. The use of MF59 adjuvant is expected to activate the CD4+ T cells and further enhance antibody production, thereby eliciting a stronger immune response compared to an unadjuvanted vaccine. Taken together, it may be possible that only with less potent influenza vaccines, a short-term negative effect of latent CMV infection is present.

The correlation of lower antibody response to the novel pandemic influenza vaccination with age points to an immunosenescence-driven weakened immune response. Typically, lower antibody responses to influenza vaccination are associated with high age (>60 years old). Interestingly, we observed already an effect of age in this group of non-elderly (18–52 years of age), although small. This effect of age was due to a lower influenza antibody response from the age of 40 years onward. It is suggested that differences between age groups to influenza vaccination responses might also explained by HA imprinting (48). HA imprinting implicates that the immune response is skewed to the group of HA antigens of the influenza strain that is first encountered during childhood. However, this was not the case and HA imprinting could be excluded as an explanation for the age differences.

Similar analyzes were performed for the effect of age and latent CMV on the seasonal influenza vaccine response in season 2010–2011. Seasonal vaccination in 2010–2011 contained the same H1N1pdm strain of the pandemic season and the antigen-drifted H3N2 strain that overlaps in serological response to great extent with previous H3N2 strains (49). Thus, both seasonal strains elicit an immunological memory response. Immunosenescence mainly affects the *de novo* immune responses (36, 37). In line with this, effects of age on an influenza vaccine response diminish after further vaccination with the same strain (34), explaining the different findings for the effect of age between the pandemic season and season 2010–2011. It was surprising to find that individuals with high anti-CMV IgG levels showed a higher influenza titer and protection rate to seasonal vaccination. We cannot exclude that these individuals might be high-antibody producers in general, as previously shown for respiratory syncytial virus and the response to other respiratory viruses (50). Also, the total group that continued to season 2010–2011 with the study was smaller ($n = 128$) and had a higher number of previous vaccinations than the group of the pandemic season ($n = 263$), complicating the adjusted analysis. Different results were obtained for using seroconversion rate instead of protection rate as definition of responder on the seasonal vaccination. A positive effect of high anti-CMV levels group was not observed on the seroconversion rate (data not shown). This shows the importance for correcting in our statistical model for these factors and strongly implies caution with interpretations of CMV-induced effects in small study groups or non-adjusted studies as reported in literature.

Important strengths of our study compared to others are the use of a novel influenza vaccine strain, the relatively large groups of study subjects in the pandemic season and the adjusted analysis with the GEE model. Since aging and latent CMV infection are thought to affect the immune system both independently and by interacting with each other, separation of these factors in analysis is crucial (51). A limitation of the study is that the study population consists of health care workers who received repeated previous influenza vaccinations. Individuals with repeated previous seasonal influenza vaccinations show in general higher pre-vaccination titers than first-time vaccinated individuals (44). Even in the pandemic season, cross reactivity was reported for the H1N1pdm strain (52, 53). Together with potential natural exposure to the H1N1pdm strain just before the study, this may explain the detectable titers before pandemic vaccination in this study. The seasonal 2009 vaccination 3 weeks before the study in the pandemic season indeed increased the pandemic pre-titer (data not shown). However, vaccine history of the past years preceding the vaccine trial of the study subjects was reported and was adjusted for in the analysis. Importantly, pre-titers did not affect the study results, since individuals in our study without detectable pre-titers

($n = 203$) for pandemic influenza vaccination showed comparable results for the effect of CMV infection for the pandemic season (data not shown).

The influenza response in humans is complex and raises the question if influenza vaccination is the best model to investigate the effect of latent CMV infection on vaccine responses A less complicated model, in which a vaccine for people that are truly naïve is used, might be a better study design for this question. However, we consider that influenza vaccination represents the most relevant because of its high societal importance. Therefore, knowledge on the effect of CMV infection on the influenza antibody response is of great importance.

In conclusion, we used a novel influenza vaccine strain to investigate the effect of age and latent CMV infection on the *de novo* immune response to influenza. We found indeed already impaired antibody responses to vaccination in adults with increasing age, but latent CMV infection did not impair the influenza virus-specific antibody response. Thereby, we show that CMV infection does not *per se* enhance the age-related impaired immunity as assumed, but if anything might give opposite effects. A model in which CMV infection boosts the immune system during adulthood, while in older adults CMV infection enhances the aging of the immune system, might be appropriate. These results are important in the decision to invest in preventing latent CMV infection in healthy individuals through strategies such as CMV vaccination.

ETHICS STATEMENT

This study was carried out in accordance with the recommendations of Good Clinical Practice with written informed consent from all subjects. All subjects gave written informed consent in accordance with the Declaration of Helsinki. The protocol was approved by the Central Committee on Research Involving Human Subjects of the Netherlands.

AUTHOR CONTRIBUTIONS

SB, DB, and JB conceptualized the study. SB, MH, and RJ executed the laboratory experiments. SB and AW performed the statistical analysis. SB, AW, DB, and JB interpreted the data and wrote the manuscript. All authors critically revised the manuscript.

FUNDING

This work was supported by the Dutch Ministry of Public Health.

REFERENCES

1. Siegrist CA, Aspinall R. B-cell responses to vaccination at the extremes of age. *Nat Rev Immunol* (2009) 9(3):185–94. doi:10.1038/nri2508
2. Tu W, Rao S. Mechanisms underlying T cell immunosenescence: aging and cytomegalovirus infection. *Front Microbiol* (2016) 7:2111. doi:10.3389/fmicb.2016.02111
3. Fulop T, Larbi A, Pawelec G. Human T cell aging and the impact of persistent viral infections. *Front Immunol* (2013) 4:271. doi:10.3389/fimmu.2013.00271
4. McElhaney JE, Kuchel GA, Zhou X, Swain SL, Haynes L. T-cell immunity to influenza in older adults: a pathophysiological framework for development of more effective vaccines. *Front Immunol* (2016) 7:41. doi:10.3389/fimmu.2016.00041
5. Loubet P, Samih-Lenzi N, Galtier F, Vanhems P, Loulergue P, Duval X, et al. Factors associated with poor outcomes among adults hospitalized for influenza in France: a three-year prospective multicenter study. *J Clin Virol* (2016) 79:68–73. doi:10.1016/j.jcv.2016.04.005
6. van Essen GA, Palache AM, Forleo E, Fedson DS. Influenza vaccination in 2000: recommendations and vaccine use in 50 developed and rapidly developing countries. *Vaccine* (2003) 21(16):1780–5. doi:10.1016/S0264-410X(03)00072-0
7. Goodwin K, Viboud C, Simonsen L. Antibody response to influenza vaccination in the elderly: a quantitative review. *Vaccine* (2006) 24(8):1159–69. doi:10.1016/j.vaccine.2005.08.105
8. Pera A, Campos C, López N, Hassouneh F, Alonso C, Tarazona R, et al. Immunosenescence: implications for response to infection and vaccination in older people. *Maturitas* (2015) 82(1):50–5. doi:10.1016/j.maturitas.2015.05.004
9. Jefferson T, Di Pietrantonj C, Al-Ansary LA, Ferroni E, Thorning S, Thomas RE. Vaccines for preventing influenza in the elderly. *Cochrane Database Syst Rev* (2010) 2:CD004876. doi:10.1002/14651858.CD004876.pub3
10. Arens R, Remmerswaal EB, Bosch JA, van Lier RA. 5(th) International Workshop on CMV and Immunosenescence – a shadow of cytomegalovirus infection on immunological memory. *Eur J Immunol* (2015) 45(4):954–7. doi:10.1002/eji.201570044
11. Pawelec G, Derhovanessian E. Role of CMV in immune senescence. *Virus Res* (2011) 157(2):175–9. doi:10.1016/j.virusres.2010.09.010
12. Cannon MJ, Schmid DS, Hyde TB. Review of cytomegalovirus seroprevalence and demographic characteristics associated with infection. *Rev Med Virol* (2010) 20(4):202–13. doi:10.1002/rmv.655
13. Stowe RP, Kozlova EV, Yetman DL, Walling DM, Goodwin JS, Glaser R. Chronic herpesvirus reactivation occurs in aging. *Exp Gerontol* (2007) 42(6):563–70. doi:10.1016/j.exger.2007.01.005
14. Korndewal MJ, Mollema L, Tcherniaeva I, van der Klis F, Kroes AC, Oudesluys-Murphy AM, et al. Cytomegalovirus infection in the Netherlands: seroprevalence, risk factors, and implications. *J Clin Virol* (2015) 63:53–8. doi:10.1016/j.jcv.2014.11.033
15. Cannon MJ, Hyde TB, Schmid DS. Review of cytomegalovirus shedding in bodily fluids and relevance to congenital cytomegalovirus infection. *Rev Med Virol* (2011) 21(4):240–55. doi:10.1002/rmv.695
16. Bhattacharyya MK, Lustig AJ. Telomere dynamics in genome stability. *Trends Biochem Sci* (2006) 31(2):114–22. doi:10.1016/j.tibs.2005.12.001
17. Lustig A, Liu HB, Metter EJ, An Y, Swaby MA, Elango P, et al. Telomere shortening, inflammatory cytokines, and anti-cytomegalovirus antibody follow distinct age-associated trajectories in humans. *Front Immunol* (2017) 8:1027. doi:10.3389/fimmu.2017.01027
18. Wikby A, Johansson B, Olsson J, Löfgren S, Nilsson BO, Ferguson F. Expansions of peripheral blood CD8 T-lymphocyte subpopulations and an association with cytomegalovirus seropositivity in the elderly: the Swedish NONA immune study. *Exp Gerontol* (2002) 37(2–3):445–53. doi:10.1016/S0531-5565(01)00212-1
19. Hadrup SR, Strindhall J, Køllgaard T, Seremet T, Johansson B, Pawelec G, et al. Longitudinal studies of clonally expanded CD8 T cells reveal a repertoire shrinkage predicting mortality and an increased number of dysfunctional cytomegalovirus-specific T cells in the very elderly. *J Immunol* (2006) 176(4):2645–53. doi:10.4049/jimmunol.176.4.2645
20. Appay V, Rowland-Jones SL. Lessons from the study of T-cell differentiation in persistent human virus infection. *Semin Immunol* (2004) 16(3):205–12. doi:10.1016/j.smim.2004.02.007
21. McElhaney JE, Zhou X, Talbot HK, Soethout E, Bleackley RC, Granville DJ, et al. The unmet need in the elderly: how immunosenescence, CMV infection,

co-morbidities and frailty are a challenge for the development of more effective influenza vaccines. *Vaccine* (2012) 30(12):2060–7. doi:10.1016/j.vaccine.2012.01.015

22. Saurwein-Teissl M, Lung TL, Marx F, Gschösser C, Asch E, Blasko I, et al. Lack of antibody production following immunization in old age: association with CD8(+)CD28(-) T cell clonal expansions and an imbalance in the production of Th1 and Th2 cytokines. *J Immunol* (2002) 168(11):5893–9. doi:10.4049/jimmunol.168.11.5893
23. Wald A, Selke S, Magaret A, Boeckh M. Impact of human cytomegalovirus (CMV) infection on immune response to pandemic 2009 H1N1 influenza vaccine in healthy adults. *J Med Virol* (2013) 85(9):1557–60. doi:10.1002/jmv.23642
24. Turner JE, Campbell JP, Edwards KM, Howarth LJ, Pawelec G, Aldred S, et al. Rudimentary signs of immunosenescence in cytomegalovirus-seropositive healthy young adults. *Age (Dordr)* (2014) 36(1):287–97. doi:10.1007/s11357-013-9557-4
25. Trzonkowski P, Mysliwska J, Szmit E, Wieckiewicz J, Lukaszuk K, Brydak LB, et al. Association between cytomegalovirus infection, enhanced proinflammatory response and low level of anti-hemagglutinins during the anti-influenza vaccination – an impact of immunosenescence. *Vaccine* (2003) 21(25–26):3826–36. doi:10.1016/S0264-410X(03)00309-8
26. Frasca D, Diaz A, Romero M, Landin AM, Blomberg BB. Cytomegalovirus (CMV) seropositivity decreases B cell responses to the influenza vaccine. *Vaccine* (2015) 33(12):1433–9. doi:10.1016/j.vaccine.2015.01.071
27. Derhovanessian E, Maier AB, Hähnel K, McElhaney JE, Slagboom EP, Pawelec G. Latent infection with cytomegalovirus is associated with poor memory CD4 responses to influenza A core proteins in the elderly. *J Immunol* (2014) 193(7):3624–31. doi:10.4049/jimmunol.1303361
28. Alonso Arias R, Moro-García MA, Echeverría A, Solano-Jaurrieta JJ, Suárez-García FM, López-Larrea C. Intensity of the humoral response to cytomegalovirus is associated with the phenotypic and functional status of the immune system. *J Virol* (2013) 87(8):4486–95. doi:10.1128/JVI.02425-12
29. den Elzen WP, Vossen AC, Cools HJ, Westendorp RG, Kroes AC, Gussekloo J. Cytomegalovirus infection and responsiveness to influenza vaccination in elderly residents of long-term care facilities. *Vaccine* (2011) 29(29–30): 4869–74. doi:10.1016/j.vaccine.2011.03.086
30. Haq K, Fulop T, Tedder G, Gentleman B, Garneau H, Meneilly GS, et al. Cytomegalovirus seropositivity predicts a decline in the T cell but not the antibody response to influenza in vaccinated older adults independent of type 2 diabetes status. *J Gerontol A Biol Sci Med Sci* (2016) 72(9):1163–70. doi:10.1093/gerona/glw216
31. Furman D, Jojic V, Sharma S, Shen-Orr SS, Angel CJ, Onengut-Gumuscu S, et al. Cytomegalovirus infection enhances the immune response to influenza. *Sci Transl Med* (2015) 7(281):281ra43. doi:10.1126/scitranslmed.aaa2293
32. Strindhall J, Ernerudh J, Mörner A, Waalen K, Löfgren S, Matussek A, et al. Humoral response to influenza vaccination in relation to pre-vaccination antibody titres, vaccination history, cytomegalovirus serostatus and CD4/CD8 ratio. *Infect Dis (Lond)* (2016) 48(6):436–42. doi:10.3109/23744235.2015.1135252
33. McElhaney JE, Garneau H, Camous X, Dupuis G, Pawelec G, Baehl S, et al. Predictors of the antibody response to influenza vaccination in older adults with type 2 diabetes. *BMJ Open Diabetes Res Care* (2015) 3(1):e000140. doi:10.1136/bmjdrc-2015-000140
34. Mosterín Höpping A, McElhaney J, Fonville JM, Powers DC, Beyer WEP, Smith DJ. The confounded effects of age and exposure history in response to influenza vaccination. *Vaccine* (2016) 34(4):540–6. doi:10.1016/j.vaccine.2015.11.058
35. Beyer WE, Palache AM, Sprenger MJ, Hendriksen E, Tukker JJ, Darioli R, et al. Effects of repeated annual influenza vaccination on vaccine sero-response in young and elderly adults. *Vaccine* (1996) 14(14):1331–9. doi:10.1016/S0264-410X(96)00058-8
36. Michel JP, Lang PO. Promoting life course vaccination. *Rejuvenation Res* (2011) 14(1):75–81. doi:10.1089/rej.2010.1078
37. Lang PO, Aspinall R. Immunosenescence and herd immunity: with an ever-increasing aging population do we need to rethink vaccine schedules? *Expert Rev Vaccines* (2012) 11(2):167–76. doi:10.1586/erv.11.187
38. Miller E, Hoschler K, Hardelid P, Stanford E, Andrews N, Zambon M. Incidence of 2009 pandemic influenza A H1N1 infection in England: a cross-sectional serological study. *Lancet* (2010) 375(9720):1100–8. doi:10.1016/S0140-6736(09)62126-7
39. Luytjes W, Enouf V, Schipper M, Gijzen K, Liu WM, van der Lubben M, et al. HI responses induced by seasonal influenza vaccination are associated with clinical protection and with seroprotection against non-homologous strains. *Vaccine* (2012) 30(35):5262–9. doi:10.1016/j.vaccine.2012.05.060
40. Zeger SL, Liang KY. Longitudinal data analysis for discrete and continuous outcomes. *Biometrics* (1986) 42(1):121–30. doi:10.2307/2531248
41. Wijnans L, Voordouw B. A review of the changes to the licensing of influenza vaccines in Europe. *Influenza Other Respir Viruses* (2016) 10(1):2–8. doi:10.1111/irv.12351
42. Wang GC, Dash P, McCullers JA, Doherty PC, Thomas PG. T cell receptor alphabeta diversity inversely correlates with pathogen-specific antibody levels in human cytomegalovirus infection. *Sci Transl Med* (2012) 4(128):128ra42. doi:10.1126/scitranslmed.3003647
43. Derhovanessian E, Theeten H, Hähnel K, Van Damme P, Cools N, Pawelec G. Cytomegalovirus-associated accumulation of late-differentiated CD4 T-cells correlates with poor humoral response to influenza vaccination. *Vaccine* (2013) 31(4):685–90. doi:10.1016/j.vaccine.2012.11.041
44. Huang KA, Chang SC, Huang YC, Chiu CH, Lin TY. Antibody responses to trivalent inactivated influenza vaccine in health care personnel previously vaccinated and vaccinated for the first time. *Sci Rep* (2017) 7:40027. doi:10.1038/srep40027
45. Castilla J, Martínez-Baz I, Martínez-Artola V, Reina G, Pozo F, García Cenoz M, et al. Decline in influenza vaccine effectiveness with time after vaccination, Navarre, Spain, season 2011/12. *Euro Surveill* (2013) 18(5). doi:10.2807/ese.18.05.20388-en
46. Reed RG, Greenberg RN, Segerstrom SC. Cytomegalovirus serostatus, inflammation, and antibody response to influenza vaccination in older adults: the moderating effect of beta blockade. *Brain Behav Immun* (2017) 61:14–20. doi:10.1016/j.bbi.2016.09.025
47. Chen WH, Winokur PL, Edwards KM, Jackson LA, Wald A, Walter EB, et al. Phase 2 assessment of the safety and immunogenicity of two inactivated pandemic monovalent H1N1 vaccines in adults as a component of the U.S. pandemic preparedness plan in 2009. *Vaccine* (2012) 30(28):4240–8. doi:10.1016/j.vaccine.2012.04.044
48. Gostic KM, Ambrose M, Worobey M, Lloyd-Smith JO. Potent protection against H5N1 and H7N9 influenza via childhood hemagglutinin imprinting. *Science* (2016) 354(6313):722–6. doi:10.1126/science.aag1322
49. Ann J, Papenburg J, Bouhy X, Rhéaume C, Hamelin MÈ, Boivin G. Molecular and antigenic evolution of human influenza A/H3N2 viruses in Quebec, Canada, 2009–2011. *J Clin Virol* (2012) 53(1):88–92. doi:10.1016/j.jcv.2011.09.016
50. Orange JS, Du W, Falsey AR. Therapeutic immunoglobulin selected for high antibody titer to RSV also contains high antibody titers to other respiratory viruses. *Front Immunol* (2015) 6:431. doi:10.3389/fimmu.2015.00431
51. Wertheimer AM, Bennett MS, Park B, Uhrlaub JL, Martinez C, Pulko V, et al. Aging and cytomegalovirus infection differentially and jointly affect distinct circulating T cell subsets in humans. *J Immunol* (2014) 192(5):2143–55. doi:10.4049/jimmunol.1301721
52. Wrammert J, Koutsonanos D, Li GM, Edupuganti S, Sui J, Morrissey M, et al. Broadly cross-reactive antibodies dominate the human B cell response against 2009 pandemic H1N1 influenza virus infection. *J Exp Med* (2011) 208(1):181–93. doi:10.1084/jem.20101352
53. Centers for Disease Control and Prevention. Serum cross-reactive antibody response to a novel influenza A (H1N1) virus after vaccination with seasonal influenza vaccine. *MMWR Morb Mortal Wkly Rep* (2009) 58(19):521–4.

12

Involvement of MicroRNAs in the Aging-Related Decline of CD28 Expression by Human T Cells

*Nato Teteloshvili[1†‡], Gerjan Dekkema[1‡], Annemieke M. Boots[2], Peter Heeringa[1], Pytrick Jellema[1], Debora de Jong[1], Martijn Terpstra[3], Elisabeth Brouwer[2], Graham Pawelec[4,5], Klaas Kok[3], Anke van den Berg[1], Joost Kluiver[1] and Bart-Jan Kroesen[6]**

[1] Department of Pathology and Medical Biology, University of Groningen, University Medical Center Groningen, Groningen, Netherlands, [2] Rheumatology and Clinical Immunology, University of Groningen, University Medical Center Groningen, Groningen, Netherlands, [3] Genetics, University of Groningen, University Medical Center Groningen, Groningen, Netherlands, [4] Department of Internal Medicine II, Center for Medical Research, University of Tübingen, Tübingen, Germany, [5] Cancer Solutions Program, Health Sciences North Research Institute, Sudbury, Ontario, Canada, [6] Laboratory Medicine, University of Groningen, University Medical Center Groningen, Groningen, Netherlands

***Correspondence:**
Bart-Jan Kroesen
b.j.kroesen@umcg.nl*

Loss of CD28 is a characteristic feature of T cell aging, but the underlying mechanisms of this loss are elusive. As differential expression of microRNAs (miRNAs) has been described between CD28+ and CD28− T cells, we hypothesized that altered miRNA expression contributes to the age-associated downregulation of CD28. To avoid the confounding effects of age-associated changes in the proportions of T cells at various differentiation stages *in vivo*, an experimental model system was used to study changes over time in the expression of miRNA associated with the loss of CD28 expression in monoclonal T cell populations at a lower or higher number of population doublings (PDs). This approach allows identification of age-associated miRNA expression changes in a longitudinal model. Results were validated in *ex vivo* samples. The cumulative number of PDs but not the age of the donor of the T cell clone was correlated with decreased expression of CD28. Principal component analysis of 252 expressed miRNAs showed clustering based on low and high PDs, irrespective of the age of the clone donor. Increased expression of miR-9-5p and miR-34a-5p was seen in clones at higher PDs, and miR-9-5p expression inversely correlated with CD28 expression in *ex vivo* sorted T-cells from healthy subjects. We then examined the involvement of miR-9-5p, miR-34a-5p, and the members of the miR-23a~24-2 cluster, in which all are predicted to bind to the 3′UTR of CD28, in the IL-15-induced loss of CD28 in T cells. Culture of fresh naive CD28+ T cells in the presence of IL-15 resulted in a gradual loss of CD28 expression, while the expression of miR-9-5p, miR-34a-5p, and members of the miR-23a~24-2 cluster increased. Binding of miR-9-5p, miR-34a-5p, miR-24-3p, and miR-27- 3p to the 3′UTR of CD28 was studied using luciferase reporter constructs. Functional binding to the 3′UTR was shown for miR-24-3p and miR-27a-3p. Our results indicate involvement of defined miRNAs in T cells in relation to specific characteristics of T cell aging, i.e., PD and CD28 expression.

Keywords: T cell aging, senescence, CD28, IL-15, miRNA, miR-9, miR-23a~24-2

INTRODUCTION

Full activation of naive T cells requires binding of the T cell receptor (TCR) to antigens displayed by the major histocompatibility complex on antigen-presenting cells (APCs) (known as "signal one") together with ligation of a T cell costimulatory receptor ("signal two"). The latter is archetypically mediated by CD28 on the T cell surface and CD80 or CD86 on the APC. This interaction results in complex signaling cascades which activate T cells, promote their differentiation, proliferation, and effector function, and mounts adaptive immune responses depending on clonally expanded, antigen-specific effector T cells and the subsequent generation of T cell memory (1). Costimulation *via* CD28 lowers the threshold for signaling *via* the TcR and triggers cytokine production. This allows T cells to respond to low abundance and low avidity antigens, and shapes T cell immunity by balancing the interplay between effector and regulatory T cells (1). The latter is especially important in focusing the immune response toward the pathogen, avoiding autoimmunity, and for downregulating the immune response upon pathogen clearance.

The composition and function of the T cell immune system in older people is characterized by lower proportions of naive T cells and higher proportions of memory T cells as a result of antigen exposure over the lifetime (2). Additionally, aging itself affects the characteristics of T cells within the naive and memory compartments and when these effects result in compromised functionality, these T cells can be designated "immunosenescent" (2–4). Developmentally programmed thymic involution at puberty results in an abrupt decline in the output of naive T cells, although residual thymic activity maintains the production of small numbers of such cells in most people in their 50s or 60's. The diversity of the memory T cell pool increasingly reflects pathogen exposures over the lifetime, especially its focus on maintaining immune surveillance of latent viruses, e.g., CMV, EBV, and many other pathogens (5, 6). Overall, numbers and proportions of naive T cells decline, despite partial compensation by homeostatic proliferation of these cells in the periphery, which may also contribute to their aging phenotype (7, 8). Repeated clonal expansions of memory cells on rechallenge by specific pathogens, or continuous challenges by persistent pathogens, are thought to be instrumental for the overall differences observed between T cells in younger and older individuals (9, 10). At the cellular level, T cell aging is characterized by a multitude of changes in the expression of cell surface proteins. Most notably, a gradual decline in the expression of CD28 has been reported as a characteristic feature of aged T cells, mostly but not only due to the age-associated accumulation of late-stage memory cells which do not express this coreceptor (11, 12). The exact mechanisms involved in the aging-related decline of CD28 are unknown. Dissecting the differences in CD28 expression resulting from altered proportions of naive and memory T cells with age, and the intrinsic aging process within single T cell populations is challenging. To approach this, we have employed monoclonal T cells with increasing population doublings (PDs) in culture as a longitudinal aging model to identify regulation of CD28 expression, and attempted to validate some of these in *ex vivo* sorted T-cells from healthy subjects (13, 14) Here, we report the activity of microRNAs (miRNAs) in this context.

MicroRNAs are small noncoding RNA molecules that regulate protein expression by interfering with the process of messenger RNA (mRNA) translation or by inducing mRNA degradation. miRNAs are crucially involved in T cell development, differentiation, activation, and function (15, 16). In addition, recent evidence has implicated the involvement of miRNAs in several aspects of T cell aging (15–19). However, if and how miRNAs are involved in the regulated decline of CD28 expression is unknown. High expression of the three members of the miR-23a~24-2 cluster in CD8+CD28− T cells relative to CD8+CD28+ T cells has been reported (20). Increased expression of miR-24 in CD28− T cells was associated with an increased susceptibility to cell death, which was counterbalanced by IL-15 (20). IL-15 is a homeostatic cytokine that supports survival and proliferation of naive CD28+ T cells in the absence of continuous TCR stimulation (21). Downregulation of CD28 in response to homeostatic cytokines, such as IL-15, which interact with common γ-chain receptors, has been well documented (21–23). Here, we studied the involvement of miRNAs in clonal expansion and IL-15-regulated expression of CD28 by T cells. Using T cell clones derived from healthy young and elderly donors, we observed clustering of miRNAs primarily according to the number of PDs. In addition, IL-15 induced loss of CD28 coincided with upregulation of miRNAs that interact with the 3′UTR of CD28 mRNA.

MATERIALS AND METHODS

Generation of T Cell Clones

T cell clones were generated from phytohemagglutinin-stimulated peripheral blood mononuclear cells (PBMC) by limiting dilution in the presence of IL-2 and pooled irradiated PBMC feeder cells as described previously (13, 24–26). In brief, cells to be cloned were plated at 0.45/well into 1 mm-diameter microplate wells containing 10^4 30 Gy-irradiated pooled PBMC from >20 random normal donors as feeder cells. Contents of positive wells were transferred after 1–2 weeks to 96-well 7 mm-diameter flat bottomed microtiter plate containing fresh medium and 10^5 pooled PBMC feeder cells between day 7 and 11, and to 16 mm-diameter 24-well cluster plate with 2.5×10^5 stimulators between day 12 and 16. Cultures were given fresh medium every 3 or 4 days and fresh feeder cells every 1–2 weeks thereafter. Clonal age is expressed in PD estimated by microscopic counting of the cells at each subculture and counting the number of doublings cumulatively undergone. Culture medium was the serum-free formulation X-Vivo 10 (BioWhittaker, Walkersville, MD, USA).

Three T cell clones from two healthy old and three T cell clones from one healthy young donor each at low and high PDs were selected for small RNA sequencing (n = 12 samples; three independent samples for each condition tested). Additional clones were used for the quantitative reverse-transcription-polymerase chain reaction (qRT-PCR) validation experiments (Table S1 in Supplementary Material). T-cell clones used were all CD4+. CD28 expression on T cell clones with low and high numbers of PDs was assessed by standard quantitative flow cytometry and expressed as median fluorescence intensity as reported previously (24, 25).

Primary Lymphocyte Subsets

Peripheral blood mononuclear cells were freshly isolated by density gradient centrifugation using Lymphoprep (Axis-Shield, Oslo, Norway) according to the manufacturer's protocol. Informed consent was obtained from all participants in accordance with the Declaration of Helsinki. The Medical Ethical Committee of the University Medical Center Groningen approved the study. For validation of differential miR-9-5p and miR-34a-5p expression in CD28+ versus CD28− T cells, CD3+CD28+ and CD3+CD28− cells were fluorescence-activated cell sorting (FACS) sorted from six healthy young (<30 years) and four healthy old (>60 years) subjects. For IL-15 culture experiments, CD3+CD8+CD45RO−CCR7+CD28+ T cells were FACS sorted from six healthy young (<30 years) subjects.

FACS of Human Primary Lymphocyte Subsets and Analysis of Cell Surface Markers

The following monoclonal antibodies were used: anti-CD3-e450 (OKT3), anti-CD8a-APC-e780 (OKT8) (eBioscience, Vienna, Austria), anti-CD45RO-FITC (UCHL1), anti-CCR7-PE (3D12) (BD Bioscience, Breda, Netherlands), and anti-CD28 PeCy7 (CD28.2) (Biolegend, Uithoorn, The Netherlands). Cells were sorted using a MoFlo flow cytometry cell sorter (Backman Coulter, Woerden, The Netherlands).

Expression of cell surface markers on T cells was assessed using mAbs against human CD28-PE-CY7 (CD28.2) (Biolegend), CCR7-PE (3D12), and CD45RO-FITC (UCHL1) (BD Biosciences). Cells were analyzed using a BD LSR-II Flow Cytometer and the Diva software (BD Biosciences). Data analysis was done using the Kaluza Flow Analysis Software (1.2) (Beckman Coulter).

T Cell Culture With Human Recombinant IL-15

Fluorescence-activated cell sorting-sorted CD3+CD8+CD28+CD45RO−CCR7+ (naive CD8+) T cells were suspended in RPMI medium (Lonza, Breda, The Netherlands) supplemented with 10 mg/ml gentamycin sulfate (Lonza) and 10% fetal calf serum (Thermo Scientific, Breda, The Netherlands) in a volume of 3 ml and seeded at a density of 1×10^6/ml in T25 cm flasks. A final concentration of 50 ng/ml human recombinant IL-15 (Peprotech, London, UK) was added to the cell culture at day 0 and refreshed every 5th day. On day 5, 10, and 15 of culture, cells were harvested and stained for flow cytometry analysis and/or lysed for RNA isolation. To study CD28, CD45RO, and CCR7 expression on naïve CD8+ T cells after IL-15 stimulation, CD3+CD8+CD28+CD45RO−CCR7+ T-cells were sorted as described above and stained with 10 umol/ml eF670 proliferation dye (eBioscience, Vienna, Austria). After 5, 10, and 15 days of culture in the presence of IL-15 (50 ng/ml), cells were harvested, stained, and analyzed by flow cytometer.

Culture of COS-7 Cells

COS-7 cells (African Green Monkey SV40-transformed kidney fibroblast cell line) were cultured in Dulbecco modified Eagle medium supplemented with 10% fetal bovine serum (Thermo Fisher Scientific, Breda, The Netherlands), 200 mM L-glutamine and 10 mg/ml gentamycin sulfate (Lonza, Breda, The Netherlands) at 37°C in 5% CO_2.

RNA Isolation

Total RNA was extracted using the miRNeasy Mini Kit (Qiagen, Venlo, The Netherlands) following the manufacturer's instructions. Micro Bio-SpinTM chromatography columns, supplied with Bio-Gel P-6 polyacrylamide gel matrices, were applied to maximize purity of the RNA samples (Bio-Rad laboratories). The ExperionTM RNA stdSens and HighSens analysis kits (Life Science, Bio-Rad Laboratories B.V, Veenendal, The Netherlands) were used to determine the RNA quality indicator score. The RNA concentration was measured on a NanoDrop ND-1000 Spectrophotometer (NanoDrop Technologies, Wilmington, DE, USA).

Small RNA Sequencing and Data Analysis

T cell clones with the biggest difference between low and high PDs were selected for small RNA-sequencing. Samples were barcoded and sequenced with Illumina HiSEQ 2000 flowcell (Illumina). The sequence reads were analyzed using the CLC BIO Genomic Work Bench Suite 4.5 (CLC BIO, Arhus, Denmark). Reads were mapped to the mature miRNAs using miRDeep2 (27). The number of mapped reads of each sample was normalized to 1×10^6. Normalized data were imported to GeneSpring (v.11.5.1) for analysis. A total of 252 miRNAs were present in at least 3 out of 12 samples with a read count >10. Mann–Whitney *U* test was performed to identify significantly differentially expressed miRNAs. Genesis (Release 1.7.6) was used to generate heatmaps. Raw and processed data are available *via* the Gene Expresison Omninbus, accession #GSE106619.

Quantitative RT-PCR

MicroRNA and gene expression levels were determined by qRT-PCR. cDNA synthesis for miRNAs was performed with Taqman miRNA Reverse Transcription kit using a multiplex reverse transcription approach with TaqMan microRNA Assays (Life Technologies, Carlsbad, CA, USA): for miR-9-5p (000583), miR-23a-3p (000399), miR-24-3p (000402), miR-27a-3p (000408), miR-31-5p (002279), miR-34a-5p (000426), and RNU44 (001094). RNU44 served as an endogenous control.

The qPCR reaction was performed using qPCR MasterMix Plus (Eurogentec, Liege, Belgium) and mean cycle threshold (Ct) values for all genes were quantified with the ViiA™ 7 software (Life Technologies). Relative expression levels were quantified using the $2{-}\Delta C_t$ ($\Delta C_t = C_t$ gene $- C_t$ reference gene) method.

Cloning of 3′UTR in a Luciferase Reporter Construct, Transient Transfection, and Luciferase Reporter Assays

The CD28 3′UTR was cloned into the psiCHECK2 vector (Promega, Madison, WI, USA) in two fragments, as previously described (28). CD28 3′UTR-1 (nt 870-2279 of ENST00000324106.8) was amplified from genomic DNA using primers containing an XhoI (5′) or NotI (3′) restriction site, forward: 5′-GCTCCTGC ACAGTGACTACA-3′, reverse 5′-ACCTTCTGCCTGACCACT TC-3′. CD28 3′UTR-1mut (same as above but with mutated miRNA binding sites), CD28 3′UTR-2 (nt 2534-4449), and CD28 3′UTR-2mut were ordered as minigenes (IDT, Leuven, Belgium). For both CD28 UTR-mut constructs mutations at position 2, 4, and 6 of the seed sequences were introduced at all potential miR-9-5p, -24-3p, -27-3p, and -34a-5p binding sites (based on sites indicated in **Figure 5A**). Sequences for the constructs are available on request. The inserts were sequence verified (BaseClear, Leiden, The Netherlands). COS-7 cells were transfected with 125 ng of the psiCHECK2 construct and either 50 nM hsa-miR-9-5p (PM10022), hsa-miR-24-3p (MC10737), hsa-miR-27a-3p (MC10939), hsa-miR-34a-5p (MC11030) mimics, or miRNA precursor negative control #1 (AM17110, ThermoFisher) using Saint-MIX (Synvolux products, Leiden, The Netherlands) following manufacturer's instructions. Cells were lysed 48 h after transfection and Renilla and Firefly luciferase activity was assessed using Dual-Luciferase Reporter Assay System (Promega) according to manufacturer's protocol. For each transfection, luciferase activity was measured in duplicate with the Luminoskan Ascent Microplate Luminometer (Thermo Scientific). The Renilla over Firefly (RL/FF) luciferase ratios were calculated and the RL/FF ratio of control precursor was set to one. All luciferase measurements were performed in at least three independent experiments.

Statistical Analysis

For correlation analysis between miRNA or CD28 expression and PD the Spearman test was used. Paired samples as presented in **Figures 2E,F** were analyzed using the Wilcoxon signed-rank test and for **Figures 3** and **4B,D** (Figures S3B–D,H–J in Supplementary Material) and **Figure 5** using the Friedman test with *post hoc* Dunnett's multiple comparison test. Results obtained from luciferase assay were analyzed using the paired *T*-test. Statistical analyses were performed with GraphPad Prism version 7.0 (GraphPad Software, San Diego, CA, USA).

RESULTS

PDs of T Cells Associates With Differential Expression of CD28 and miRNAs

For all 16 T cell clones, a passage at a lower number of PDs (≤40, median 29) and a passage at a high number of PDs (>40, median 56) was used (Table S1 in Supplementary Material). The Mean fluorescence intensity (MFI) of CD28 showed an inverse correlation with the number of PDs (**Figure 1**), which is in line with previous work (**Figure 1**) (14). No changes in CD28 expression were observed in the different age groups in which clones were grouped (data not shown). Small RNA sequencing was performed on the highest and lowest PD passage of 6 T cell clones. The T-cell clones used for this analysis were selected based on PD passages at the lowest and highest end of the PD spectrum.

Principal component analysis of the 252 miRNAs detected in at least 3 of 12 samples revealed a perfect separation of the

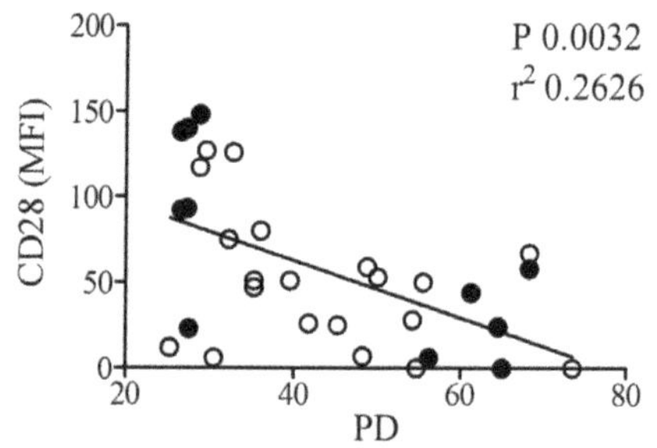

FIGURE 1 | The population doublings (PDs) of T cell clones inversely correlate with CD28 expression. CD4+ T cell clones used for small RNA sequencing (filled symbols) with high and low PD and additional T cell clones (open symbols) were fluorescence-activated cell sorting analyzed for expression of CD28. Shown is the relation between CD28 expression based on mean fluorescence intensity (MFI) and PD of the T-cell clones. For one of the clones no MFI data are available.

T cell clones in the first component based on PD (**Figure 2A**). No clustering was observed according to the age of the donor. Ten miRNAs were significantly differentially expressed between T cell clones with a low and a high number of PDs (**Figure 2B**). Five of these ten miRNAs were selected for validation based on having high expression levels and a more than 1.5-fold change in expression levels (see Table S2 in Supplementary Material). Validation was done by qRT-PCR on the 6 T cell clones that had been included for small RNA sequencing complemented with 10 additional T cell clones, also harvested at (intermediate) low and a high PD, giving a total of 32 samples (Table S1 in Supplementary Material). We observed a significant correlation for both miR-9-5p and miR-34a-5p levels with the number of PDs of the T cell clones (**Figures 2C,D**) and not for the other three miRNAs (data not shown).

Independent Validation in Primary T Cell Subsets

To further validate the association between miR-9-5p and miR-34a-5p with aged T cells and CD28 loss, we sorted CD3+ CD28+ and CD3+CD28− T cells from peripheral blood of six healthy young (<30 years) and four healthy old (>60 years) subjects. In line with the results obtained from the high and low PD T cell clones, qRT-PCR analysis revealed significantly higher levels of miR-9-5p in the CD3+CD28− T cell population as compared to the CD3+CD28+ T cells (**Figure 2E**). No significant differences were observed for miR-34a-5p (**Figure 2F**). Of note, lower relative expression levels of both miR-9-5p and miR-34a-5p were observed in the primary sorted T-cells, compared to the T-cell clones.

Upregulation of miRNAs by IL-15 in Naïve CD8+ T Cells

Regulation of CD28 expression in CD8+ T cells has been described to occur downstream of IL-15. This prompted us to investigate whether IL-15 regulated the expression levels of miR-9-5p and miR-34a-5p. We also included miR-23a-3p, miR-24-3p,

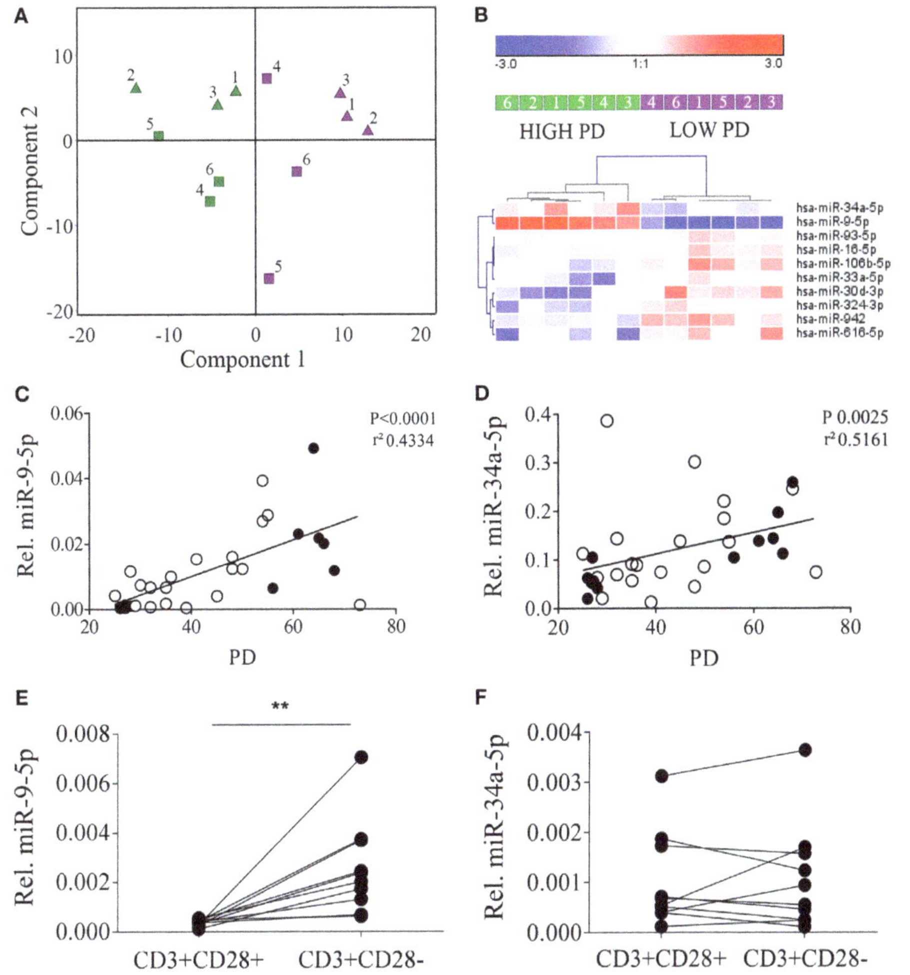

FIGURE 2 | MicroRNAs (miRNA) expression analysis in CD4+ T cell clones reveals primarily clusters according to the proliferative history of the T cell clones and partly correlates with the expression of CD28. **(A)** Principal component analysis identifies low population doublings (PDs) (purple samples) versus high PDs (green samples) as the primary identifier of biological variation for miRNA expression. Triangles indicate young and squares old donors and numbers correspond to the T cell clone numbers indicated in Table S1 in Supplementary Material. **(B)** Hierarchical clustering of the T cell clones according to low and high PDs based on the 10 most significantly differentially expressed miRNAs. Correlation between **(C)** miR-9-5p and **(D)** miR-34a-5p and the PDs of the T cell clones used in the analysis. Filled symbols denote T cell clones used in the small RNA-sequencing samples and open symbols denote additional T cell clones used to validate data from small RNA-sequencing. Significant higher expression of **(E)** miR-9-5p but not **(F)** miR-34-5p in fluorescence-activated cell sorting-sorted CD3+CD28− T cells versus CD3+CD28+ T cells. Expression levels of the miRNAs relative to the expression of RNU44 is shown. Significance (**$P \leq 0.01$) is depicted.

and miR-27a-3p all belonging to the miR-23a~24-2 cluster, in this analysis as differentially expression in CD28+ versus CD28− T cells has been previously described (20).

To this end, we first sorted naive CD8+CD28+ T cells and cultured them for 15 days in the presence of IL-15 (Figure S1 in Supplementary Material). Culturing naive CD8+CD28+ T cells in the presence of IL-15 resulted in a shift to a memory phenotype as shown by a gain of CD45RO expression and a concomitant decrease in the expression of CCR7 (**Figures 3A,B**) and CD3 (data not shown). In line with the literature (21–23), we observed a significant downregulation of CD28 expression by naive T cells in response to IL-15. The percentage of CD28+ T cells decreased to 36% after 15 days culture in the presence of IL-15 (**Figure 3C**). Next to the decrease in the percentage of CD28+ T cells, also the expression of CD28 per cell was measured by the MFI decreased significantly (**Figure 3D**).

Association Between miRNA Binding to the 3′UTR of CD28 and CD28 Expression

Next we studied whether IL-15-induced downregulation of CD28 was directly related to cell division. Analysis of sorted naïve T-cells stained with a proliferation dye revealed a progressive downregulation of CD28, both in terms of percentage positive cells and expression level, directly related to the number of cell divisions. Cells that did not divide retained CD28 expression. Similarly, cell division also correlated with acquiring a memory phenotype, as denoted by a loss of CCR7 and gain of CD45RO

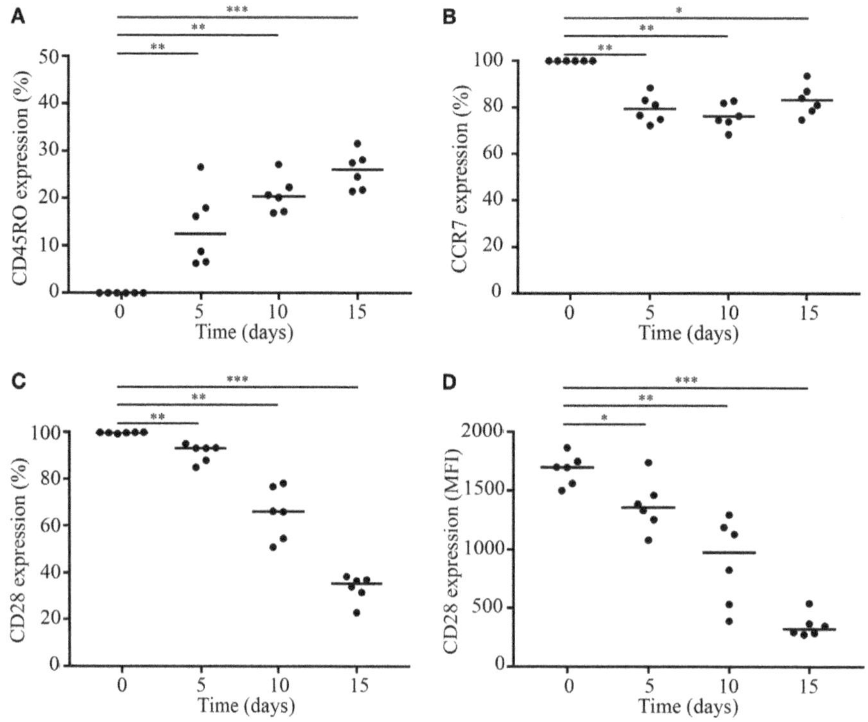

FIGURE 3 | IL-15 induces loss of CD28 by naive CD8+ T cells. Fluorescence-activated cell sorting-sorted naive CD8+CD45RO−CCR7+CD28+ T cells were cultured in the presence of IL-15 (50 ng/ml). Directly after sorting and after 5, 10, and 15 days of culture, expression of **(A)** CD45RO, **(B)** CCR7, and **(C,D)** CD28 was assessed. MFI = median fluorescence intensity. Significance (*$p < 0.05$, **$p < 0.01$, ***$p < 0.001$) is depicted. $N = 6$.

expression. These differences were most pronounced at day 15, but were also seen after 5 and 10 days stimulation with IL-15 (Figures S2 and S3 in Supplementary Material).

Expression levels of the five selected miRNAs were assessed directly after sorting cells and after 5, 10, and 15 days of culture in the presence of IL-15. Expression of miR-9-5p, miR-34a-5p, miR-23a-3p, miR-24-3p, and miR-27a-3p increased over the 15 days of culture with similar kinetics for miR-34a-3p (**Figure 4B**) and the members of the miR-23a~24-2 family (**Figures 4C–E**). MiR-9-5p levels increased already at day 5, although to a lower extend (**Figure 4A**). Absolute expression levels significantly differed between the miRNAs with miR-24-3p having the highest and miR-9-5p the lowest expression levels. As a control, we tested the expression of a randomly selected unrelated miRNA (miR-31-5p), which did not significantly change as a result of stimulation with IL-15 (**Figure 4F**).

Next, we identified putative miRNA binding sites in the 3′UTR of the CD28 mRNA. Using the Targetscan miRNA binding site prediction algorithm as well as manual searches for 6-, 7-, and 8-mer seed binding sites we identified two binding sites for miR-9-5p, miR-23a-3p, and miR-34a-5p and three binding sites for miR-24-3p and miR-27a-3p (**Figure 5A**). The presence of binding sites for these IL-15 responsive miRNAs in the 3′UTR of the CD28 transcript suggests a direct regulation. Two consecutive regions covering the 3′UTR of CD28 were cloned in a luciferase reporter construct for analysis to assess direct binding of miR-9-5p, miR-34a-5p, and the two most abundant members of the miR-23a~24-2 family (miR-24-3p and miR-27a-3p). In addition, we also generated CD28 3′UTR constructs in which the binding sites of the four miRNAs were mutated. COS-7 cells were transiently transfected with these constructs and specific miRNAs or control mimics. Luciferase assays using the wild-type (WT) CD28 3′UTR regions indicated binding of miR-9-5p, miR-24-3p, and miR-27a-3p to CD28-UTR-1 and of miR-24-3p to CD28-UTR-2 (**Figures 5A,B**). Comparison of WT to mutated constructs indicated that the relative R/F ratio of miR-27a-3p alone and in combination with miR-24-3p was reduced, albeit not significant (p-value = 0.11, p-value = 0.058, **Figure 5C**). For CD28-UTR-2 a reduced relative R/F ratio was observed for miR-24-3p and miR-34a-5p (p-value = 0.0062, p-value = 0.012, **Figure 5C**). Together these data suggest that miR-24-3p and miR-27a-3p are the most important miRNAs for direct regulation of CD28 expression.

DISCUSSION

Loss of CD28 is regarded as a hallmark of T cell aging (11, 14). To study T cell aging, various *in vitro* models have been applied, among which are T cell clones and IL-15 treatment of naive CD28+ T cells (21–24). We showed an inverse correlation between both miR-9-5p levels and miR-34a-5p, and CD28 expression in T cell clones with low and high PDs, in aged primary T cells and in IL-15 exposed naive T cells. In the latter model, we also showed IL-15 induced upregulation of the members of the miR-23a~24-2 cluster. Luciferase reporter assays showed

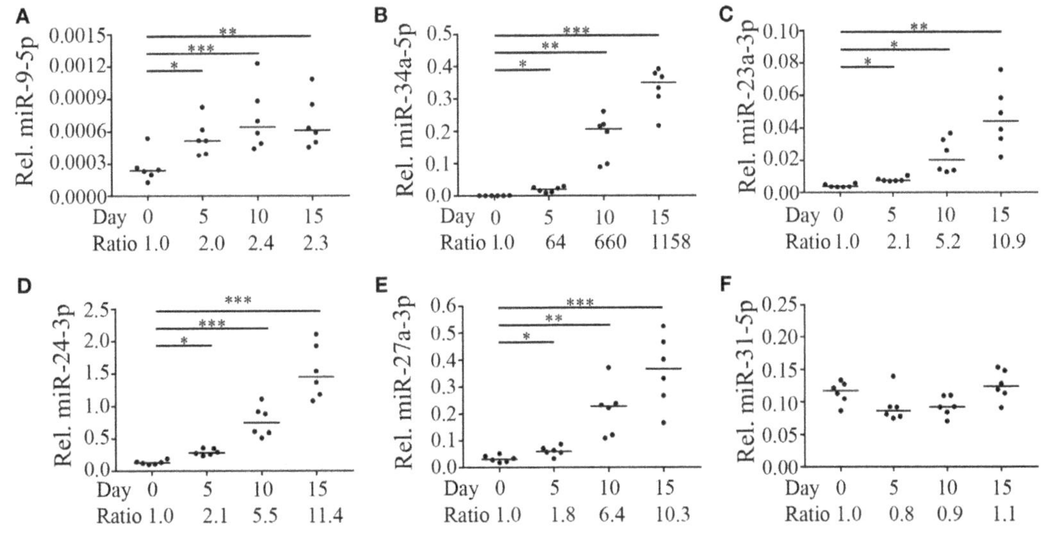

FIGURE 4 | Expression of miR-9-5p, miR-34a-5p, and miR-23a~24-2 cluster in CD8+ naive T cells is regulated by IL-15. Fluorescence-activated cell sorting-sorted naive CD8+CD45RO−CCR7+CD28+ T cells were cultured in the presence of IL-15 (50 ng/ml). Directly after sorting and after 5, 10, and 15 days of culture, expression levels of **(A)** miR-9-5p, **(B)** miR-34a-5p, **(C)** miR-23a-3p, **(D)** miR-24-3p, **(E)** miR-27a-3p (all three part of the miR-23a~24-2 cluster), and **(F)** as a non-IL-15-responsive control, miR-31-5p were assessed by RT-qPCR. Expression levels of the microRNAs (miRNAs) relative to the expression of RNU44 are shown. Significance (*$p < 0.05$, **$p < 0.01$, ***$p < 0.001$) is depicted. $N = 6$.

targeting of the 3′UTR of the CD28 transcript by miR-24 and miR-27a, indicating miRNA dependent regulation of CD28 expression upon T cell aging.

The negative correlation between the number of PDs and the expression level of CD28 in T cell clones is consistent with their previously reported senescent phenotype (13, 14). We showed a clear PD-associated difference in miRNA expression levels in T cell clones, which was independent of the age of the T cell donor. These observations are consistent with previous findings showing an overall immune-biological similarity between T cell clones from centenarian and young adults (26, 29) and confirm that centenarian-derived T cell clones are, *per se*, not functionally compromised. We identified 10 miRNAs with a significant differential expression pattern in T cell clones with low and high number of PDs and confirmed an association with the number of PDs for miR-9-5p and miR-34a-5p. For miR-9-5p, we validated higher miR-9-5p levels in primary CD28− T cells as compared to CD28+ T cells isolated from both young and old subjects.

In a second model system used in this study, we assessed the kinetics of miR-9-5p and miR-34a expression in naive CD28+ T cells in response to IL-15. IL-15 expression increases with age and maintains survival of effector CD8+ T-cells. Increased expression of IL-15 in aged individuals has been implicated in the loss of CD28 expression by T-cells (6). In line with literature findings, culture of naïve CD8+ T cells with IL-15 induced a memory phenotype and concomitant gradual downregulation of CD28 in the proliferating cell fraction. We show that IL-15 mediated downregulation of CD28 by naïve CD8+CD28+ T cells is associated with a concomitant upregulation of miR-9-5p, miR-34a-5p, and the three members of the miR-23a~24-2 cluster. This confirms the previously reported high expression of the members of the miR-23a~24-2 cluster in CD28− T cells compared to CD28+ T cells (20). It remains to be established whether IL-15 induced miRNA expression involves other cytokines besides IL-15, such as TNF-a, which has also been implicated in the regulation of CD28 expression (30, 31).

Aging-related changes in expression of cell surface receptors are not restricted to CD28. Specifically, CD3γ regulated modulation of the TcR/CD3 complex has been reported in relation to aging (32). Downregulation of CD28 expression in our study was not seen as a result of stimulation by common γ-chain interacting cytokines *per se*, as culturing T cells in the presence of IL-4 did not induce downregulation of CD28 expression (data not shown). However, implication of the epigenome in the aging immune signature of memory CD8 T cells, involving silencing of the IL-7R gene and IL-7 signaling, has been described previously (33, 34).

As a mechanism to explain IL-15 induced loss of CD28 expression, we propose involvement of miRNAs targeting of the 3′UTR of the CD28 transcript. Indeed, several potential binding sites of miR-9-5p, miR-34a-5p, and miR-23a~24-2 cluster members are present in the 3′UTR of CD28. Using a luciferase reporter assay we confirmed binding of miR-24-3p and miR-27a-3p to the 3′UTR of the CD28 transcript, thus providing evidence for their functional involvement in the regulation of CD28 expression upon induction by IL-15.

We initiated our search for aging associated miRNAs with CD4+ T-cell clones. This allowed us to analyze both high and low PD samples of the same T cell clone. Because CD28 expression is regulated more profoundly in CD8+ T cells and previous studies have been conducted specifically using CD8+ T cells, we subsequently used sorted naïve CD8+ T cells to study IL-15 stimulation induced regulation of miRNAs and CD28 expression. We confirmed differential expression for miR-9-5p and miR-34a-5p. Between the various experimental settings, we noted considerable differences

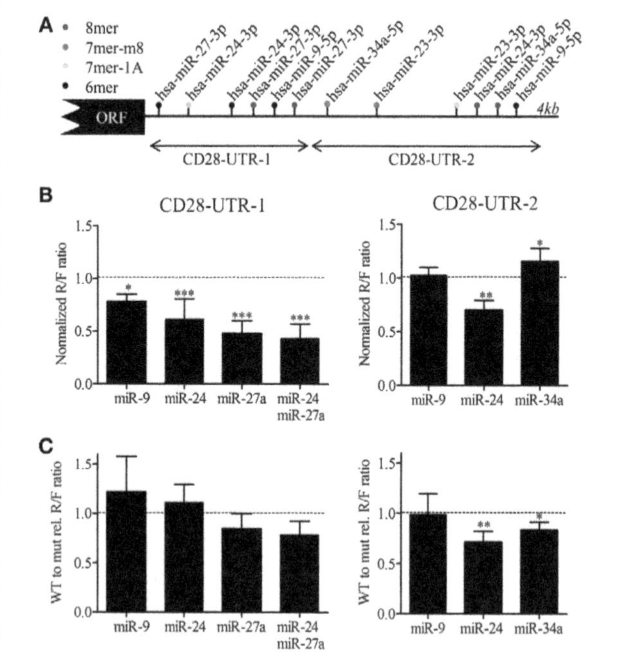

FIGURE 5 | MicroRNAs (miRNAs) binding site analysis of the CD28 3′UTR. **(A)** Schematic overview of the predicted miRNA binding sites for miR-9-5p, miR-34a-5p, and members of the miR-23a~miR-24-2 cluster in the 3′UTR of CD28 (ENST00000324106.8). Binding sites were identified using the Targetscan prediction algorithm (release 7.1) in combination with a manual search for 6mers. The arrow indicates the two regions that were cloned in the luciferase reporter constructs. 8mer: exact match to positions 2–8 of the mature miRNA followed by an A, 7mer-m8: exact match to positions 2–8 of the mature miRNA, 7mer-A1: exact match to positions 2–7 of the mature miRNA followed by an A and 6mer: exact match to positions 2–7 of the mature miRNA. **(B)** Binding analysis of miR-9-5p, miR-24-3p, and miR-27a-3p to the proximal part of the CD28 3′UTR (CD28-UTR-1, left) and of miR-9-5p, miR-24-3p, and miR-34a-5p to the distal part (CD28-UTR-2 right). Cos-7 cells were transfected with psi-Check-2 construct harboring each fragment of the 3′UTR of CD28 **(A)** in combination with control precursor, or the miRNA(s) as indicated. The Renilla (R) over Firefly (F) luciferase ratio set to one for the control precursor transfected cells is shown. **(C)** The normalized R/F ratio of the wild-type CD28 UTR region relative (rel) to the normalized R/F ratio of the same region with mutated binding sites for the tested miRNAs. Significance (*$p < 0.05$, **$p < 0.01$, ***$p < 0.001$) is depicted. Each luciferase experiment was measured in duplicate and each experiment was performed at a minimum of three independent experiments.

in the expression level of the miRNAs studied. Expression of miRNAs is cell type dependent and might, as such, explain differences observed between the various experimental settings.

We used a luciferase reporter system to verify functional binding of miR-9-5p miR-24-3p, miR-27a-3p and miR-34a-5p to the 3′UTR of CD28. Two approaches were followed, the first using WT 3′UTR constructs in combination with miRNA precursor overexpression and the second using 3′UTR constructs in which seed sequences of the miRNAs had been mutated. The combined analysis indicated that miR-24-3p and miR-27a-3p was the most effective in binding to the 3′UTR of CD28. It should be noted that results were obtained using COS-7 cells and it remains to be determined whether these results can be translated to T-cells. However, transducing T-cells directly with these constructs is not only technically complicated but also induces unpredictable activation-associated physiological changes.

The aging-related decline in CD28 expression is observed in human T cells but not in rodents. Notably, two of three miR-27a binding sites are missing in the 3′UTR of mouse CD28. On the other hand, the 3′UTR of mouse CD28 has one additional miR-24 binding site compared to the 3′UTR of human CD28. Such differences, but also other differences including higher or lower miRNA or target gene levels can explain differences in miRNA-mediated CD28 regulation between humans and rodents.

In conclusion, our results provide evidence for involvement of miRNAs in the process of replication-associated aging and IL-15-mediated regulation of CD28 expression. The data support a positive feedback loop in which IL-15 induces loss of CD28 and induction of miR-9 as well as the members of the miR-23a~24-2 cluster during T cell aging. The induced loss of CD28 and associated senescent phenotype of aged T cells may be stabilized or further enhanced by induction of the IL-15-induced miRNAs.

ETHICS STATEMENT

Informed consent was obtained from all participants in accordance with the Declaration of Helsinki. The study was approved by the Medical Ethical Committee (METC) of the University Medical Center Groningen.

AUTHOR CONTRIBUTIONS

NT and GD performed experiments, prepared the data, and were involved in writing. PH supervised experiments and revised the manuscript. MT, PJ, and DJ performed experiments. EB, GP, and KK supervised the project and revised the manuscript. GP provided the T cell clones. AvdB, JK, AB, and B-JK initiated and supervised the project and the experiments and wrote the manuscript.

ACKNOWLEDGMENTS

The authors would like to thank R. J. vd Leij, G. Mesander, J. Teunis, T. Bijma, and M. Zygmund for the outstanding technical support. The authors thank the UMCG Genomics Coordination center, the UG Center for Information Technology and their sponsors BBMRI-NL & TarGet for storage and compute infrastructure. We would like to thank the Center for Information Technology of the University of Groningen for their support and for providing access to the Peregrine high-performance computing cluster. The authors are grateful to all young and elderly volunteers for participating in the study.

FUNDING

Study was supported by unrestricted funds from the Jan Kornelis de Cock Foundation and the Groningen University Institute for Drug Exploration.

FIGURE S1 | Sorting strategy of CD8+CD45RO−CCR7+CD28+T cells.

FIGURE S2 | Loss of CD28 expression after 15 days culture with IL-15. Fluorescence-activated cell sorting-sorted naïve CD8+CD45RO−CCR7+CD28+ T cells were stained with proliferation dye to study CD28 expression after proliferation upon IL-15 stimulation (50 ng/ml). Proliferation of the naïve CD8 T cells was assessed after 15 days of culture. **(A)** Gate setting for the identification of the population doublings (PDs). Within the different PDs, **(B,E)** expression of CD28 per generation, **(C)** CD28 expression per cell per generation, **(D,F)** CD45RO, and **(F)** CCR7 expression was assessed. MFI = median fluorescence intensity. Significance ($^*p < 0.05$, $^{**}p < 0.01$) is depicted. $N = 3$.

FIGURE S3 | Loss of CD28 expression after 5 and 10 days culture with IL-15. Fluorescence-activated cell sorting-sorted naïve CD8+CD45RO−CCR7+ CD28+ T cells were stained with proliferation dye to study CD28 expression after proliferation upon IL-15 stimulation (50 ng/ml). Proliferation of the naïve CD8 T cells was assessed after **(A–F)** 5 and **(G–L)** 10 days of culture. **(A,G)** Gate setting for the identification of the population doublings (PDs). Within the different PDs **(B,E,H,K)** expression of CD28 per generation, **(C,I)** CD28 expression per cell per generation, **(D,F,J,L)** CD45RO and **(F,L)** CCR7 expression was assessed. MFI = median fluorescence intensity. Significance ($^*p < 0.05$, $^{**}p < 0.01$) is depicted. N = 3.

REFERENCES

1. Esensten JH, Helou YA, Chopra G, Weiss A, Bluestone JA. CD28 costimulation: from mechanism to therapy. *Immunity* (2016) 44(5):973–88. doi:10.1016/j.immuni.2016.04.020
2. Vallejo AN. CD28 extinction in human T cells: altered functions and the program of T-cell senescence. *Immunol Rev* (2005) 205:158–69. doi:10.1111/j.0105-2896.2005.00256.x
3. Pawelec G. Does the human immune system ever really become “senescent”? *F1000Res* (2017) 6. doi:10.12688/f1000research.11297.1
4. Kennedy RB, Ovsyannikova IG, Haralambieva IH, Oberg AL, Zimmermann MT, Grill DE, et al. Immunosenescence-related transcriptomic and immunologic changes in older individuals following influenza vaccination. *Front Immunol* (2016) 7:450. doi:10.3389/fimmu.2016.00450
5. Fulop T, Larbi A, Pawelec G. Human T cell aging and the impact of persistent viral infections. *Front Immunol* (2013) 4:271. doi:10.3389/fimmu.2013.00271
6. Pangrazzi L, Naismith E, Meryk A, Keller M, Jenewein B, Trieb K, et al. Increased IL-15 production and accumulation of highly differentiated CD8+ effector/memory T cells in the bone marrow of persons with cytomegalovirus. *Front Immunol* (2017) 8:715. doi:10.3389/fimmu.2017.00715
7. Goronzy JJ, Fang F, Cavanagh MM, Qi Q, Weyand CM. Naive T cell maintenance and function in human aging. *J Immunol* (2015) 194(9):4073–80. doi:10.4049/jimmunol.1500046
8. van der Geest KS, Abdulahad WH, Teteloshvili N, Tete SM, Peters JH, Horst G, et al. Low-affinity TCR engagement drives IL-2-dependent post-thymic maintenance of naive CD4+ T cells in aged humans. *Aging Cell* (2015) 14(5):744–53. doi:10.1111/acel.12353
9. Lopez-Otin C, Blasco MA, Partridge L, Serrano M, Kroemer G. The hallmarks of aging. *Cell* (2013) 153(6):1194–217. doi:10.1016/j.cell.2013.05.039
10. Boyd SD, Liu Y, Wang C, Martin V, Dunn-Walters DK. Human lymphocyte repertoires in ageing. *Curr Opin Immunol* (2013) 25(4):511–5. doi:10.1016/j.coi.2013.07.007
11. Sansoni P, Vescovini R, Fagnoni F, Biasini C, Zanni F, Zanlari L, et al. The immune system in extreme longevity. *Exp Gerontol* (2008) 43(2):61–5. doi:10.1016/j.exger.2007.06.008
12. Muller L, Pawelec G. As we age: does slippage of quality control in the immune system lead to collateral damage? *Ageing Res Rev* (2015) 23(Pt A):116–23. doi:10.1016/j.arr.2015.01.005
13. Pawelec G, Rehbein A, Haehnel K, Merl A, Adibzadeh M. Human T-cell clones in long-term culture as a model of immunosenescence. *Immunol Rev* (1997) 160:31–42. doi:10.1111/j.1600-065X.1997.tb01025.x
14. Adibzadeh M, Pohla H, Rehbein A, Pawelec G. Long-term culture of monoclonal human T lymphocytes: models for immunosenescence? *Mech Ageing Dev* (1995) 83(3):171–83. doi:10.1016/0047-6374(95)01625-A
15. Teteloshvili N, Smigielska-Czepiel K, Kroesen BJ, Brouwer E, Kluiver J, Boots AM, et al. T-cell activation induces dynamic changes in miRNA expression patterns in CD4 and CD8 T-cell subsets. *Microrna* (2015) 4(2):117–22. doi:10.2174/2211536604666150819194636
16. Bektas A, Schurman SH, Sen R, Ferrucci L. Human T cell immunosenescence and inflammation in aging. *J Leukoc Biol* (2017) 102(4):977–88. doi:10.1189/jlb.3RI0716-335R
17. Virts EL, Thoman ML. Age-associated changes in miRNA expression profiles in thymopoiesis. *Mech Ageing Dev* (2010) 131(11–12):743–8. doi:10.1016/j.mad.2010.09.008
18. Ohyashiki M, Ohyashiki JH, Hirota A, Kobayashi C, Ohyashiki K. Age-related decrease of miRNA-92a levels in human CD8+ T-cells correlates with a reduction of naive T lymphocytes. *Immun Ageing* (2011) 8(1):11. doi:10.1186/1742-4933-8-11
19. Hackl M, Brunner S, Fortschegger K, Schreiner C, Micutkova L, Muck C, et al. miR-17, miR-19b, miR-20a, and miR-106a are down-regulated in human aging. *Aging Cell* (2010) 9(2):291–6. doi:10.1111/j.1474-9726.2010.00549.x
20. Brunner S, Herndler-Brandstetter D, Arnold CR, Wiegers GJ, Villunger A, Hackl M, et al. Upregulation of miR-24 is associated with a decreased DNA damage response upon etoposide treatment in highly differentiated CD8(+) T cells sensitizing them to apoptotic cell death. *Aging Cell* (2012) 11(4):579–87. doi:10.1111/j.1474-9726.2012.00819.x
21. Alves NL, Hooibrink B, Arosa FA, van Lier RA. IL-15 induces antigen-independent expansion and differentiation of human naive CD8+ T cells in vitro. *Blood* (2003) 102(7):2541–6. doi:10.1182/blood-2003-01-0183
22. Borthwick NJ, Lowdell M, Salmon M, Akbar AN. Loss of CD28 expression on CD8(+) T cells is induced by IL-2 receptor gamma chain signalling cytokines and type I IFN, and increases susceptibility to activation-induced apoptosis. *Int Immunol* (2000) 12(7):1005–13. doi:10.1093/intimm/12.7.1005
23. Chiu WK, Fann M, Weng NP. Generation and growth of CD28nullCD8+ memory T cells mediated by IL-15 and its induced cytokines. *J Immunol* (2006) 177(11):7802–10. doi:10.4049/jimmunol.177.11.7802
24. Pawelec G, Kempf J, Larbi A, Barnett Y. Clonal culture models of T cell senescence. In: Fulop T, Franceschi C, Hirokawa K, Pawelec G, editors. *Handbook of Immunosenescence: Basic Understanding and Clinical Implications*. Cham: Springer International Publishing (2017). p. 1–15.
25. Pawelec G, Barnett Y. Ageing and senescence in immune cells in vitro and in vivo. In: Rattan SIS, Hayflick L, editors. *Cellular Ageing and Replicative Senescence*. Cham: Springer International Publishing (2016). p. 85–95.
26. Pawelec G, Barnett Y, Mariani E, Solana R. Human CD4+ T cell clone longevity in tissue culture: lack of influence of donor age or cell origin. *Exp Gerontol* (2002) 37(2–3):265–9. doi:10.1016/S0531-5565(01)00192-9
27. Friedlander MR, Mackowiak SD, Li N, Chen W, Rajewsky N. miRDeep2 accurately identifies known and hundreds of novel microRNA genes in seven animal clades. *Nucleic Acids Res* (2012) 40(1):37–52. doi:10.1093/nar/gkr688
28. Gibcus JH, Tan LP, Harms G, Schakel RN, de Jong D, Blokzijl T, et al. Hodgkin lymphoma cell lines are characterized by a specific miRNA expression profile. *Neoplasia* (2009) 11(2):167–76. doi:10.1593/neo.08980
29. Mazzatti DJ, Pawelec G, Longdin R, Powell JR, Forsey RJ. SELDI-TOF-MS ProteinChip array profiling of T-cell clones propagated in long-term culture identifies human profilin-1 as a potential bio-marker of immunosenescence. *Proteome Sci* (2007) 5:7. doi:10.1186/1477-5956-5-7
30. Qian JX, Lee SM, Suen Y, Knoppel E, van de Ven C, Cairo MS. Decreased interleukin-15 from activated cord versus adult peripheral blood mononuclear cells and the effect of interleukin-15 in upregulating antitumor immune activity and cytokine production in cord blood. *Blood* (1997) 90(8):3106–17.

31. Bryl E, Vallejo AN, Weyand CM, Goronzy JJ. Down-regulation of CD28 expression by TNF-alpha. *J Immunol* (2001) 167(6):3231–8. doi:10.4049/jimmunol.167.6.3231
32. Boding L, Bonefeld CM, Nielsen BL, Lauritsen JP, von Essen MR, Hansen AK, et al. TCR down-regulation controls T cell homeostasis. *J Immunol* (2009) 183(8):4994–5005. doi:10.4049/jimmunol.0901539
33. Moskowitz DM, Zhang DW, Hu B, Le Saux S, Yanes RE, Ye Z, et al. Epigenomics of human CD8 T cell differentiation and aging. *Sci Immunol* (2017) 2(8):eaag0192. doi:10.1126/sciimmunol.aag0192
34. Ucar D, Marquez EJ, Chung CH, Marches R, Rossi RJ, Uyar A, et al. The chromatin accessibility signature of human immune aging stems from CD8(+) T cells. *J Exp Med* (2017) 214(10):3123–44. doi:10.1084/jem.20170416

Debunking the Myth of Exercise-Induced Immune Suppression: Redefining the Impact of Exercise on Immunological Health Across the Lifespan

John P. Campbell and James E. Turner**

Department for Health, University of Bath, Bath, United Kingdom

***Correspondence:**
John P. Campbell
j.campbell@bath.ac.uk;
James E. Turner
j.e.turner@bath.ac.uk

Epidemiological evidence indicates that regular physical activity and/or frequent structured exercise reduces the incidence of many chronic diseases in older age, including communicable diseases such as viral and bacterial infections, as well as non-communicable diseases such as cancer and chronic inflammatory disorders. Despite the apparent health benefits achieved by leading an active lifestyle, which imply that regular physical activity and frequent exercise enhance immune competency and regulation, the effect of a single bout of exercise on immune function remains a controversial topic. Indeed, to this day, it is perceived by many that a vigorous bout of exercise can temporarily suppress immune function. In the first part of this review, we deconstruct the key pillars which lay the foundation to this theory—referred to as the "open window" hypothesis—and highlight that: (i) limited reliable evidence exists to support the claim that vigorous exercise heightens risk of opportunistic infections; (ii) purported changes to mucosal immunity, namely salivary IgA levels, after exercise do not signpost a period of immune suppression; and (iii) the dramatic reductions to lymphocyte numbers and function 1–2 h after exercise reflects a transient and time-dependent redistribution of immune cells to peripheral tissues, resulting in a heightened state of immune surveillance and immune regulation, as opposed to immune suppression. In the second part of this review, we provide evidence that frequent exercise enhances—rather than suppresses—immune competency, and highlight key findings from human vaccination studies which show heightened responses to bacterial and viral antigens following bouts of exercise. Finally, in the third part of this review, we highlight that regular physical activity and frequent exercise might limit or delay aging of the immune system, providing further evidence that exercise is beneficial for immunological health. In summary, the over-arching aim of this review is to rebalance opinion over the perceived relationships between exercise and immune function. We emphasize that it is a misconception to label any form of acute exercise as immunosuppressive, and, instead, exercise most likely improves immune competency across the lifespan.

Keywords: exercise, physical activity, upper respiratory tract infections, open window hypothesis, infection susceptibility, ageing, immunosenescence, immune competency

INTRODUCTION

Lifelong physical activity[1] is a potent means of reducing the risk of non-communicable diseases including cancer, cardiovascular disease, and other chronic inflammatory disorders (1). Evidence also shows that a physically active lifestyle diminishes the risk of contracting a range of communicable diseases including viral and bacterial infections (2–6). In contrast to the widely accepted long-term health benefits that are achieved by regular physical activity, which imply that immune competency and regulation are improved by frequent exercise bouts, the effect of a single bout of exercise on immune function remains hotly disputed. Undeniably, acute vigorous exercise has a profound effect on the phenotypic makeup and functional capacity of the immune system. Indeed, the behavior of almost all immune cell populations in the bloodstream is altered in some way during and after exercise (7, 8). However, for decades, it has been widely accepted that these changes result in a temporary decline in immune competency in the hours following exercise. In the first part of this review, we re-interpret these data and strive to dispel the misconception that an acute bout of exercise is detrimental to immunological health. In the second part of this article, we demonstrate that rather than suppressing immunity, contemporary evidence shows that an acute bout of exercise improves immune surveillance, for example leading to enhanced antibacterial and antiviral immunity. Finally, in the third part of this article, we summarize recent data suggesting that regular physical activity and frequent exercise, which reduces systemic inflammatory activity and improves aspects of immune function, also leads to alterations in classical biomarkers of an aging immune system. These changes could be interpreted as limiting or delaying immunological aging (9–13).

PART A: IS IT TIME TO CLOSE THE SHUTTERS ON THE "OPEN-WINDOW" HYPOTHESIS? A BOUT OF EXERCISE DOES NOT SUPPRESS IMMUNE COMPETENCY

A prevailing myth has formed in the literature that participating in an acute bout of aerobic exercise, particularly if it is vigorous and prolonged, can be detrimental to immune competency. The foundations of this belief lay in research publications emanating from the 1980s and 1990s, reviewed extensively elsewhere (7, 8, 14). Findings from these early studies led to three principles of exercise immunology being formed, which have, until now, generally been unchallenged in the literature: (i) infection risk is increased after an acute bout of prolonged and vigorous aerobic exercise; (ii) acute bouts of vigorous exercise can lead to a temporary reduction to salivary IgA levels culminating in a higher risk of opportunistic infections; and (iii) transient decreases in the number of peripheral blood immune cells, which occurs in the hours following vigorous exercise, represents a period of immune suppression. Over the years, these collective observations have coalesced and led to the creation of the so-called "open-window" hypothesis, which purports that the immune system is compromised in the hours after vigorous exercise, leading to an increased risk of opportunistic infections in the days thereafter. To this day, the "open window" hypothesis continues to be discussed (15), despite the existence of contradictory evidence. Here, in the first part of this review, we aim to dispel the "open-window" hypothesis by revisiting key research studies and highlighting that limited evidence exists to support each of the three pillars that lay its foundation.

Exercise and Opportunistic Infections

It has been speculated for over a century that participation in physical activity heightens the risk of opportunistic infections (16). However, deeper investigation into the relationship between exercise and infection susceptibility did not take place until the end of the twentieth century. At this juncture, the principle focus of many of these studies in the late 1980s and early 1990s was to determine whether infection incidence was increased in elite and recreational athletes in the weeks following mass participation distance running events. One of the first studies from this era found that one third of 150 runners participating in the 1982 Two Oceans 56 km ultramarathon in Cape Town South Africa self-reported symptoms of upper respiratory tract infections (URTIs; symptoms = runny nose, sore throat, sneezing) within 2 weeks of the race (17). The control group, who were age matched and shared a home with another of the race competitors, reported only half the amount of URTIs in the same period (17). Similar observations were made in an often-cited larger study of the 1987 Los Angeles Marathon (18). Of 2,311 respondents who had completed the marathon and whom did not report an infection in the week prior to the race, 12.9% reported an infection in the week after the race compared to only 2.2% of individuals who withdrew from the race for reasons other than illness (odds ratio of infection in runners versus non-runners = 5.9). A separate study conducted around the same time found that shorter duration running events, such as 5, 10 km, and half-marathons (21 km) did not appear to elicit an increased incidence of self-reported URTIs (19), thereby suggesting that URTI symptoms are increased only when the duration of the exercise is long.

A fundamental limitation of each of the aforementioned studies is that none of the self-reported infections were clinically confirmed by laboratory analyses (e.g., molecular or microbiological techniques, such as polymerase chain reaction or bacterial cultures). As a consequence, it was questioned whether the

[1] "Physical activity" refers to activities undertaken during leisure time, at home, as part of employment, or for transport purposes. "Exercise" is a component of physical activity within the leisure time domain and refers to physical activities that are planned, structured, repetitive, and undertaken for the purpose of improving or maintaining components of physical fitness and/or sporting performance. When individuals are referred to as being "active" or "inactive," the description infers that these people undertake (or fail to undertake) a defined level of exercise or physical activity (e.g., age-specific physical activity recommendations, such as those published by the World Health Organisation). In this review, the term "exercise" will generally be used to describe the effects that active behaviours have on immune competency. Individuals described as being "sedentary" accumulate prolonged periods of behaviour eliciting low energy expenditure (e.g. sitting and lying).

self-reported URTIs in these studies represented genuine infections. Clarifying this issue, a study employing nasopharyngeal and throat swabs in athletes who reported URTI symptoms over a 5-month period—including periods of competition—found that few of the self-reported infections were of bacterial, viral, chlamydial, or mycoplasmal nature (20). Indeed, of 37 episodes of URTI reported by athletes in this study, only 11 of these (30%) had a positive laboratory diagnosis. These findings place the previously discussed marathon studies in a different light (17, 18) and open the possibility that many of the URTIs reported were a symptom of other non-infectious causes. Indeed, of the of the non-infectious "URTIs" reported by Spence et al. (20), and likely captured elsewhere (17, 18), it is proposed that these symptoms are a result of other causes, including allergy and asthma, non-specific mucosal inflammation, or airway epithelial cell trauma due to increased ventilation or exposure to cold air (21). In the few cases of clinically confirmed URTIs, these appear to be from viruses—in particular rhinoviruses (i.e., the "common cold")—rather than bacterial infection (20, 22), which is in line with the typical incidence and etiology of infections at the population level (23).

In the previously discussed clinical laboratory study of infection incidence in athletes (20), it is notable that the proportion of athletes with a confirmed infection during the 5-month period was as follows: 2/20 controls (10%), 3/31 (10%) recreational athletes, and 6/32 (19%) elite athletes. Although this study was small, these data appear to align with observations from earlier self-report studies which found that the incidence of URTI symptoms was higher in those with the fastest race time and those who had completed a greater training volume pre-race (17, 18). These early observations contributed to the formulation of the "J-shaped curve" (24). This hypothesis infers that those who undertake an excessive volume of exercise, over a period of weeks and months, sometimes referred to as "over-training" or "intensified training" (25, 26), are at a greater risk of infections (24). In this scenario, other factors present *prior* to an acute bout of exercise, such as psychological stress and anxiety (27–29), or nutritional deficiencies (30) which are known to impact immune regulation, are likely to impact immune competency and contribute to the risk of genuine URTIs, rather than the acute and transient immune changes that arise *after* the acute bout of exercise itself; these acute immunological changes arising after acute exercise are discussed later in this article (see Part A: "Is it Time to Close the Shutters on the "Open-Window" Hypothesis? A Bout of Exercise Does Not Suppress Immune Competency"; and see "Exercise and Salivary IgA and Changes to Lymphocyte Frequency and Functional Capacity in the Hours After Acute Exercise").

Moreover, we contend that attendance at any mass participation event—whether it is a marathon or otherwise—is likely to increase the risk of acquiring novel infectious pathogens, which are in abundance due to the mass gathering of people. For example, it has been shown that around 40% of individuals attending the Hajj—a crowded religious event in Saudi Arabia—self-report an URTI (31). In this study, there was a greater risk of infection among those with the longest exposure to crowds (31). Thus, it is important to consider that other underlying factors, often not measured in the context of exercise and illness studies, likely play a greater role in infection risk than exercise participation *per se*. For example, recently, it has been demonstrated that air travel is a significant predictor of illness symptoms in athletes (32). Infections linked to air travel are exacerbated by long-haul flights crossing multiple time zones, implicating many other factors known to influence immune function, including exposure to hypobaric hypoxia, radiation, temperature changes, sleep disruption, fatigue, altered or inadequate diet, dehydration, and psychological stress (32–34).

Contrary to the aforementioned reports that exercise heightens infection incidence, it is often overlooked that other studies indicate that exercise participation may in fact *reduce* the incidence of infections. For example, a recent prospective cohort study of 1,509 Swedish men and women aged 20–60 years found that higher physical activity levels were associated with a lower incidence of self-reported URTIs (35). A much smaller but very detailed analysis of illness records kept by 11 elite endurance athletes over a period of 3–16 years showed that the total number of training hours per year was inversely correlated with sickness days reported (36). Similarly, another study of swimmers monitored for 4 years found that national level athletes had higher incidence of infections than more elite international level athletes (37). Finally, studies of ultramarathon runners, who undertake the largest volume of exercise among athletes, have shown that these individuals report fewer days missed from school or work due to illness compared to the general population. For example, the mean number of sickness days reported over 12 months was 1.5 days in a study of 1,212 ultramarathon runners and 2.8 days in a study of 489 ultramarathon runners (38, 39). These studies compared their findings to data from the United States Department of Health and Human Services report in 2009, showing that the general population report on average 4.4 illness days each year. Thus, a number of studies challenge the "J-shaped curve," indicating that athletes undertaking the largest training loads, become ill less frequently than athletes competing at, and training at, a lower level. These findings have previously been conceptualized by extending the "J-shaped curve" into an "S-shaped curve," thereby suggesting that very elite athletes are better adapted to the demands of their training (40). Given the nature of their design, very few of these reports—akin to many of the aforementioned studies showing increased infection risk among athletes following mass participation endurance events—used appropriate laboratory diagnostics to confirm an infection. However, despite their limitations, it is important to highlight that there are as many epidemiological studies showing that regular exercise *reduces* infections as there are studies showing exercise *increases* infections, and that these studies are often overlooked in the exercise immunology literature.

It should also be considered whether the commonly reported "increased frequency" of illness symptoms among athletic populations or those taking part in sporting events is indeed more frequent than among the general population. For example, large studies have reported that approximately 7–10% of athletes competing in the Olympic Games report symptoms of illness during the competition weeks (41, 42). However, accumulating evidence suggests the incidence of infection among athletes is not substantially different to other populations. For example, in a telephone survey of 2011 adults considered to represent the general population in the USA, 24% experienced a cold during a 4-week period, which is a similar timeframe to many international sporting competitions (43). In another telephone survey of 4,051 adults in the USA, 72% experienced at least 1 non-influenza related URTI over 12 months, and on average, experienced 2 infections annually (44). In a year-long Internet-based monitoring study of 627 individuals over 14 years of age in Germany, weekly acute respiratory illness rates were 2.7–8.2%, manifesting in 1.3–3.2 episodes annually (45). Thus, evidence suggests that the frequency of illness episodes in athletic communities is similar to the general population annually.

In the context of exercise participation in older age, it would appear to be counterintuitive that the incidence of URTI symptoms appears to be inversely correlated with age: it has been shown that URTI symptoms are more common in younger rather than older runners (18). While, once more, this aforementioned study did not confirm infections by laboratory analyses, it is notable that if acute exercise does suppress immune competency, it might be expected that older adults—whom typically have inferior immune function—would be at greatest risk of exercise-induced immune suppression. Rather than exercise *per se,* again, a more likely explanation for differences in illness symptoms between groups of athletes are other factors present before competing, such as fatigue, nutritional deficiency, psychological stress, or environmental exposures. On the other hand, proponents of the "open-window" hypothesis could portend that experienced athletes have higher tolerance of the symptoms associated with URTI, and/or have developed coping methods or strategies to reduce symptoms. Alternatively, experienced athletes may have evolved strategies to reduce infection risk by adopting good practice (e.g., sleep, diet, hygiene) before, during and following attendance at a mass participation event.

Separately, it has also been questioned whether illness symptoms—even if confirmed to be infectious—are a result of encountering a novel pathogen. For example, over a decade ago, some studies suggested that reactivation of latent viruses—such as *Epstein Barr Virus* which had most likely infected the host during childhood—was responsible for illness symptoms after exercise (46, 47). Although these studies suggest new pathogens were not to blame, it was interpreted that exercise-induced immune suppression had resulted in loss of viral control. However, herpes viruses can reactivate even with a fully functioning immune system, for example, in response to adrenergic activity, reactive oxygen species and inflammatory cytokines (48–50), all of which increase during exercise. Moreover, recent evidence appears to discount herpes virus involvement in causing symptoms of illness, by showing that individuals previously infected with *Cytomegalovirus*, or those infected with both *Epstein Barr Virus* and *Cytomegalovirus*, exhibited a lower incidence of illness symptoms than individuals not latently infected (51).

Taken together, evidence that participation in an acute bout of vigorous exercise leads to heightened infection incidence remains spurious. If symptoms of URTI are observed after a bout of vigorous exercise, the cause is unlikely to be infectious. However, if infection or immune impairment is confirmed, their trigger is more likely to be the physical, nutritional, and psychological wellbeing of the individual prior to undertaking the single bout of acute vigorous exercise. In the context of mass participation sporting events, it is likely that increased exposure to pathogens, or the influence of environmental factors that can affect immune function (e.g., travel, sleep disruption) most likely explain genuine infections. Thus, we conclude that it is unlikely that vigorous and prolonged exercise heighten the risk of infections and should not be considered a deterrent to those seeking to become more physically active.

Exercise and Salivary IgA

A second mainstay of exercise immunology that has received considerable attention over the last three decades is the assessment of exercise-induced changes to mucosal immunity, principally *via* measurement of IgA levels in saliva (52). Given that IgA is the most abundant immunoglobulin in mucosal secretions and that its principle role is the inhibition of invading pathogens, isolated changes to salivary IgA following exercise has been considered of some importance in light of the purportedly higher risk of infections among athletes (7, 8).

One of the earliest and most cited papers in this research area found that IgA was reduced by 20% after 2–3 h of cross-country skiing (53). Another study found that this effect is transient, whereby salivary IgA concentrations decreased immediately after 2 h of intensive cycling exercise, and remained low in samples collected 1 h post-exercise, but returned to normal levels within 24 h (54). A criticism of these studies at that time was that the absolute IgA levels reported did not adequately control for the amount of saliva produced, and thus these results may misrepresent IgA secretion. Although some studies measuring IgA secretory rate (IgA protein concentration multiplied by saliva flow rate) support the early findings with IgA concentration, others have shown profoundly contradictory results. For example, in alignment with prior observations, it was found in trained runners that IgA secretion rate decreased by 25% from pre-marathon to 90 min post-marathon (55). Likewise, in a separate study, a 20% reduction in IgA secretion rate was observed in elite athletes after a 2-h rowing exercise session (56). Several other studies of similar design reported analogous findings (57–59); however, contradictory findings are also in abundance but are much less cited in the literature. Indeed, an elegant study exploring the effects of different exercise intensities, including moderate- and high-intensity exercise to exhaustion, found that although saliva flow rate decreased, IgA secretion rate actually increased in response to both of the exercise bouts. In the words of the authors, exercise to exhaustion has an "*effect on the quantity of saliva, but not the quality of saliva*" (60). Many other studies have also reported that exercise does not elicit a decrease in IgA secretion rates following exercise (61–66).

Any subtle isolated changes to IgA that occur after exercise appear to be clinically insignificant as it would appear that the increased incidence of URTI symptoms that has been purported following vigorous and prolonged exercise is unrelated to salivary immunoglobulin status. A longitudinal field study of participants in the Comrades Marathon (86.5 km ultramarathon) in South

Africa found that salivary IgA levels in the 4 weeks prior to the race, and 2 weeks following the race, were unrelated to the incidence of self-reported URTI (67). In the aforementioned study, it was found that symptoms of URTI were highest 4 weeks prior to the marathon, and URTI symptoms seemed to re-appear within many of the same athletes 1 or 2 weeks post-marathon. This study did not confirm the re-emergence of infections by laboratory testing, but if this was indeed demonstrated in future studies, it again shows that acute exercise participation *per se* does not heighten risk of opportunistic infections. In this case, an underlying infection, not resolved prior to exercise participation, or some other idiosyncrasy, is perhaps to blame. Such conclusions appear to be supported by evidence from athletes who report the most frequent illness symptoms. For example, these individuals exhibit mostly anti-inflammatory cytokine responses when whole blood, collected at rest, is cultured *ex vivo* with antigens from diphtheria, tetanus, acellular pertussis, poliomyelitis, and hemophilus influenza type b (68, 69). These findings suggest the immune system may be functionally altered by underlying illness, or is already different in these "illness-prone" athletes prior to infection, rather than exercise affecting immune function *per se*.

A flaw in studies investigating the link between mucosal immunity and purported exercise-induced infection risk is that oral health status is rarely adequately evaluated. Salivary IgA is heavily involved in host-bacterial ecology and mucosal homeostasis (70, 71). As optimal oral health is rare in adults—with nearly all exhibiting caries, gingivitis or periodontitis—profound between-person IgA variation has been reported, which is dependent on oral health status (71). Moreover, periodontal diseases are complex and multifactorial, and as a result, studies report large fluctuations in IgA levels relative to disease status between persons, probably due to the bespoke ecological makeup of different host mucosa (71). In addition, oral disease is a common problem in athlete populations (72), which is likely to be caused by high volume and frequent carbohydrate consumption, and in some, a neglect of oral hygiene, perhaps due to practical constraints. Thus, changes to oral inflammatory status has not been adequately considered, and emerging salivary biomarkers of oral inflammation, such as immunoglobulin-free light chains (73), may offer a means of controlling for this confounder. As highlighted elsewhere (70), salivary IgA is also highly vulnerable to short-term variation, in particular, due to circadian rhythms, typically peaking in the morning, and falling thereafter (74). As salivary IgA secretion is controlled by the parasympathetic and sympathetic nervous system, psychological stress also plays a powerful role in regulating IgA levels (75). Animal models suggest that salivary IgA levels could vary up to 27-fold within the same host over a short period of time (76). Salivary IgA levels are also affected by factors such as sex differences (77), diet, ethnicity, disease, medications, tobacco, and phase of the menstrual cycle, as reviewed elsewhere (71). To overcome some of these variations in salivary IgA, it is often the case that studies evaluate only secretory IgA (sIgA; i.e., IgA containing the secretory component) as this represents IgA produced by local mucosal plasma cells, and not IgA from the bloodstream transported *via* crevicular fluid. While this approach may reduce some confounding error, most IgA in saliva contains the secretory component and is, itself, subject to large variation; extensively reviewed elsewhere (78). Given these many considerations, we propose that longitudinal measurement of salivary IgA, as an isolated measure of immune competency within a single host, and even more so between persons, depicts too confusing a picture, and it is ambitious to say that any subtle changes to salivary IgA following exercise reflects immune suppression and a heightened risk of opportunistic infections. Given the limitations of salivary IgA measurement, research is being undertaken to explore mucosal IgA in other biofluids, and a recent study has shown links between reduced tear IgA levels and infection incidence (79). Others have moved toward more comprehensive oral immunity panels (80), and such strategies could benefit further from an integrative approach that, in addition to immune parameters, incorporates full dental examination, oral inflammation biomarkers, and host mucosal ecology.

Changes to Lymphocyte Frequency and Functional Capacity in the Hours After Acute Exercise

One of the most reproduced findings in human exercise physiology is the profound and transient time-dependent change that arises to the phenotypic composition and functional capacity of lymphocytes in the peripheral bloodstream in response to a single bout of exercise (8). During vigorous aerobic exercise, it is commonly observed that peripheral blood lymphocyte frequency—and, concomitantly, the functional capacity of the lymphocyte pool—is dramatically increased, leading to the concept that, during exercise, exercise appears to "stimulate" the immune system. On the other hand, in the hours following exercise, it is typically observed that total peripheral blood lymphocyte frequency—and the functional capacity of the lymphocyte pool—is decreased below pre-exercise levels, leading some to propose that exercise induces a short-term window of immune suppression (termed the "open-window" hypothesis). The purpose of this part of our review is to outline that it is a misconception to state that the "reductions" to lymphocyte frequency and function, that arise in the hours following acute exercise, reflects immune suppression, and instead we emphasize that during this post-exercise period, the immune system is in a heightened state of immune surveillance and regulation.

Transient Changes to Blood Lymphocyte Frequency in the Hours Following Exercise

The classic biphasic response of lymphocytes to acute steady state vigorous exercise lasting for around at least 45–60 minutes, is first characterized by a dramatic lymphocytosis. This response is typified by a dramatic influx of natural killer cells, which rise by up to 10-fold, and $CD8^+$ T cells which increase to a lesser—but still profound—extent by approximately 2.5-fold (81). This exercise intensity-dependent mobilization is driven in part by increased shear forces and blood pressure during exercise causing a non-specific flushing of the marginal pools (82) but, moreover, is principally governed by adrenergic stimulation of beta-2-adrenergic receptors on the surface of lymphocytes, arising from adrenaline released during exercise, causing endothelial detachment and subsequent recirculation of lymphocytes into the bloodstream (83–85). Indeed, the lymphocyte mobilization response observed during exercise appears to broadly mirror the differential expression of beta-2 adrenergic receptors on lymphocytes: natural killer cells > CD8+ T cells > B cells > CD4+ T cells, including regulatory T cells (81, 86–88). Upon exercise cessation, the classic biphasic exercise response is next characterized by a dramatic decrease in the frequency of lymphocytes in the bloodstream. This nadir is typically observed approximately 1–2 h post-exercise when the lymphocyte numerical count is lower than pre-exercise levels; lymphocyte frequency normally returns to pre-exercise levels within 24 h (87, 89, 90). The lymphopenia that occurs 1–2 h later is exercise intensity dependent and the most profound reductions during this period are typically observed among natural killer cells and CD8+ T cells (90). Akin to purported reductions to salivary IgA, discussed earlier, it was perceived that the numerical decline of blood lymphocytes that arises during this time represented "double jeopardy" (89), temporarily exposing an individual to impaired immune competency and concomitantly providing an "open-window" for opportunistic infections (91, 92).

Rather than suppressing immune competency however, a more contemporary viewpoint is that this acute and transient lymphopenia 1–2 h after exercise is beneficial to immune surveillance and regulation. Indeed, in what appears to be a highly specialized and systematic response, it is widely proposed that exercise redeploys immune cells to peripheral tissues (e.g., mucosal surfaces) to conduct immune surveillance. Here, these immune cells are thought to identify and eradicate other cells infected with pathogens, or those that have become damaged or malignant, termed the acute stress/exercise immune-enhancement hypothesis (93). A seminal study by Kruger and colleagues, using fluorescent cell tracking in rodents, found that T cells are redeployed in large numbers to peripheral tissues including the gut and lungs, and to the bone marrow following exercise (84, 94). In line with Dhabhar's theory, it is hypothesized that this redistribution reflects heightened immune surveillance in sites where pathogens are likely to be encountered during and after exercise (i.e., lungs, gut). This response has also been proposed to maintain immune homeostasis *via* augmented regulatory activities (12). In this context, evidence implies that bone marrow homing and subsequent apoptosis of senescent T cells stimulates the production or mobilization of new progenitor cells into the periphery (95), which has been hypothesized as an exercise-induced means of maintaining a younger immune system (12), discussed later in Part C "Does Exercise and Regular Physical Activity Influence Immunological Ageing." Links between exercise-induced apoptosis and lymphopenia have in the past been interpreted as detrimental, with speculation that apoptosis could be responsible for the fall in lymphocyte number in the hours after exercise (96, 97). Other studies have reported increased lymphocyte apoptosis immediately after exercise (i.e., as a result of the large mobilization of cells) but not in the hours following exercise during lymphopenia (98–100). Although the magnitude of lymphocyte apoptosis reported in studies is dependent on the measurement technique, typically <10% of lymphocytes undergo post-exercise apoptosis (96, 97). Given the 30–60% decrease in lymphocyte numbers post-exercise (89, 101, 102), apoptosis could be a small contributor to exercise-induced lymphopenia, but this process of cell death is likely to be beneficial given the stimulation of progenitor cells from the bone marrow (95).

While it has not been shown in humans that exercise—in line with rodent models—causes the redistribution of immune cells to peripheral tissues, further support for a coordinated, exercise-induced immune surveillance response elicited by lymphopenia, is revealed by studying the phenotypic characteristics of the cells that preferentially mobilize and subsequently extravasate out of the circulation after exercise. With regard to natural killer cells—the most exercise-responsive lymphocyte subset—CD56^{dim} cells are preferentially redeployed rather than their CD56^{bright} counterparts (81). CD56^{dim} cells are a mature subset of natural killer cells which have exclusive migratory potential for non-lymphoid tissue and potent effector capabilities, including the capacity to produce high amounts of perforin and granzyme, whereas CD56^{bright} cells are a more immature regulatory cell subset (103) and reside in secondary lymphoid organs, typified by their cell-surface expression of CD62L and CCR7 (104). CD56^{dim} natural killer cells can be further dissected, into cells with highly potent effector function based on loss of NKG2A and expression of killer immunoglobulin-like receptors and CD57 (105, 106). In a recent study, it was shown that these natural killer cells, which are capable of rapid effector functions, are preferentially redistributed after exercise (107, 108). Synergistically, T cells also appear to exert heterogeneous but highly coordinated responses to acute exercise. Indeed, it is consistently observed that discrete populations of CD8+ but not CD4+ T cell subsets are redeployed by exercise. For some time, there was confusion pertaining to the exact behavior of CD8+ T cells in response to exercise. Rather than losing or gaining markers of adhesion or activation—as evaluated elsewhere (8)—these changes represent a uniform redeployment of a preferentially mobilized group of memory cells. In a flurry of studies about a decade ago, it was shown that exercise selectively mobilizes memory CD8+ T cells with a phenotypic propensity for homing to peripheral tissues—typified for example by CD11, and not CCR7 or CD62L expression—and the distinctive capacity to mount rapid effector functions (81, 109–111). This response presumably facilitates the detection and elimination of neoplastic, stressed or infected cells in synergy with natural killer cells, as proposed elsewhere (112). Aligned with the immune surveillance theory of Burnet and Thomas, reviewed elsewhere (113), these results imply that sentinel cells of the immune system are redeployed by exercise-induced perturbations to stress hormones, to exert effector functions against neoplastic, stressed, or infected cells in the hours following exercise. This process, which occurs daily in a natural diurnal process (114), orchestrated subtly by stress hormones (115, 116), appears to be primed in response to exercise, leading to enhanced immune surveillance (117). Principles of the acute stress/exercise immune-enhancement hypothesis continue to be investigated. For example, it has recently been shown that acute exercise does not preferentially mobilize CD8+ T cells and natural killer cells with the capacity for skin-homing (118). However, skin-homing in this context is a role that may be fulfilled by exercise-responsive mucosal-associated invariant T cells (119); but further work is needed in this area.

A key example illustrating how exercise-induced immune cell redistribution is beneficial to host health can be found in the rapidly emerging field of exercise oncology. Indeed, a recent seminal study demonstrated inhibition of tumor onset and disease progression across a range of tumor models in voluntarily active rodents (112). In this work, natural killer cell infiltration was significantly increased in tumors from active versus inactive rodents, leading to the conclusion that the presence of natural killer cells (but perhaps also T cells) in tumor sites, redeployed by adrenaline during exercise stress, "provides a spark" for tumor elimination, in what could be considered a form of "exercise immunotherapy" (112, 120). Importantly, administration of propranolol—a beta 2 adrenergic blocker—abolished the adrenaline-induced redistribution of immune cells, and nullified the anti-tumor effect of exercise on neoplastic growth (112). While these studies are limited to rodents, there is growing evidence that exercise may promote anti-cancer effects in humans. For example, in a key study recently conducted in humans, it was shown that natural killer cells with a highly mature effector phenotype are preferentially redistributed after exercise, and have the capacity to exert augmented cytotoxicity against myeloma and lymphoma cells *in vitro* (107, 108). In light of these results, research is now being conducted to harness the beneficial impact of acute exercise on lymphocyte kinetics for the purposes of cancer immunotherapy (121). It is beyond the scope of this review to discuss other findings in this exciting field and we briefly conclude that the aforementioned studies imply that exercise-induced lymphocytosis, and the lymphopenia that follows, is beneficial to the immune system's capacity to identify and neutralize damaged and neoplastic cells in peripheral tissues. Furthermore, in the context of neoplastic growth, this process may be directly responsible for reduced incidence of cancer among physically active people across the lifespan (122). Further comprehensive discussion of the role of exercise and lymphocyte kinetics in anti-tumor responses can be found elsewhere (117). Clearly more research is needed in this area, and a shift in focus toward investigating the benefits—rather than purported detrimental effects—of exercise on health, is no doubt underway and will be a key focus for exercise immunologists in the coming years.

Transient Changes to Blood Lymphocyte Function in the Hours Following Exercise

A common misinterpretation, brought about by the exercise-induced reductions to blood lymphocyte frequency in the hours following exercise, is the observation that the functional capacity of immune cells in the peripheral blood is reduced in the hours following vigorous exercise. As measurements of cell function in peripheral blood are entirely dependent on the cells present at the time of sampling, a change to the composition of the cells in blood in the hours after exercise—as outlined in the section; "Transient Changes to Blood Lymphocyte Frequency in the Hours Following Exercise"—will consequently lead to parallel changes in overall cell function, indicated by the performance of the sampled cells being assayed. For example, among CD8$^+$ T cells, subsets that exhibit strong effector function (e.g., CD45 RA$^+$CD27$^-$CD28$^-$CCR7$^-$CD62L$^-$CD57$^+$), substantially increase during exercise (81, 123). Thus, during exercise, blood is predominantly occupied by cells capable of responding strongly (i.e., IFN-gamma production) to *in vitro* stimuli, and therefore, many studies have shown an increase in IFN-gamma production by cells isolated close to the exercise stimulus. In the hours following exercise, the same effector CD8$^+$ T cells are subsequently redeployed to peripheral tissues, and, as such, this results in the blood having fewer cells capable of responding strongly to *in vitro* stimuli, thus explaining the commonly reported decrease in cellular function post-exercise. These effects have been neatly demonstrated approximately two decades ago when it was shown that IFN-gamma production by stimulated CD8$^+$ T cells is reduced 2 h after completing a prolonged 2.5 h bout of cycling (124). Importantly, it was shown that this reduced capacity to produce IFN-gamma was due to a reduced number of IFN-gamma-positive CD8$^+$ T cells in peripheral blood at the same time-point (124, 125).

The same principles apply to other cell functions, such as *in vitro* proliferation in response to mitogenic stimuli. However, with this measurement in particular, the commonly reported increase in T cell proliferation immediately after acute bouts of exercise is also strongly influenced by laboratory processes and *in vitro* assay conditions (e.g., blood processing, temperature, mitogen selection) (126). A recent meta-analysis of 24 studies concluded that lymphocyte proliferation is suppressed following acute bouts of exercise, and that a greater magnitude of suppression is caused by exercise lasting longer than 1 h, regardless of exercise intensity (127). However, this meta-analysis did not examine the most important determinant of cell function following exercise: the time-dependent changes in the cellular composition of the samples assayed. Thus, findings such as these should be interpreted with caution if analyses did not differentiate between studies collecting samples immediately after exercise or in the hours following.

As with research focusing on T cells, a similar group of studies citing reductions to natural killer cell cytotoxicity following acute exercise, reviewed elsewhere (128), did not always take into account dramatic shifts in the constitutional makeup of the natural killer cell compartment, which is known to change in response to exercise (81). Once more, changes to the functional capacity of the total natural killer cell pool are likely to have been misrepresented, given that many of these cells, with potent effector functions, are redistributed to peripheral tissues following exercise cessation. The principles discussed herein regarding lymphocyte function are also broadly applicable to the assessment of function in other cells, such as neutrophils and monocytes; the response of these cells to exercise is beyond the scope of this article and is reviewed elsewhere (8).

Taken together, it is important to emphasize that statements such as "*acute intensive exercise elicits a depression of several aspects of acquired immune function*" and "*prolonged bouts of heavy exertion reduce the normal functioning of all major immune cell subtypes*" mentioned elsewhere (8, 15) should be interpreted with caution. We conclude that the results of studies exploring the effects of acute exercise on cell function must be considered very carefully in light of the time-dependent changes in the cellular composition of blood that typically arise following a vigorous bout.

Summary: Exercise Induces Lymphocyte Immune Surveillance Not Immune Suppression

In summary, strong evidence implies that a reduction in the frequency and function of lymphocytes (and other immune cells) in peripheral blood in the hours following vigorous and prolonged exercise does not reflect immune suppression. Instead, the observed lymphopenia represents a heightened state of immune surveillance and immune regulation driven by a preferential mobilization of cells to peripheral tissues. As such, nutritional interventions, which have been employed to dampen the magnitude of exercise lymphopenia (124, 129) are unlikely to reduce the incidence of infections, but interventions that augment exercise-induced lymphocyte trafficking may provide benefits (130).

PART B: REGULAR PHYSICAL ACTIVITY AND FREQUENT EXERCISE AUGMENT ASPECTS OF IMMUNE COMPETENCY ACROSS THE LIFESPAN

Contrary to a commonly held belief—outlined in Part A "Is it Time to Close the Shutters on the "Open Window" Hypothesis? A Bout of Exercise Does Not Suppress Immune Competency?"—that acute vigorous exercise can suppress aspects of immune function, an increasingly large body of research indicates that both single bouts of exercise, or frequent participation in regular exercise, can act as an adjuvant to stimulate the immune system. Numerous methods exist to assess the effects of behavioral interventions on immunity (131) but arguably the optimal means of evaluating global immune competency at a systems level is *via* assessment of the immune response to *in vivo* challenge, ideally with a novel and clinically recognized pathogen, for example *via* vaccination (132). Thus, here, in the first section of Part B "Regular Physical Activity and Frequent Exercise Augment Aspects of Immune Competency Across the Lifespan," we focus on the influence that exercise has on immune responses to antigenic challenge, which requires a coordinated response from most, if not all, innate and adaptive immune system components. In light of the age-associated decline in immune competence with aging—caused in part by underlying changes to the numerical, phenotypic, and functional capacity of almost all innate and adaptive immune cells—the second section of Part B "Regular Physical Activity and Frequent Exercise Augment Aspects of Immune Competency Across the Lifespan," will evaluate the impact aging has on the immune benefits that can be attained from exercise throughout the lifespan. A detailed discussion of immunological aging processes and the influence that an active lifestyle has on established biomarkers of an aging immune system is covered in Part C "Does exercise and Regular Physical Activity Influence Immunological Ageing?" of this article.

Exercise and Immune Responses to Experimental *In Vivo* Challenge Across the Lifespan

In a research context, the most clinically relevant model to assess *in vivo* challenge in a controlled manner is *via* vaccination. Vaccine administration assesses the integrated capacity of the immune system to recognize and process antigen, leading to antigen neutralization. In a clinical research context, vaccination responses are principally quantified clinically in two ways, either *via* antibody production from antigen-specific plasma cells or *via* cytokine responses—typically IFN-gamma production—from T cells stimulated with cognate antigen.

Vaccination: Effects of a Single Exercise Bout

Evidence from an array of studies, evaluated recently in a comprehensive review elsewhere (9), indicates that a single acute bout of exercise appears to enhance immune responses to vaccination in both younger and older individuals. The majority of studies to date have examined muscle-damaging upper arm resistance exercise performed close to the time of vaccination which is administered shortly after the regimen into exercised muscle. However, other modes of exercise, including acute bouts of whole body aerobic activity, have also been investigated. Six of the eight trials identified in the aforementioned review indicated a statistically significant exercise-induced enhancement of immune responses against constituent antigens contained within the vaccine administered (133–138). It is notable that in five of these studies, statistically significant benefits were found where the vaccine strains appeared to have lower immunogenicity (9). For example, it was shown in a trial of 133 young adults, approximately 20 years of age, receiving either a full- or half-dose Pneumovax-23 (a pneumococcal vaccine), that those who exercised at the time of receiving the half-dose vaccine had heightened responses to five of the eleven pneumococcal strains contained in the vaccine, whereas no differences were observed for the other six strains; and no benefits of exercise were observed for the full-dose vaccine (137). As such, given the potential effectiveness of exercise as an adjuvant in situations where vaccine immunogenicity is low, studying the effects of exercise on antibody responses in older adults—whom typically exhibit impaired responses—has received considerable attention. In one recent study, it was found that antibody responses in women 55–75 years of age, were significantly improved when moderate-intensity aerobic exercise was performed immediately prior to vaccination; however, no beneficial effects were found in men (138). Another trial reported no benefits of a single 45-min bout of moderate-intensity walking exercise on the immune response to influenza and pneumococcal vaccination in women around 47 years of age (139). Finally, a very recent study found no effect of a bout of resistance exercise on antibody responses to influenza vaccination in adults approximately 73 years of age (140). It is possible that a number of factors including immunological aging, biological sex and variations in sex hormone levels, and perhaps latent infections (e.g., herpes viruses) (141–143) limit the immunostimulatory effects of exercise, and many studies have not adequately controlled for these factors. Alternatively, in light of the mechanisms proposed in the acute stress/exercise immune-enhancement hypothesis (93), it is plausible that more intensive exercise may be needed to elicit enhanced vaccine responses. Despite null findings, it is important to point out that few, if any, studies investigating the effects of acute exercise on vaccination responses have reported exercise-induced *impairment* to immune responses, and rather, these studies report that exercise has no effect, or in some cases a beneficial effect, on the immune response to vaccination in older adults.

Vaccination: Effects of Frequent Exercise Bouts

Data from vaccine studies exploring the effects of regular physical activity or frequent exercise training on the immune response to vaccination provides robust support for the argument that exercise enhances, rather than suppresses immunity. Indeed, at least eight studies have demonstrated heightened vaccination responses in older adults, typically over 60 years of age, who are physically active (144–151). For example, an early study categorized adults aged 62 years or older, into one of three groups: active (undertaking at least 20 min of vigorous exercise three or more times per week), moderately active (undertaking regular exercise but with lower intensity, frequency, and/or duration), or sedentary (non-exercisers). Two weeks after influenza vaccination, it was shown that serum anti-influenza IgG and IgM titers were higher in active versus sedentary adults, and so too were peripheral blood mononuclear cell responses to antigen-specific stimulation (144). In addition, a recent study has shown that men aged 65–85 years, who regularly undertook moderate or vigorous exercise training, exhibited higher antibody responses compared to inactive controls in response to an influenza vaccine (151). Data linking habitual levels of physical activity to enhanced immune competency in humans are supported by evidence from animal studies, and show that the immunological benefits of exercise may be particularly beneficial in enhancing otherwise poor responses in older age (152).

Interpreting Data From Vaccine Trials

A major criticism of vaccine and exercise trials conducted in humans is that many solely focus on the maximal antibody titer following vaccination, and it is not practical to follow-up with investigations into infection incidence as a gauge of protection status following vaccination (153). As such, it is unknown whether differences observed with absolute antibody titers, or the amount of IFN-gamma produced from stimulated T cells, between exercise and control groups, is representative of clinically meaningful benefits in terms of protection from infections. Three elegant studies in rodents imply that benefits, beyond antibody titer, may be brought about by acute exercise. In one of these studies, it was found that antibody responses to influenza exposure were *lower* in rodents that exercised around the time of exposure, compared to those that did not exercise, yet, exercised mice were still protected and did not exhibit any signs of infection upon re-exposure to the virus (154). Moreover, in an earlier study by the same authors, it was found that mice undertaking an acute bout of exercise before being expose to influenza exhibited a lower severity of infection and had enhanced viral clearance and lower inflammation in the lungs in the days following (155). Thus, it may be the case that exercise enhances immune responses, beyond those captured using maximal antibody titer as an endpoint. In accordance with this view, an elegant rodent study conducted by an independent group (156) found that mice exercised for 20–30 min at moderate intensity 4 h after intranasal influenza exposure had a substantially higher survival rate (18 of 22 survived; 82%) when compared to mice that did not exercise after influenza exposure (10 of 23 survived; 43%).

Contact Sensitivity Reactions and Acute Exercise Bouts

More recent studies have examined the effects of acute exercise on immune competency using other *in vivo* models of immune challenge that, in principle, also assess the coordinated efforts of immune system components. These studies have employed contact-sensitivity reactions by topically applying to skin, the dendritic cell and T cell stimulant (or attractant) diphenylcyclopropenone (DPCP), and the non-specific inflammatory stimulant, croton oil (157, 158). For example, in studies of young adults (approximately 20–30 years of age), by applying a primary sensitizing dose of DPCP 20 min after 2 h of moderate-intensity treadmill running, and assessing recall challenge 4 weeks later, it has been concluded that this form of exercise impairs both the induction of T cell immunity and the memory response (159, 160). Thirty minutes of moderate- or vigorous-intensity running had no effect, and no forms of exercise modulated the non-specific inflammatory challenge in response to croton oil (159, 160). Although these findings are biologically interesting, the clinical relevance of exercise-induced change is unclear, in part, because the process of DPCP-induced immune modulation is not well defined (158) unlike the immune response to antigen administration by vaccination.

Summary: Exercise Enhances Immune Responses to *In Vivo* Antigenic Challenge

We conclude that there is growing evidence from a powerful array of studies in humans and rodents, indicating that exercise enhances, or at least does not suppress immune responses to *in vivo* challenge in younger and older individuals. These observations—which contradict those predicated by the "open-window" hypothesis—support the contention that an acute bout of exercise has no detrimental immune consequences for health. Thus, exercise should be encouraged, particularly for older adults who are at greatest risk of infections and who may obtain the greatest exercise-induced benefits to immune competency; an overview of the impact of aging on the immunological benefits that can be attained from exercise is described next.

Does Aging Influence the Immunological Benefits of Exercise and Regular Physical Activity?

Effect of a Single Exercise Bout

Research investigating the effects of exercise on immune function has sought to establish whether the observed benefits, as outlined earlier in young adults, such as exercise-induced immune cell mobilisation, that has been implicated in protection against cancer, is also applicable to older adults. For example, it has been reported that the magnitude of T cell mobilization in response to acute vigorous exercise is smaller in older (65 ± 1 years) compared to younger (22 ± 1 years) adults (161, 162). However, in this study, it was also shown that following exercise, the magnitude of T cell proliferation in response to mitogens was smaller in young adults, whereas a similar exercise-induced stimulation of natural killer cell cytotoxicity was observed for both groups (161, 162). It is beyond the scope of this review to fully critique investigations examining the influence of single exercise bouts on the function of different immune cells, with comparisons made between younger and older individuals across the lifespan; we refer the reader to comprehensive reviews on this topic (163–165). Nevertheless, it is important to point out that many studies in this area are difficult to interpret: at the time of their publication, the influence of *Cytomegalovirus* infection on the magnitude of exercise-induced immune responses was not known and was therefore not considered (123, 166). Moreover, while the magnitude of change to lymphocyte kinetics is likely to be important for detecting and eliminating viral and bacterial infections and neoplastic cells, this process is complex to study, and comparisons between younger and older people is difficult, partly due to other age-associated changes that influence the physiological response to exercise, such as the decline in fitness (e.g., sarcopenia, cardiorespiratory fitness) with age. It is likely that some, or all of these factors impact upon on the efficacy of exercise as an adjuvant to vaccination responses in older adults, outlined earlier in the section "Exercise and Immune Responses to Experimental *In Vivo* Challenge Across the Lifespan." In light of the challenge interpreting the clinical relevance of the aforementioned lymphocyte kinetics studies, from here onward, we briefly evaluate the impact of regular physical activity or frequent exercise bouts on immune competency across the lifespan, using measurements in samples collected from participants at rest.

Frequent Bouts of Exercise

Immune competency at rest has been assessed in cross-sectional studies, comparing elderly individuals differentiated by physical activity level or cardiorespiratory fitness, or by examining immune function before and after structured exercise training interventions. For example, it has commonly been reported among the elderly, that the most active participants, compared to those who are least active, show the highest T cell proliferation and cytokine production in response to mitogens (163–165). Fewer studies have assessed innate immune competency, but higher natural killer cell cytotoxicity has been consistently shown among the elderly who are active compared to less active age-matched controls (163–165). Recent studies have expanded measurements into other innate immune cells such as neutrophils. For example, a recent cross-sectional study of 211 elderly adults, showed that neutrophils from the 20 most active participants, compared to the 20 least active participants, migrated toward interleukin (IL)-8 with greater chemotactic accuracy, but there were no differences in chemotactic speed (167). In addition, a recent exercise training study has shown in both young and middle-aged adults, that 10 weeks of moderate-intensity continuous cycling training, or high-intensity interval cycling training, improve neutrophil and monocyte phagocytosis and oxidative burst irrespective of age (168). Improvements in these common measurements of immune competency, however, are not always consistent in longitudinal studies employing exercise training interventions, with around half of studies reporting improvements, and half reporting no change (163–165). One reason for this could be because the dramatic effects of *Cytomegalovirus* on driving immunological aging was not considered by most of these studies, and it is feasible that results would be different when examining individuals who are latently infected compared to those who are seronegative. Importantly however, no studies report impaired immune competency from increased participation in structured exercise. Altogether, we conclude that despite declines in fitness and immune competency, aging does not appear to negate the immunological benefits that can be attained from exercise, and indeed, frequent participation in exercise across the lifespan may lead to immune benefits, even in older age.

PART C: DOES EXERCISE AND REGULAR PHYSICAL ACTIVITY INFLUENCE IMMUNOLOGICAL AGEING?

Since the first exercise immunology research in the early 1900s, and the substantial increase in scientific interest from the late 1980s and early 1990s (169), studies examining interaction between immune function and lifestyle factors such as exercise and physical activity have become common. Although a few exercise studies published in the last 10–15 years have investigated some immunological processes relevant to aging, health, and disease, the theme of exercise-induced "immune suppression" continues to influence the design of new studies or at least features in the interpretation of findings and is often justified or contextualized with relevance to self-reported illness symptoms among athletes. As outlined in Part A "Is it Time to Close the Shutters on the "Open-Window" Hypothesis? A Bout of Exercise Does Not Suppress Immune Competency," there is limited reliable evidence to show that exercise heightens risk of opportunistic infections, but there is, however, a growing body of evidence to show that exercise enhances, rather than suppresses, immune competency, as summarized in Part B: "Regular Physical Activity and Frequent Exercise Augment Aspects of Immune Competency Across the Lifespan." The beneficial effects of exercise on immune function are likely to be greatest for elderly people exhibiting the age-associated deterioration of immune competency, also referred to as immunosenescence. Moreover, preliminary evidence suggests that physical activity and regular structured exercise may even limit or delay immunological aging. Here, in Part C: "Does Exercise and Regular Physical Activity Influence Immunological Ageing?" we evaluate whether an active lifestyle influences immunosenescence.

The Aging Immune System

Aging is associated with profound changes to the numerical, phenotypic, and functional capacity of almost all innate and adaptive immune cells, resulting in altered immune responses. Some innate immune cells exhibit numerical, phenotypic, and functional alterations with aging, whereas others appear to be less affected (170).

For example, the numbers and functions of eosinophils, basophils, and mast cells appear to be largely unchanged with aging, or at least, there is not a clear effect of age based on the limited current literature (170). Neutrophil numbers often increase with aging, but these cells exhibit diminished phagocytosis and impaired chemotaxis, although chemokinesis is maintained (170). Natural killer cells increase with aging, driven by an accumulation of cytotoxic $CD56^{dim}$ cells but a decline in regulatory $CD56^{bright}$ cells, and overall, cytokine production and cytotoxicity are less on a per cell basis (170). Other innate lymphocytes, such as invariant CD1d-restricted natural killer T cells (iNKT cells), which represent <1% of the T cell pool, decline in number but age-associated changes to their function have not been established (171). Monocyte numbers are stable with aging, but classical cells ($CD14^{++}CD16^{-}$) decline, and intermediate ($CD14^{+}CD16^{+}$) and non-classical ($CD14^{+}CD16^{++}$) cells increase, but overall, monocyte cytokine production is impaired (170, 172). These changes with blood monocytes are thought to be mirrored by tissue-resident macrophages, whereby classically activated M1 cells decline, and alternatively activated M2 cells accumulate (173). However, alterations in tissue-resident cells with advancing age are very likely to be a result of adipose tissue accumulation and dysfunction that also occurs in parallel with aging (174, 175). Indeed, inflamed adipose tissue attracts macrophages with cell-surface characteristics similar to M2 alternatively activated cells—often assumed to be anti-inflammatory. However, despite their cell-surface phenotype, these cells are potent producers of inflammatory cytokines in adipose tissue, and likely drive age- and obesity-associated inflammation (176–179). Thus, the M1/M2 paradigm for macrophages is likely to be an over-simplification (180, 181). It is unknown if other, primarily tissue-resident cells, are affected by adipose tissue dysfunction, but with aging, the number and function of dendritic cells have been reported to decrease in the skin and mucosal membranes (170). There is also an age-associated increase in myeloid-derived suppressor cells—a heterogeneous population of granulocytes, macrophages, and dendritic cells—that may impair aspects of immune function by producing reactive oxygen species and inhibitory cytokines (182).

Within the adaptive immune system, there are substantial changes to the numbers, function, and phenotype of T cells with aging. Among the broad population of $CD4^{+}$ T-helper cells, aging is associated with a predominance of Th2 (i.e., IL-4 and IL-10), and Th17-producing cells (i.e., IL-17-producing cells that are associated with autoimmune disease), whereas there is a decline in cells with a Th1 profile [i.e., IFN-gamma- and tumor necrosis factor-alpha (TNF-alpha)-producing cells] (183, 184). With aging, the numbers and proportions of antigen-inexperienced $CD4^{+}$ and $CD8^{+}$ T cells decreases (e.g., $CD27^{+}CD28^{+}CD45RA^{+}$ $CD57^{-}CD62L^{+}CCR7^{+}KLRG1^{-}$ naïve cells) (185, 186). In parallel, the numbers and proportions of antigen-experienced $CD4^{+}$ and $CD8^{+}$ T cells increases (e.g., $CD27^{-}CD28^{-}CD45RA^{+}CD57^{+}CD$ $62L^{-}CCR7^{-}KLRG1^{+}$ memory cells), and these cells are potent producers of inflammatory cytokines (185, 186). These changes are driven by lower hematopoietic stem cell numbers, thymic involution resulting in reduced output of antigen-naïve T cells, and infection with latent viruses, in particular *Cytomegalovirus* (185, 187). With aging, T cells that express natural killer cell-associated cell-surface proteins (NKT-like cells) also accumulate, exhibiting similar changes to their phenotype, functional properties, and specificities as with the broader population of $CD4^{+}$ and $CD8^{+}$ T cells (171). There is an age-associated decline in the total number of γδ T cells; however age *per se*, in the absence of chronic infections, is associated with a decline in Vδ2 cells (60–80% of γδ T cells), whereas Vδ1 (15–20% γδ T cells) remain stable (188). Some evidence suggests that γδ T cell proliferative responses are impaired with aging, perhaps due to increased susceptibility of Vδ2 cells to apoptosis (189, 190). Natural regulatory T cells increase with aging whereas inducible regulatory T cells decrease, but it is unclear if their function is affected (191). As with T cells, aging is associated with a decline in the numbers and proportions of naïve B cells, an accumulation of memory B cells with limited specificities, and impaired plasma cell antibody production (192).

Several robust and accepted hallmarks of immunosenescence have been established, especially within the adaptive immune system. For example, low numbers and proportions of naïve T cells (in particular $CD8^{+}$ T cells) and high numbers and proportions of memory T cells (especially late-stage differentiated $CD8^{+}$ T cells) are well established biomarkers (185, 186, 193, 194). In addition, a cluster of parameters, revealed in longitudinal studies of octogenarians and nonagenarians from an isolated population in Sweden, have been referred to as the immune risk profile (195–197). Biomarkers included low numbers and proportions of B cells, high numbers and proportions of late-stage differentiated $CD8^{+}$ T cells (i.e., $CD27^{-}CD28^{-}$), poor T cell proliferation in response to mitogens, a CD4:CD8 ratio of <1.0, infection with *Cytomegalovirus* and high plasma IL-6, which together, predicted greater all-cause mortality at 2-, 4-, and 6-year follow-up (195, 197–200). Indeed, the age-associated increase in systemic inflammation, referred to as "inflammageing" is another principle observation among aging and longevity studies (201, 202). Subsequently, high levels of IL-6, TNF-alpha, and C-reactive protein, have been associated with shorter survival (203–205). Overall, it is well established that elderly individuals exhibit impaired immune responses to *in vivo* challenge with novel antigens (143, 206, 207) and these individuals are subsequently thought to be at increased risk of infection. Encouragingly however, as outlined in Part B: "Regular Physical Activity and Frequent Exercise Augment Aspects of Immune Competency Across the Lifespan" exercise can be a potent stimulus of immune function, including the response to vaccination, and some evidence suggests that exercise might delay or limit the age-associated decline in immune competency.

Relationships Between Exercise and Regular Physical Activity With Hallmarks of an Aging Adaptive Immune System

As summarized in Part B: "Regular Physical Activity and Frequent Exercise Augment Aspects of Immune Competency Across the Lifespan" many studies have examined the influence of regular physical activity or frequent structured exercise on the function of the adaptive immune system with aging (163–165). Here, we focus on recent studies that have examined relationships between exercise, physical activity or cardiorespiratory fitness, and the numbers and proportions of $CD4^{+}$ and $CD8^{+}$ naïve and memory

T cells, as hallmarks of immunosenescence. Indeed, a small number of studies have investigated whether the characteristics of the T cell pool are influenced by an active lifestyle. There is a larger body of evidence in young adults, typically between 18 and 30 years, compared to older adults, hereafter considered as being over 40 years of age due to the characteristics of studies published to date. If an active lifestyle can be linked with a smaller accumulation of memory T cells, and a smaller decline in naïve T cells, then in young adults, one interpretation might be that exercise prevents, or at least delays immunosenescence, whereas in older adults, these associations could be interpreted as countering or limiting the development of an age-associated immune profile.

Experimental Evidence in Young People: Can Exercise Prevent or Delay Aging of the Adaptive Immune System?

The characteristics of the T cell pool have been examined in 16 young adults (50% male; 18 ± 2 years) classified as being very active (well-trained soccer players self-reporting 9–12 h of exercise per week) and compared to 16 young adults (50% male; 19 ± 2 years) classified as being untrained (individuals self-reporting 2–3 h of exercise per week). Untrained individuals showed the highest proportions of $CD4^+$ and $CD8^+$ memory T cells, and the lowest proportions of $CD8^+$ naïve T cells, defined on the basis of CD57 and CD28 expression (208). Although these results suggest that regular exercise might limit the age-associated accumulation of memory T cells and decline in naïve T cells, the effects were strongly influenced by sex: only untrained males exhibited high proportions of memory T cells and low proportions of naïve cells compared to trained males, and these effects were driven by changes in the $CD4^+$ T cell pool (208). Extending these findings by examining a female-only population of young adults, the same authors compared 13 well-trained soccer players (self-reporting around 12 h of exercise per week; 20 ± 2 years) to 13 untrained controls (self-reporting around 3 h of exercise per week; 21 ± 2 years) (209). Trained females exhibited a greater proportion of $CD8^+$ naïve T cells compared to untrained females, but these associations did not remain statistically significant after controlling for body fat percentage (trained 21.7 ± 4.0 versus untrained 25.1 ± 4.1%, $p < 0.05$) (209). Indeed, very few studies have considered whether relationships between an active lifestyle and markers of an aging immune system could be influenced by other factors, such as body composition. Recently, a very small study of 15 males aged 30 ± 4 years, categorized participants using a combination of gold standard methods for measuring physiological and lifestyle variables (210). Three groups were formed (sedentary, active, and very active) on the basis of objectively assessed habitual physical activity, directly measured cardiorespiratory fitness, and body composition assessed with dual energy X-ray absorptiometry (210). This work showed that sedentary individuals had higher proportions of memory $CD4^+$ T cells expressing CD45RO and PD-1, supporting the results of other published studies that have not taken body composition into consideration.

It should be emphasized, that among younger adults in particular, mixed results have been reported when investigating links between an active lifestyle and hallmarks of an aging immune system. Most investigations have been cross-sectional in design, or have made observations between groups over short periods. For example, one study has shown that national standard triathletes (age range 18–36 years, $n = 19$), appear to exhibit impaired thymic output, assessed by T cell receptor excision circle levels (211). Among $CD4^+$ and $CD8^+$ T cells, these athletes had lower absolute numbers of naïve cells and higher absolute numbers of memory cells compared to age-matched less active controls ($n = 16$), as shown by CD45RA, CD45RO, and CD27 expression (211). Similar observations have been made by examining individuals in the third decade of life, showing that endurance athletes, compared to less active controls, appear to exhibit slightly larger accumulations of memory T cells and slightly fewer naïve T cells, defined by CD45RA and CCR7 expression (212). Thus, it appears that among younger individuals (i.e., less than 40 years of age), if exercise is undertaken at very extreme volumes, such as more than 5–10 times the amount of physical activity recommended each week (i.e., 12–25 h per week), this might contribute toward a small decline in naïve T cells and a small increase in memory T cells. It is possible that these changes are due to reactivation of latent viruses, which could be independent of immune function, and driven by exercise-induced adrenergic activity, oxidative stress and inflammatory cytokines (48–50). However, these results might also be explained by fluctuations in cell numbers and cell sub-populations in peripheral blood over time. Such changes have been interpreted as being linked to exercise training load (213, 214), but it is also conceivable that these changes occur due to seasonal variation, as has been shown in non-exercise contexts (215, 216).

Experimental Evidence in Older People: Can Exercise Limit or Counter Aging of the Adaptive Immune System?

Although most studies have examined associations between biomarkers of an aging adaptive immune system in young adults, other studies have made measurements across a broader range of ages. For example, one study examined 102 men ranging in age from 18 to 61 years (mean 39 ± 6 years) (217). It was shown that the proportion of the $CD4^+$ and $CD8^+$ T cell pool comprising of memory cells (defined as $KLRG1^+CD57^+$ or $KLRG1^+CD28-$) was inversely correlated with cardiorespiratory fitness, which is largely indicative of an active lifestyle (217). The age-associated decrease of naïve T cells (defined as $KLRG1^-CD57^-$ or $KLRG1^-CD28^+$) and increase in memory T cells did not withstand statistical adjustment for cardiorespiratory fitness, but remained significant after adjusting statistically for body composition and *Cytomegalovirus* infection (217). Thus, it was concluded that fitter individuals exhibit a smaller age-associated decline of naïve T cells and a smaller accumulation of memory T cells.

As with work examining relationships between an active lifestyle and hallmarks of an aging adaptive immune system in young and middle-aged adults, similar associations have been shown in an older population of 61 men aged 65–85 years (218). In this study, participants self-reported to be "untrained" ($n = 15$), or to lead a "moderate" training lifestyle ($n = 16$;

taking part in team sports or running less than 6 km two to three times per week), or an "intense" training lifestyle ($n = 15$; running approximately 10 km at least 5 days per week). These categories were confirmed with a validated physical activity questionnaire and by measurement of cardiorespiratory fitness. Both training groups exhibited a lower proportion of CD4$^+$ and CD8$^+$ memory cells (defined as CD45RA$^+$CCR7$^-$), but these associations were largest and only statistically significant among men leading an "intense" training lifestyle, suggesting a dose–response effect of exercise. Although findings were less clear when examining other cell subpopulations based on CD45RA and CCR7 expression, and there were no effects of exercise when examining CD28$^-$ cells, men in the "trained" groups had T cells with the longest telomeres (218). Another recent study compared 125 adults (55–79 years of age) who maintained a high level of cycling throughout life to 75 age-matched inactive controls (219). Within the CD4$^+$ and CD8$^+$ T cell pool, the frequency of naive cells (defined as CD45RA$^+$) was greater, and the frequency of memory cells (defined as CD45RA-) was lower among cyclists. Extended phenotyping revealed that CD4$^+$ and CD8$^+$ CCR7-CD45RA$^+$ accumulation was less among cyclists, but no differences were found for CD28-CD57$^+$ cells. Cyclists also exhibited higher frequencies of recent thymic emigrants and regulatory B cells, lower Th17 polarization, and in plasma, higher IL-7 and lower IL-6 (219). Despite these findings, suggesting a beneficial effect of leading an active lifestyle on immunosenescence among older adults, there is some inconsistency in the literature. For example, comparing elderly athletes ($n = 12$, approximately 74 years of age) to less active age-matched controls ($n = 26$), there were no differences in thymic output, the proportions of naïve or memory CD4$^+$ and CD8$^+$ T cells (defined with CD45RA and CCR7 expression), or T cell activation in response to anti-CD3 stimulation (212). Most investigations of T cell immunosenescence and lifestyle among healthy elderly adults have had cross-sectional study designs. Longitudinal studies, or randomized and controlled trials of exercise training are lacking and might yield promising results. For example, one study has compared 6 months of exercise training in men and women ($n = 28$, aged 61–76 years) to a similar group who maintained their current lifestyle ($n = 20$, aged 62–79 years) (220). Using a simple immunophenotyping strategy, the results showed that the proportion of CD4$^+$ T cells expressing CD28 increased in the exercise group after 6 months, but not in those who maintained their lifestyle (220).

Summary of Experimental Evidence

In summary, evidence shows that the characteristics of the T cell pool appear to be influenced by leading an active lifestyle, determined by exercise training, physical activity level, or cardiorespiratory fitness. It seems that among both the young and elderly, an active lifestyle is generally linked to lower numbers and proportions of memory T cells and higher numbers and proportions of naïve T cells (10). This summary is partly supported by a recent systematic review, concluding that regular structured exercise increases the number of naïve T cells in peripheral blood at rest (221). Altogether, findings from recent studies examining relationships between an active lifestyle and the characteristics of the T cell pool—as robust and accepted biomarkers of immunosenescence—support observations from some cross-sectional and longitudinal studies, showing that other measures of immune competency, which typically decline with aging, can be improved with physical activity or regular structured exercise (163–165). However, further research is needed in this area that employs precise lifestyle measurements (e.g., using wearable technology to assess physical activity, and dual energy X-ray absorptiometry to measure body composition) and more robust measurements of immune competency (e.g., absolute cell counts rather than proportions, measurements of cell function, and *in vivo* antigen challenges) while controlling for factors that drive immunosenescence (e.g., inflammation and *Cytomegalovirus* infection).

Mechanisms

Links between a physically active lifestyle with lower numbers or proportions of memory T cells, and higher numbers or proportions of naïve T cells, have been hypothesized as being driven by the acute effects of exercise bouts. For example, it has been suggested that repeated bouts of exercise might prevent or delay immunological aging by limiting the accumulation of CD4$^+$ and CD8$^+$ antigen-experienced memory T cell clones, repopulating blood with antigen-inexperienced naïve T cells (11, 12). In this hypothesis, it is proposed that memory T cells are frequently mobilized into blood during regular bouts of exercise, followed by an extravasation to peripheral tissues, where these cells are exposed to pro-apoptotic stimuli, such as reactive oxygen species, glucocorticoids, and cytokines (11, 12). Subsequently, it is proposed that the number of naïve T cells increases as part of a negative feedback loop governing the number of naïve and memory cells in the immune system, which is bolstered by exercise-induced thymopoiesis and extra-thymic T cell development (11, 12). Supporting the mechanisms proposed in this hypothesis, many investigations have shown that memory T cells are mobilized into the circulation during exercise, followed by extravasation out of the bloodstream in the hours following (81, 123). In addition, studies in mice show that lymphocyte apoptosis occurs post-exercise in tissues thought to be the homing destination of mobilized cells (222). Although some T cells mobilized by exercise might be resistant to apoptosis, given that *Cytomegalovirus*-specific CD8$^+$ T cells express high levels of Bcl-2 (223), other work has shown that *Cytomegalovirus*-specific CD8$^+$ T cells, are equally as susceptible to Fas-induced apoptosis as the total pool of CD8$^+$ T cells (224). Further, irrespective of virus specificity, studies have shown that T cells expressing cell-surface proteins such as CD57 and KLRG1 are more susceptible to H_2O_2-induced apoptosis than total lymphocytes and naïve T cells (225, 226). Thus, the concept of exercise directly countering memory T cell accumulation is supported by evidence from human and animal studies.

It is unknown whether triggering apoptosis among expanded clones of memory T cells specific for viruses such as *Cytomegalovirus* is advantageous. For example, in a transplant setting, *Cytomegalovirus* disease occurs when T cells fail to provide antiviral control (227) and a robust pro-inflammatory response to *Cytomegalovirus* has been associated with longer survival in the elderly (228). However, it remains to be determined what proportion of the T cell pool needs to be specific for *Cytomegalovirus* to limit viral reactivation. Infection with *Cytomegalovirus* results in approximately 10% of the $CD4^+$ and $CD8^+$ T cell pool becoming specific for this virus (229), although large inter-individual differences exist. For example, it has been reported that 23% of the $CD8^+$ T cell pool can become specific for a single *Cytomegalovirus* epitope (223). Traditionally, it has been considered disadvantageous for such a large proportion of the T cell pool to be specific for one virus. This view is linked to another age- or infection-associated change that occurs in parallel—a fall in the numbers and proportions of naïve cells—which has been interpreted as limiting capacity to engage novel antigens. These interpretations are based upon two assumptions. First, there is an upper limit to the size of the immune system, and second, thymic output is negligible after adolescence (230). Thus, it has been proposed that antigen-inexperienced naïve T cells could be "used up" due to ongoing differentiation into antigen-experienced memory T cells that "fill up" immunological "space" (230). It has also been proposed that this accumulation of antigen-experienced memory T cells leads to "squeezing out" of T cells targeting less dominant viruses leading to loss of viral control (231). This concept of a fixed amount of immunological space has since been debated (232, 233) and thymic output is now known to persist, albeit reduced, up until around 70 years of age (234). However, even if removal of some memory T cells is not essential for maintaining an effective T cell pool, assuming these cells contribute to systemic inflammation, their removal might limit "inflammageing" (230). Despite uncertainties over the susceptibility of memory T cells to undergo apoptosis, or whether it is advantageous to stimulate their removal, it seems that exercise-induced immune cell death in the tissues has relevance to other processes. For example, apoptotic cells and cell debris stimulates hematopoietic stem cell mobilization into blood (95) perhaps promoting trafficking to the thymus or extrathymic sites facilitating output of naïve T cells (235). Additional support for exercise stimulating production of naïve T cells is provided by work showing that contracting skeletal muscle produces IL-7 (236) which might increase thymic mass and function (237).

A physically active lifestyle might also counter T cell immunosenescence indirectly, perhaps by limiting adipose tissue accumulation and dysfunction that occurs with aging and obesity (174, 238, 239). Indeed, obesity has been linked with impaired lymphocyte proliferation (240), shorter leukocyte telomere length (241), and a skewing of the T cell pool toward a regulatory and Th2-phenotype (242). In addition, large expansions of differentiated $\alpha\beta$ T cells and $\gamma\delta$ T cells have been shown among people with obesity, with $\gamma\delta$ T cells exhibiting impaired antiviral function (243–245). It is generally accepted that repeated stimulation with antigens from *Cytomegalovirus* drives immunosenescence (185, 186, 193, 194). With obesity, adipose tissue is the primary source of pro-inflammatory cytokines and reactive oxygen species (174, 246) which can reactivate *Cytomegalovirus* directly (48, 49). Thus, exercise might limit T cell immunosenescence by decreasing visceral and subcutaneous adipose tissue (238), providing a potent anti-inflammatory and anti-oxidative stimulus (247, 248). In turn, lower systemic inflammation and better redox balance might limit viral reactivation, reducing stimulation with antigens from viruses such as *Cytomegalovirus*. In addition, T cell dysfunction might also be prevented, in part, by limiting reactive oxygen species production (249).

In summary, leading a physically active lifestyle appears to limit the age-associated changes to the cellular composition of the adaptive immune system, but the mechanisms are yet to be determined. Exercise might counter the expansion of memory T cells directly, which is desirable assuming these cells contribute to systemic inflammation and not all are required to control latent viruses. Limiting the expansion of memory T cells also assumes the "size" of the immune system is fixed, the capacity to produce antigen-naïve T cells is limited, and these constraints contribute to immune decline in the elderly. However, exercise might affect memory T cell accumulation indirectly, by reducing viral reactivation, or preventing T cell senescence, by controlling adipose tissue deposition and dysfunction that drives inflammation and oxidative stress with aging and obesity.

CONCLUDING REMARKS

Contemporary evidence from epidemiological studies shows that leading a physically active lifestyle reduces the incidence of communicable (e.g., bacterial and viral infections) and non-communicable diseases (e.g., cancer), implying that immune competency is enhanced by regular exercise bouts. However, to this day, research practice, academic teaching, and even physical activity promotion and prescription continues to consider a prevailing myth that exercise can temporarily suppress immune function. We have critically reviewed related evidence, and conclude that regular physical activity and frequent exercise are beneficial, or at the very least, are not detrimental to immunological health. We summarize that (i) limited reliable evidence exists to support the claim that exercise suppresses cellular or soluble immune competency, (ii) exercise *per se* does not heighten the risk of opportunistic infections, and (iii) exercise can enhance *in vivo* immune responses to bacterial, viral, and other antigens. In addition, we present evidence showing that regular physical activity and frequent exercise might limit or delay immunological aging. We conclude that leading an active lifestyle is likely to be beneficial, rather than detrimental, to immune function, which may have implications for health and disease in older age.

AUTHOR CONTRIBUTIONS

JC and JT contributed equally toward literature searching and retrieval, the ideas and interpretation of the studies described, drafting and revision of the manuscript, and approval of the final version to be published. JT and JC both agreed to be accountable for the work in ensuring that questions related to the accuracy or integrity of any part of the work are appropriately investigated and resolved.

REFERENCES

1. Warburton DER, Bredin SSD. Health benefits of physical activity: a systematic review of current systematic reviews. *Curr Opin Cardiol* (2017) 32(5): 541–56. doi:10.1097/HCO.0000000000000437
2. Pape K, Ryttergaard L, Rotevatn TA, Nielsen BJ, Torp-Pedersen C, Overgaard C, et al. Leisure-time physical activity and the risk of suspected bacterial infections. *Med Sci Sports Exerc* (2016) 48(9):1737–44. doi:10.1249/MSS.0000000000000953
3. Kostka T, Berthouze SE, Lacour J, Bonnefoy M. The symptomatology of upper respiratory tract infections and exercise in elderly people. *Med Sci Sports Exerc* (2000) 32(1):46–51. doi:10.1097/00005768-200001000-00008
4. Leveille SG, Gray S, LaCroix AZ, Ferrucci L, Black DJ, Guralnik JM. Physical inactivity and smoking increase risk for serious infections in older women. *J Am Geriatr Soc* (2000) 48(12):1582–8. doi:10.1111/j.1532-5415.2000.tb03867.x
5. Romaniszyn D, Pobiega M, Wojkowska-Mach J, Chmielarczyk A, Gryglewska B, Adamski P, et al. The general status of patients and limited physical activity as risk factors of methicillin-resistant *Staphylococcus aureus* occurrence in long-term care facilities residents in Krakow, Poland. *BMC Infect Dis* (2014) 14:271. doi:10.1186/1471-2334-14-271
6. Baik I, Curhan GC, Rimm EB, Bendich A, Willett WC, Fawzi WW. A prospective study of age and lifestyle factors in relation to community-acquired pneumonia in US men and women. *Arch Intern Med* (2000) 160(20):3082–8. doi:10.1001/archinte.160.20.3082
7. Walsh NP, Gleeson M, Pyne DB, Nieman DC, Dhabhar FS, Shephard RJ, et al. Position statement. Part two: maintaining immune health. *Exerc Immunol Rev* (2011) 17:64–103.
8. Walsh NP, Gleeson M, Shephard RJ, Gleeson M, Woods JA, Bishop NC, et al. Position statement. Part one: immune function and exercise. *Exerc Immunol Rev* (2011) 17:6–63.
9. Pascoe AR, Fiatarone Singh MA, Edwards KM. The effects of exercise on vaccination responses: a review of chronic and acute exercise interventions in humans. *Brain Behav Immun* (2014) 39:33–41. doi:10.1016/j.bbi.2013.10.003
10. Turner JE. Is immunosenescence influenced by our lifetime "dose" of exercise? *Biogerontology* (2016) 17(3):581–602. doi:10.1007/s10522-016-9642-z
11. Simpson RJ, Guy K. Coupling aging immunity with a sedentary lifestyle: has the damage already been done? – a mini-review. *Gerontology* (2010) 56(5):449–58. doi:10.1159/000270905
12. Simpson RJ. Aging, persistent viral infections, and immunosenescence: can exercise "make space"? *Exerc Sport Sci Rev* (2011) 39(1):23–33. doi:10.1097/JES.0b013e318201f39d
13. Turner JE, Brum PC. Does regular exercise counter T cell immunosenescence reducing the risk of developing cancer and promoting successful treatment of malignancies? *Oxid Med Cell Longev* (2017) 2017:4234765. doi:10.1155/2017/4234765
14. Mackinnon LT. *Advances in Exercise Immunology*. Champaign, IL: Human Kinetics (1999). xii, 363 p.
15. Peake JM, Neubauer O, Walsh NP, Simpson RJ. Recovery of the immune system after exercise. *J Appl Physiol (1985)* (2017) 122(5):1077–87. doi:10.1152/japplphysiol.00622.2016
16. Cowles WN. Fatigue as a contributory cause of pneumonias. *Boston Med Surg J* (1918) 179:555. doi:10.1056/NEJM191810311791801
17. Peters EM, Bateman ED. Ultramarathon running and upper respiratory tract infections. An epidemiological survey. *S Afr Med J* (1983) 64(15):582–4.
18. Nieman DC, Johanssen LM, Lee JW, Arabatzis K. Infectious episodes in runners before and after the Los Angeles Marathon. *J Sports Med Phys Fitness* (1990) 30(3):316–28.
19. Nieman DC, Johanssen LM, Lee JW. Infectious episodes in runners before and after a roadrace. *J Sports Med Phys Fitness* (1989) 29(3):289–96.
20. Spence L, Brown WJ, Pyne DB, Nissen MD, Sloots TP, McCormack JG, et al. Incidence, etiology, and symptomatology of upper respiratory illness in elite athletes. *Med Sci Sports Exerc* (2007) 39(4):577–86. doi:10.1249/mss.0b013e31802e851a
21. Gleeson M. Immune function in sport and exercise. *J Appl Physiol (1985)* (2007) 103(2):693–9. doi:10.1152/japplphysiol.00008.2007
22. Cox AJ, Gleeson M, Pyne DB, Callister R, Hopkins WG, Fricker PA. Clinical and laboratory evaluation of upper respiratory symptoms in elite athletes. *Clin J Sport Med* (2008) 18(5):438–45. doi:10.1097/JSM.0b013e318181e501
23. Makela MJ, Puhakka T, Ruuskanen O, Leinonen M, Saikku P, Kimpimaki M, et al. Viruses and bacteria in the etiology of the common cold. *J Clin Microbiol* (1998) 36(2):539–42.
24. Nieman DC. Exercise, infection, and immunity. *Int J Sports Med* (1994) 15(Suppl 3):S131–41. doi:10.1055/s-2007-1021128
25. Meeusen R, Duclos M, Foster C, Fry A, Gleeson M, Nieman D, et al. Prevention, diagnosis and treatment of the overtraining syndrome: joint consensus statement of the European College of Sport Science (ECSS) and the American College of Sports Medicine (ACSM). *Eur J Sport Sci* (2013) 13(1):1–24. doi:10.1080/17461391.2012.730061
26. Meeusen R, Duclos M, Foster C, Fry A, Gleeson M, Nieman D, et al. Prevention, diagnosis, and treatment of the overtraining syndrome: joint consensus statement of the European College of Sport Science and the American College of Sports Medicine. *Med Sci Sports Exerc* (2013) 45(1):186–205. doi:10.1249/MSS.0b013e318279a10a
27. Edwards JP, Walsh NP, Diment PC, Roberts R. Anxiety and perceived psychological stress play an important role in the immune response after exercise. *Exerc Immunol Rev* (2018) 24:26–34.
28. Glaser R, Kiecolt-Glaser JK. Stress-induced immune dysfunction: implications for health. *Nat Rev Immunol* (2005) 5(3):243–51. doi:10.1038/nri1571
29. Kohut ML, Lee W, Martin A, Arnston B, Russell DW, Ekkekakis P, et al. The exercise-induced enhancement of influenza immunity is mediated in part by improvements in psychosocial factors in older adults. *Brain Behav Immun* (2005) 19(4):357–66. doi:10.1016/j.bbi.2004.12.002
30. Bermon S, Castell LM, Calder PC, Bishop NC, Blomstrand E, Mooren FC, et al. Consensus statement immunonutrition and exercise. *Exerc Immunol Rev* (2017) 23:8–50.
31. Choudhry AJ, Al-Mudaimegh KS, Turkistani AM, Al-Hamdan NA. Hajj-associated acute respiratory infection among hajjis from Riyadh. *East Mediterr Health J* (2006) 12(3–4):300–9.
32. Svendsen IS, Taylor IM, Tonnessen E, Bahr R, Gleeson M. Training-related and competition-related risk factors for respiratory tract and gastrointestinal infections in elite cross-country skiers. *Br J Sports Med* (2016) 50(13):809–15. doi:10.1136/bjsports-2015-095398
33. Gleeson M. Immunological aspects of sport nutrition. *Immunol Cell Biol* (2016) 94(2):117–23. doi:10.1038/icb.2015.109
34. Schwellnus MP, Derman WE, Jordaan E, Page T, Lambert MI, Readhead C, et al. Elite athletes travelling to international destinations >5 time zone differences from their home country have a 2-3-fold increased risk of illness. *Br J Sports Med* (2012) 46(11):816–21. doi:10.1136/bjsports-2012-091395
35. Fondell E, Lagerros YT, Sundberg CJ, Lekander M, Balter O, Rothman KJ, et al. Physical activity, stress, and self-reported upper respiratory tract infection. *Med Sci Sports Exerc* (2011) 43(2):272–9. doi:10.1249/MSS.0b013e3181edf108
36. Martensson S, Nordebo K, Malm C. High training volumes are associated with a low number of self-reported sick days in elite endurance athletes. *J Sports Sci Med* (2014) 13(4):929–33.
37. Hellard P, Avalos M, Guimaraes F, Toussaint JF, Pyne DB. Training-related risk of common illnesses in elite swimmers over a 4-yr period. *Med Sci Sports Exerc* (2015) 47(4):698–707. doi:10.1249/MSS.0000000000000461
38. Hoffman MD, Krishnan E. Health and exercise-related medical issues among 1,212 ultramarathon runners: baseline findings from the Ultrarunners Longitudinal TRAcking (ULTRA) study. *PLoS One* (2014) 9(1):e83867. doi:10.1371/journal.pone.0083867
39. Hoffman MD, Fogard K. Demographic characteristics of 161-km ultramarathon runners. *Res Sports Med* (2012) 20(1):59–69. doi:10.1080/15438627.2012.634707
40. Malm C. Susceptibility to infections in elite athletes: the S-curve. *Scand J Med Sci Sports* (2006) 16(1):4–6. doi:10.1111/j.1600-0838.2005.00499.x
41. Derman W, Schwellnus M, Jordaan E. Clinical characteristics of 385 illnesses of athletes with impairment reported on the WEB-IISS system during the London 2012 Paralympic Games. *PM R* (2014) 6(8 Suppl):S23–30. doi:10.1016/j.pmrj.2014.05.016
42. Bonini M, Gramiccioni C, Fioretti D, Ruckert B, Rinaldi M, Akdis C, et al. Asthma, allergy and the Olympics: a 12-year survey in elite athletes.

Curr Opin Allergy Clin Immunol (2015) 15(2):184–92. doi:10.1097/ACI.0000000000000149
43. Bramley TJ, Lerner D, Sames M. Productivity losses related to the common cold. *J Occup Environ Med* (2002) 44(9):822–9. doi:10.1097/00043764-200209000-00004
44. Fendrick AM, Monto AS, Nightengale B, Sarnes M. The economic burden of non-influenza-related viral respiratory tract infection in the United States. *Arch Intern Med* (2003) 163(4):487–94. doi:10.1001/archinte.163.4.487
45. Bayer C, Remschmidt C, an der Heiden M, Tolksdorf K, Herzhoff M, Kaersten S, et al. Internet-based syndromic monitoring of acute respiratory illness in the general population of Germany, weeks 35/2011 to 34/2012. *Euro Surveill* (2014) 19(4):1–11. doi:10.2807/1560-7917.ES2014.19.4.20684
46. Gleeson M, Pyne DB, Austin JP, Lynn Francis J, Clancy RL, McDonald WA, et al. Epstein-Barr virus reactivation and upper-respiratory illness in elite swimmers. *Med Sci Sports Exerc* (2002) 34(3):411–7. doi:10.1097/00005768-200203000-00005
47. Cox AJ, Gleeson M, Pyne DB, Saunders PU, Clancy RL, Fricker PA. Valtrex therapy for Epstein-Barr virus reactivation and upper respiratory symptoms in elite runners. *Med Sci Sports Exerc* (2004) 36(7):1104–10. doi:10.1249/01.MSS.0000131957.40985.2B
48. Speir E. Cytomegalovirus gene regulation by reactive oxygen species. Agents in atherosclerosis. *Ann N Y Acad Sci* (2000) 899:363–74. doi:10.1111/j.1749-6632.2000.tb06200.x
49. Docke WD, Prosch S, Fietze E, Kimel V, Zuckermann H, Klug C, et al. Cytomegalovirus reactivation and tumour necrosis factor. *Lancet* (1994) 343(8892):268–9. doi:10.1016/S0140-6736(94)91116-9
50. Prösch S, Wendt CEC, Reinke P, Priemer C, Oppert M, Krüger DH, et al. A novel link between stress and human cytomegalovirus (HCMV) infection: sympathetic hyperactivity stimulates HCMV activation. *Virology* (2000) 272:357–65. doi:10.1006/viro.2000.0367
51. He CS, Handzlik M, Muhamad A, Gleeson M. Influence of CMV/EBV serostatus on respiratory infection incidence during 4 months of winter training in a student cohort of endurance athletes. *Eur J Appl Physiol* (2013) 113(10):2613–9. doi:10.1007/s00421-013-2704-x
52. Bishop NC, Gleeson M. Acute and chronic effects of exercise on markers of mucosal immunity. *Front Biosci (Landmark Ed)* (2009) 14:4444–56. doi:10.2741/3540
53. Tomasi TB, Trudeau FB, Czerwinski D, Erredge S. Immune parameters in athletes before and after strenuous exercise. *J Clin Immunol* (1982) 2(3):173–8. doi:10.1007/BF00915219
54. Mackinnon LT, Chick TW, van As A, Tomasi TB. Decreased secretory immunoglobulins following intense endurance exercise. *Sports Train Med Rehabil* (1989) 1:209–18. doi:10.1080/15438628909511878
55. Nieman DC, Henson DA, Fagoaga OR, Utter AC, Vinci DM, Davis JM, et al. Change in salivary IgA following a competitive marathon race. *Int J Sports Med* (2002) 23(1):69–75. doi:10.1055/s-2002-19375
56. Nehlsen-Cannarella SL, Nieman DC, Fagoaga OR, Kelln WJ, Henson DA, Shannon M, et al. Saliva immunoglobulins in elite women rowers. *Eur J Appl Physiol* (2000) 81(3):222–8. doi:10.1007/s004210050034
57. Palmer FM, Nieman DC, Henson DA, McAnulty SR, McAnulty L, Swick NS, et al. Influence of vitamin C supplementation on oxidative and salivary IgA changes following an ultramarathon. *Eur J Appl Physiol* (2003) 89(1):100–7. doi:10.1007/s00421-002-0756-4
58. Steerenberg PA, van Asperen IA, van Nieuw Amerongen A, Biewenga A, Mol D, Medema GJ. Salivary levels of immunoglobulin A in triathletes. *Eur J Oral Sci* (1997) 105(4):305–9. doi:10.1111/j.1600-0722.1997.tb00245.x
59. Nieman DC, Dumke CI, Henson DA, McAnulty SR, McAnulty LS, Lind RH, et al. Immune and oxidative changes during and following the western states endurance run. *Int J Sports Med* (2003) 24(7):541–7. doi:10.1055/s-2003-42018
60. Blannin AK, Robson PJ, Walsh NP, Clark AM, Glennon L, Gleeson M. The effect of exercising to exhaustion at different intensities on saliva immunoglobulin A, protein and electrolyte secretion. *Int J Sports Med* (1998) 19(8):547–52. doi:10.1055/s-2007-971958
61. Killer SC, Svendsen IS, Gleeson M. The influence of hydration status during prolonged endurance exercise on salivary antimicrobial proteins. *Eur J Appl Physiol* (2015) 115(9):1887–95. doi:10.1007/s00421-015-3173-1
62. Allgrove JE, Gomes E, Hough J, Gleeson M. Effects of exercise intensity on salivary antimicrobial proteins and markers of stress in active men. *J Sports Sci* (2008) 26(6):653–61. doi:10.1080/02640410701716790
63. Sari-Sarraf V, Reilly T, Doran DA. Salivary IgA response to intermittent and continuous exercise. *Int J Sports Med* (2006) 27(11):849–55. doi:10.1055/s-2006-923777
64. Reid MR, Drummond PD, Mackinnon LT. The effect of moderate aerobic exercise and relaxation on secretory immunoglobulin A. *Int J Sports Med* (2001) 22(2):132–7. doi:10.1055/s-2001-11347
65. Davison G. Innate immune responses to a single session of sprint interval training. *Appl Physiol Nutr Metab* (2011) 36(3):395–404. doi:10.1139/h11-033
66. Walsh NP, Blannin AK, Clark AM, Cook L, Robson PJ, Gleeson M. The effects of high-intensity intermittent exercise on saliva IgA, total protein and alpha-amylase. *J Sports Sci* (1999) 17(2):129–34. doi:10.1080/026404199366226
67. Peters EM, Shaik J, Kleinveldt N. Upper respiratory tract infection symptoms in ultramarathon runners not related to immunoglobulin status. *Clin J Sport Med* (2010) 20(1):39–46. doi:10.1097/JSM.0b013e3181cb4086
68. Gleeson M, Bishop N, Oliveira M, McCauley T, Tauler P, Muhamad AS. Respiratory infection risk in athletes: association with antigen-stimulated IL-10 production and salivary IgA secretion. *Scand J Med Sci Sports* (2012) 22(3):410–7. doi:10.1111/j.1600-0838.2010.01272.x
69. Gleeson M, Bishop N, Oliveira M, Tauler P. Influence of training load on upper respiratory tract infection incidence and antigen-stimulated cytokine production. *Scand J Med Sci Sports* (2013) 23(4):451–7. doi:10.1111/j.1600-0838.2011.01422.x
70. Brandtzaeg P. Secretory immunity with special reference to the oral cavity. *J Oral Microbiol* (2013) 5:1–24. doi:10.3402/jom.v5i0.20401
71. Marcotte H, Lavoie MC. Oral microbial ecology and the role of salivary immunoglobulin A. *Microbiol Mol Biol Rev* (1998) 62(1):71–109.
72. Needleman I, Ashley P, Petrie A, Fortune F, Turner W, Jones J, et al. Oral health and impact on performance of athletes participating in the London 2012 Olympic Games: a cross-sectional study. *Br J Sports Med* (2013) 47(16):1054–8. doi:10.1136/bjsports-2013-092891
73. Heaney JL, Gleeson M, Phillips AC, Taylor IM, Drayson MT, Goodall M, et al. Salivary immunoglobulin free light chains: reference ranges and responses to exercise in young and older adults. *Exerc Immunol Rev* (2016) 22:28–41.
74. Li TL, Gleeson M. The effect of single and repeated bouts of prolonged cycling and circadian variation on saliva flow rate, immunoglobulin A and alpha-amylase responses. *J Sports Sci* (2004) 22(11–12):1015–24. doi:10.1080/02640410410001716733
75. Engeland CG, Hugo FN, Hilgert JB, Nascimento GG, Junges R, Lim HJ, et al. Psychological distress and salivary secretory immunity. *Brain Behav Immun* (2016) 52:11–7. doi:10.1016/j.bbi.2015.08.017
76. Deslauriers N, Oudghiri M, Seguin J, Trudel L. The oral immune system: dynamics of salivary immunoglobulin production in the inbred mouse. *Immunol Invest* (1986) 15(4):339–49. doi:10.3109/08820138609052953
77. Booth CK, Dwyer DB, Pacque PF, Ball MJ. Measurement of immunoglobulin A in saliva by particle-enhanced nephelometric immunoassay: sample collection, limits of quantitation, precision, stability and reference range. *Ann Clin Biochem* (2009) 46(Pt 5):401–6. doi:10.1258/acb.2009.008248
78. Brandtzaeg P. Do salivary antibodies reliably reflect both mucosal and systemic immunity? *Ann N Y Acad Sci* (2007) 1098:288–311. doi:10.1196/annals.1384.012
79. Hanstock HG, Walsh NP, Edwards JP, Fortes MB, Cosby SL, Nugent A, et al. Tear fluid SIgA as a noninvasive biomarker of mucosal immunity and common cold risk. *Med Sci Sports Exerc* (2016) 48(3):569–77. doi:10.1249/MSS.0000000000000801
80. Gleeson M, Pyne DB, Elkington LJ, Hall ST, Attia JR, Oldmeadow C, et al. Developing a multi-component immune model for evaluating the risk of respiratory illness in athletes. *Exerc Immunol Rev* (2017) 23:52–64.
81. Campbell JP, Riddell NE, Burns VE, Turner M, van Zanten JJ, Drayson MT, et al. Acute exercise mobilises CD8+ T lymphocytes exhibiting an effector-memory phenotype. *Brain Behav Immun* (2009) 23(6):767–75. doi:10.1016/j.bbi.2009.02.011
82. Shephard RJ. Adhesion molecules, catecholamines and leucocyte redistribution during and following exercise. *Sports Med* (2003) 33(4):261–84. doi:10.2165/00007256-200333040-00002

83. Benschop RJ, Nijkamp FP, Ballieux RE, Heijnen CJ. The effects of beta-adrenoceptor stimulation on adhesion of human natural killer cells to cultured endothelium. *Br J Pharmacol* (1994) 113(4):1311–6. doi:10.1111/j.1476-5381.1994.tb17141.x
84. Kruger K, Lechtermann A, Fobker M, Volker K, Mooren FC. Exercise-induced redistribution of T lymphocytes is regulated by adrenergic mechanisms. *Brain Behav Immun* (2008) 22(3):324–38. doi:10.1016/j.bbi.2007.08.008
85. Dimitrov S, Lange T, Born J. Selective mobilization of cytotoxic leukocytes by epinephrine. *J Immunol* (2010) 184(1):503–11. doi:10.4049/jimmunol.0902189
86. Turner JE, Spielmann G, Wadley AJ, Aldred S, Simpson RJ, Campbell JP. Exercise-induced B cell mobilisation: preliminary evidence for an influx of immature cells into the bloodstream. *Physiol Behav* (2016) 164(Pt A):376–82. doi:10.1016/j.physbeh.2016.06.023
87. Kruger K, Alack K, Ringseis R, Mink L, Pfeifer E, Schinle M, et al. Apoptosis of T-cell subsets after acute high-intensity interval exercise. *Med Sci Sports Exerc* (2016) 48(10):2021–9. doi:10.1249/MSS.0000000000000979
88. Clifford T, Wood MJ, Stocks P, Howatson G, Stevenson EJ, Hilkens CMU. T-regulatory cells exhibit a biphasic response to prolonged endurance exercise in humans. *Eur J Appl Physiol* (2017) 117(8):1727–37. doi:10.1007/s00421-017-3667-0
89. Shek PN, Sabiston BH, Buguet A, Radomski MW. Strenuous exercise and immunological changes: a multiple-time-point analysis of leukocyte subsets, CD4/CD8 ratio, immunoglobulin production and NK cell response. *Int J Sports Med* (1995) 16(7):466–74. doi:10.1055/s-2007-973039
90. Shinkai S, Shore S, Shek PN, Shephard RJ. Acute exercise and immune function. Relationship between lymphocyte activity and changes in subset counts. *Int J Sports Med* (1992) 13(6):452–61. doi:10.1055/s-2007-1021297
91. Kakanis MW, Peake J, Brenu EW, Simmonds M, Gray B, Hooper SL, et al. The open window of susceptibility to infection after acute exercise in healthy young male elite athletes. *Exerc Immunol Rev* (2010) 16:119–37.
92. Pedersen BK, Ullum H. NK cell response to physical activity: possible mechanisms of action. *Med Sci Sports Exerc* (1994) 26(2):140–6. doi:10.1249/00005768-199402000-00003
93. Dhabhar FS. Effects of stress on immune function: the good, the bad, and the beautiful. *Immunol Res* (2014) 58(2–3):193–210. doi:10.1007/s12026-014-8517-0
94. Kruger K, Mooren FC. T cell homing and exercise. *Exerc Immunol Rev* (2007) 13:37–54.
95. Mooren FC, Kruger K. Apoptotic lymphocytes induce progenitor cell mobilization after exercise. *J Appl Physiol (1985)* (2015) 119(2):135–9. doi:10.1152/japplphysiol.00287.2015
96. Mars M, Govender S, Weston A, Naicker V, Chuturgoon A. High intensity exercise: a cause of lymphocyte apoptosis? *Biochem Biophys Res Commun* (1998) 249(2):366–70. doi:10.1006/bbrc.1998.9156
97. Mooren FC, Lechtermann A, Volker K. Exercise-induced apoptosis of lymphocytes depends on training status. *Med Sci Sports Exerc* (2004) 36(9):1476–83. doi:10.1249/01.MSS.0000139897.34521.E9
98. Mooren FC, Bloming D, Lechtermann A, Lerch MM, Volker K. Lymphocyte apoptosis after exhaustive and moderate exercise. *J Appl Physiol* (2002) 93(1):147–53. doi:10.1152/japplphysiol.01262.2001
99. Tanimura Y, Shimizu K, Tanabe K, Otsuki T, Yamauchi R, Matsubara Y, et al. Exercise-induced oxidative DNA damage and lymphocytopenia in sedentary young males. *Med Sci Sports Exerc* (2008) 40(8):1455–62. doi:10.1249/MSS.0b013e31817242cf
100. Simpson RJ, Florida-James GD, Whyte GP, Black JR, Ross JA, Guy K. Apoptosis does not contribute to the blood lymphocytopenia observed after intensive and downhill treadmill running in humans. *Res Sports Med* (2007) 15(3):157–74. doi:10.1080/15438620701405339
101. Shephard RJ, Shek PN. Effects of exercise and training on natural killer cell counts and cytolytic activity: a meta-analysis. *Sports Med* (1999) 28(3):177–95. doi:10.2165/00007256-199928030-00003
102. Hansen JB, Wilsgard L, Osterud B. Biphasic changes in leukocytes induced by strenuous exercise. *Eur J Appl Physiol Occup Physiol* (1991) 62(3):157–61. doi:10.1007/BF00643735
103. Freud AG, Caligiuri MA. Human natural killer cell development. *Immunol Rev* (2006) 214:56–72. doi:10.1111/j.1600-065X.2006.00451.x
104. Poli A, Michel T, Theresine M, Andres E, Hentges F, Zimmer J. CD56bright natural killer (NK) cells: an important NK cell subset. *Immunology* (2009) 126(4):458–65. doi:10.1111/j.1365-2567.2008.03027.x
105. Bjorkstrom NK, Riese P, Heuts F, Andersson S, Fauriat C, Ivarsson MA, et al. Expression patterns of NKG2A, KIR, and CD57 define a process of CD56dim NK-cell differentiation uncoupled from NK-cell education. *Blood* (2010) 116(19):3853–64. doi:10.1182/blood-2010-04-281675
106. Lopez-Verges S, Milush JM, Pandey S, York VA, Arakawa-Hoyt J, Pircher H, et al. CD57 defines a functionally distinct population of mature NK cells in the human CD56dimCD16+ NK-cell subset. *Blood* (2010) 116(19):3865–74. doi:10.1182/blood-2010-04-282301
107. Bigley AB, Rezvani K, Chew C, Sekine T, Pistillo M, Crucian B, et al. Acute exercise preferentially redeploys NK-cells with a highly-differentiated phenotype and augments cytotoxicity against lymphoma and multiple myeloma target cells. *Brain Behav Immun* (2014) 39:160–71. doi:10.1016/j.bbi.2013.10.030
108. Bigley AB, Rezvani K, Pistillo M, Reed J, Agha N, Kunz H, et al. Acute exercise preferentially redeploys NK-cells with a highly-differentiated phenotype and augments cytotoxicity against lymphoma and multiple myeloma target cells. Part II: impact of latent cytomegalovirus infection and catecholamine sensitivity. *Brain Behav Immun* (2015) 49:59–65. doi:10.1016/j.bbi.2014.12.027
109. Simpson RJ, Florida-James GD, Cosgrove C, Whyte GP, Macrae S, Pircher H, et al. High-intensity exercise elicits the mobilization of senescent T lymphocytes into the peripheral blood compartment in human subjects. *J Appl Physiol (1985)* (2007) 103(1):396–401. doi:10.1152/japplphysiol.00007.2007
110. Simpson RJ, Cosgrove C, Ingram LA, Florida-James GD, Whyte GP, Pircher H, et al. Senescent T-lymphocytes are mobilised into the peripheral blood compartment in young and older humans after exhaustive exercise. *Brain Behav Immun* (2008) 22(4):544–51. doi:10.1016/j.bbi.2007.11.002
111. Simpson RJ, Cosgrove C, Chee MM, McFarlin BK, Bartlett DB, Spielmann G, et al. Senescent phenotypes and telomere lengths of peripheral blood T-cells mobilized by acute exercise in humans. *Exerc Immunol Rev* (2010) 16:40–55.
112. Pedersen L, Idorn M, Olofsson GH, Lauenborg B, Nookaew I, Hansen RH, et al. Voluntary running suppresses tumor growth through epinephrine- and IL-6-dependent NK cell mobilization and redistribution. *Cell Metab* (2016) 23(3):554–62. doi:10.1016/j.cmet.2016.01.011
113. Kim R, Emi M, Tanabe K. Cancer immunoediting from immune surveillance to immune escape. *Immunology* (2007) 121(1):1–14. doi:10.1111/j.1365-2567.2007.02587.x
114. Scheiermann C, Kunisaki Y, Frenette PS. Circadian control of the immune system. *Nat Rev Immunol* (2013) 13(3):190–8. doi:10.1038/nri3386
115. Suzuki K, Hayano Y, Nakai A, Furuta F, Noda M. Adrenergic control of the adaptive immune response by diurnal lymphocyte recirculation through lymph nodes. *J Exp Med* (2016) 213(12):2567–74. doi:10.1084/jem.20160723
116. Dimitrov S, Benedict C, Heutling D, Westermann J, Born J, Lange T. Cortisol and epinephrine control opposing circadian rhythms in T cell subsets. *Blood* (2009) 113(21):5134–43. doi:10.1182/blood-2008-11-190769
117. Hojman P. Exercise protects from cancer through regulation of immune function and inflammation. *Biochem Soc Trans* (2017) 45(4):905–11. doi:10.1042/BST20160466
118. Turner JE, Wadley AJ, Aldred S, Fisher JP, Bosch JA, Campbell JP. Intensive exercise does not preferentially mobilize skin-homing T cells and NK cells. *Med Sci Sports Exerc* (2016) 48(7):1285–93. doi:10.1249/MSS.0000000000000914
119. Hanson ED, Danson E, Nguyen-Robertson CV, Fyfe JJ, Stepto NK, Bartlett DB, et al. Maximal exercise increases mucosal associated invariant T cell frequency and number in healthy young men. *Eur J Appl Physiol* (2017) 117(11):2159–69. doi:10.1007/s00421-017-3704-z
120. Gross E, Sunwoo JB, Bui JD. Cancer immunosurveillance and immunoediting by natural killer cells. *Cancer J* (2013) 19(6):483–9. doi:10.1097/PPO.0000000000000005
121. Simpson RJ, Bigley AB, Agha N, Hanley PJ, Bollard CM. Mobilizing immune cells with exercise for cancer immunotherapy. *Exerc Sport Sci Rev* (2017) 45(3):163–72. doi:10.1249/JES.0000000000000114
122. Moore SC, Lee IM, Weiderpass E, Campbell PT, Sampson JN, Kitahara CM, et al. Association of leisure-time physical activity with risk of 26 types of

cancer in 1.44 million adults. *JAMA Intern Med* (2016) 176(6):816–25. doi:10.1001/jamainternmed.2016.1548
123. Turner JE, Aldred S, Witard OC, Drayson MT, Moss PM, Bosch JA. Latent cytomegalovirus infection amplifies CD8 T-lymphocyte mobilisation and egress in response to exercise. *Brain Behav Immun* (2010) 24(8):1362–70. doi:10.1016/j.bbi.2010.07.239
124. Lancaster GI, Khan Q, Drysdale PT, Wallace F, Jeukendrup AE, Drayson MT, et al. Effect of prolonged exercise and carbohydrate ingestion on type 1 and type 2 T lymphocyte distribution and intracellular cytokine production in humans. *J Appl Physiol (1985)* (2005) 98(2):565–71. doi:10.1152/japplphysiol.00754.2004
125. Starkie RL, Rolland J, Febbraio MA. Effect of adrenergic blockade on lymphocyte cytokine production at rest and during exercise. *Am J Physiol Cell Physiol* (2001) 281(4):C1233–40. doi:10.1152/ajpcell.2001.281.4.C1233
126. Siedlik JA, Deckert JA, Benedict SH, Bhatta A, Dunbar AJ, Vardiman JP, et al. T cell activation and proliferation following acute exercise in human subjects is altered by storage conditions and mitogen selection. *J Immunol Methods* (2017) 446:7–14. doi:10.1016/j.jim.2017.03.017
127. Siedlik JA, Benedict SH, Landes EJ, Weir JP, Vardiman JP, Gallagher PM. Acute bouts of exercise induce a suppressive effect on lymphocyte proliferation in human subjects: a meta-analysis. *Brain Behav Immun* (2016) 56:343–51. doi:10.1016/j.bbi.2016.04.008
128. Zimmer P, Schenk A, Kieven M, Holthaus M, Lehmann J, Lovenich L, et al. Exercise induced alterations in NK-cell cytotoxicity – methodological issues and future perspectives. *Exerc Immunol Rev* (2017) 23:66–81.
129. McFarlin BK, Venable AS, Carpenter CK, Henning AL, Stephan O. Oral supplementation with baker's yeast beta glucan is associated with altered monocytes, T cells and cytokines following a bout of strenuous exercise. *Front Physiol* (2017) 8:786. doi:10.3389/fphys.2017.00786
130. Witard OC, Turner JE, Jackman SR, Kies AK, Jeukendrup AE, Bosch JA, et al. High dietary protein restores overreaching induced impairments in leukocyte trafficking and reduces the incidence of upper respiratory tract infection in elite cyclists. *Brain Behav Immun* (2014) 39:211–9. doi:10.1016/j.bbi.2013.10.002
131. Albers R, Bourdet-Sicard R, Braun D, Calder PC, Herz U, Lambert C, et al. Monitoring immune modulation by nutrition in the general population: identifying and substantiating effects on human health. *Br J Nutr* (2013) 110(Suppl 2):S1–30. doi:10.1017/S0007114513001505
132. Burns VE, Gallagher S. Antibody response to vaccination as a marker of in vivo immune function in psychophysiological research. *Neurosci Biobehav Rev* (2010) 35(1):122–6. doi:10.1016/j.neubiorev.2010.01.005
133. Edwards KM, Burns VE, Reynolds T, Carroll D, Drayson M, Ring C. Acute stress exposure prior to influenza vaccination enhances antibody response in women. *Brain Behav Immun* (2006) 20(2):159–68. doi:10.1016/j.bbi.2005.07.001
134. Edwards KM, Burns VE, Allen LM, McPhee JS, Bosch JA, Carroll D, et al. Eccentric exercise as an adjuvant to influenza vaccination in humans. *Brain Behav Immun* (2007) 21(2):209–17. doi:10.1016/j.bbi.2006.04.158
135. Edwards KM, Burns VE, Adkins AE, Carroll D, Drayson M, Ring C. Meningococcal A vaccination response is enhanced by acute stress in men. *Psychosom Med* (2008) 70(2):147–51. doi:10.1097/PSY.0b013e318164232e
136. Edwards KM, Campbell JP, Ring C, Drayson MT, Bosch JA, Downes C, et al. Exercise intensity does not influence the efficacy of eccentric exercise as a behavioural adjuvant to vaccination. *Brain Behav Immun* (2010) 24(4):623–30. doi:10.1016/j.bbi.2010.01.009
137. Edwards KM, Pung MA, Tomfohr LM, Ziegler MG, Campbell JP, Drayson MT, et al. Acute exercise enhancement of pneumococcal vaccination response: a randomised controlled trial of weaker and stronger immune response. *Vaccine* (2012) 30(45):6389–95. doi:10.1016/j.vaccine.2012.08.022
138. Ranadive SM, Cook M, Kappus RM, Yan H, Lane AD, Woods JA, et al. Effect of acute aerobic exercise on vaccine efficacy in older adults. *Med Sci Sports Exerc* (2014) 46(3):455–61. doi:10.1249/MSS.0b013e3182a75ff2
139. Long JE, Ring C, Drayson M, Bosch J, Campbell JP, Bhabra J, et al. Vaccination response following aerobic exercise: can a brisk walk enhance antibody response to pneumococcal and influenza vaccinations? *Brain Behav Immun* (2012) 26(4):680–7. doi:10.1016/j.bbi.2012.02.004
140. Edwards KM, Pascoe AR, Fiatarone-Singh MA, Singh NA, Kok J, Booy R. A randomised controlled trial of resistance exercise prior to administration of influenza vaccination in older adults. *Brain Behav Immun* (2015) 49:e24–5. doi:10.1016/j.bbi.2015.06.102
141. Furman D, Hejblum BP, Simon N, Jojic V, Dekker CL, Thiebaut R, et al. Systems analysis of sex differences reveals an immunosuppressive role for testosterone in the response to influenza vaccination. *Proc Natl Acad Sci U S A* (2014) 111(2):869–74. doi:10.1073/pnas.1321060111
142. Trigunaite A, Dimo J, Jorgensen TN. Suppressive effects of androgens on the immune system. *Cell Immunol* (2015) 294(2):87–94. doi:10.1016/j.cellimm.2015.02.004
143. Haq K, McElhaney JE. Immunosenescence: influenza vaccination and the elderly. *Curr Opin Immunol* (2014) 29:38–42. doi:10.1016/j.coi.2014.03.008
144. Kohut ML, Cooper MM, Nickolaus MS, Russell DR, Cunnick JE. Exercise and psychosocial factors modulate immunity to influenza vaccine in elderly individuals. *J Gerontol A Biol Sci Med Sci* (2002) 57(9):M557–62. doi:10.1093/gerona/57.9.M557
145. Kohut ML, Arntson BA, Lee W, Rozeboom K, Yoon KJ, Cunnick JE, et al. Moderate exercise improves antibody response to influenza immunization in older adults. *Vaccine* (2004) 22(17–18):2298–306. doi:10.1016/j.vaccine.2003.11.023
146. Smith TP, Kennedy SL, Fleshner M. Influence of age and physical activity on the primary in vivo antibody and T cell-mediated responses in men. *J Appl Physiol (1985)* (2004) 97(2):491–8. doi:10.1152/japplphysiol.01404.2003
147. Schuler PB, Leblanc PA, Marzilli TS. Effect of physical activity on the production of specific antibody in response to the 1998–99 influenza virus vaccine in older adults. *J Sports Med Phys Fitness* (2003) 43(3):404.
148. Grant RW, Mariani RA, Vieira VJ, Fleshner M, Smith TP, Keylock KT, et al. Cardiovascular exercise intervention improves the primary antibody response to keyhole limpet hemocyanin (KLH) in previously sedentary older adults. *Brain Behav Immun* (2008) 22(6):923–32. doi:10.1016/j.bbi.2008.01.006
149. Woods JA, Keylock KT, Lowder T, Vieira VJ, Zelkovich W, Dumich S, et al. Cardiovascular exercise training extends influenza vaccine seroprotection in sedentary older adults: the immune function intervention trial. *J Am Geriatr Soc* (2009) 57(12):2183–91. doi:10.1111/j.1532-5415.2009.02563.x
150. Yang Y, Verkuilen J, Rosengren KS, Mariani RA, Reed M, Grubisich SA, et al. Effects of a traditional Taiji/Qigong curriculum on older adults' immune response to influenza vaccine. *Med Sport Sci* (2008) 52:64–76. doi:10.1159/000134285
151. de Araujo AL, Silva LC, Fernandes JR, Matias Mde S, Boas LS, Machado CM, et al. Elderly men with moderate and intense training lifestyle present sustained higher antibody responses to influenza vaccine. *Age (Dordr)* (2015) 37(6):105. doi:10.1007/s11357-015-9843-4
152. Kapasi ZF, Catlin PA, Joyner DR, Lewis ML, Schwartz AL, Townsend EL. The effects of intense physical exercise on secondary antibody response in young and old mice. *Phys Ther* (2000) 80(11):1076–86.
153. Grande AJ, Reid H, Thomas EE, Nunan D, Foster C. Exercise prior to influenza vaccination for limiting influenza incidence and its related complications in adults. *Cochrane Database Syst Rev* (2016) (8):CD011857. doi:10.1002/14651858.CD011857.pub2
154. Warren K, Thompson N, Wannemuehler M, Kohut M. Antibody and CD8+ T cell memory response to influenza A/PR/8/34 infection is reduced in treadmill-exercised mice, yet still protective. *J Appl Physiol (1985)* (2013) 114(10):1413–20. doi:10.1152/japplphysiol.01355.2012
155. Sim YJ, Yu S, Yoon KJ, Loiacono CM, Kohut ML. Chronic exercise reduces illness severity, decreases viral load, and results in greater anti-inflammatory effects than acute exercise during influenza infection. *J Infect Dis* (2009) 200(9):1434–42. doi:10.1086/606014
156. Lowder T, Padgett DA, Woods JA. Moderate exercise protects mice from death due to influenza virus. *Brain Behav Immun* (2005) 19(5):377–80. doi:10.1016/j.bbi.2005.04.002
157. Nosbaum A, Vocanson M, Rozieres A, Hennino A, Nicolas JF. Allergic and irritant contact dermatitis. *Eur J Dermatol* (2009) 19(4):325–32. doi:10.1684/ejd.2009.0686
158. Gulati N, Suarez-Farinas M, Fuentes-Duculan J, Gilleaudeau P, Sullivan-Whalen M, Correa da Rosa J, et al. Molecular characterization of human skin response to diphencyprone at peak and resolution phases: therapeutic insights. *J Invest Dermatol* (2014) 134(10):2531–40. doi:10.1038/jid.2014.196

159. Diment BC, Fortes MB, Edwards JP, Hanstock HG, Ward MD, Dunstall HM, et al. Exercise intensity and duration effects on in vivo immunity. *Med Sci Sports Exerc* (2015) 47(7):1390–8. doi:10.1249/MSS.0000000000000562
160. Harper Smith AD, Coakley SL, Ward MD, Macfarlane AW, Friedmann PS, Walsh NP. Exercise-induced stress inhibits both the induction and elicitation phases of in vivo T-cell-mediated immune responses in humans. *Brain Behav Immun* (2011) 25(6):1136–42. doi:10.1016/j.bbi.2011.02.014
161. Ceddia MA, Price EA, Kohlmeier CK, Evans JK, Lu Q, McAuley E, et al. Differential leukocytosis and lymphocyte mitogenic response to acute maximal exercise in the young and old. *Med Sci Sports Exerc* (1999) 31(6):829–36. doi:10.1097/00005768-199906000-00011
162. Woods JA, Evans JK, Wolters BW, Ceddia MA, McAuley E. Effects of maximal exercise on natural killer (NK) cell cytotoxicity and responsiveness to interferon-alpha in the young and old. *J Gerontol A Biol Sci Med Sci* (1998) 53(6):B430–7. doi:10.1093/gerona/53A.6.B430
163. Simpson RJ, Lowder TW, Spielmann G, Bigley AB, LaVoy EC, Kunz H. Exercise and the aging immune system. *Ageing Res Rev* (2012) 11(3):404–20. doi:10.1016/j.arr.2012.03.003
164. Kohut ML, Senchina DS. Reversing age-associated immunosenescence via exercise. *Exerc Immunol Rev* (2004) 10:6–41.
165. Woods JA, Lowder TW, Keylock KT. Can exercise training improve immune function in the aged? *Ann N Y Acad Sci* (2002) 959:117–27. doi:10.1111/j.1749-6632.2002.tb02088.x
166. Simpson RJ, Bigley AB, Spielmann G, LaVoy EC, Kunz H, Bollard CM. Human cytomegalovirus infection and the immune response to exercise. *Exerc Immunol Rev* (2016) 22:8–27.
167. Bartlett DB, Fox O, McNulty CL, Greenwood HL, Murphy L, Sapey E, et al. Habitual physical activity is associated with the maintenance of neutrophil migratory dynamics in healthy older adults. *Brain Behav Immun* (2016) 56:12–20. doi:10.1016/j.bbi.2016.02.024
168. Bartlett DB, Shepherd SO, Wilson OJ, Adlan AM, Wagenmakers AJM, Shaw CS, et al. Neutrophil and monocyte bactericidal responses to 10 weeks of low-volume high-intensity interval or moderate-intensity continuous training in sedentary adults. *Oxid Med Cell Longev* (2017) 2017:8148742. doi:10.1155/2017/8148742
169. Shephard RJ. Development of the discipline of exercise immunology. *Exerc Immunol Rev* (2010) 16:194–222.
170. Hazeldine J, Lord JM. Innate immunesenescence: underlying mechanisms and clinical relevance. *Biogerontology* (2015) 16(2):187–201. doi:10.1007/s10522-014-9514-3
171. Peralbo E, Alonso C, Solana R. Invariant NKT and NKT-like lymphocytes: two different T cell subsets that are differentially affected by ageing. *Exp Gerontol* (2007) 42(8):703–8. doi:10.1016/j.exger.2007.05.002
172. Ziegler-Heitbrock L, Ancuta P, Crowe S, Dalod M, Grau V, Hart DN, et al. Nomenclature of monocytes and dendritic cells in blood. *Blood* (2010) 116(16):e74–80. doi:10.1182/blood-2010-02-258558
173. Goh J, Ladiges WC. Exercise enhances wound healing and prevents cancer progression during aging by targeting macrophage polarity. *Mech Ageing Dev* (2014) 139:41–8. doi:10.1016/j.mad.2014.06.004
174. Kanneganti TD, Dixit VD. Immunological complications of obesity. *Nat Immunol* (2012) 13(8):707–12. doi:10.1038/ni.2343
175. Garg SK, Delaney C, Shi H, Yung R. Changes in adipose tissue macrophages and T cells during aging. *Crit Rev Immunol* (2014) 34(1):1–14. doi:10.1615/CritRevImmunol.2013006833
176. Kratz M, Coats BR, Hisert KB, Hagman D, Mutskov V, Peris E, et al. Metabolic dysfunction drives a mechanistically distinct proinflammatory phenotype in adipose tissue macrophages. *Cell Metab* (2014) 20(4):614–25. doi:10.1016/j.cmet.2014.08.010
177. Bourlier V, Zakaroff-Girard A, Miranville A, De Barros S, Maumus M, Sengenes C, et al. Remodeling phenotype of human subcutaneous adipose tissue macrophages. *Circulation* (2008) 117(6):806–15. doi:10.1161/CIRCULATIONAHA.107.724096
178. Zeyda M, Farmer D, Todoric J, Aszmann O, Speiser M, Gyori G, et al. Human adipose tissue macrophages are of an anti-inflammatory phenotype but capable of excessive pro-inflammatory mediator production. *Int J Obes (Lond)* (2007) 31(9):1420–8. doi:10.1038/sj.ijo.0803632
179. Xu X, Grijalva A, Skowronski A, van Eijk M, Serlie MJ, Ferrante AW Jr. Obesity activates a program of lysosomal-dependent lipid metabolism in adipose tissue macrophages independently of classic activation. *Cell Metab* (2013) 18(6):816–30. doi:10.1016/j.cmet.2013.11.001
180. Chavez-Galan L, Olleros ML, Vesin D, Garcia I. Much more than M1 and M2 macrophages, there are also CD169(+) and TCR(+) macrophages. *Front Immunol* (2015) 6:263. doi:10.3389/fimmu.2015.00263
181. Mills CD. Anatomy of a discovery: m1 and m2 macrophages. *Front Immunol* (2015) 6:212. doi:10.3389/fimmu.2015.00212
182. Bueno V, Sant'Anna OA, Lord JM. Ageing and myeloid-derived suppressor cells: possible involvement in immunosenescence and age-related disease. *Age (Dordr)* (2014) 36(6):9729. doi:10.1007/s11357-014-9729-x
183. Shearer GM. Th1/Th2 changes in aging. *Mech Ageing Dev* (1997) 94(1–3):1–5.
184. Schmitt V, Rink L, Uciechowski P. The Th17/Treg balance is disturbed during aging. *Exp Gerontol* (2013) 48(12):1379–86. doi:10.1016/j.exger.2013.09.003
185. Fulop T, Larbi A, Pawelec G. Human T cell aging and the impact of persistent viral infections. *Front Immunol* (2013) 4:271. doi:10.3389/fimmu.2013.00271
186. Pawelec G. Hallmarks of human "immunosenescence": adaptation or dysregulation? *Immun Ageing* (2012) 9(1):15. doi:10.1186/1742-4933-9-15
187. Geiger H, de Haan G, Florian MC. The ageing haematopoietic stem cell compartment. *Nat Rev Immunol* (2013) 13(5):376–89. doi:10.1038/nri3433
188. Roux A, Mourin G, Larsen M, Fastenackels S, Urrutia A, Gorochov G, et al. Differential impact of age and cytomegalovirus infection on the gamma-delta T cell compartment. *J Immunol* (2013) 191(3):1300–6. doi:10.4049/jimmunol.1202940
189. Colonna-Romano G, Aquino A, Bulati M, Lio D, Candore G, Oddo G, et al. Impairment of gamma/delta T lymphocytes in elderly: implications for immunosenescence. *Exp Gerontol* (2004) 39(10):1439–46. doi:10.1016/j.exger.2004.07.005
190. Michishita Y, Hirokawa M, Guo YM, Abe Y, Liu J, Ubukawa K, et al. Age-associated alteration of gammadelta T-cell repertoire and different profiles of activation-induced death of Vdelta1 and Vdelta2 T cells. *Int J Hematol* (2011) 94(3):230–40. doi:10.1007/s12185-011-0907-7
191. Jagger A, Shimojima Y, Goronzy JJ, Weyand CM. Regulatory T cells and the immune aging process: a mini-review. *Gerontology* (2014) 60(2):130–7. doi:10.1159/000355303
192. Siegrist CA, Aspinall R. B-cell responses to vaccination at the extremes of age. *Nat Rev Immunol* (2009) 9(3):185–94. doi:10.1038/nri2508
193. Appay V, Sauce D. Naive T cells: the crux of cellular immune aging? *Exp Gerontol* (2014) 54:90–3. doi:10.1016/j.exger.2014.01.003
194. Pawelec G. Immunosenenescence: role of cytomegalovirus. *Exp Gerontol* (2013) 54:1–5. doi:10.1016/j.exger.2013.11.010
195. Wikby A, Maxson P, Olsson J, Johansson B, Ferguson FG. Changes in CD8 and CD4 lymphocyte subsets, T cell proliferation responses and non-survival in the very old: the Swedish longitudinal OCTO-immune study. *Mech Ageing Dev* (1998) 102(2–3):187–98. doi:10.1016/S0047-6374(97)00151-6
196. Pawelec G, Ferguson FG, Wikby A. The SENIEUR protocol after 16 years. *Mech Ageing Dev* (2001) 122(2):132–4. doi:10.1016/S0047-6374(00)00240-2
197. Wikby A, Johansson B, Ferguson F, Olsson J. Age-related changes in immune parameters in a very old population of Swedish people: a longitudinal study. *Exp Gerontol* (1994) 29(5):531–41. doi:10.1016/0531-5565(94)90036-1
198. Wikby A, Nilsson BO, Forsey R, Thompson J, Strindhall J, Lofgren S, et al. The immune risk phenotype is associated with IL-6 in the terminal decline stage: findings from the Swedish NONA immune longitudinal study of very late life functioning. *Mech Ageing Dev* (2006) 127(8):695–704. doi:10.1016/j.mad.2006.04.003
199. Wikby A, Ferguson F, Forsey R, Thompson J, Strindhall J, Lofgren S, et al. An immune risk phenotype, cognitive impairment, and survival in very late life: impact of allostatic load in Swedish octogenarian and nonagenarian humans. *J Gerontol A Biol Sci Med Sci* (2005) 60(5):556–65. doi:10.1093/gerona/60.5.556
200. Olsson J, Wikby A, Johansson B, Lofgren S, Nilsson BO, Ferguson FG. Age-related change in peripheral blood T-lymphocyte subpopulations and cytomegalovirus infection in the very old: the Swedish longitudinal OCTO immune study. *Mech Ageing Dev* (2000) 121(1–3):187–201. doi:10.1016/S0047-6374(00)00210-4
201. Franceschi C, Bonafe M, Valensin S, Olivieri F, De Luca M, Ottaviani E, et al. Inflamm-aging. An evolutionary perspective on immunosenescence. *Ann N Y Acad Sci* (2000) 908:244–54. doi:10.1111/j.1749-6632.2000.tb06651.x

202. Franceschi C, Capri M, Monti D, Giunta S, Olivieri F, Sevini F, et al. Inflammaging and anti-inflammaging: a systemic perspective on aging and longevity emerged from studies in humans. *Mech Ageing Dev* (2007) 128(1):92–105. doi:10.1016/j.mad.2006.11.016
203. Giovannini S, Onder G, Liperoti R, Russo A, Carter C, Capoluongo E, et al. Interleukin-6, C-reactive protein, and tumor necrosis factor-alpha as predictors of mortality in frail, community-living elderly individuals. *J Am Geriatr Soc* (2011) 59(9):1679–85. doi:10.1111/j.1532-5415.2011.03570.x
204. Baune BT, Rothermundt M, Ladwig KH, Meisinger C, Berger K. Systemic inflammation (interleukin 6) predicts all-cause mortality in men: results from a 9-year follow-up of the MEMO Study. *Age (Dordr)* (2011) 33(2): 209–17. doi:10.1007/s11357-010-9165-5
205. Bruunsgaard H, Ladelund S, Pedersen AN, Schroll M, Jorgensen T, Pedersen BK. Predicting death from tumour necrosis factor-alpha and interleukin-6 in 80-year-old people. *Clin Exp Immunol* (2003) 132(1):24–31. doi:10.1046/j.1365-2249.2003.02137.x
206. McElhaney JE, Kuchel GA, Zhou X, Swain SL, Haynes L. T-cell immunity to influenza in older adults: a pathophysiological framework for development of more effective vaccines. *Front Immunol* (2016) 7:41. doi:10.3389/fimmu.2016.00041
207. Frasca D, Blomberg BB. Aging, cytomegalovirus (CMV) and influenza vaccine responses. *Hum Vaccin Immunother* (2016) 12(3):682–90. doi:10.1080/21645515.2015.1105413
208. Brown FF, Bigley AB, Sherry C, Neal CM, Witard OC, Simpson RJ, et al. Training status and sex influence on senescent T-lymphocyte redistribution in response to acute maximal exercise. *Brain Behav Immun* (2014) 39:152–9. doi:10.1016/j.bbi.2013.10.031
209. Brown FF, Bigley AB, Ross JC, LaVoy EC, Simpson RJ, Galloway SD. T-lymphocyte populations following a period of high volume training in female soccer players. *Physiol Behav* (2015) 152(Pt A):175–81. doi:10.1016/j.physbeh.2015.09.027
210. Gustafson MP, DiCostanzo AC, Wheatley CM, Kim CH, Bornschlegl S, Gastineau DA, et al. A systems biology approach to investigating the influence of exercise and fitness on the composition of leukocytes in peripheral blood. *J Immunother Cancer* (2017) 5:30. doi:10.1186/s40425-017-0231-8
211. Prieto-Hinojosa A, Knight A, Compton C, Gleeson M, Travers PJ. Reduced thymic output in elite athletes. *Brain Behav Immun* (2014) 39:75–9. doi:10.1016/j.bbi.2014.01.004
212. Moro-Garcia MA, Fernandez-Garcia B, Echeverria A, Rodriguez-Alonso M, Suarez-Garcia FM, Solano-Jaurrieta JJ, et al. Frequent participation in high volume exercise throughout life is associated with a more differentiated adaptive immune response. *Brain Behav Immun* (2014) 39:61–74. doi:10.1016/j.bbi.2013.12.014
213. Teixeira AM, Rama L, Carvalho HM, Borges G, Carvalheiro T, Gleeson M, et al. Changes in naive and memory T-cells in elite swimmers during a winter training season. *Brain Behav Immun* (2014) 39:186–93. doi:10.1016/j.bbi.2014.01.002
214. Cosgrove C, Galloway SD, Neal C, Hunter AM, McFarlin BK, Spielmann G, et al. The impact of 6-month training preparation for an Ironman triathlon on the proportions of naive, memory and senescent T cells in resting blood. *Eur J Appl Physiol* (2012) 112(8):2989–98. doi:10.1007/s00421-011-2273-9
215. Dopico XC, Evangelou M, Ferreira RC, Guo H, Pekalski ML, Smyth DJ, et al. Widespread seasonal gene expression reveals annual differences in human immunity and physiology. *Nat Commun* (2015) 6:7000. doi:10.1038/ncomms8000
216. Goldinger A, Shakhbazov K, Henders AK, McRae AF, Montgomery GW, Powell JE. Seasonal effects on gene expression. *PLoS One* (2015) 10(5): e0126995. doi:10.1371/journal.pone.0126995
217. Spielmann G, McFarlin BK, O'Connor DP, Smith PJ, Pircher H, Simpson RJ. Aerobic fitness is associated with lower proportions of senescent blood T-cells in man. *Brain Behav Immun* (2011) 25(8):1521–9. doi:10.1016/j.bbi.2011.07.226
218. Silva LC, de Araujo AL, Fernandes JR, Matias Mde S, Silva PR, Duarte AJ, et al. Moderate and intense exercise lifestyles attenuate the effects of aging on telomere length and the survival and composition of T cell subpopulations. *Age (Dordr)* (2016) 38(1):24. doi:10.1007/s11357-016-9879-0
219. Duggal NA, Pollock RD, Lazarus NR, Harridge S, Lord JM. Major features of immunesenescence, including reduced thymic output, are ameliorated by high levels of physiacl activity in adulthood. *Aging Cell* (2018). doi:10.1111/acel.12750
220. Shimizu K, Kimura F, Akimoto T, Akama T, Tanabe K, Nishijima T, et al. Effect of moderate exercise training on T-helper cell subpopulations in elderly people. *Exerc Immunol Rev* (2008) 14:24–37.
221. Cao Dinh H, Beyer I, Mets T, Onyema OO, Njemini R, Renmans W, et al. Effects of physical exercise on markers of cellular immunosenescence: a systematic review. *Calcif Tissue Int* (2017) 100(2):193–215. doi:10.1007/s00223-016-0212-9
222. Kruger K, Frost S, Most E, Volker K, Pallauf J, Mooren FC. Exercise affects tissue lymphocyte apoptosis via redox-sensitive and Fas-dependent signaling pathways. *Am J Physiol Regul Integr Comp Physiol* (2009) 296(5):R1518–27. doi:10.1152/ajpregu.90994.2008
223. Khan N, Shariff N, Cobbold M, Bruton R, Ainsworth JA, Sinclair AJ, et al. Cytomegalovirus seropositivity drives the CD8 T cell repertoire toward greater clonality in healthy elderly individuals. *J Immunol* (2002) 169(4):1984–92. doi:10.4049/jimmunol.169.4.1984
224. Mueller YM, De Rosa SC, Hutton JA, Witek J, Roederer M, Altman JD, et al. Increased CD95/Fas-induced apoptosis of HIV-specific CD8(+) T cells. *Immunity* (2001) 15(6):871–82. doi:10.1016/S1074-7613(01)00246-1
225. Wang JS, Lin CT. Systemic hypoxia promotes lymphocyte apoptosis induced by oxidative stress during moderate exercise. *Eur J Appl Physiol* (2010) 108(2):371–82. doi:10.1007/s00421-009-1231-2
226. Takahashi A, Hanson MG, Norell HR, Havelka AM, Kono K, Malmberg KJ, et al. Preferential cell death of CD8+ effector memory (CCR7-CD45RA-) T cells by hydrogen peroxide-induced oxidative stress. *J Immunol* (2005) 174(10):6080–7. doi:10.4049/jimmunol.174.10.6080
227. Stocchi R, Ward KN, Fanin R, Baccarani M, Apperley JF. Management of human cytomegalovirus infection and disease after allogeneic bone marrow transplantation. *Haematologica* (1999) 84(1):71–9.
228. Derhovanessian E, Maier AB, Hahnel K, Zelba H, de Craen AJ, Roelofs H, et al. Lower proportion of naive peripheral CD8+ T cells and an unopposed pro-inflammatory response to human cytomegalovirus proteins in vitro are associated with longer survival in very elderly people. *Age (Dordr)* (2013) 35(4):1387–99. doi:10.1007/s11357-012-9425-7
229. Sylwester AW, Mitchell BL, Edgar JB, Taormina C, Pelte C, Ruchti F, et al. Broadly targeted human cytomegalovirus-specific CD4+ and CD8+ T cells dominate the memory compartments of exposed subjects. *J Exp Med* (2005) 202(5):673–85. doi:10.1084/jem.20050882
230. Franceschi C, Bonafe M, Valensin S. Human immunosenescence: the prevailing of innate immunity, the failing of clonotypic immunity, and the filling of immunological space. *Vaccine* (2000) 18(16):1717–20. doi:10.1016/S0264-410X(99)00513-7
231. Akbar AN, Fletcher JM. Memory T cell homeostasis and senescence during aging. *Curr Opin Immunol* (2005) 17(5):480–5. doi:10.1016/j.coi.2005.07.019
232. van Leeuwen EM, Koning JJ, Remmerswaal EB, van Baarle D, van Lier RA, ten Berge IJ. Differential usage of cellular niches by cytomegalovirus versus EBV- and influenza virus-specific CD8+ T cells. *J Immunol* (2006) 177(8): 4998–5005. doi:10.4049/jimmunol.177.8.4998
233. Huster KM, Stemberger C, Gasteiger G, Kastenmuller W, Drexler I, Busch DH. Cutting edge: memory CD8 T cell compartment grows in size with immunological experience but nevertheless can lose function. *J Immunol* (2009) 183(11):6898–902. doi:10.4049/jimmunol.0902454
234. Ferrando-Martinez S, Franco JM, Ruiz-Mateos E, Hernandez A, Ordonez A, Gutierrez E, et al. A reliable and simplified sj/beta-TREC ratio quantification method for human thymic output measurement. *J Immunol Methods* (2010) 352(1–2):111–7. doi:10.1016/j.jim.2009.11.007
235. Radtke F, MacDonald HR, Tacchini-Cottier F. Regulation of innate and adaptive immunity by Notch. *Nat Rev Immunol* (2013) 13(6):427–37. doi:10.1038/nri3445
236. Haugen F, Norheim F, Lian H, Wensaas AJ, Dueland S, Berg O, et al. IL-7 is expressed and secreted by human skeletal muscle cells. *Am J Physiol Cell Physiol* (2010) 298(4):C807–16. doi:10.1152/ajpcell.00094.2009
237. Fry TJ, Mackall CL. The many faces of IL-7: from lymphopoiesis to peripheral T cell maintenance. *J Immunol* (2005) 174(11):6571–6. doi:10.4049/jimmunol.174.11.6571
238. Tchernof A, Despres JP. Pathophysiology of human visceral obesity: an update. *Physiol Rev* (2013) 93(1):359–404. doi:10.1152/physrev.00033.2011
239. Trim W, Turner JE, Thompson D. Parallels in immunometabolic adipose tissue dysfunction with ageing and obesity. *Front Immunol* (2018) 9:169. doi:10.3389/fimmu.2018.00169

240. Nieman DC, Henson DA, Nehlsen-Cannarella SL, Ekkens M, Utter AC, Butterworth DE, et al. Influence of obesity on immune function. *J Am Diet Assoc* (1999) 99(3):294–9. doi:10.1016/S0002-8223(99)00077-2
241. Muezzinler A, Zaineddin AK, Brenner H. Body mass index and leukocyte telomere length in adults: a systematic review and meta-analysis. *Obes Rev* (2014) 15(3):192–201. doi:10.1111/obr.12126
242. van der Weerd K, Dik WA, Schrijver B, Schweitzer DH, Langerak AW, Drexhage HA, et al. Morbidly obese human subjects have increased peripheral blood CD4+ T cells with skewing toward a Treg- and Th2-dominated phenotype. *Diabetes* (2012) 61(2):401–8. doi:10.2337/db11-1065
243. Alam I, Larbi A, Pawelec G. Nutritional status influences peripheral immune cell phenotypes in healthy men in rural Pakistan. *Immun Ageing* (2012) 9(1):16. doi:10.1186/1742-4933-9-16
244. Spielmann G, Johnston CA, O'Connor DP, Foreyt JP, Simpson RJ. Excess body mass is associated with T cell differentiation indicative of immune ageing in children. *Clin Exp Immunol* (2014) 176(2):246–54. doi:10.1111/cei.12267
245. Costanzo AE, Taylor KR, Dutt S, Han PP, Fujioka K, Jameson JM. Obesity impairs gammadelta T cell homeostasis and antiviral function in humans. *PLoS One* (2015) 10(3):e0120918. doi:10.1371/journal.pone.0120918
246. Aroor AR, DeMarco VG. Oxidative stress and obesity: the chicken or the egg? *Diabetes* (2014) 63(7):2216–8. doi:10.2337/db14-0424
247. Gleeson M, Bishop NC, Stensel DJ, Lindley MR, Mastana SS, Nimmo MA. The anti-inflammatory effects of exercise: mechanisms and implications for the prevention and treatment of disease. *Nat Rev Immunol* (2011) 11(9): 607–15. doi:10.1038/nri3041
248. Radak Z, Chung HY, Goto S. Systemic adaptation to oxidative challenge induced by regular exercise. *Free Radic Biol Med* (2008) 44(2):153–9. doi:10.1016/j.freeradbiomed.2007.01.029
249. Henson SM, Lanna A, Riddell NE, Franzese O, Macaulay R, Griffiths SJ, et al. p38 signaling inhibits mTORC1-independent autophagy in senescent human CD8(+) T cells. *J Clin Invest* (2014) 124(9):4004–16. doi:10.1172/JCI75051

14

Septic Shock and the Aging Process: A Molecular Comparison

Fabiano Pinheiro da Silva and Marcel Cerqueira César Machado*

Laboratório de Emergências Clínicas, Faculdade de Medicina FMUSP, Universidade de São Paulo, São Paulo, Brazil

***Correspondence:**
Fabiano Pinheiro da Silva
pinheirofabiano@hotmail.com

Aging is a continuous process promoted by both intrinsic and extrinsic factors that each trigger a multitude of molecular events. Increasing evidence supports a central role for inflammation in this progression. Here, we discuss how the low-grade chronic inflammation that characterizes aging is tightly interconnected with other important aspects of this process, such as DNA damage, mitochondrial dysfunction, and epigenetic changes. Similarly, inflammation also plays a critical role in many morbid conditions that affect patients who are admitted to Intensive Care. Although the inflammatory response is low grade and persistent in healthy aging while it is acute and severe in critically ill states, we hypothesize that both situations have important interconnections. Here, we performed an extensive review of the literature to investigate this potential link. Because sepsis is the most extensively studied disease and is the leading cause of death in Critical Care, we focus our discussion on comparing the inflammatory profile of healthy older people with that of patients in septic shock to explain why we believe that both situations have synergistic effects, leading to critically ill aged patients having a worse prognosis when compared with critically ill young patients.

Keywords: aging, systemic inflammation, immunity, sepsis, critical care

INTRODUCTION

Over time, improved health conditions have led to a steady growth in the older population, resulting in a substantial increase in the number of critically ill-aged patients. In addition, advanced age is associated with a worse outcome in all of the most frequent critical care conditions (1).

Chronic, low-grade, systemic inflammation, and the deregulation of several innate and acquired immune responses have been reported in seniors (2). The signaling pathways implicated in this scenario, called inflammaging, create a complex network (3–7) that is probably triggered and perpetuated by prolonged exposure to varied exogenous and endogenous factors, such as infection, tissue injury, DNA damage, mitochondrial dysfunction, intestinal barrier failure, and dysbiosis (8–10) and may contribute to the increased risk of acute illnesses, disability, and death in this population (11). Indeed, inappropriate inflammation and metabolic stress lead to the accumulation of senescent cells, which are characterized by transcriptional and epigenetic alterations that determine cell cycle arrest, as well as aberrant mRNA production and maturation, chromatin structure changes, and impaired proteostasis (12, 13). Moreover, emergency myelopoiesis and the persistence of immature myeloid cell progenitors have been shown to be significant contributors to dysfunctional inflammation in sepsis and are emerging in aging research (14, 15).

Pathogen-associated molecular patterns are molecules shared by many microorganisms, but not found in mammals, that are recognized by the immune system and activate cell defense. Several host factors are also able to alarm the immune system, even in sterile conditions. Indeed, persistent or recurrent contact with microbes (16), as well as with non-infectious danger signals, induce the production of damage-associated molecular patterns (DAMPs), which accumulate during aging (17). Examples include adenosine triphosphate, high mobility group box 1 protein, oxidized lipoproteins, heat shock proteins, and urate and cholesterol crystals. These DAMPs are able to activate membrane receptors and cytosolic receptors (including inflammasomes) or act directly at the nuclear level, inducing gene transcription (16, 18). Moreover, accumulating evidence suggests that mitochondrial and genomic DNA and histones also activate danger signals and induce systemic protection (19). For example, levels of circulating cell-free DNA, presumably released from damaged or dying cells, are increased in older adults (20) and are associated with both mortality and the magnitude of the inflammatory response (21–23). Similarly, critical inflammatory conditions, such as sepsis, are also characterized by high levels of circulating host DNA (24, 25).

Many nucleic acid molecular sensors have been found (26). CpG-enriched DNA, such as mitochondrial and bacterial DNA, are mostly recognized by TLR9 (21, 27), but other systems to detect not only mitochondrial and microbial DNA but also the nuclear DNA that migrates to the cytosol under pathologic conditions have been described (28–31). Furthermore, inside the nucleus, a sophisticated system of DNA sensors is able to detect DNA damage and activate immune signaling (31). In parallel, harmful DNA coming from pathogens, apoptotic cells, or DNA replication byproducts can be directly degraded by DNases to avoid the excessive activation of immune cascades (31).

Enduring Permanent Aggression: From Mitochondrial Dysfunction to Genomic Instability

Aging is accompanied by a decline in mitochondrial function in all tissues; however, some tissues, such as the muscles, are particularly affected (32). Beyond their function in bioenergetics, growing research suggests that mitochondria participate in many other mechanisms that are deregulated in senescence (33). Indeed, mitochondria are important organelles in the maintenance of stem cells (12), the activation of the unfolded protein response (34), the regulation of innate and adaptive immune pathways (35, 36), and the modulation of the metabolic profile of the cell (32). As such, mitochondria are deeply integrated into cellular homeostasis (37).

Similarly, mitochondrial dysfunction is a common finding in a wide range of patients in critical care conditions (38–41). Pro-inflammatory mediators and oxidative stress impair the function of the respiratory chain enzyme complexes and damage the mitochondrial structure, including their genes (42, 43). While the genomic DNA can be affected in a similar manner, the mitochondrial DNA is likely more vulnerable to this type of damage due to its close location to the electron transport chain, its lack of protective histones, the limited efficiency of the mtDNA repair mechanisms, and the fact that, like bacterial DNA, it exclusively contains coding regions (44, 45). However, a single-cell contains thousands of mitochondrial genomes, and mutations of all of them in the same gene are unlikely, putting the nuclear genome at a higher risk (46). An excellent publication from Patananan et al. describes the current challenges to therapeutically modifying the mitochondrial genome and the important concept of heteroplasmy (47). Furthermore, emerging evidence suggests that DNA damage activates signaling from the nucleus to the mitochondria, creating complex networks that are crucial for mitochondria maintenance (48).

The genetic lesions arising from DNA damage include point mutations, translocations, gains, losses, strand breaks, and telomere shortening. DNA lesions occur frequently, even under physiological conditions (49). These genetic changes have a well-established impact on the aging process and have been largely investigated as both a cause and consequence of chronic low-grade inflammation. The same process may occur in the critically ill; however, it seems to occur over a short-time period and be massive in this population, while it is low-grade and persistent during aging.

The occurrence of DNA damage induces further immune activation, promoting a vicious circle with disastrous consequences (50). Indeed, there is increasing evidence pointing to reciprocal interactions between DNA damage, DNA repair, and the immune system (51). In the short term, depending on the intensity of damage or the presence of deficient DNA repair responses (52–54), genotoxic stress has the potential to induce aberrant cell responses, apoptosis, organ failure, and immunosuppression (19, 43). The occurrence and magnitude of acute DNA lesions in the setting of severe systemic inflammation, however, remain to be confirmed. In the long term, these plausible DNA mutations and deletions can significantly impact patient quality of life and predispose the survivors of inflammatory catastrophes to several morbid consequences. In this regard, a recent publication from our group showed that sepsis induces telomere shortening (55), confirming that inflammation affects telomere length (56) and that stress-induced premature senescence is a telomere-dependent process (57). Despite that, however, the other evidence in the literature addressing this topic is controversial and/or indirect. The phenotype of sepsis survivors, for example, resembles accelerated aging, and sepsis survivors suffer from a higher risk of additional morbidities, such as cardiovascular disease, cognitive impairment, tumor progression, and possibly death, for years following the sepsis event (58–60).

Since genomic instability is a hallmark of aging, genetic damage secondary to severe infection or other causes of critical illnesses may have a larger impact in seniors than in young patients. We believe that this is a critical factor that partially explains the worse outcome of older people, compared with the young, when affected by overwhelming inflammatory syndromes.

Redox reactions generate oxidatively modified signaling biomolecules that are crucial for the generation of appropriate innate and adaptive cell responses (35) and for many other fundamental biological processes (61–63). Reactive oxygen and nitrogen species have important physiological effects and display various well-established specific signaling functions, but they need to be tightly regulated; otherwise, they can generate significant tissue damage (64). Oxidative damage occurs to a larger extent both in older people and in the presence of acute or chronic inflammatory processes. It can lead to substantial DNA damage and significantly contribute to genomic instability and mitochondrial dysfunction. A DNA microarray study performed by our group found that the oxidative phosphorylation and the mitochondrial dysfunction pathways were the most-enriched pathways in septic patients of advanced age when compared with the young septic group (65).

The Epigenetic Code: An Additional Layer of Complexity

Epigenetic changes involve various histone marks, DNA methylation, nucleosome positioning, and mechanisms governed by non-coding RNAs that are able to repress or activate transcription (66). Epigenetic alterations are important aspects in the regulation of aging, linking environmental factors with the genetic profile (67). We believe epigenetic modifications may be implicated in the global modifications to the cell response that manifest during the evolution of catastrophic inflammatory processes, especially those caused by overwhelming infection. In support of this hypothesis, a recent publication reported that sepsis in humans induces selective and precise chromatin modifications in distinct promoter regions of immunologically relevant genes (68). Cellular dysfunction secondary to genetic and epigenetic changes in the course of major inflammatory syndromes may be stochastic and partially reversible, even though some organs and tissues appear to be more strongly affected. Moreover, DNA regions that are robustly activated are likely more influenced since they are less protected than the heterochromatin. Unfortunately, this topic remains obscure in the critically ill. However, it could potentially explain, for example, the long-term cognitive impairment that is frequently detected in survivors of septic shock and other intriguing findings, such as the phenomenon of endotoxin tolerance (69).

There is a significant interconnection between the DNA damage response and epigenetic changes. DNA damage is a serious threat to cell viability, compromising the integrity of both the genome and the epigenome. The DNA damage response can lead to significant alterations in chromatin structure, affecting chromatin components and epigenetic marks, with major implications for cell metabolism (70). As stated by López-León and Goya, "aging seems to be characterized by a progressive depression of the transcriptional activity of chromatin" (71); this has been partially attributed to a reduction in DNA methylation and an altered chromatin architecture (72). The end result of epigenetic changes is aberrant gene expression, reactivation of transposable elements, and genomic instability (73).

There is increasing evidence that together with the above discussed factors, microRNAs and long non-coding RNAs also play a key role in fundamental epigenetic processes, with important implications for the aging process and various morbid states (74–76).

Aging and Critical Illnesses: From Low-grade to Explosive Inflammation

The treatment of critically ill aged patients is challenging. Older people frequently exhibit atypical symptomatology, due to comorbidities and dysfunctions throughout all body systems that are related to the aging process (77).

Sepsis is a disease of the elderly. The incidence of sepsis increases exponentially with age, and sepsis-associated long-term sequelae particularly affect older patients. Sepsis survivors are at substantial risk for poor quality of life, functional disability, and cognitive impairment. As advances in medicine and quality of life extend the life expectancy worldwide, a growing number of aged patients need critical care (78). A recent study demonstrated a significant rise in survivorship after sepsis in the United States, caused by a rising incidence of sepsis rather than improvements in its case fatality rate, generating a substantial population burden of aged patients with disabilities (79).

The reason for the higher susceptibility to infection and increased mortality in older adults remains in debate (80). The basal inflammatory state found in healthy seniors suggests that aged people possess a limited capacity to control inflammation. Similarly, the critically ill are frequently affected by overwhelming inflammatory syndromes, where the host response is the major cause of damage. Examples include diseases such as septic shock, severe acute pancreatitis, burns, trauma, ischemia reperfusion injuries, and hemorrhages. As discussed earlier, the chronic low-grade inflammation in the elderly and the explosive inflammation in the critically ill share several commonalities. We propose that, together, these processes may have synergistic effects, leading to a worse outcome (**Figure 1**).

Notably, these synergistic effects have interesting peculiarities. A study performed by our group found that older people are as immunocompetent as young individuals regarding the cytokines, chemokines, and growth factors produced in response to devastating infections. After our analysis of several inflammatory mediators in the plasma of critically ill individuals, we were unable to find any reason that could serve to better explain why the aged show an increased susceptibility and mortality to septic shock (81). As detailed in the section below, this phenomenon can be partially explained by the fact that aged people probably display a prolonged inflammatory systemic response under acute stress conditions, when compared with the systemic response of the young, even though both groups share the same ability to trigger and sustain the same intensity of inflammatory signaling in the acute phase (81). Moreover, in a study performed in rats, we were able to demonstrate that despite a similar systemic response, aged rats show increased intestinal gene expression levels of TNFα, α-defensin 5, and α-defensin 7, when compared with young rats (82). Similarly, other work from our group demonstrated greater gene expression levels of COX-2 and intercellular junction proteins in the guts of aged rats with acute pancreatitis when compared with young rats in the same conditions, suggesting that, in situations of intestinal damage, the young animals are better able to restore intestinal barrier integrity (83). The results of these studies strongly suggest that the inflammatory response of the elderly is compartmentalized, with significant differences in the inflammatory profile depending on the organ under investigation.

For many years, the catastrophic systemic inflammation associated with many critical care diseases has been attributed to a massive and transient activation of the innate immune system, followed by a period of immunosuppression (84, 85). Seminal high-throughput gene expression studies performed

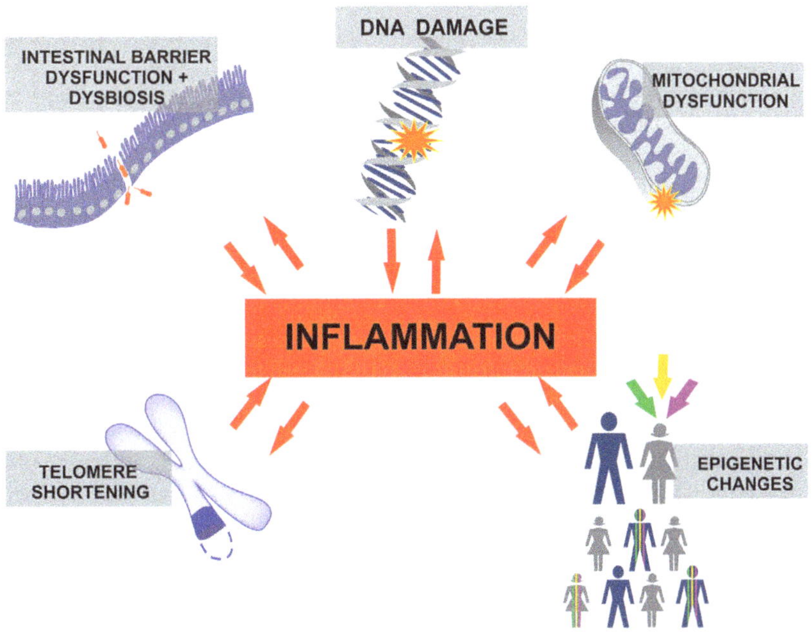

FIGURE 1 | The inflammation that characterizes healthy aging and the inflammatory processes in several critical care conditions differ in duration and intensity, but both involve similar molecular interconnections where inflammation plays a central role.

in septic patients by the Wong group, however, challenge this theory. Indeed, instead of the classical biphasic curve, they have consistently detected an elliptical curve, formed by the persistent activation of innate immune genes in conjunction with widespread repression of gene programs corresponding to the adaptive immune system (86–88). Confirming these findings, a similar pattern was found in trauma patients (89), suggesting that infectious and non-infectious systemic inflammation in the critically ill may involve analogous cell responses. Notably, more recent studies are finding subtle differences in the transcriptional program of different acute stress conditions and even in different subsets of the same morbid process (90).

Maintenance of the Intestinal Epithelial Barrier and the Human Microbiome

The intestinal mucosal barrier is a fundamental line of defense against undesirable luminal contents, such as microorganisms, toxins, and antigens, preventing their entrance into the bloodstream. It is mostly composed of epithelial cells, immune components, and mucus. Some researchers also consider the microbiome as part of the intestinal barrier (9, 91), since it helps to maintain the integrity of the intestinal barrier, providing nutrients and protecting against pathogens.

Aged people are in a persistent systemic inflammatory state that may be partially attributed to increased bacterial translocation, secondary to intestinal barrier dysfunction (92). As people age, the intestinal barrier weakens, partially due to decreased levels of tight junctions connecting epithelial cells, and the enteric immune system becomes ineffective (93). Indeed, higher plasma levels of lipopolysaccharide can be detected in the blood of older subjects, when compared with young individuals (94, 95). Furthermore, there is a shift in the intestinal microbiome after the age of 65, with an increased abundance of Bacteroidetes phyla (96) and a reduction in the capacity of the microbiota to carry out metabolic processes, such as short-chain fatty acid production (97). We propose that these previous alterations to the intestinal barrier in the elderly are probably exacerbated during systemic inflammation processes. In support of this idea, Zhang et al. recently demonstrated that neutrophil activation and aging are both affected by the intestinal microbiota and that depletion of the microbiome with broad-spectrum antibiotics significantly reduces the number of circulating aged neutrophils, ameliorating inflammation-related organ damage in a model of endotoxin shock (98). Another recent publication showed that germ-free mice do not display the increase in circulating cytokines that is a hallmark of aging and that co-housing germ-free mice with old, but not young, conventionally raised mice reconstitutes this phenotype; the authors concluded that, in mice, intestinal permeability increases with age due to microbial dysbiosis (99). Taken together, these observations suggest that the increased mortality of aged patients in critical care conditions is probably due to a prolonged systemic inflammatory response, at least partially caused by increased bacterial translocation and defective bacterial clearance (100).

Microbiome studies are challenging because there is extensive inter-individual variability, even among healthy subjects. Genetic, lifestyle, and environmental factors, such as diet, physical activity, geography, and exposure to xenobiotics, all cause substantial modifications to the intestinal microbiome. However, despite this extensive interindividual variability, specialists agree on the existence of a global human core microbiota (101, 102).

Commensal bacteria have much shorter generation times than humans and consequently undergo rapid evolutionary changes, adapting quickly to environmental changes. Unfortunately, external forces sometimes shape a microbiome that is detrimental to the host, a state called dysbiosis. Once established, dysbiosis can exert profound effects on the immune system, creating a feedback loop in which host factors and the microbiome (cell components and metabolites) regulate each other, perpetuating the dysbiotic state (103). It is well established that the intestinal microbiota is severely modified during critical illnesses. However, it remains unclear which change occurs first.

The causal mechanisms of dysbiosis in the critically ill are not completely understood, but they likely result from many intrinsic and extrinsic factors, such as widespread antibiotics use, hypoxic injury, inflammation, intestinal dysmotility, epithelial barrier disruption, vasopressors treatment, and sedation (104). The intestinal microbiome of the critically ill differs substantially from that of healthy individuals and is characterized by lower phylogenetic diversity, commensal microbe loss, and pathobiont overgrowth (105, 106).

CONCLUDING REMARKS

Older adults in critical care conditions develop a peculiar inflammatory response, which is associated with poorer outcomes. Current treatments are unspecific and mainly rely on life support techniques. Novel strategies are under investigation (99), and Personalized Medicine has been widely discussed to improve care of the critically ill (107); however, to a large extend, these proposals still remain experimental and hypothetical, without impacting clinical applications. Thus, manipulation of the inflammatory storms that are so frequent in Critical Care remains a challenging task, filled with negative results and nebulous findings. Prolonged hospital stays, recurrent infections, decrepitude, and malnutrition characterize the critically ill population as a whole, but particularly apply to the subset composed of aged adults.

By the other hand, impressive advances in the molecular biology of aging are emerging. Biomarkers of aging have been extensively investigated to guide tailored treatments of the aging process, as well as to detect individuals that age faster (108). Despite the current challenges (109–111), *in vivo* partial cellular reprogramming (112), direct reprogramming (109), and epigenetic interventions (67) are tentative highways for drug development and captivating platforms to reach this goal. Indeed, the rapid advancement of scientific knowledge in this field provides hope that, in a not-so-distant future, sophisticated medical technologies to delay and even reverse normal aging might be available.

AUTHOR CONTRIBUTIONS

FPS conceived and wrote the manuscript. MCCM contributed with suggestions and ideas.

ACKNOWLEDGMENTS

English editing was performed by Edanz.

REFERENCES

1. Joyce MF, Reich JA. Critical care issues of the geriatric patient. *Anesthesiol Clin* (2015) 33(3):551–61. doi:10.1016/j.anclin.2015.05.009
2. Shaw AC, Joshi S, Greenwood H, Panda A, Lord JM. Aging of the innate immune system. *Curr Opin Immunol* (2010) 22(4):507–13. doi:10.1016/j.coi.2010.05.003
3. Ruan Q, Qian F, Yu Z. Effects of polymorphisms in immunity-related genes on the immune system and successful aging. *Curr Opin Immunol* (2014) 29:49–55. doi:10.1016/j.coi.2014.04.003
4. Johnson SC, Dong X, Vijg J, Suh Y. Genetic evidence for common pathways in human age-related diseases. *Aging Cell* (2015) 14(5):809–17. doi:10.1111/acel.12362
5. Ter Horst R, Jaeger M, Smeekens SP, Oosting M, Swertz MA, Li Y, et al. Host and environmental factors influencing individual human cytokine responses. *Cell* (2016) 167(4):1111–1124e1113. doi:10.1016/j.cell.2016.10.018
6. Xia S, Zhang X, Zheng S, Khanabdali R, Kalionis B, Wu J, et al. An update on inflamm-aging: mechanisms, prevention, and treatment. *J Immunol Res* (2016) 2016:8426874. doi:10.1155/2016/8426874
7. Fulop T, Witkowski JM, Le Page A, Fortin C, Pawelec G, Larbi A. Intracellular signalling pathways: targets to reverse immunosenescence. *Clin Exp Immunol* (2017) 187(1):35–43. doi:10.1111/cei.12836
8. Goldberg EL, Dixit VD. Drivers of age-related inflammation and strategies for healthspan extension. *Immunol Rev* (2015) 265(1):63–74. doi:10.1111/imr.12295
9. Cesar Machado MC, da Silva FP. Intestinal barrier dysfunction in human pathology and aging. *Curr Pharm Des* (2016) 22(30):4645–50. doi:10.2174/1381612822666160510125331
10. He S, Sharpless NE. Senescence in health and disease. *Cell* (2017) 169(6):1000–11. doi:10.1016/j.cell.2017.05.015
11. High KP, Akbar AN, Nikolich-Zugich J. Translational research in immune senescence: assessing the relevance of current models. *Semin Immunol* (2012) 24(5):373–82. doi:10.1016/j.smim.2012.04.007
12. Lopez-Otin C, Blasco MA, Partridge L, Serrano M, Kroemer G. The hallmarks of aging. *Cell* (2013) 153(6):1194–217. doi:10.1016/j.cell.2013.05.039
13. Kirkland JL, Tchkonia T. Cellular senescence: a translational perspective. *EBioMedicine* (2017) 21:21–8. doi:10.1016/j.ebiom.2017.04.013
14. Flores RR, Clauson CL, Cho J, Lee BC, McGowan SJ, Baker DJ, et al. Expansion of myeloid-derived suppressor cells with aging in the bone marrow of mice through a NF-kappaB-dependent mechanism. *Aging Cell* (2017) 16(3):480–7. doi:10.1111/acel.12571
15. Mathias B, Delmas AL, Ozrazgat-Baslanti T, Vanzant EL, Szpila BE, Mohr AM, et al. Human myeloid-derived suppressor cells are associated with chronic immune suppression after severe sepsis/septic shock. *Ann Surg* (2017) 265(4):827–34. doi:10.1097/SLA.0000000000001783
16. Kang JW, Kim SJ, Cho HI, Lee SM. DAMPs activating innate immune responses in sepsis. *Ageing Res Rev* (2015) 24(Pt A):54–65. doi:10.1016/j.arr.2015.03.003
17. Kapetanovic R, Bokil NJ, Sweet MJ. Innate immune perturbations, accumulating DAMPs and inflammasome dysregulation: a ticking time bomb in ageing. *Ageing Res Rev* (2015) 24(Pt A):40–53. doi:10.1016/j.arr.2015.02.005
18. Feldman N, Rotter-Maskowitz A, Okun E. DAMPs as mediators of sterile inflammation in aging-related pathologies. *Ageing Res Rev* (2015) 24 (Pt A):29–39. doi:10.1016/j.arr.2015.01.003
19. Poliezhaieva T, Ermolaeva MA. DNA damage in protective and adverse inflammatory responses: friend of foe? *Mech Ageing Dev* (2017) 165 (Pt A):47–53. doi:10.1016/j.mad.2016.06.004
20. Bandaranayake T, Shaw AC. Host resistance and immune aging. *Clin Geriatr Med* (2016) 32(3):415–32. doi:10.1016/j.cger.2016.02.007

21. Zhang Q, Raoof M, Chen Y, Sumi Y, Sursal T, Junger W, et al. Circulating mitochondrial DAMPs cause inflammatory responses to injury. *Nature* (2010) 464(7285):104–7. doi:10.1038/nature08780
22. Nakahira K, Haspel JA, Rathinam VA, Lee SJ, Dolinay T, Lam HC, et al. Autophagy proteins regulate innate immune responses by inhibiting the release of mitochondrial DNA mediated by the NALP3 inflammasome. *Nat Immunol* (2011) 12(3):222–30. doi:10.1038/ni.1980
23. Jylhava J, Jylha M, Lehtimaki T, Hervonen A, Hurme M. Circulating cell-free DNA is associated with mortality and inflammatory markers in nonagenarians: the Vitality 90+ Study. *Exp Gerontol* (2012) 47(5):372–8. doi:10.1016/j.exger.2012.02.011
24. Rhodes A, Cecconi M. Cell-free DNA and outcome in sepsis. *Crit Care* (2012) 16(6):170. doi:10.1186/cc11508
25. Hamaguchi S, Akeda Y, Yamamoto N, Seki M, Yamamoto K, Oishi K, et al. Origin of circulating free DNA in sepsis: analysis of the CLP mouse model. *Mediators Inflamm* (2015) 2015:614518. doi:10.1155/2015/614518
26. Gasser S, Zhang WY, Tan NY, Tripathi S, Suter MA, Chew ZH, et al. Sensing of dangerous DNA. *Mech Ageing Dev* (2016) 165(Pt A):33–46. doi:10.1016/j.mad.2016.09.001
27. Magna M, Pisetsky DS. The alarmin properties of DNA and DNA-associated nuclear proteins. *Clin Ther* (2016) 38(5):1029–41. doi:10.1016/j.clinthera.2016.02.029
28. Ablasser A, Goldeck M, Cavlar T, Deimling T, Witte G, Rohl I, et al. cGAS produces a 2'-5'-linked cyclic dinucleotide second messenger that activates STING. *Nature* (2013) 498(7454):380–4. doi:10.1038/nature12306
29. Xiao TS, Fitzgerald KA. The cGAS-STING pathway for DNA sensing. *Mol Cell* (2013) 51(2):135–9. doi:10.1016/j.molcel.2013.07.004
30. Liu L, Yang M, Kang R, Dai Y, Yu Y, Gao F, et al. HMGB1-DNA complex-induced autophagy limits AIM2 inflammasome activation through RAGE. *Biochem Biophys Res Commun* (2014) 450(1):851–6. doi:10.1016/j.bbrc.2014.06.074
31. Nakad R, Schumacher B. DNA damage response and immune defense: links and mechanisms. *Front Genet* (2016) 7:147. doi:10.3389/fgene.2016.00147
32. Sun N, Youle RJ, Finkel T. The mitochondrial basis of aging. *Mol Cell* (2016) 61(5):654–66. doi:10.1016/j.molcel.2016.01.028
33. Hill S, Van Remmen H. Mitochondrial stress signaling in longevity: a new role for mitochondrial function in aging. *Redox Biol* (2014) 2:936–44. doi:10.1016/j.redox.2014.07.005
34. Durieux J, Wolff S, Dillin A. The cell-non-autonomous nature of electron transport chain-mediated longevity. *Cell* (2011) 144(1):79–91. doi:10.1016/j.cell.2010.12.016
35. Mills EL, Kelly B, O'Neill LAJ. Mitochondria are the powerhouses of immunity. *Nat Immunol* (2017) 18(5):488–98. doi:10.1038/ni.3704
36. Sancho D, Enamorado M, Garaude J. Innate immune function of mitochondrial metabolism. *Front Immunol* (2017) 8:527. doi:10.3389/fimmu.2017.00527
37. Bohovych I, Khalimonchuk O. Sending out an SOS: mitochondria as a signaling hub. *Front Cell Dev Biol* (2016) 4:109. doi:10.3389/fcell.2016.00109
38. Wendel M, Heller AR. Mitochondrial function and dysfunction in sepsis. *Wien Med Wochenschr* (2010) 160(5–6):118–23. doi:10.1007/s10354-010-0766-5
39. Galley HF. Oxidative stress and mitochondrial dysfunction in sepsis. *Br J Anaesth* (2011) 107(1):57–64. doi:10.1093/bja/aer093
40. Chakraborty M, Hickey AJ, Petrov MS, Macdonald JR, Thompson N, Newby L, et al. Mitochondrial dysfunction in peripheral blood mononuclear cells in early experimental and clinical acute pancreatitis. *Pancreatology* (2016) 16(5):739–47. doi:10.1016/j.pan.2016.06.659
41. Picca A, Lezza AMS, Leeuwenburgh C, Pesce V, Calvani R, Landi F, et al. Fueling inflamm-aging through mitochondrial dysfunction: mechanisms and molecular targets. *Int J Mol Sci* (2017) 18(5):ii:E933. doi:10.3390/ijms18050933
42. Suliman HB, Carraway MS, Piantadosi CA. Postlipopolysaccharide oxidative damage of mitochondrial DNA. *Am J Respir Crit Care Med* (2003) 167(4):570–9. doi:10.1164/rccm.200206-518OC
43. Kozlov AV, Lancaster JR Jr, Meszaros AT, Weidinger A. Mitochondria-meditated pathways of organ failure upon inflammation. *Redox Biol* (2017) 13:170–81. doi:10.1016/j.redox.2017.05.017
44. Ozawa T. Mitochondrial genome mutation in cell death and aging. *J Bioenerg Biomembr* (1999) 31(4):377–90. doi:10.1023/A:1005479920097
45. Van Remmen H, Richardson A. Oxidative damage to mitochondria and aging. *Exp Gerontol* (2001) 36(7):957–68. doi:10.1016/S0531-5565(01)00093-6
46. Lieber MR, Karanjawala ZE. Ageing, repetitive genomes and DNA damage. *Nat Rev Mol Cell Biol* (2004) 5(1):69–75. doi:10.1038/nrm1281
47. Patananan AN, Wu TH, Chiou PY, Teitell MA. Modifying the mitochondrial genome. *Cell Metab* (2016) 23(5):785–96. doi:10.1016/j.cmet.2016.04.004
48. Fang EF, Scheibye-Knudsen M, Chua KF, Mattson MP, Croteau DL, Bohr VA. Nuclear DNA damage signalling to mitochondria in ageing. *Nat Rev Mol Cell Biol* (2016) 17(5):308–21. doi:10.1038/nrm.2016.14
49. Lindahl T. The intrinsic fragility of DNA (Nobel Lecture). *Angew Chem Int Ed Engl* (2016) 55(30):8528–34. doi:10.1002/anie.201602159
50. Ermolaeva MA, Schumacher B. Systemic DNA damage responses: organismal adaptations to genome instability. *Trends Genet* (2014) 30(3):95–102. doi:10.1016/j.tig.2013.12.001
51. Ioannidou A, Goulielmaki E, Garinis GA. DNA damage: from chronic inflammation to age-related deterioration. *Front Genet* (2016) 7:187. doi:10.3389/fgene.2016.00187
52. Bauer NC, Corbett AH, Doetsch PW. The current state of eukaryotic DNA base damage and repair. *Nucleic Acids Res* (2015) 43(21):10083–101. doi:10.1093/nar/gkv1136
53. Gaillard H, Aguilera A. Transcription as a threat to genome integrity. *Annu Rev Biochem* (2016) 85:291–317. doi:10.1146/annurev-biochem-060815-014908
54. Chatterjee N, Walker GC. Mechanisms of DNA damage, repair, and mutagenesis. *Environ Mol Mutagen* (2017) 58(5):235–63. doi:10.1002/em.22087
55. Oliveira NM, Rios EC, de Lima TM, Victorino VJ, Barbeiro H, Pinheiro da Silva F, et al. Sepsis induces telomere shortening: a potential mechanism responsible for delayed pathophysiological events in sepsis survivors? *Mol Med* (2016) 22:886–91. doi:10.2119/molmed.2016.00225
56. Zhang J, Rane G, Dai X, Shanmugam MK, Arfuso F, Samy RP, et al. Ageing and the telomere connection: an intimate relationship with inflammation. *Ageing Res Rev* (2016) 25:55–69. doi:10.1016/j.arr.2015.11.006
57. de Magalhães JP, Passos JF. Stress, cell senescence and organismal ageing. *Mech Ageing Dev* (2017). doi:10.1016/j.mad.2017.07.001
58. Mota JM, Leite CA, Souza LE, Melo PH, Nascimento DC, de-Deus-Wagatsuma VM, et al. Post-sepsis state induces tumor-associated macrophage accumulation through CXCR4/CXCL12 and favors tumor progression in mice. *Cancer Immunol Res* (2016) 4(4):312–22. doi:10.1158/2326-6066.CIR-15-0170
59. Shankar-Hari M, Ambler M, Mahalingasivam V, Jones A, Rowan K, Rubenfeld GD. Evidence for a causal link between sepsis and long-term mortality: a systematic review of epidemiologic studies. *Crit Care* (2016) 20:101. doi:10.1186/s13054-016-1276-7
60. Shankar-Hari M, Rubenfeld GD. Understanding long-term outcomes following sepsis: implications and challenges. *Curr Infect Dis Rep* (2016) 18(11):37. doi:10.1007/s11908-016-0544-7
61. Forman HJ. Redox signaling: an evolution from free radicals to aging. *Free Radic Biol Med* (2016) 97:398–407. doi:10.1016/j.freeradbiomed.2016.07.003
62. Wang X, Hai C. Novel insights into redox system and the mechanism of redox regulation. *Mol Biol Rep* (2016) 43(7):607–28. doi:10.1007/s11033-016-4022-y
63. Sies H, Berndt C, Jones DP. Oxidative stress. *Annu Rev Biochem* (2017) 86:715. doi:10.1146/annurev-biochem-061516-045037
64. Adams L, Franco MC, Estevez AG. Reactive nitrogen species in cellular signaling. *Exp Biol Med (Maywood)* (2015) 240(6):711–7. doi:10.1177/1535370215581314
65. Vieira da Silva Pellegrina D, Severino P, Vieira Barbeiro H, Maziero Andreghetto F, Tadeu Velasco I, Possolo, et al. Septic shock in advanced age: transcriptome analysis reveals altered molecular signatures in neutrophil granulocytes. *PLoS One* (2015) 10(6):e0128341. doi:10.1371/journal.pone.0128341
66. Booth LN, Brunet A. The aging epigenome. *Mol Cell* (2016) 62(5):728–44. doi:10.1016/j.molcel.2016.05.013
67. Benayoun BA, Pollina EA, Brunet A. Epigenetic regulation of ageing: linking environmental inputs to genomic stability. *Nat Rev Mol Cell Biol* (2015) 16(10):593–610. doi:10.1038/nrm4048
68. Weiterer S, Uhle F, Lichtenstern C, Siegler BH, Bhuju S, Jarek M, et al. Sepsis induces specific changes in histone modification patterns in human monocytes. *PLoS One* (2015) 10(3):e0121748. doi:10.1371/journal.pone.0121748
69. Collins PE, Carmody RJ. The regulation of endotoxin tolerance and its impact on macrophage activation. *Crit Rev Immunol* (2015) 35(4):293–323. doi:10.1615/CritRevImmunol.2015015495
70. Dabin J, Fortuny A, Polo SE. Epigenome maintenance in response to DNA damage. *Mol Cell* (2016) 62(5):712–27. doi:10.1016/j.molcel.2016.04.006
71. López-Leon M, Goya RG. The emerging view of aging as a reversible epigenetic process. *Gerontology* (2017) 63(5):426–31. doi:10.1159/000477209

72. Sen P, Shah PP, Nativio R, Berger SL. Epigenetic mechanisms of longevity and aging. *Cell* (2016) 166(4):822–39. doi:10.1016/j.cell.2016.07.050
73. Pal S, Tyler JK. Epigenetics and aging. *Sci Adv* (2016) 2(7):e1600584. doi:10.1126/sciadv.1600584
74. Flynn RA, Chang HY. Long noncoding RNAs in cell-fate programming and reprogramming. *Cell Stem Cell* (2014) 14(6):752–61. doi:10.1016/j.stem.2014.05.014
75. Kim DH, Marinov GK, Pepke S, Singer ZS, He P, Williams B, et al. Single-cell transcriptome analysis reveals dynamic changes in lncRNA expression during reprogramming. *Cell Stem Cell* (2015) 16(1):88–101. doi:10.1016/j.stem.2014.11.005
76. Victoria B, Nunez Lopez YO, Masternak MM. MicroRNAs and the metabolic hallmarks of aging. *Mol Cell Endocrinol* (2017) 455:131–47. doi:10.1016/j.mce.2016.12.021
77. Clifford KM, Dy-Boarman EA, Haase KK, Maxvill K, Pass SE, Alvarez CA. Challenges with diagnosing and managing sepsis in older adults. *Expert Rev Anti Infect Ther* (2016) 14(2):231–41. doi:10.1586/14787210.2016.1135052
78. Liang SY. Sepsis and other infectious disease emergencies in the elderly. *Emerg Med Clin North Am* (2016) 34(3):501–22. doi:10.1016/j.emc.2016.04.005
79. Iwashyna TJ, Cooke CR, Wunsch H, Kahn JM. Population burden of long-term survivorship after severe sepsis in older Americans. *J Am Geriatr Soc* (2012) 60(6):1070–7. doi:10.1111/j.1532-5415.2012.03989.x
80. Kale SS, Yende S. Effects of aging on inflammation and hemostasis through the continuum of critical illness. *Aging Dis* (2011) 2(6):501–11.
81. Pinheiro da Silva F, Zampieri FG, Barbeiro DF, Barbeiro HV, Goulart AC, Torggler Filho F, et al. Septic shock in older people: a prospective cohort study. *Immun Ageing* (2013) 10(1):21. doi:10.1186/1742-4933-10-21
82. Cunha DM, Koike MK, Barbeiro DF, Barbeiro HV, Hamasaki MY, Coelho Neto GT, et al. Increased intestinal production of alpha-defensins in aged rats with acute pancreatic injury. *Exp Gerontol* (2014) 60:215–9. doi:10.1016/j.exger.2014.11.008
83. Barbeiro DF, Koike MK, Coelho AM, da Silva FP, Machado MC. Intestinal barrier dysfunction and increased COX-2 gene expression in the gut of elderly rats with acute pancreatitis. *Pancreatology* (2016) 16(1):52–6. doi:10.1016/j.pan.2015.10.012
84. Bone RC. Sir Isaac Newton, sepsis, SIRS, and CARS. *Crit Care Med* (1996) 24(7):1125–8. doi:10.1097/00003246-199607000-00010
85. Hotchkiss RS, Karl IE. The pathophysiology and treatment of sepsis. *N Engl J Med* (2003) 348(2):138–50. doi:10.1056/NEJMra021333
86. Tang BM, Huang SJ, McLean AS. Genome-wide transcription profiling of human sepsis: a systematic review. *Crit Care* (2010) 14(6):R237. doi:10.1186/cc9392
87. Wong HR. Genome-wide expression profiling in pediatric septic shock. *Pediatr Res* (2013) 73(4 Pt 2):564–9. doi:10.1038/pr.2013.11
88. Maslove DM, Wong HR. Gene expression profiling in sepsis: timing, tissue, and translational considerations. *Trends Mol Med* (2014) 20(4):204–13. doi:10.1016/j.molmed.2014.01.006
89. Xiao W, Mindrinos MN, Seok J, Cuschieri J, Cuenca AG, Gao H, et al. A genomic storm in critically injured humans. *J Exp Med* (2011) 208(13):2581–90. doi:10.1084/jem.20111354
90. Severino P, Silva E, Baggio-Zappia GL, Brunialti MK, Nucci LA, Junior OR, et al. Gene expression profiling of mononuclear cells from patients with sepsis secondary to community-acquired pneumonia. *Genom Data* (2014) 2:332–4. doi:10.1016/j.gdata.2014.10.004
91. Peterson LW, Artis D. Intestinal epithelial cells: regulators of barrier function and immune homeostasis. *Nat Rev Immunol* (2014) 14(3):141–53. doi:10.1038/nri3608
92. Man AL, Gicheva N, Nicoletti C. The impact of ageing on the intestinal epithelial barrier and immune system. *Cell Immunol* (2014) 289(1–2):112–8. doi:10.1016/j.cellimm.2014.04.001
93. Lustgarten MS. Classifying aging as a disease: the role of microbes. *Front Genet* (2016) 7:212. doi:10.3389/fgene.2016.00212
94. Qian F, Wang X, Zhang L, Chen S, Piecychna M, Allore H, et al. Age-associated elevation in TLR5 leads to increased inflammatory responses in the elderly. *Aging Cell* (2012) 11(1):104–10. doi:10.1111/j.1474-9726.2011.00759.x
95. Ghosh S, Lertwattanarak R, Garduno Jde J, Galeana JJ, Li J, Zamarripa F, et al. Elevated muscle TLR4 expression and metabolic endotoxemia in human aging. *J Gerontol A Biol Sci Med Sci* (2015) 70(2):232–46. doi:10.1093/gerona/glu067
96. Claesson MJ, Cusack S, O'Sullivan O, Greene-Diniz R, de Weerd H, Flannery E, et al. Composition, variability, and temporal stability of the intestinal microbiota of the elderly. *Proc Natl Acad Sci U S A* (2011) 108(Suppl 1):4586–91. doi:10.1073/pnas.1000097107
97. Woodmansey EJ, McMurdo ME, Macfarlane GT, Macfarlane S. Comparison of compositions and metabolic activities of fecal microbiotas in young adults and in antibiotic-treated and non-antibiotic-treated elderly subjects. *Appl Environ Microbiol* (2004) 70(10):6113–22. doi:10.1128/AEM.70.10.6113-6122.2004
98. Zhang D, Chen G, Manwani D, Mortha A, Xu C, Faith JJ, et al. Neutrophil ageing is regulated by the microbiome. *Nature* (2015) 525(7570):528–32. doi:10.1038/nature15367
99. Thevaranjan N, Puchta A, Schulz C, Naidoo A, Szamosi JC, Verschoor CP, et al. Age-associated microbial dysbiosis promotes intestinal permeability, systemic inflammation, and macrophage dysfunction. *Cell Host Microbe* (2017) 21(4):455–466e454. doi:10.1016/j.chom.2017.03.002
100. Nacionales DC, Szpila B, Ungaro R, Lopez MC, Zhang J, Gentile LF, et al. A detailed characterization of the dysfunctional immunity and abnormal myelopoiesis induced by severe shock and trauma in the aged. *J Immunol* (2015) 195(5):2396–407. doi:10.4049/jimmunol.1500984
101. Falony G, Joossens M, Vieira-Silva S, Wang J, Darzi Y, Faust K, et al. Population-level analysis of gut microbiome variation. *Science* (2016) 352(6285):560–4. doi:10.1126/science.aad3503
102. Zhernakova A, Kurilshikov A, Bonder MJ, Tigchelaar EF, Schirmer M, Vatanen T, et al. Population-based metagenomics analysis reveals markers for gut microbiome composition and diversity. *Science* (2016) 352(6285):565–9. doi:10.1126/science.aad3369
103. Levy M, Kolodziejczyk AA, Thaiss CA, Elinav E. Dysbiosis and the immune system. *Nat Rev Immunol* (2017) 17(4):219–32. doi:10.1038/nri.2017.7
104. Haak BW, Wiersinga WJ. The role of the gut microbiota in sepsis. *Lancet Gastroenterol Hepatol* (2017) 2(2):135–43. doi:10.1016/S2468-1253(16)30119-4
105. Dickson RP. The microbiome and critical illness. *Lancet Respir Med* (2016) 4(1):59–72. doi:10.1016/S2213-2600(15)00427-0
106. McDonald D, Ackermann G, Khailova L, Baird C, Heyland D, Kozar R, et al. Extreme dysbiosis of the microbiome in critical illness. *mSphere* (2016) 1(4):e199–196. doi:10.1128/mSphere.00199-16
107. Pinheiro da Silva F, Cesar Machado MC. Personalized medicine for sepsis. *Am J Med Sci* (2015) 350(5):409–13. doi:10.1097/MAJ.0000000000000558
108. Sebastiani P, Thyagarajan B, Sun F, Schupf N, Newman AB, Montano M, et al. Biomarker signatures of aging. *Aging Cell* (2017) 16(2):329–38. doi:10.1111/acel.12557
109. Srivastava D, DeWitt N. In vivo cellular reprogramming: the next generation. *Cell* (2016) 166(6):1386–96. doi:10.1016/j.cell.2016.08.055
110. von Joest M, Bua Aguin S, Li H. Genomic stability during cellular reprogramming: mission impossible? *Mutat Res* (2016) 788:12–6. doi:10.1016/j.mrfmmm.2016.01.001
111. Marion RM, Blasco MA. Long live partial reprogramming. *Circ Res* (2017) 120(9):1381–3. doi:10.1161/CIRCRESAHA.117.310594
112. Ocampo A, Reddy P, Martinez-Redondo P, Platero-Luengo A, Hatanaka F, Hishida T, et al. In vivo amelioration of age-associated hallmarks by partial reprogramming. *Cell* (2016) 167(7):1719–1733e1712. doi:10.1016/j.cell.2016.11.052

15

Parallels in Immunometabolic Adipose Tissue Dysfunction with Ageing and Obesity

*William Trim, James E. Turner and Dylan Thompson**

Department for Health, University of Bath, Bath, United Kingdom

Correspondence:
Dylan Thompson
d.thompson@bath.ac.uk

Ageing, like obesity, is often associated with alterations in metabolic and inflammatory processes resulting in morbidity from diseases characterised by poor metabolic control, insulin insensitivity, and inflammation. Ageing populations also exhibit a decline in immune competence referred to as immunosenescence, which contributes to, or might be driven by chronic, low-grade inflammation termed "inflammageing". In recent years, animal and human studies have started to uncover a role for immune cells within the stromal fraction of adipose tissue in driving the health complications that come with obesity, but relatively little work has been conducted in the context of immunometabolic adipose function in ageing. It is now clear that aberrant immune function within adipose tissue in obesity—including an accumulation of pro-inflammatory immune cell populations—plays a major role in the development of systemic chronic, low-grade inflammation, and limiting the function of adipocytes leading to an impaired fat handling capacity. As a consequence, these changes increase the chance of multiorgan dysfunction and disease onset. Considering the important role of the immune system in obesity-associated metabolic and inflammatory diseases, it is critically important to further understand the interplay between immunological processes and adipose tissue function, establishing whether this interaction contributes to age-associated immunometabolic dysfunction and inflammation. Therefore, the aim of this article is to summarise how the interaction between adipose tissue and the immune system changes with ageing, likely contributing to the age-associated increase in inflammatory activity and loss of metabolic control. To understand the potential mechanisms involved, parallels will be drawn to the current knowledge derived from investigations in obesity. We also highlight gaps in research and propose potential future directions based on the current evidence.

Keywords: adipose, ageing, immunometabolism, obesity, inflammageing, immunosenescence

INTRODUCTION

Metabolically driven inflammation is a hallmark of cardiovascular disease and type-II diabetes mellitus (1). Several organs including the liver, the skeletal muscle, and the gut have a role in the generation and progression of these diseases. However, it has become clear that adipose tissue accumulation, sometimes within and around these organs, is a major driving force for metabolic and inflammatory dysfunction (1–3). Obesity, defined herein as a body mass index (BMI; $\geq$30 kg/m^2), leads to extensive adipose tissue deposition and negative health consequences, due to chronic caloric overconsumption and an excessively sedentary lifestyle (4, 5). Globally, over 2.1 billion adults were overweight (BMI $\geq$ 25 to $<$30 kg/m^2) or obese in 2014 (6). This number has been steadily increasing with global age-standardised mean BMI scores increasing by 0.4 and 0.5 kg/m^2 each decade in men and women, respectively (7).

Obesity is characterised by poor metabolic control, oxidative stress, mitochondrial dysfunction, impaired immune function, and chronic, low-grade inflammation (8–13). In particular, it is well established that adipose tissue in obesity is a potent contributor to chronic, low-grade systemic inflammation, which can result in multiorgan dysfunction. One of the main factors associated with obesity-induced adipose tissue inflammation is dysregulation of the immune cell populations within the tissue stromal fraction, which contribute to the propagation of a pro-inflammatory microenvironment that spills over into the circulation and other organs (1, 14).

In contrast to obesity-centric research, the role of immunometabolic adipose tissue dysfunction in human ageing has been largely unexplored. In older people, many biological systems and processes become dysregulated (15). Indeed, age-associated immunological dysregulation potently modulates systemic inflammation, multiorgan dysfunction, and longevity (16–18). Moreover, molecular modulation of adipose tissue inflammatory and metabolic processes influences longevity in animal models, suggesting that adipose tissue may play an important role in the ageing process (19, 20). Further, in humans, an age-associated redistribution of adiposity towards the abdominal cavity occurs independently of obesity (21, 22). However, the role of adipose-resident immune cells and the interplay between metabolic and inflammatory processes in ageing adipose tissue is poorly characterised.

The aim of this review is to summarise the immunological alterations that take place in adipose tissue with obesity and ageing, with the aim to improve understanding of the role for adipose tissue immunometabolic dysfunction in age- and obesity-associated disease. This review first evaluates evidence showing obesity-specific immunological alterations in adipose tissue, which will then be used as a basis for understanding the potential role of adipose tissue immunological alterations in the pathophysiology of age-associated diseases.

THE IMMUNE SYSTEM AND INFLAMMATION

The immune system protects the host against viruses, bacteria, fungi, parasites, and tumours through a complex integration of innate and adaptive defences. The innate immune system provides a first line of defence, comprising physical barriers such as the skin and chemical barriers on surfaces exposed to the environment, preventing pathogens entering the body. In addition, the innate immune system has cellular defences, including monocytes, macrophages, natural killer (NK) cells, mast cells, neutrophils, eosinophils, basophils, and dendritic cells. Some cells possess characteristics of both the innate and adaptive immune system. For example, the small population of innate lymphocytes that are cluster of differentiation (CD) 1d restricted referred to as invariant natural killer T cell (iNKT) and other T-cells that express NK cell-associated surface proteins (NKT-like cells). Professional antigen-presenting cells link the two arms of the immune system. For example, dendritic cells act as tissue sentinels and, upon antigen encounter, travel from peripheral tissues (e.g., places in contact with the external environment; like the digestive system and dermis) to the lymph nodes where they activate cells of the adaptive immune system: B-cells and T-cells (23, 24). T-cells comprise 60–75% of all lymphocytes and originate from the bone marrow, maturing in the thymus, and circulate in blood as either antigen-naive or antigen-experienced cells (25). B-cells comprise 5–15% of all lymphocytes and elicit their effector functions, including their memory response, *via* soluble immunoglobulins (Igs), which can neutralise toxins or flag pathogens and target cells for elimination by other cells of the immune system such as macrophages and NK-cells (24).

In response to injury or infection, a local immune response is initiated, characterised by swelling, heat, and pain. One of the first local changes is an increase in blood flow facilitating an influx of acute-phase reactants, such as C-reactive protein, and an accumulation of innate and then adaptive immune cells for pathogen elimination and tissue repair. However, alterations to the tissue microenvironment and local stimuli can result in uncontrolled inflammation. Such alterations to the anti-inflammatory or pro-inflammatory milieu can disrupt systemic homeostasis and metabolic demand, perpetuating the inflammatory response that has profound health implications. A degree of inflammation within adipose tissue is central to tissue remodelling, as many of the cells, cytokines, and pro-oxidants produced at normal levels, regulate tissue homeostasis (26). However, prolongation of this normally transient and well-controlled process drives chronic, low-grade systemic inflammation that is central to the impaired health with obesity and ageing.

ADIPOSE TISSUE INFLAMMATION AND METABOLIC DISEASE

Impairments in adipose tissue function associated with structural and functional changes to the tissue results in the propagation of abnormal and often pro-inflammatory secretory profiles from adipocytes and cells of the stromal fraction. This association was first understood when murine obesity was linked with increased production of the inflammatory, insulin desensitising cytokine: tumour necrosis factor-α (TNF-α) (27). In the context of obesity, adipose tissue dysfunction is promoted by a chronic positive energy imbalance. Similar metabolic impairments are also observed in other conditions characterised by adipose tissue dysfunction, including ageing and lipodystrophy. Consequently, the similarities between these conditions allow for comparisons to be made to better understand the processes involved (28–30).

To date, a variety of stimuli for immunometabolic deterioration within adipose tissue have been proposed. These include increased gut-derived antigens (e.g., lipopolysaccharide), stimulation of immune cells by dietary or endogenously derived lipids, adipocyte hypertrophy—leading to apoptosis, necrosis, fibrosis, and hypoxia—and adipocyte dysfunction from mechanical stress (31). Collectively, these alterations impact various aspects of adipose tissue function, including changes to local blood flow, which impairs the endocrine potential of the tissue; changes to the extracellular matrix, which instigates monocyte infiltration to manage tissue remodelling; and adoption of a pro-inflammatory and pro-oxidative microenvironment, which act to recruit immune cells driving their pro-inflammatory polarisation (32–35). Moreover, the dysfunction of preadipocytes (adipocyte stem cell precursors) induced by a pro-inflammatory and pro-oxidative microenvironment inhibits the healthy turnover of adipose tissue, potentiated by, and impacting upon, impaired endothelial function, which exacerbates local hypoxia (34–36). The net result of these disturbances is the aberrant secretion of adipokines, which, *via* paracrine and endocrine means, impact appetite, bone health, metabolic health, and systemic inflammation through the activation of pro-inflammatory signal cascades [i.e., nuclear factor κB (NFκB), NLR family pyrin domain containing 3 (NLRP-3), and *c*-Jun *N*-terminal kinases (JNKs) signalling] (1, 37). Adipose tissue immunometabolic dysfunction also impacts the ability of adipocytes to buffer lipids. This dysfunction leads to the shunting of lipids towards non-adipose tissues, including the liver, the skeletal muscle, and the heart, promoting tissue-specific insulin resistance and inflammation, triggering β-cell, and metabolic dysfunction (1, 38, 39).

METHODOLOGICAL CONSIDERATIONS IN ADIPOSE TISSUE IMMUNOLOGICAL RESEARCH

Adipose tissue is an immunometabolically active organ in a constant state of flux (40). Therefore, assessment of adipose tissue function is a difficult task, and the nature of sampling tissue means the available data tend to represent a snap-shot of adipose physiology and function. In the context of the current review, this means that the assessment of adipose cellular composition at a given point in time will not necessarily provide a full and complete picture of the events that have led to the characterised phenotype. In human research, adipose tissue samples are often collected under fasting conditions, and very little information is available in the post-prandial state where much of the day is spent, which potently alters adipose tissue immunometabolic status (41). Furthermore, in human studies, the adipose tissue sampling methodology (e.g., surgical versus aspiration biopsies) may influence some outcomes (42). In mice, both the breed and inconsistency in whether animals are fasted or fed has the potential to influence their metabolic profile (43). Some investigations have adopted arteriovenous difference blood sampling techniques to sample the blood flowing across the subcutaneous adipose depots in an attempt to understand the dynamic behaviour of the tissue (44). This methodology allows for a greater understanding of how adipose tissue responds, in real-time, potentially giving a more complete picture of adipose tissue functionality.

Adipose tissue is distributed throughout the body with site-specific physiological properties. In humans, abdominal subcutaneous and visceral adipose tissue differ substantially in function and cellularity, and considerable depot differences are also apparent between gluteofemoral and abdominal adipose tissues, which is particularly relevant when comparing males and females due to sex-specific adipose tissue distribution (45, 46). In mice, different adipose tissue depots also possess unique physiological properties both between and within specific depots. Although beyond the scope of this review, differences include adipocyte size and expandability in response to high-fat overfeeding, control of lipolysis, and fatty acid and leukocyte composition (47, 48). Most investigations of adipose tissue immunology have been conducted with animal models, with considerably less work with humans. Although differences in adipose tissue biology between humans and animals is beyond the scope of this review, it is important to recognise that human adipose tissue is, indeed, very different to that of animals such as mice in terms of functionality, physiology, distribution, and make-up (i.e., quantities of brown and white adipose tissue, respectively) (49).

To assess the constituents of the adipose tissue stromal fraction, many approaches have been employed, including immunohistochemistry, analysis of gene expression and protein level, and flow cytometry. Each method has benefits and drawbacks, which are summarised in **Table 1**. For example, it has been shown that immunohistochemistry yields reproducible results, but with flow cytometry, the recovery of macrophages after tissue digestion can be a possible source of variation (50). However, there is good agreement between flow cytometric analysis of adipose tissue cellular composition and the expression mRNA for key cell surface markers across a range of adiposities in humans (**Figure 1**) (35). Moreover, differences between studies in the selection of cell markers, coupled with lack of consensus over cell identification strategies, make direct comparison between studies complex and could feasibly explain conflicting results.

The mode of reporting assessments of cellular composition also requires consideration. Reporting proportional representation of cell types within the stromal fraction versus absolute cell counts can produce different findings. For instance, a proportional decline in certain populations in relation to total stromal cell yields may be a consequence of an expansion of another cell population within the tissue instead of an absolute decline in specific cell numbers. For example, one report showed that, compared to older mice, young mice exhibited around twice as many macrophages in adipose tissue when expressed as a percentage of the total stromal yield. However, these age-related differences were not seen when data were expressed per gram of adipose tissue (51). In summary, when interpreting the results of different studies, it must be considered whether the laboratory methods and data presentation/expression could in-part explain discrepant results, especially when interpreting cell counts and/or proportions within adipose tissue.

TRADITIONAL CONCEPTS IN ADIPOSE TISSUE IMMUNOLOGY: AN INFLAMMATORY ROLE FOR MONOCYTES AND MACROPHAGES

Macrophages were first discovered within adipose tissue forming multinucleated crown-like structures of ~15 cells clustering around dead or dying adipocytes in obese C57/BL6J mice (52). In young obese mice and humans, these structures have been shown to comprise 90% of all adipose tissue macrophages (53). Macrophages are the main leukocyte in the adipose stromal fraction of young, non-obese mice and humans, comprising

TABLE 1 | Appraisal of three commonly utilised methods of assessing the cells of the adipose tissue stromal fraction.

Method	Benefits	Drawbacks
Immunohistochemistry	– Small amount of tissue required – Information on cell locality – Intact undisturbed tissue sample – Long-term storage – Some sample remains available for future analysis	– Manual counting is subject to investigator bias – Time consuming for manual counting – Limited to 2 or 3 antibodies per tissue slice
Flow cytometry	– Commonly 10–12 antibodies can be used in parallel – Thousands of cells analysed from one sample – Absolute cell counts can be determined – Isotype control and fluorescence minus one tubes can be added to an experiment to minimise the influence of subjectivity when gating populations	– Extensive processing required to extract the stromal fraction possibly leading to artefacts – Possibility for selective cell type loss with processing – Cell autofluorescence complicates gating of some populations (i.e., macrophages) – Large (>300 mg) tissue sample required – Small margin for bias when gating cell populations
Gene and protein expression (RT-PCR and Western blot)	– Very little tissue required – Little processing of the tissue required prior to freezing – Long-term storage – Some sample remains available for future analysis	– Requires isolation of a specific marker not expressed on any other cell type – Cannot be multiplexed by examining multiple markers on cell types

RT-PCR, reverse transcription polymerase chain reaction.

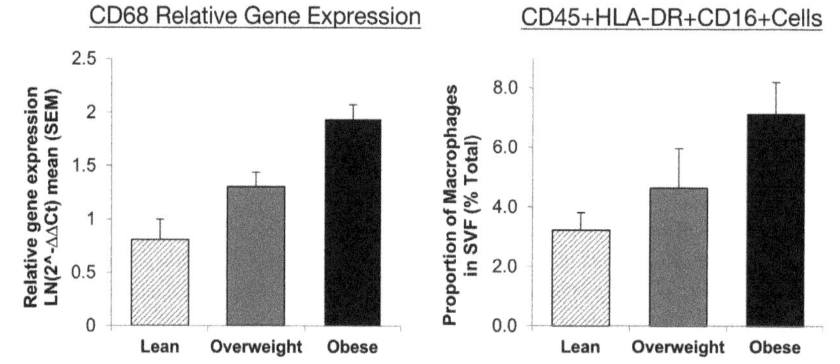

FIGURE 1 | Agreement between RT-PCR and flow cytometric assessment of macrophage abundance in lean, overweight, and obese individuals subcutaneous abdominal adipose tissue. Relative gene expression of CD68 was used to identify macrophages (n = 30) and presented as mean $2^{-\Delta\Delta Ct}$ ± SEM. Proportions of macrophages in the adipose tissue SVF as a percentage of total cells (n = 17). Macrophages were identified as CD45+HLA-DR+CD16+ cells. Presented with permission from Travers et al. (35). Abbreviations: CD, cluster of differentiation; HLA-DR, human leukocyte antigen-antigen D related; RT-PCR, reverse transcription polymerase chain reaction; SVF, stromal vascular fraction.

4–15% of total stromal cell count (54, 55). Macrophage content increases with adiposity, and the accumulation is greatest in visceral depots in humans (55, 56). Adipose tissue macrophages are derived from monocytes, which differentiate in response to growth factors, including macrophage colony-stimulating factor and granulocyte–macrophage colony-stimulating factor (57, 58). Monocytes, defined by their cell surface expression of CD14 and CD16 (see **Table 2**), circulate in peripheral blood until they migrate into adipose tissue primarily in response to chemokine (C-C motif) ligand-2 (CCL-2)—also known as monocyte chemoattractant protein 1 (MCP-1)—released from adipose tissue (57, 59). MCP-1 promotes the local proliferation of adipose-resident macrophages, contributing to the large accumulation of these cells with obesity (60). Monocytes also enter the adipose microcirculation in response to adipocyte-derived cell-stress markers, including CCL-5, also known as regulated on activation, normal T-cell expressed and secreted (RANTES), interleukin (IL)-6, interferon-γ (IFN-γ), and TNF-α (61). Production of these signals, which enhances macrophage accumulation, also polarises macrophages into highly inflammatory, classically activated cells, referred to herein as M1-like macrophages to be consistent with the reporting of data in the studies we summarise. However, we acknowledge that the M1 and M2 classification of macrophages is simplistic and becoming outdated[1] (see **Table 2**).

[1]Traditionally, macrophages have been categorised as M1 (classically activated, often thought to be pro-inflammatory) and M2 (alternatively activated, often thought to be anti-inflammatory). It is now understood that this is an oversimplification of macrophage phenotype. However, much of the available research in adipose tissue, especially in mice, has maintained the M1 and M2 categorisation. In this article, for consistency and ease of comparing studies, the terms "M1-like" and "M2-like" will be used. Within adipose tissue, it is now accepted that tissue-resident macrophages have a tissue-remodelling and pro-inflammatory phenotype, representing an intermediate population in mice and humans (i.e., cells that display an M2-like surface expression profile while demonstrating an M1-like secretory profile and function) (33, 63, 79, 170, 246, 247, 248, 249). Therefore, the role of macrophages in expanded and/or dysfunctional adipose tissue is likely to be far more complex than originally envisaged.

TABLE 2 | Adipose tissue macrophage phenotypic classifications in humans.

Type	Cell surface expression profile	Secretion profile	Function
M1-like *"classically activated"*	CD14+CD16++ CD11c+CD31+CD44+CD45+CD206−HLA-DR+	TNF-α, IL-6, IL-8, IL-1β, NO	Pro-inflammatory, pro-oxidative, antimicrobial, pathogen clearance
Intermediate population	CD14+CD16+ CD11c+CD45+CD206+	TNF-α, IL-6, IL-8	Pro-inflammatory and pro-oxidative, tissue remodelling
M2-like *"alternatively activated"*	CD14++ CD16+ CD45+CD163+CD206+	IL-10, TGF-β	Anti-inflammatory, fibrosis, tissue surveillance, angiogenesis

Text in italics and quotes emphasises other common terms to describe these cells. Intermediate population refers to adipose tissue macrophages expressing M2-like surface markers (e.g., CD206), while demonstrating an M1-like pro-inflammatory function. Expression pattern of CD14 and CD16 is best established on monocytes rather than macrophages. It is important to note that macrophage populations within adipose tissue can express markers of alternatively activated cells (e.g., CD206+) while also imparting a pro-inflammatory, classically activated function within the tissue, highlighting the spectrum of macrophage polarity within adipose tissue.

CD, cluster of differentiation; HLA-DR, human leukocyte antigen-antigen D related; IL, interleukin; NO, nitric oxide; TGF-β, transforming growth factor-beta; TNF-α, tumour necrosis factor-α.

It has been consistently shown that there is a positive relationship between the number of macrophages in adipose tissue and the degree of whole-body insulin resistance in mice and humans (35, 62, 63). Moreover, TNF-α—which is primarily produced by macrophages in adipose tissue—is a potent inhibitor of insulin signalling and an activator of NFκB signalling (27, 64). In obese and inflamed adipose tissue, NFκB is activated by the fatty acid chaperone—Fetuin-A—interacting with the lipid-sensing toll-like receptor 4 (TLR-4) on the macrophage cell surface (65–67). In the commonly studied 3T3-L1 adipocyte cell line, TNF-α has been shown to directly impact insulin signalling by inactivating insulin receptor substrate 1 (IRS-1) through p44/42 mitogen-activated protein kinase (MAPK) activation (68). Chronic activation of pro-inflammatory stress sensors and signalling pathways: p44/42, JNK, p38, and MAPK by TNF-α derived from subcutaneous adipose-resident macrophages indirectly stimulates lipolysis in adipocytes, impairing lipid handling capacity (69–71). It has also been observed, *in vitro*, that monocytes incubated with palmitate—an abundant saturated fatty acid—exhibit upregulated IL-6 and TNF-α mRNA (72). Further, upon macrophage–adipocyte co-culture, there is a substantial increase in macrophage-derived TNF-α and IL-1β (65). As TNF-α, IL-6, and IL-1β stimulate a feed-forward activation of NFκB and JNK, this leads to IRS-1 phosphorylation at serine residues rather than tyrosine, perpetuating insulin signalling impairments (73). Another factor influencing macrophage function in adipose tissue is hypoxia brought about by adipocyte expansion, without concurrent angiogenesis, impairing oxygen supply (74, 75). Hypoxia potentiates the palmitate-induced pro-inflammatory and pro-oxidative polarisation of human macrophages, while hypoxia-inducible factor-1α (HIF-1α) can directly induce pro-inflammatory M1-like macrophage polarisation and pro-inflammatory cytokine productions (76, 77). Macrophage-derived reactive oxygen species produced as a result of hypoxia may also impair lipid and glucose metabolic control through the S-nitrosylation of the peroxisome proliferator-activated receptor-γ (PPAR-γ) nuclear receptor (78).

Macrophages are considered central regulators of fibrosis and may also increase progenitor cell deposition into the extracellular matrix as a means of protecting hypertrophic adipocytes from rupturing (59). M2-like macrophages possess a pro-fibrotic potential and are, therefore, recruited into the adipose tissue in response to "danger signals" (i.e., cytokines, acute-phase proteins, and stress signal cascades) released from hypertrophic adipocytes (79). However, the exposure of macrophages to hormones, cytokines, chemokines, and fatty acids found within dysfunctional adipose tissue encourages them to adopt a pro-inflammatory phenotype potentiating metabolic deteriorations and inflammation (80, 81). In human obesity, perhaps counter intuitively based on the simple macrophage phenotyping, it is the M2-like, and not M1-like, macrophages, with a tumour-associated genetic signature and remodelling phenotype that correlates with obesity in subcutaneous adipose tissue (33). Another stimulus that might influence macrophage infiltration into adipose tissue is endoplasmic reticulum stress, which promotes a pro-inflammatory microenvironment through the initiation of the unfolded protein response. In mice, increased fatty acid-mediated oxidative stress upregulates pro-inflammatory cytokine expression, which, in humans, is also initiated by elevated TNF-α and IL-1β (82, 83). Endoplasmic reticulum stress responses involving the inositol-requiring enzyme 1α and CCAAT-enhancer-binding protein homologous protein direct pro-inflammatory, M1-like macrophage polarisation in adipose tissue (84, 85). Finally, it is unknown whether macrophages initiate inflammatory responses in adipose tissue or whether other cells present stimulate macrophage accumulation and dysfunction. For example, some studies in mice indicate that macrophages infiltrate adipose tissue in the absence of other leukocytes, whereas other studies show that different leukocyte subsets are central to macrophage accumulation (86).

Recent evidence has indicated that a unique adipose-resident macrophage population exists. In mice fed a high-fat diet, a population of sympathetic neuron-associated macrophages accumulate within visceral adipose tissue. This macrophage population regulates adipocyte exposure to norepinephrine by sequestering and degrading norepinephrine released into the adipose tissue interstitium. This process is brought about by the selective expression of the norepinephrine transporter, *SLC6A2*, and genes controlling norepinephrine-degradation such as monoamine oxidase-A by these macrophages (87). However, unlike other adipose-resident macrophage populations, these sympathetic neuron-associated macrophages do not increase within obese adipose tissue *via* proliferative mechanisms, but instead appear to infiltrate the tissue selectively (87). Given that catecholamines increase lipolytic rate in adipocytes *via* adrenergic receptors triggering the downstream hydrolysis of triglycerides, selective knockout of these sympathetic neuron-associated macrophages protects against high-fat diet-induced obesity, in mice. Moreover, the capacity to buffer regional norepinephrine releases, which in healthy adipose tissue may act as a protective mechanism to avoid the dangerous effects of chronic exposure to norepinephrine, is also sufficient to modulate overall sympathetic tone in murine adipose tissue, influencing whole-body metabolism (88).

In summary, a number of factors including adipose tissue cellular composition and secretions plus broader anatomical and physiological characteristics of the tissue have been found to modulate metabolic and inflammatory processes and influence macrophage phenotype and function. However, due to adipose sampling in humans being a "snap-shot" of the dynamic changes that the tissue undergoes with obesity, further work is required to fully understand these interactions. A summary of the likely interactions between adipocytes and adipose-resident macrophages with obesity is presented in **Figure 2**.

A BROADER PERSPECTIVE ON ADIPOSE TISSUE IMMUNOLOGY

Adipose tissue dysfunction is the result of a complex interaction between all cell types within the tissue. Understanding this interplay has been the subject of intensive investigation, which will first be discussed in the context of obesity as a foundation for understanding the function of adipose tissue with ageing. The following sections will summarise research examining different immune cell populations in adipose tissue in the context of obesity, considering cells of the weight of evidence (most to least) supporting their role within dysfunctional adipose tissue.

Neutrophils in Obesity-Associated Adipose Tissue Dysfunction

In mice fed a high-fat diet, the accumulation of neutrophils (identified in mice as Ly6g+CD11b+) occurs in visceral, but not subcutaneous, adipose tissue after 3 days (89). Neutrophils

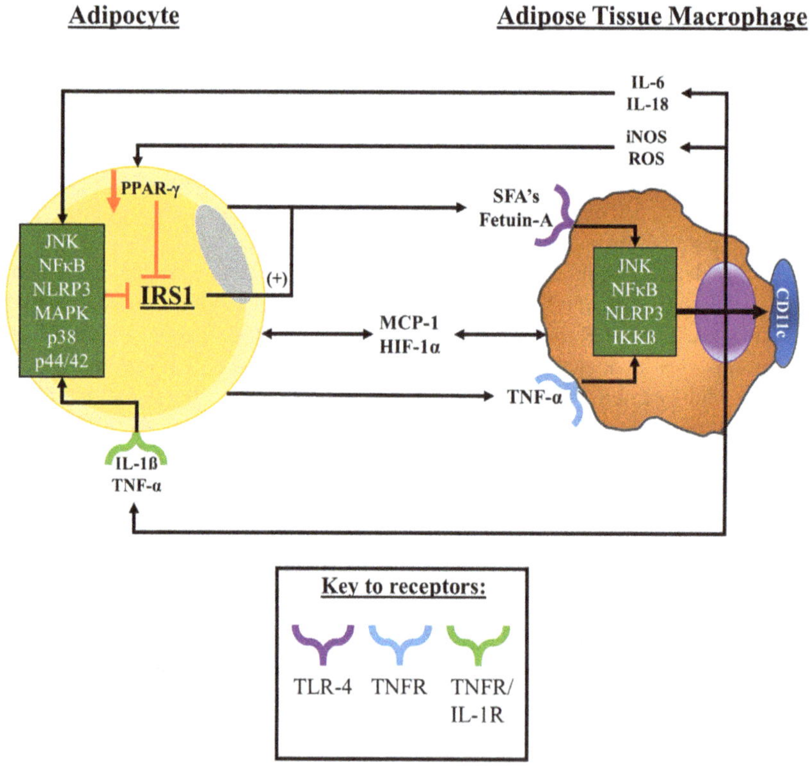

FIGURE 2 | Adipocyte–macrophage interactions with obesity. With obesity, adipocytes expand promoting a state of proinflammation, ER stress, and tissue hypoxia, promoting adipocyte apoptosis/necrosis. Upon these changes in obese adipose tissue macrophages are signalled into the tissue by hypoxic, chemokine, and cytokine signals to surround dysfunctional adipocytes. Macrophages in obese adipose tissue release, and are exposed to, TNF-α and MCP-1—among other factors, including SFAs—which collectively promote the activation of a variety of stress signalling cascades. Consequently, adipose-resident macrophages adopt a pro-inflammatory secretory profile and upregulate their surface expression of CD11c. As a result, adipocytes become exposed to secreted factors such as TNF-α and MCP-1, exacerbating the pro-inflammatory microenvironment of the tissue and potentiating the activation of stress signal cascades within adipocytes. These interactions promote a feed-forward recruitment of monocytes into the tissue and their pro-inflammatory polarisation as well as impairing tissue insulin sensitivity that potentially promotes the release of FFAs into the microenvironment. Abbreviations: CD, cluster of differentiation; ER, endoplasmic reticulum; FFAs, free-fatty acids; HIF-1α, hypoxia-inducible factor-1α; IKKβ, inhibitor of nuclear factor kappa B kinase subunit beta; IL, interleukin; IL-1R, interleukin-1 receptor; iNOS, inducible nitric oxide synthase; IRS-1, insulin receptor substrate 1; JNK, c-Jun *N*-terminal kinases; MAPK, mitogen-activated protein kinase; MCP-1, monocyte chemoattractant protein 1; NFκB, nuclear factor kappa B; NLRP-3, NLR family pyrin domain containing 3; PPAR-γ, peroxisome proliferator-activated receptor gamma; ROS, reactive oxygen species; SFAs, saturated fatty acids; TNFR, tumour necrosis factor receptor; TNF-α, tumour necrosis factor-α.

are 20-fold more abundant in adipose tissue from mice fed a high-fat diet compared to chow-fed mice, accounting for ~2% of total stromal cells (89–91). The accumulation of neutrophils in adipose tissue in obese mice leads to elevated elastase production (89). *In vitro* experiments have shown that increased exposure to elastase can contribute to IRS-1 downregulation, resulting in impaired glucose tolerance and insulin resistance (92). Further, systemic and intraperitoneal glucose tolerance has been shown to be impaired in mice injected with elastase compared to those treated with an elastase inhibitor. Neutrophil-derived elastase also imparts pro-inflammatory actions on murine intraperitoneal macrophages *via* TLR-4 signalling, upregulating *TNF-α, IL-1β,* and *IL-6* gene expression, potentially resulting in a feed-forward recruitment of neutrophils and M1-like macrophages into adipose tissue (89).

In humans, immunohistochemical analyses (CD66b+ staining) have shown neutrophils to accumulate in the microvasculature of adipose tissue with increasing adiposity, correlating with elevated NFκB and cyclooxygenase-2 (COX-2) staining (93). Further, it has also been suggested that elevated chemokine (C-X-C motif) ligand (CXCL)-2 release from obese adipose tissue may promote neutrophil infiltration (94). However, in humans at least, several questions remain unanswered. For example, whether neutrophil accumulation is an early step in adipose tissue dysfunction and to what extent neutrophils modulate ongoing inflammatory responses with adipose tissue.

NK-Cells in Obesity-Associated Adipose Tissue Dysfunction

Comprehensive investigations in mice have suggested that a population of NK-cells, uniquely expressing the IL-6 receptor alpha and colony-stimulating factor 1 receptor (IL6Ra+Csf1r+), induced *via* IL-6/STAT-3 (signal transducer and activator of transcription-3) signalling, accumulate with obesity within visceral adipose tissue (95). Ablation of IL6Ra+Csf1r+ NK-cells improves insulin and glucose control and reduces overall adiposity, adipocyte size, macrophage infiltration, and macrophage crown-like structures (95). It has been suggested that IL-15 and aberrant leptin secretion with obesity might instigate an adipose-specific NK-cell expansion and activation in response to high-fat diet overfeeding, stimulating NK-cell IFN-γ, TNF-α, and MCP-1 production, negatively impacting whole-body insulin sensitivity (96–98).

In humans with obesity and type-II diabetes, activated NK-cells accumulate in visceral and subcutaneous abdominal adipose tissue, producing IFN-γ and TNF-α (99–101). Moreover, the increase in IL6Ra+ NK-cells in peripheral blood of people with obesity suggests that obese dysfunctional adipose tissue may cause a pro-inflammatory NK-cell population expansion that spills out into the circulation (95). It has been proposed that adipose-resident macrophages produce CCL-3, CCL-4, and CXCL-10, stimulating the recruitment of NK-cells into adipose tissue, whereupon macrophage-derived IL-15 promotes NK-cell proliferation and activation (102). Once within adipose tissue, NK-cell modulation of MCP-1 expression could potentiate macrophage recruitment and proliferation (60), and finally, through an upregulation of NK-cell-derived TNF-α and IFN-γ, NK-cells may guide M1-like macrophage polarisation. Therefore, NK-cells may be pivotal in the generation of obesity-associated immunometabolic adipose tissue dysfunction.

B-Cells in Obesity-Associated Adipose Tissue Dysfunction

In lean murine visceral adipose tissue, B-cells constitute 10% of the stromal fraction, increasing to 20% in response to high-fat overfeeding, and this accumulation has been reported to occur before macrophage infiltration (103). B-cell localisation around macrophage clusters may be central to their functional relevance within adipose tissue in obesity, suggesting a role in steering macrophage functionality, perhaps *via* LTB4/leukotriene-B4 receptor 1 (LTB4R1) signalling. LTB4/LTB4R1 signalling promotes leukocyte infiltration into tissues, influences cytokine production, and is increased in obese murine visceral adipose tissue B-cells (103). In support, B-cells promote visceral adipose tissue macrophage recruitment and TNF-α production, *in vivo* and *in vitro,* in mice fed a high-fat diet (104). Moreover, B-cells have also been linked with the accumulation and differentiation of IFN-γ-producing CD4+ and CD8+ T-cells within murine visceral adipose tissue (103, 105). Indeed, CD8+ T-cells have been shown to produce 30% less IFN-γ in B-cell-deficient mice fed a high-fat diet suggesting a role for B-cells in T-cell activation (104, 105). B-cells may also promote the expansion of a senescent population of CD4+CD153+PD-1+ T-cells in murine visceral adipose tissue that, in turn, secrete osteopontin that promotes B-cell IgG production and suppresses IL-10 secretion (105, 106).

In obese human subcutaneous adipose tissue, B-cells comprise <4% of all stromal cells, but localise around macrophage crown-like structures and in the perivascular space (107). In obese human adipose tissue, a ~3-fold increase in the expression of the B-cell marker *B220* mRNA has been reported (108), although flow cytometric analysis of human subcutaneous adipose tissue has shown that very few B-cells are present in adipose tissue (109). Contradictory findings could be an artefact of methodology, indicating that further work in humans, employing a combination of methodological approaches, is warranted. In summary, B-cells may play a role in the early stages of obesity-induced adipose tissue dysfunction, modulating the functions of other cells within the stromal fraction, promoting a pro-inflammatory microenvironment.

T-Cells in Obesity-Associated Adipose Tissue Dysfunction

Within lean human adipose tissue, T-cells represent ~10% of the stromal fraction (one-third CD8+ T-cells and two-thirds CD4+ T-cells). More than half of the CD4+ T-cell compartment within murine adipose tissue are regulatory T-cells (110). Studies in humans have shown that T-cells are recruited into adipose tissue in response to adipocyte-derived CCL-20 binding to CCL-6 on the surface of T-cells, as well as CCR-5 to RANTES interactions (109, 111, 112). Moreover, adipose-resident T-cells display a visceral adipose tissue-specific antigen-driven expansion, suggesting a signal within the tissue promotes their clonal expansion. A potential signal has been suggested to derive from B-cells, which may infiltrate or respond to dysfunctional adipose tissue earlier than T-cells (105, 113, 114). T-cells typically exhibit a differentiated or activated phenotype shown by low-surface expression of CD62L and high expression of CD25 in murine and human adipose tissue, respectively (35, 113).

CD8+ Cytotoxic T-Cells in Obesity-Associated Adipose Tissue Dysfunction

In mice fed a high-fat diet, CD8+ T-cells are the predominant T-cell subpopulation to accumulate in adipose tissue. The early selective recruitment of CD8+ cells into visceral adipose tissue in mice occurs in parallel with a reduction in blood CD8+ T-cells in the first 2 weeks of overfeeding (113). Mouse models also show that adipose-resident CD8+ T-cells have an activated CD62L−CD44+ effector phenotype, which is brought about, *in situ*, by MCP-1 release from adipocytes (113, 115). Co-culturing CD8+ T-cells with obese murine adipocytes has been shown to initiate, potentiate, and maintain the inflammatory response by instigating the infiltration of macrophages towards adipocytes, followed by their activation by CD8+ T-cell-derived MCP-1 (113). Moreover, selective depletion of CD8+ T-cells in obese mice has been shown to improve metabolic health and reduce local tissue and serum levels of IL-6 and TNF-α (113).

In obese humans, CD8A mRNA expression is increased in visceral adipose tissue (113, 116), whilst in subcutaneous adipose tissue CD8+ T-cells adopt an activated phenotype compared to blood (35, 109). As serum MCP-1 is substantially elevated in patients with type-II diabetes and is a potent activator of CD8+ T-cells, MCP-1 may be a cause of elevated adipose tissue CD8+ T-cell activation with obesity or metabolic disease (115, 117). The stimulus for CD8+ T-cell migration into obese adipose tissue is yet to be confirmed *in vivo*, in humans, although significantly elevated CCL-20 release by obese adipose tissue has been observed *in vitro* (109). In the circulation, CD8+ T-cells from obese individuals express elevated levels of TNF-α, IFN-γ, and RANTES. Importantly, IFN-γ has been found to inhibit insulin-mediated upregulation of fatty acid synthase (FAS) and lipoprotein lipase and was associated with a downregulation of phosphatidylinositol 3-kinase regulatory subunit alpha expression (a key component of insulin signalling) (109). These observations suggest a modulatory capacity for CD8+ T-cells in adipose tissue metabolic health by influencing insulin-mediated triglyceride storage (109).

CD4+ Helper T-Cells (Th Cells) in Obesity-Associated Adipose Tissue Dysfunction

CD4+ T-cells accumulate within human subcutaneous adipose tissue with obesity, exhibiting an activated CD25+ phenotype (35). Recent findings suggest that circulating CD4+ T-cells adopt an effector memory (CXCR-3+CD62L−) phenotype with human obesity in response to a metabolically driven adaptation within T-cells *via* the p110δ subunit of phosphoinositide 3-kinase (PI3K) (118). Indeed, lipid activation of this subunit is also associated with sustained activation of T-cells, indicating that dendritic cell-independent, metabolically driven activation could drive chronic activation within adipose tissue (119, 120). The Th cell balance has the potential to play an important role in adipose tissue inflammatory disorders. For example, in mice, IFN-γ secretion is increased mainly as a consequence of Th cell (Th-1) cell predominance within visceral adipose tissue upon high-fat diet overfeeding (112, 114). The direct effect of IFN-γ in obesity induced by a high-fat diet includes impaired insulin signalling and the promotion of macrophage infiltration and crown-like formations *via* MCP-1 (121). In addition, IFN-γ from Th-1 cells instigates CXCL-10 release from 3T3-L1 adipocytes, providing a positive feedback recruitment loop (122). Moreover, IFN-γ secretion, when combined with TNF-α, can lead to chronic activation of NFκB signalling (123). However, Th-2 cells could serve to promote M2-like macrophage maturation through their production of IL-4 and IL-13 (124). Human and murine research indicates that CD4+ T-cells within both visceral and subcutaneous adipose tissue not only control their own recruitment, activation, and differentiation but are also influenced by other tissue-resident immune cells (i.e., B-cells) and adipocytes. Consequently, CD4+ T-cells have both direct and indirect roles in obesity-associated adipose tissue immunometabolic dysfunction.

Regulatory T-Cells in Obesity-Associated Adipose Tissue Dysfunction

Regulatory T-cells represent more than half of all CD4+ T-cells in lean murine adipose tissue, and in obesity, regulatory T-cells accumulate around macrophages, produce IL-4 and IL-10, and promote Th-2 T-cell polarisation (110). Regulatory T-cells also suppress adipocyte-derived inflammatory markers and restore metabolic health by promoting translocation of glucose transporter-4 to the cell membrane, countering the effects of TNF-α. However, adipose-resident regulatory T-cells appear to decline with increasing duration of obesity in mice (125). It is thought that the decline in regulatory T-cell numbers is a result of IFN-γ-induced impairments in proliferative capacity in visceral adipose (125). These changes occur in parallel with insulin resistance in mice and humans (110, 113, 114). In human obesity—which occurs over a much longer time-span than in mice—it has been shown that there is a substantial increase in regulatory T-cells within subcutaneous adipose tissue, and this could be a compensatory mechanism to counter adipose tissue inflammation (35). However, a proportional decline in regulatory T-cells has also been reported within the adipose tissue stromal fraction in obesity (126). These observations suggest that regulatory T-cells may limit ongoing pro-inflammatory events that occur with obesity-induced adipose tissue dysfunction. However, it is possible that with chronic local inflammation, regulatory T-cell proliferation is impaired and numbers decline.

iNKT Cells in Obesity-Associated Adipose Tissue Dysfunction

Within lean human and murine adipose tissue, iNKT cells typically express low levels of CD4 and NK1.1 and secrete large amounts of IL-4 and IL-10, demonstrating an anti-inflammatory capacity (127). Indeed, with obesity, iNKT cells may initially provide an anti-inflammatory function to limit the ongoing pro-inflammatory response driven by other infiltrating leukocytes.

However, with obesity, iNKT cells decline substantially although the reason for this decline is unclear (127). Further, in mice, iNKT cell accumulation in adipose tissue is limited with adipocyte CD1d knockout and, in turn, these animals exhibit a poor metabolic profile (128). However, it has been suggested that CD1d knockout models may reduce IFN-γ production, independent of iNKT cells (128). In addition, recent investigations have shown that iNKT cells have a role in adipocyte browning and modulating regulatory T-cell responses in mice, promoting the anti-inflammatory actions of regulatory T-cells (129, 130). In non-obese humans, visceral adipose tissue is also enriched with iNKT cells, and these cells exhibit a distinct Th-2 cytokine profile (131, 132). However, with obesity, the proportion of iNKT cells within the adipose tissue stromal fraction declines substantially, in tandem with the development of metabolic syndrome and inflammation, as observed in obese mice (128, 131, 132). In summary, iNKT cells likely assist in the regulation of a healthy adipose tissue microenvironment in a similar way to regulatory T-cells and eosinophils (see Eosinophils in Obesity-Associated Adipose Tissue Dysfunction). Therefore, a reduction in iNKT cells with obesity might contribute to the diminished anti-inflammatory signals within dysfunctional adipose tissue.

Dendritic Cells in Obesity-Associated Adipose Tissue Dysfunction

Dendritic cells accumulate in adipose tissue of mice fed a high-fat diet and likely contribute to the pro-inflammatory microenvironment *via* macrophage recruitment and IL-6 production (133, 134). Myeloid dendritic cells may also promote Th cells to adopt a Th-1 phenotype, which contribute to IFN-γ production (133, 135–137). However, in mice, both the flow cytometric analyses and knockout models commonly utilised are subject to criticism due to their non-specificity for "true" dendritic cells (133, 138). It has recently been shown that type-I IFN signalling is pivotal to the development of obesity-associated metabolic disease in mice, and therefore, plasmacytoid dendritic cells have been implicated in diet-induced obesity (139). Indeed, in mice fed a high-fat diet, plasmacytoid dendritic cells have been shown to increase ~3-fold, possibly as a result of elevated recruitment and activation with obesity by the adipokine, chemerin. In turn, dendritic cell accumulation has been suggested to enhance type-I IFN signalling, leading to IFN-β-induced MCP-1 production and macrophage recruitment/proliferation (60, 133, 139–143). In humans, distinct CD1c+ myeloid dendritic cell populations have been identified within subcutaneous, but not visceral adipose tissue, and the number of these cells correlates positively with BMI (138). Moreover, dietary lipids modulate the abundance of dendritic cells within lymphoid structures in adipose tissue, and as dendritic cells communicate with other lymphoid cells *via* lipid-derived molecules, dendritic cells may modulate adipose tissue immunometabolic responses (144, 145).

Eosinophils in Obesity-Associated Adipose Tissue Dysfunction

Eosinophils in the abdominal adipose tissue of mice have a role in improving insulin sensitivity and stimulating anti-inflammatory responses through the production of IL-4 (146–148). Mice fed a high-fat diet exhibit a decline in eosinophil numbers within adipose tissue (147). In addition, eosinophils have been estimated to produce up to 90% of the IL-4 found within murine adipose tissue, promoting M2-like macrophage polarisation and tyrosine hydroxylase expression. In turn, macrophage tyrosine hydroxylase expression drives the production of catecholamines by macrophages, triggering the expression of uncoupling protein 1 in white adipose tissue (148–150). Moreover, it has been shown that mice fed a high-fat diet and injected with eosinophils intravenously do not accumulate adipose-resident macrophages (147). Further, obese eosinophil knockout mice demonstrate significantly greater degrees of insulin resistance compared to wild-type mice (147).

Mast Cells in Obesity-Associated Adipose Tissue Dysfunction

Obesity in mice is associated with an accumulation of mast cells in adipose tissue and higher levels of tryptase in serum—a granule released by mast cells (151). In mice fed a high-fat diet, mast cells have been reported to accumulate in visceral adipose tissue and may contribute to the development of obesity through the stimulation of adipocyte protease expression, promoting microvessel growth, enabling leukocyte infiltration, and adipose tissue expansion (151, 152). In humans with obesity and type-II diabetes, pharmacological stabilisation of mast cells to prevent degranulation leads to improvements in a number of parameters, including glycosylated haemoglobin, fasting blood glucose, total cholesterol, low-density lipoprotein, triglycerides, and high-density lipoprotein, independent of changes to BMI (153). Therefore, despite contradictory findings in murine research, study on humans indicates a potential role for mast cell dysregulation in the aetiology of metabolic diseases. However, whether this is a result of adipose-resident mast cells specifically is yet to be established.

Summary of the Cellular Changes Associated with Obesity-Induced Adipose Tissue Dysfunction

Adipose tissue dysfunction with obesity is associated with changes to the numbers and/or function of a variety of immune cells. With this ongoing immunological dysregulation, adipose tissue adopts a pro-inflammatory bias, dramatically impacting the metabolic health of the tissue. Consequently, dysfunctional adipose tissue influences whole-body immunometabolic health contributing to the generation of diseases including type-II diabetes and cardiovascular diseases. A summary of obesity-associated changes to adipose tissue-resident immune cell populations is presented in **Figure 3**.

IMMUNOLOGICAL AGEING AND ADIPOSE TISSUE

Most physiological systems become dysfunctional with ageing due to accumulations of cellular changes that contribute to the onset of disease. Nine hallmarks of ageing have been proposed characterising age-associated whole-body dysfunction, which include genomic instability, telomere attrition, epigenetic alterations, loss of proteostasis, dysregulated nutrient sensing, mitochondrial dysfunction, cellular senescence, stem cell exhaustion, and altered intracellular communication (15). The physiological stresses induced by obesity also cause a range of cellular and whole-body deteriorations that underpin the pathophysiology of adipose tissue accumulation and dysfunction. Many of these obesity-associated changes overlap with the hallmarks of ageing; thus, it has been proposed that obesity could be considered an accelerated model of ageing (13, 28, 154, 155).

Ageing is associated with a decline in immune function, referred to as immunosenescence, which is thought to contribute to chronic, low-grade inflammation or "inflammageing" (16, 156–159). The broader consequences of an ageing immune system are increased susceptibility to infections and cancer in combination with weaker responses to novel antigens, including those administered by vaccination (160). Immunosenescence is best characterised and most marked among cells of the adaptive immune system. However, a common general observation is that lymphoid cell numbers decline (along with their proliferative capacity), whereas myeloid cell numbers typically increase, but only some innate immune cells exhibit age-associated dysfunction (156). The most robust hallmarks of immunosenescence are alterations to the T-cell pool in peripheral blood. These changes are, in-part, not only due to thymic involution limiting the output of naive T-cells but also due to a lifetime of antigen exposure, which drives the differentiation of naive T-cells into memory T-cells (160). Thus, ageing is associated with an accumulation of pro-inflammatory effector memory T-cells and a decline in naive T-cells in peripheral blood (160–162).

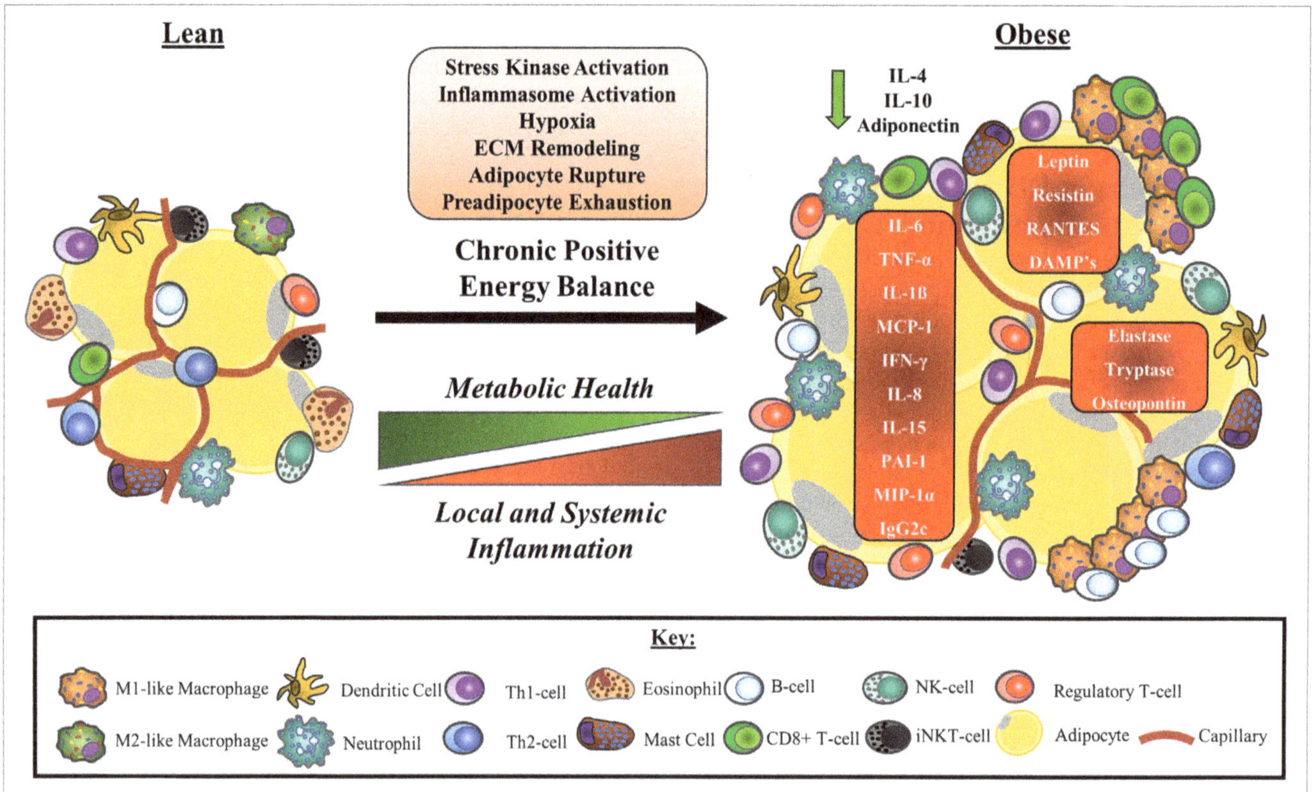

FIGURE 3 | A model of obesity-driven immunological changes within adipose tissue. Under a chronic state of positive energy balance, adipose tissue undergoes a multitude of changes that include the hypertrophic expansion of adipocytes without concurrent angiogenic responses. The consequences of these adaptations include local tissue hypoxia as a result of reduced tissue blood flow and impaired oxygen delivery. The rapid expansion of adipocytes also leads to unstable adipocytes prone to rupturing, releasing their lipid contents. This instability is further exacerbated by an exhaustion of the preadipocytes required to facilitate adipose tissue expansion. The net result of these physiological changes to adipocytes is the release of DAMPs and other signalling molecules that initiate stress kinase activation and promote monocyte infiltration to manage the remodelling of the ECM. Neutrophils are the first cells to accumulate in adipose tissue, followed by a range of other immune cells, most notably, B-cells, CD8+ T-cells, and M1-like/intermediate, or "double-negative" (CD11c–CD206–) macrophages that surround unstable adipocytes in crown-like structures. As a consequence, a Th-1 cell and M1-like macrophage secretion profile predominated and some anti-inflammatory immune cells such as eosinophils and iNKT-cells leave the tissue. Other anti-inflammatory cells, including regulatory T-cells, may increase to compensate. Pro-inflammatory cytokines and adipokines dominate the tissue microenvironment potentiating the activation of stress kinases and inflammasomes. Local inflammation reduces adipose tissue insulin sensitivity, impairing metabolic health and promoting ectopic lipid deposition. Pro-inflammatory adipose tissue contributes to the chronic, low-grade inflammation characteristic of obesity, and metabolic disease. Abbreviations: CD, cluster of differentiation marker; DAMP, damage-associated molecular pattern; ECM, extracellular matrix; IFN-γ, interferon gamma; Ig, immunoglobulin; IL, interleukin; iNKT-cell, invariant natural killer T cell; MCP-1, monocyte chemotactic protein 1 (CCL-2); MIP-1α, macrophage inflammatory protein 1 alpha (CCL-3); PAI-1, plasminogen activator inhibitor 1; RANTES, regulated on activation, normal T-cell expressed and secreted (CCL-5); Th cell, helper T cell; TNF-α, tumour necrosis factor-α.

Obesity, as with ageing, is associated with increased susceptibility to infections and an inability to mount effective immune responses to novel antigens (163–166). Thus, obesity might promote immunological decline through several mechanisms, with dysfunctional adipose tissue as a potential-driving factor. For example, obesity might exacerbate immunosenescence by promoting activation and differentiation of immune cells passing through the adipose tissue microvasculature, which could have implications for the phenotype and function of cells found in peripheral blood and other tissues. In addition, immune cell accumulation in adipose tissue promotes differentiation into pro-inflammatory cytokine-producing cells, which likely drives inflammageing. Exacerbated inflammation influence processes early in the immune response to novel pathogens, such as antigen recognition, processing, and presentation, but might also impair the ability to control latent or chronic infections and undergo processes such as wound healing. Experimental evidence supports some of these ideas, suggesting that adipose tissue dysfunction in obesity promotes immunological ageing (105).

Although there is less research specifically examining adipose tissue in the context ageing compared to obesity, a role for adipose tissue in late-onset disease development has been established. Ageing is associated with increased abdominal and ectopic adipose tissue accumulation, which is linked with the onset of frailty and cardiometabolic disease (167). Moreover, organelle stress and the accumulation of senescent cells (p16INK4a+) within adipose tissue that secrete IL-6, IL-8, and TNF-α further contribute to a pro-inflammatory, dysfunctional adipose tissue with age (168, 169). However, comparatively little is understood about immune cell populations within aged adipose tissue, especially in humans. Thus, the remaining sections will review literature examining the accumulation of different immune cells in adipose tissue with ageing, beginning with cells where there is most evidence, followed by cells that have been examined least.

Macrophages in Aged Adipose Tissue

Very few studies have investigated the effects of ageing on adipose tissue macrophage populations to date; however, the available data support a role for macrophages in age-associated adipose tissue dysfunction. This concept is discussed below and summarised in **Figure 4**. In visceral adipose tissue from old non-obese mice, it has been shown that the absolute numbers of adipose-resident macrophages do not increase substantially but may decline in proportions given the expanded stromal vascular fraction with age. However, with age, visceral adipose tissue macrophages have a predominantly pro-inflammatory, so-called "double-negative" (CD11c−CD206−) phenotype producing IL-6 and TNF-α and down regulating *PPAR-γ* (51, 170). Furthermore, peritoneal macrophages cultured with adipose-derived conditioned media induces M1-like polarisation, indicating that the products of adipose tissue have a direct impact on immune cells (170). Age-associated adipocyte-derived inflammation likely comes about by the activation of the NFκB signalling pathway (51). As a result, NFκB activation may act as a stimulus for the pro-inflammatory polarisation of adipose tissue macrophages, supporting the idea that changes within adipose tissue, independent from total adipose tissue mass, drive age-associated adipose tissue inflammation (171). These observations in mice likely correspond to those made in obese adipose tissue from humans (**Figure 1**) but experimental evidence is limited at present. Moreover, another study in middle-aged (11 months old) mice suggests that the proportions of "double-negative" (CD11c−CD206−) and M2-like macrophages are largely unaltered, whereas M1-like macrophages decline slightly when compared to young murine visceral adipose tissue (172). Note that these 11-month-old mice are representative of humans aged 30–40 years (173).

Sympathetic neuron-associated, catecholamine-degrading macrophages which impair lipolysis have also been reported to accumulate in aged murine visceral adipose tissue (175). With obesity, these sympathetic neuron-associated macrophages appear to infiltrate the tissue selectively (87). However, with ageing, these cells appear to accumulate in adipose tissue *via* proliferative mechanisms, *in situ* (175). The metabolic effects of these cells are due to NLRP-3 activation, which upregulates growth differentiation factor 3 (GDF3) expression within macrophages (175). GDF3 interacts with adipocytes to inhibit lipolysis and stimulates the expression of enzymes that oxidise and remove catecholamines (87, 175). Therefore, in the context of ageing, sympathetic neuron-associated macrophages likely regulate whole-body metabolism, inhibiting lipolytic signalling and free-fatty acid mobilisation as with obesity, contributing to immunometabolic dysfunction both locally and systemically.

In humans, only one study has investigated how ageing influences adipose tissue macrophages. Metabolically healthy Pima Indians, aged 18–44 years, were assessed for insulin sensitivity and subcutaneous adipose tissue macrophage content. Adipose tissue macrophage number increased until ~31–33 years old, plateauing or slightly declining thereafter, but with ageing, adopted an activated phenotype as shown by plasminogen activator inhibitor 1 and *CD11c* mRNA expression (**Figure 4**). The expression of these two macrophage activation markers was also associated with a decline in insulin sensitivity, independent of adiposity. Further, a negative relationship was observed between advancing age and whole-body insulin sensitivity ($r = -0.23$, $P = 0.07$). These findings suggest that although adipose-resident macrophages may decline or plateau in middle age, activation of these cells might impart an insulin-desensitising effect (174). Although this study offers the only direct assessment of adipose-resident macrophage populations with advancing age in humans, there are several factors that should be considered. For example, this study provides data up until middle age only and was conducted in a specific population with unique metabolic, genetic, and lifestyle characteristics. In addition, examining adipose-resident macrophages using gene expression and immunohistochemical analysis has some limitations (see **Table 1**).

The stimulus for age-associated macrophage pro-inflammatory polarisation is unclear, but endoplasmic reticulum stress, as shown in obese adipose tissue and adipose tissue macrophages, has been implicated. For example, it has been shown in aged murine adipose tissue stromal cells that endoplasmic reticulum stress promotes an inflammatory environment, elevating IL-6, MCP-1, and TNF-α production within adipose tissue, potentially in response to altered autophagy (176, 177). Ageing is associated

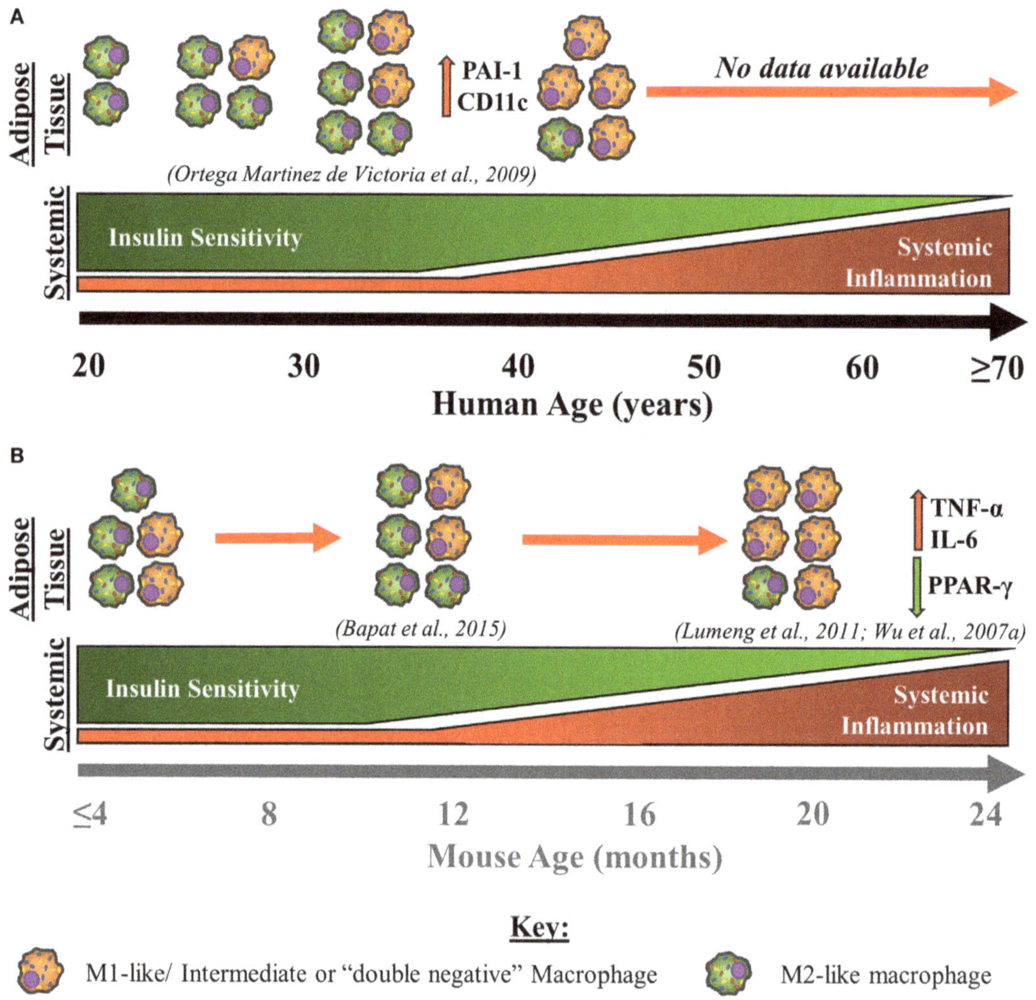

FIGURE 4 | Age-associated changes in adipose tissue macrophages and immunometabolic health in humans **(A)** and mice **(B)**. This schematic is a theoretical representation based on the limited empirical evidence that is available. With advancing age in humans **(A)**, subcutaneous adipose tissue macrophage content increases steadily until 31–33 years whereupon numbers slightly decline, until 45 years old (174). Although absolute adipose tissue macrophage content declines from around the age 31–33 years old until 45 years old, at least, the presence of more pro-inflammatory activated macrophages [M1-like/intermediate, or "double-negative" (CD11c–CD206–) macrophages] increases, which is associated with a decline in insulin sensitivity. With advancing age, insulin sensitivity continues to decline, while low-grade systemic inflammation begins to steadily increase from middle age into old age. With advancing age in mice **(B)**, an increase in pro-inflammatory macrophages within visceral adipose tissue that produce TNF-α and IL-6 and have downregulated PPAR-γ expression is also observed up to 18–24 months, at least (51, 170). Further, in middle-aged mice (44 weeks old), "double-negative" (CD11c–CD206–) and M2-like macrophages are largely unchanged or are modestly elevated, while M1-like macrophages exhibit a slight decline (172). Therefore, it is theorised that there is a continued pro-inflammatory macrophage activation/polarisation with advancing age in humans, independent of changes in absolute counts within the adipose tissue. Further, the same pattern of events appears to occur within murine adipose tissue, although the age at which this shift to a pro-inflammatory bias occurs is unknown. The similarities between data from aged mice and humans indicate that macrophages adopt a predominantly pro-inflammatory M1-like/intermediate, or "double-negative" (CD11c–CD206–) phenotype into old age, contributing to the increased systemic inflammation and impaired metabolic health exhibited by older individuals. Abbreviations: CD, cluster of differentiation marker; IL, interleukin; PAI-1, plasminogen activator inhibitor 1; PPAR-γ, peroxisome proliferator-activated receptor gamma; TNF-α, tumour necrosis factor-α.

with decreased vascularisation as a result of impaired angiogenesis, supporting local hypoxia, which might drive adipose tissue macrophage accumulation (36, 178–180). Ageing is also associated with reductions in the mitochondrial cytochrome *c* oxidase subunit 5B (COX5B) component of complex IV within adipocytes, which represses HIF-1α (181). Therefore, reductions in COX5B in human visceral adipose tissue with age both elevates HIF-1α and intracellular lipid storage as a result of decreased fatty acid oxidation, promoting adipocyte enlargement, *in vitro* (181). If this hypertrophic expansion was to continue, stress signals prompting macrophage infiltration could be released, as is observed in obesity (53, 79, 182).

Regulatory T-Cells in Aged Adipose Tissue

As with obesity, regulatory T-cells increase in the adipose tissue of old compared to young mice (110, 170, 172). The expanded population of these regulatory T-cells is transcriptionally more closely related to adipose-resident conventional T-cells than splenic regulatory T-cells (i.e., selective enrichment for *PPAR-γ* gene expression, among others), indicating that their characteristics may be driven, in part, by their location within the adipose tissue (172). However, unlike in obesity, an increase in regulatory T-cells in aged murine adipose tissue is linked with a decline in metabolic function independent of macrophage accumulation (172). These observations indicate that, in aged adipose tissue, a reduction in regulatory T-cells may be protective, because the immune profile of adipose tissue regulatory T-cell knockout mice is shifted towards those of young mice (172). Moreover, *ex vivo* adipose tissue basal glucose uptake was nearly twice as high for adipose-resident regulatory T-cell knockout mice compared to control tissues, supporting a causal association between adipose tissue regulatory T-cells and age-associated insulin resistance (172).

Although it is unclear whether the function of regulatory T-cells with ageing in humans is impaired, studies in aged mice indicate that these cells retain their suppressive capacity (172, 183). As a degree of inflammation is essential for the maintenance of healthy adipose tissue, the substantial increase in adipose tissue regulatory T-cells combined with the retention of their suppressive capacity may be an indication of overcompensation, impacting the immunometabolic properties of aged murine adipose tissue (26, 172). Although the observations concerning regulatory T-cells within aged murine adipose tissue provide evidence that age- and obesity-associated insulin insensitivity may be orchestrated by unique immune cell populations, further work in the adipose tissue of older humans is required to better understand this immunometabolic interplay. Additional work in older mice is also warranted as the animals examined by Bapat et al. (172) were substantially younger than those examined in other studies investigating age-associated adipose tissue immunological dysfunction (51, 170, 172) (see **Figure 4**). Nonetheless, recent evidence offers some support for a non-obesity-dependent regulatory T-cell-driven, late-onset metabolic deterioration, called type-IV diabetes (172).

B-Cells in Aged Adipose Tissue

It has been shown that the visceral adipose tissue of obese, old mice is enriched with a specific B-cell population compared to young, obese mice, and these cells differ from splenic B-cells (184). Co-culturing splenic B-cells with visceral adipocytes from old, obese mice caused B-cells to adopt an age-associated phenotype (184). These B-cells, which had been altered by adipose tissue, had higher levels of basal inflammation and NFκB protein within the nuclear extract, as has been shown with peripheral blood B-cells from older humans (185). In addition, the visceral adipose tissue of old mice has also been shown to be enriched with IgG2c (a mouse-specific IgG isoform), an observation that has also been made in obese mice (104, 184). It was proposed by Frasca and Blomberg (184) that increased hypoxia and *CCL-2* expression, along with increased adipocyte-derived TNF-α, IFN-γ, IL-6, and IL-21, prompted an obesity-driven accumulation of pro-inflammatory B-cells, which is exacerbated with ageing (184). Nonetheless, it should be noted that older mice in this study were heavier than younger mice and had more visceral adiposity. Thus, it is difficult to tease apart the effects of ageing or obesity in this work. Other evidence suggests that metabolic secretions released from dysfunctional adipose tissue with age, rather than typical pro-inflammatory factors, contribute to B-cell dysfunction. For example, it has been shown that incubation of B-cells from young mice with leptin induces STAT-3 signalling within B-cells, leading to TNF-α and IL-6 production, possibly contributing to the elevated production of these cytokines in aged murine adipose tissue (51, 171, 186).

CD4+ Th Cells and CD8+ Cytotoxic T-Cells in Aged Adipose Tissue

CD4+ T-cells within the visceral adipose tissue of obese mice display an "aged" phenotype and accumulate 4-fold with obesity (105, 170). High-fat overfeeding in mice causes an accumulation of CD4+ T-cells in the visceral adipose tissue expressing markers associated with senescence such as CD153+PD-1+CD44^{high}CD4+ T-cells in visceral adipose tissue. These cells secrete osteopontin, causing local inflammation (105). Moreover, CD4+ T-cells expressing markers such as CD153 also accumulate in the circulation with age in mice, perhaps linking changes in blood to changes in adipose tissue, or *vice versa* (187). Compared to the 4-fold increase in CD4+ T-cells in aged murine visceral adipose tissue, CD8+ T-cells exhibit a 7-fold increase, in parallel with an increase in *CCR-5* gene expression, which is involved in the migration and homing of effector T-cells (170, 188). However, whether adipose tissue CD8+ cells impart a pro-inflammatory function with age is unclear. CD8+ T-cells within aged adipose tissue have not been studied in isolation; although when adipose tissue stromal cells from aged mice were cultured *ex vivo*, no difference was found in the production of IFN-γ compared to young mice (170). Although there was a greater production of TNF-α from aged murine adipose tissue, this was attributed to macrophages (170). It is, therefore, currently unclear what role CD8+ T-cells play in aged adipose tissue. Furthermore, it is unclear what signal promotes this CD8+ T-cell expansion within aged adipose tissue and whether this contributes to, or merely reflects, the increased CD8:CD4 T-cell ratio in the circulation of older individuals (189).

Under-investigated Cells in Aged Adipose Tissue

Neutrophils, eosinophils, mast cells, dendritic cells, NK-cells, and iNKT cells have a role in obesity-associated adipose tissue dysfunction. Indeed, obesity is associated with alterations in the numbers, proportions and functions of many cell types, either resulting in a pro-inflammatory change (i.e., neutrophils, mast cells, dendritic cells, NK-cells) or an anti-inflammatory change (i.e., eosinophils and iNKT cells). These alterations contribute towards, or occur in response to, the immunometabolic dysfunction within adipose tissue caused by obesity. However, currently, there is no direct evidence for a similar role for these cells within adipose tissue in an ageing context.

Although no research has specifically examined neutrophils in aged adipose tissue in mice or humans, elevated *COX-2* mRNA has been shown in visceral adipose tissue from older mice, which may indicate neutrophil activation in response to elevated basal prostaglandin E2 (PGE_2) expression (51, 93, 190, 191). Moreover, neutrophils migrate through tissues secreting proteases (e.g., elastase) in response to homing signals including, among others, leptin, and aberrant secretion of this adipokine with age may promote neutrophil entry into adipose tissue (192–195). Neutrophils also demonstrate misdirected chemotaxis, with ageing, which, if neutrophils were signalled into adipose tissue in response to aberrant leptin secretions, would potentially exacerbate damage to the tissue, as membrane-bound proteases would be released over a wider area (196). In obese adipose tissue, increased elastase release by tissue-resident neutrophils impacts upon the metabolic health of adipose tissue by interacting with IRS-1 and TLR-4 signalling, impairing insulin sensitivity (89, 92, 197, 198). Therefore, using obesity as a model, neutrophil degranulation as a result of impaired navigation through the adipose tissue may contribute to age-associated adipose tissue dysfunction.

Mast cell and eosinophil numbers and function in adipose tissue has not been investigated in an ageing context. With eosinophils, considering that the number of these cells do not change with ageing in the circulation, it might be speculated that the same is true in adipose tissue (199). However, in obesity, the decline in adipose tissue eosinophils in mice might promote a pro-inflammatory macrophage predominance due to less eosinophil-derived IL-4 and IL-10. Subsequently, a loss of eosinophil-derived anti-inflammatory signals could contribute to fewer M2-like macrophages and the increase in M1-like or "double-negative" (CD11c−CD206−) macrophages with ageing in visceral adipose tissue. If mast cells are shown to be present in aged adipose tissue, the reported increase in PGE_2 within aged murine adipose tissue may promote mast cell degranulation, considering that PGE_2 inhibits the release of mediators that limit mast cell activation (51, 200).

Although no research has examined dendritic cells in adipose tissue with ageing, some evidence suggests that the pro-inflammatory profile of aged murine adipose tissue, as shown by high gene expression for IL-6, TNF-α, and PGE_2, could influence dendritic cell function (51). PGE_2 augments IL-23 production in aged murine and human dendritic cells, promoting Th-17 responses, while a pro-inflammatory aged adipose tissue microenvironment could promote NFκB activation within dendritic cells, as is seen in obese adipose tissue (138, 201–205). Dendritic cells from the circulation of older individuals may also have the potential to guide pro-on within adipose tissue due to increased intracellular IL-6 and TNF-α and increased expression of co-stimulatory and activation markers, as is observed in the context of obesity (133, 137, 158, 206). Nonetheless, these observations have yet to be investigated within aged adipose tissue and can, therefore, only represent speculative mechanisms at present.

We are unaware of any research that has investigated the role of NK-cells in aged adipose tissue. However, in mice, aberrant leptin secretions have been suggested to drive specifically activated $CD56^{dim}$ NK-cell polarisation, contributing to elevated TNF-α production and metabolic impairments (95, 96, 194). As well as leptin, the elevated TNF-α within aged murine adipose tissue may also serve to recruit NK-cells as TNF-α is essential for NK-cell recruitment into other organs such as the liver (207). It remains unclear whether the aberrant secretory profile of aged adipose tissue influences NK-cell function. However, as circulating $CD56^{dim}$ NK-cells accumulate in the blood of older people, if these cells were recruited into adipose tissue by TNF-α, leptin, or another yet to be established signal, they may contribute towards pro-inflammatory macrophage polarisation (102, 208–212).

Adipose tissue iNKT-cells have not been investigated with ageing, but considering that IL-4- and IL-10-producing NK1.1+iNKT-cells decline with obesity (127), it is possible that ageing has similar effects. However, given endogenous lipid antigens derived from adipocytes influence the secretion profile of iNKT-cells (127, 213, 214), then interactions between adipocytes and iNKT-cells might contribute towards iNKT-cell dysregulation in aged adipose tissue. For example, loading glycolipids into the CD1d receptor on adipocytes is mediated by intracellular ceramides (127), and sphingolipid ceramide content is higher in adipose tissue from old mice compared to young (51). Thus, in principle, enhanced ceramide-mediated glycolipid loading within aged adipocytes might drive overactivation of iNKT-cells with ageing.

SUMMARY, CONSIDERATIONS, AND FUTURE DIRECTIONS

Poor metabolic control, insulin resistance, inflammation, and impaired immune function are hallmarks of ageing and also characteristics of obesity. In addition, as outlined in this review, individuals who are obese, or elderly, exhibit similar immunological profiles in adipose tissue (**Tables 3–6**). Given the overlap between obesity and ageing, it is likely that changes to the numbers and function of some immune cells within obese and aged adipose—especially macrophages—contribute to dysfunction of this tissue. Moreover, it is possible that alterations to the immune profile of obese adipose tissue accelerate local and whole-body ageing. Finally, changes to the numbers and function of some immune cells within obese, and likely aged adipose tissue, whether a cause or consequence of adipose tissue dysfunction, may also underpin the development of metabolic diseases, as shown with obesity. However, there is limited work in an ageing context.

Improving our understanding of the interactions between ageing and adipose tissue dysfunction may help with the development of therapeutic and preventative strategies to improve longevity and quality of life in ageing populations. For example, with obesity, immunological dysregulation in adipose tissue is a well-established contributor to type-II diabetes and has consequently been a target for strategies such as caloric restriction, physical activity, and pharmacological manipulation. Caloric restriction imparts beneficial effects on metabolic control and blunts the production of pro-inflammatory cytokines from obese, murine adipose tissue (232, 233). Caloric restriction in older mice also delays ageing, in part due to beneficial effects on adipose tissue metabolic health and function (234). Moreover, in obese women, short- (1 month) and long-term (6 months) caloric restriction promotes an anti-inflammatory profile in abdominal, subcutaneous adipose tissue and reduces total adipose tissue

TABLE 3 | A comparison of the change in abundance for select immune cell subsets within adipose tissue with age and obesity compared to young and lean, respectively.

	Immune cells within adipose tissue			
	Ageing	**Ageing references**	**Obesity**	**Obesity references**
CD8+ T-cells	↑	(170)	↑	(113)
CD4+ T-cells	↑ ← →	(170)	↑	(35, 105)
Regulatory T-cells	↑(?)	(172)	↑/↓	(35, 125)
B-cells	↑(?)	(184)	↑	(104, 107)
Macrophages				
M1-like/intermediate/DN	↑	(51, 170)	↑	(63, 87)
M2-like	↓	(174, 175)	↓	(35, 65)
Eosinophils	?		↓	(147)
Mast cells	?		↑(?)	(151, 152, 215)
NK cells	?		↑	(95, 97)
iNKT cells	?		↓	(128, 132)
Neutrophils	?		↑	(89, 93)
Dendritic cells	?		↑	(133, 139)

↓, decrease; ↑, increase; ← →, little or no change or equivocal data; ?, unclear or no evidence; CD, cluster of differentiation marker; DN, double-negative macrophage (CD11c–CD206–); iNKT cell, invariant natural killer T cell; NK-cell, natural killer cell.

TABLE 4 | Changes to adipose tissue and adipocytes with age and obesity compared to young and lean, respectively.

	Broader Tissue-Specific Changes			
	Ageing	**Ageing references**	**Obesity**	**Obesity references**
Adipocyte size	↑	(216)	↑	(31)
Endoplasmic reticulum stress	↑	(176, 177)	↑	(82, 85)
Mitochondrial dysfunction	↑	(181)	↑	(217)
Stem cell exhaustion	↑	(13)	↑	(13)
Tissue blood flow	↓	(180)	↓	(36, 178)
Tissue hypoxia	↑		↑	

↓, decrease; ↑, increase.

TABLE 5 | Changes in the soluble factors produced and/or released by adipose tissue (adipocytes and cells of the stromal fraction) with age and obesity compared to young and lean, respectively.

	Soluble and secreted factors within adipose tissue			
	Ageing	**Ageing references**	**Obesity**	**Obesity references**
IL-6	↑	(171)	↑	(218)
MCP-1	↑	(170)	↑	(60)
TNF-α	↑	(51)	↑	(27)
IFN-γ	← →	(170)	↑	(113)
IL-10	← →	(170)	↓	(219)
IL-1β	↑	(51)	↑	(79)
Adiponectin	↓← →	(220)	↓	(221)
Leptin	↑	(192, 193)	↑	(222)

↓, decrease; ↑, increase; ← →, little or no change or equivocal data; IFN-γ, interferon gamma; IL, interleukin; MCP-1, monocyte chemotactic protein 1; TNF-α, tumour necrosis factor-α.

macrophage content (235, 236). Physical activity can reduce systemic inflammation, targeting dysregulated chemokine and adipokine secretory patterns in mice and humans (40, 237–239).

TABLE 6 | Changes in the expression of proteins within adipose tissue (adipocytes and cells of the stromal fraction) with age and obesity compared to young and lean, respectively.

	Proteins expressed within adipose tissue			
	Ageing	**Ageing references**	**Obesity**	**Obesity references**
CCR-2	↑	(170)	↑	(223)
CCR-5	↑	(170)	↑	(111, 112)
CCR-7	↓	(170)	↓	(224)
CX3CR-1	↓	(170)	↑ ← →	(225–228)
CXCR-3	↑	(170)	↑	(229)
PGE_2	↑	(51)	↑	(230)
PPAR-γ	↓	(51)	↑	(231)

↓, decrease; ↑, increase; ← →, little or no change or equivocal data; CCR, (C-C motif) chemokine receptor; CX3CR-1, (C-X3-C motif) chemokine receptor 1; CXCR-3, (C-X-C motif) chemokine receptor 3; PGE_2, prostaglandin E2; PPAR-γ, peroxisome proliferator-activated receptor gamma.

In parallel, physical activity also limits the accumulation of immune cells such as CD8+ T-cells—potentially by attenuating RANTES/CCR-5 signalling within human adipose tissue (237). Moreover, physical activity reduces neutrophil number and elastase expression, as well as shifting macrophages to an M2-like phenotype within the adipose tissue of mice fed a high-fat diet (237, 240, 241). In addition, exercise might limit, or delay immunosenescence by inducing an anti-inflammatory/anti-oxidative microenvironment within aged adipose tissue, limiting non-specific activation of T-cells and propagation of inflammation, by dampening adipose tissue-derived signals (242–244). Finally, pharmacological therapies (e.g., the PPAR-γ agonists rosiglitazone) promote M2-like macrophage repolarisation after high-fat overfeeding in mice (245). Further, PPAR signalling overlaps with the network of longevity genes, and PPAR-γ2 (adipocyte specific)-deficient mice have a considerably reduced lifespan, possibly mediated by the anti-inflammatory effects on adipose tissue macrophages (19, 20, 245). Therefore, targeting immunological dysregulation in adipose tissue might promote healthy ageing.

In conclusion, obesity is a useful model to develop our understanding of age-associated adipose tissue dysfunction. There is now an improved appreciation of how this metabolically and immunologically active tissue influences ageing and immunometabolic disease(s). The available evidence indicates that age-associated adipose tissue dysfunction occurs irrespective of changes in adipose tissue masses, and this dysfunction appears to play an active role in the pathophysiology of ageing. Moreover, the accumulation of predominantly pro-inflammatory immune cells in obese adipose tissue exacerbates the immunometabolic dysfunction of the tissue and might act as a potent stimulus for accelerating ageing in obesity. Importantly, countermeasures that target inflammation within dysfunctional adipose tissue offer promise to reduce the burden of obesity- and age-associated immunometabolic diseases.

AUTHOR CONTRIBUTIONS

All authors contributed equally to this work.

ACKNOWLEDGMENTS

We thank Dr. Frankie Brown and Lauren Struszczak for their helpful comments during the preparation of this manuscript.

FUNDING

This work was supported by funding from the BBSRC (BB/N004809/1) and the University of Bath.

REFERENCES

1. Hotamisligil GS. Inflammation, metaflammation and immunometabolic disorders. *Nature* (2017) 542(7640):177–85. doi:10.1038/nature21363
2. Hotamisligil GS. Inflammation and metabolic disorders. *Nature* (2006) 444(7121):860–7. doi:10.1038/nature05485
3. Lumeng CN, Saltiel AR. Inflammatory links between obesity and metabolic disease. *J Clin Invest* (2011) 121(6):2111–7. doi:10.1172/jci57132
4. de Ferranti S, Mozaffarian D. The perfect storm: obesity, adipocyte dysfunction, and metabolic consequences. *Clin Chem* (2008) 54(6):945–55. doi:10.1373/clinchem.2007
5. Gonzalez-Muniesa P, Martinez-Gonzalez MA, Hu FB, Despres JP, Matsuzawa Y, Loos RJF, et al. Obesity. *Nat Rev Dis Primers* (2017) 3:17034. doi:10.1038/nrdp.2017.34
6. World Health Organisation. *Obesity and overweight.* (2015). Available from: http://www.who.int/mediacentre/factsheets/fs311/en/
7. Finucane MM, Stevens GA, Cowan M, Danaei G, Lin JK, Paciorek CJ, et al. National, regional, and global trends in body mass index since 1980: systematic analysis of health examination surveys and epidemiological studies with 960 country-years and 9.1 million participants. *Lancet* (2011) 377(9765):557–67. doi:10.1016/S0140-6736(10)62037-5
8. Ballou SP, Kushner I. Chronic inflammation in older people: recognition, consequences, and potential intervention. *Clin Geriatr Med* (1997) 13(4):653–69.
9. Paolisso G, Rizzo MR, Mazziotti G, Tagliamonte MR, Gambardella A, Rotondi M, et al. Advancing age and insulin resistance: role of plasma tumor necrosis factor-alpha. *Am J Physiol* (1998) 275(2 Pt 1):E294–9.
10. Bruunsgaard H, Andersen-Ranberg K, Jeune B, Pedersen AN, Skinhoj P, Pedersen BK. A high plasma concentration of TNF-alpha is associated with dementia in centenarians. *J Gerontol A Biol Sci Med Sci* (1999) 54(7):M357–64. doi:10.1093/gerona/54.7.M357
11. Bartlett DB, Firth CM, Phillips AC, Moss P, Baylis D, Syddall H, et al. The age-related increase in low-grade systemic inflammation (inflammaging) is not driven by cytomegalovirus infection. *Aging Cell* (2012) 11(5):912–5. doi:10.1111/j.1474-9726.2012.00849.x
12. Pararasa C, Bailey CJ, Griffiths HR. Ageing, adipose tissue, fatty acids and inflammation. *Biogerontology* (2015) 16(2):235–48. doi:10.1007/s10522-014-9536-x
13. Pérez LM, Pareja-Galeano H, Sanchis-Gomar F, Emanuele E, Lucia A, Gálvez BG. 'Adipaging': aging and obesity share biological hallmarks related to a dysfunctional adipose tissue. *J Physiol* (2016) 594(12):3187–207. doi:10.1113/JP271691
14. Hotamisligil GS. Foundations of immunometabolism and implications for metabolic health and disease. *Immunity* (2017) 47(3):406–20. doi:10.1016/j.immuni.2017.08.009
15. Lopez-Otin C, Blasco MA, Partridge L, Serrano M, Kroemer G. The hallmarks of aging. *Cell* (2013) 153(6):1194–217. doi:10.1016/j.cell.2013.05.039
16. Franceschi C, Bonafe M, Valensin S, Olivieri F, De Luca M, Ottaviani E, et al. Inflamm-aging. An evolutionary perspective on immunosenescence. *Ann N Y Acad Sci* (2000) 908:244–54. doi:10.1111/j.1749-6632.2000.tb06651.x
17. Calçada D, Vianello D, Giampieri E, Sala C, Castellani G, de Graaf A, et al. The role of low-grade inflammation and metabolic flexibility in aging and nutritional modulation thereof: a systems biology approach. *Mech Ageing Dev* (2014) 136–137:138–47. doi:10.1016/j.mad.2014.01.004
18. Arai Y, Martin-Ruiz CM, Takayama M, Abe Y, Takebayashi T, Koyasu S, et al. Inflammation, but not telomere length, predicts successful ageing at extreme old age: a longitudinal study of semi-supercentenarians. *EBioMedicine* (2015) 2(10):1549–58. doi:10.1016/j.ebiom.2015.07.029
19. Picard F, Guarente L. Molecular links between aging and adipose tissue. *Int J Obes Relat Metab Disord* (2005) 29(Suppl 1):S36–9. doi:10.1038/sj.ijo.0802912
20. Argmann C, Dobrin R, Heikkinen S, Auburtin A, Pouilly L, Cock T-A, et al. Pparγ2 is a key driver of longevity in the mouse. *PLoS Genet* (2009) 5(12):e1000752. doi:10.1371/journal.pgen.1000752
21. Schwartz RS, Shuman WP, Bradbury VL, Cain KC, Fellingham GW, Beard JC, et al. Body fat distribution in healthy young and older men. *J Gerontol* (1990) 45(6):M181–5. doi:10.1093/geronj/45.6.M181
22. JafariNasabian P, Inglis JE, Reilly W, Kelly OJ, Ilich JZ. Aging human body: changes in bone, muscle and body fat with consequent changes in nutrient intake. *J Endocrinol* (2017) 234(1):R37–51. doi:10.1530/joe-16-0603
23. Huang FP, Platt N, Wykes M, Major JR, Powell TJ, Jenkins CD, et al. A discrete subpopulation of dendritic cells transports apoptotic intestinal epithelial cells to T cell areas of mesenteric lymph nodes. *J Exp Med* (2000) 191(3):435–44. doi:10.1084/jem.191.3.435
24. Parkin J, Cohen B. An overview of the immune system. *Lancet* (2001) 357(9270):1777–89. doi:10.1016/S0140-6736(00)04904-7
25. Zuniga-Pflucker JC. T-cell development made simple. *Nat Rev Immunol* (2004) 4(1):67–72. doi:10.1038/nri1257
26. Wernstedt Asterholm I, Tao C, Morley TS, Wang QA, Delgado-Lopez F, Wang ZV, et al. Adipocyte inflammation is essential for healthy adipose tissue expansion and remodeling. *Cell Metab* (2014) 20(1):103–18. doi:10.1016/j.cmet.2014.05.005
27. Hotamisligil GS, Shargill NS, Spiegelman BM. Adipose expression of tumor necrosis factor-alpha: direct role in obesity-linked insulin resistance. *Science* (1993) 259(5091):87–91. doi:10.1126/science.7678183
28. Tchkonia T, Morbeck DE, Von Zglinicki T, Van Deursen J, Lustgarten J, Scrable H, et al. Fat tissue, aging, and cellular senescence. *Aging Cell* (2010) 9(5):667–84. doi:10.1111/j.1474-9726.2010.00608.x
29. Fiorenza CG, Chou SH, Mantzoros CS. Lipodystrophy: pathophysiology and advances in treatment. *Nat Rev Endocrinol* (2011) 7(3):137–50. doi:10.1038/nrendo.2010.199
30. Goossens GH, Blaak EE. Adipose tissue dysfunction and impaired metabolic health in human obesity: a matter of oxygen? *Front Endocrinol* (2015) 6:55. doi:10.3389/fendo.2015.00055
31. Reilly SM, Saltiel AR. Adapting to obesity with adipose tissue inflammation. *Nat Rev Endocrinol* (2017) 13(11):633–43. doi:10.1038/nrendo.2017.90
32. Hosogai N, Fukuhara A, Oshima K, Miyata Y, Tanaka S, Segawa K, et al. Adipose tissue hypoxia in obesity and its impact on adipocytokine dysregulation. *Diabetes* (2007) 56(4):901. doi:10.2337/db06-0911
33. Bourlier V, Zakaroff-Girard A, Miranville A, Barros S, Maumus M, Sengenes C, et al. Remodeling phenotype of human subcutaneous adipose tissue macrophages. *Circulation* (2008) 117(6):806–15. doi:10.1161/circulationaha.107.724096
34. Lafontan M. Adipose tissue and adipocyte dysregulation. *Diabetes Metab* (2014) 40(1):16–28. doi:10.1016/j.diabet.2013.08.002
35. Travers RL, Motta AC, Betts JA, Bouloumie A, Thompson D. The impact of adiposity on adipose tissue-resident lymphocyte activation in humans. *Int J Obes (Lond)* (2015) 39(5):762–9. doi:10.1038/ijo.2014.195
36. Pasarica M, Sereda OR, Redman LM, Albarado DC, Hymel DT, Roan LE, et al. Reduced adipose tissue oxygenation in human obesity: evidence for rarefaction, macrophage chemotaxis, and inflammation without an angiogenic response. *Diabetes* (2009) 58(3):718–25. doi:10.2337/db08-1098
37. Donath MY, Shoelson SE. Type 2 diabetes as an inflammatory disease. *Nat Rev Immunol* (2011) 11(2):98–107. doi:10.1038/nri2925
38. Karpe F, Dickmann JR, Frayn KN. Fatty acids, obesity, and insulin resistance: time for a reevaluation. *Diabetes* (2011) 60(10):2441–9. doi:10.2337/db11-0425
39. McQuaid SE, Hodson L, Neville MJ, Dennis AL, Cheeseman J, Humphreys SM, et al. Downregulation of adipose tissue fatty acid trafficking in obesity: a driver for ectopic fat deposition? *Diabetes* (2011) 60(1):47–55. doi:10.2337/db10-0867

40. Thompson D, Karpe F, Lafontan M, Frayn K. Physical activity and exercise in the regulation of human adipose tissue physiology. *Physiol Rev* (2012) 92(1):157–91. doi:10.1152/physrev.00012.2011
41. Travers RL, Motta AC, Betts JA, Thompson D. Adipose tissue metabolic and inflammatory responses to a mixed meal in lean, overweight and obese men. *Eur J Nutr* (2017) 56(1):375–85. doi:10.1007/s00394-015-1087-7
42. Mutch DM, Tordjman J, Pelloux V, Hanczar B, Henegar C, Poitou C, et al. Needle and surgical biopsy techniques differentially affect adipose tissue gene expression profiles. *Am J Clin Nutr* (2009) 89(1):51–7. doi:10.3945/ajcn.2008.26802
43. Jensen TL, Kiersgaard MK, Sørensen DB, Mikkelsen LF. Fasting of mice: a review. *Lab Anim* (2013) 47(4):225–40. doi:10.1177/0023677213501659
44. Thompson D, Manolopoulos K, Bouloumie A. Arterio-venous differences in peripheral blood mononuclear cells across human adipose tissue and the effect of adrenaline infusion. *Int J Obes (Lond)* (2012) 36(9):1256–8. doi:10.1038/ijo.2011.219
45. Karpe F, Pinnick KE. Biology of upper-body and lower-body adipose tissue—link to whole-body phenotypes. *Nat Rev Endocrinol* (2015) 11(2):90–100. doi:10.1038/nrendo.2014.185
46. Manolopoulos KN, Karpe F, Frayn KN. Gluteofemoral body fat as a determinant of metabolic health. *Int J Obes (Lond)* (2010) 34(6):949–59. doi:10.1038/ijo.2009.286
47. Caesar R, Manieri M, Kelder T, Boekschoten M, Evelo C, Müller M, et al. A combined transcriptomics and lipidomics analysis of subcutaneous, epididymal and mesenteric adipose tissue reveals marked functional differences. *PLoS One* (2010) 5(7):e11525. doi:10.1371/journal.pone.0011525
48. Cinti S. The adipose organ at a glance. *Dis Model Mech* (2012) 5(5):588–94. doi:10.1242/dmm.009662
49. Chusyd DE, Wang D, Huffman DM, Nagy TR. Relationships between rodent white adipose fat pads and human white adipose fat depots. *Front Nutr* (2016) 3:10. doi:10.3389/fnut.2016.00010
50. Morgan-Bathke M, Harteneck D, Jaeger P, Sondergaard E, Karwoski R, Espinosa, et al. Comparison of methods for analyzing human adipose tissue macrophage content. *Obesity (Silver Spring)* (2017) 25(12):2100–7. doi:10.1002/oby.22012
51. Wu D, Ren Z, Pae M, Guo W, Cui X, Merrill AH, et al. Aging up-regulates expression of inflammatory mediators in mouse adipose tissue. *J Immunol* (2007) 179(7):4829–39. doi:10.4049/jimmunol.179.7.4829
52. Weisberg SP, McCann D, Desai M, Rosenbaum M, Leibel RL, Ferrante AW. Obesity is associated with macrophage accumulation in adipose tissue. *J Clin Invest* (2003) 112(12):1796–808. doi:10.1172/jci200319246
53. Cinti S, Mitchell G, Barbatelli G, Murano I, Ceresi E, Faloia E, et al. Adipocyte death defines macrophage localization and function in adipose tissue of obese mice and humans. *J Lipid Res* (2005) 46(11):2347–55. doi:10.1194/jlr.M500294-JLR200
54. Curat CA, Miranville A, Sengenès C, Diehl M, Tonus C, Busse R, et al. From blood monocytes to adipose tissue-resident macrophages: induction of diapedesis by human mature adipocytes. *Diabetes* (2004) 53(5):1285–92. doi:10.2337/diabetes.53.5.1285
55. Harman-Boehm I, Bluher M, Redel H, Sion-Vardy N, Ovadia S, Avinoach E, et al. Macrophage infiltration into omental versus subcutaneous fat across different populations: effect of regional adiposity and the comorbidities of obesity. *J Clin Endocrinol Metab* (2007) 92(6):2240–7. doi:10.1210/jc.2006-1811
56. Curat CA, Wegner V, Sengenes C, Miranville A, Tonus C, Busse R, et al. Macrophages in human visceral adipose tissue: increased accumulation in obesity and a source of resistin and visfatin. *Diabetologia* (2006) 49(4):744–7. doi:10.1007/s00125-006-0173-z
57. Geissmann F, Manz MG, Jung S, Sieweke MH, Merad M, Ley K. Development of monocytes, macrophages, and dendritic cells. *Science* (2010) 327(5966):656–61. doi:10.1126/science.1178331
58. Wang C, Yu X, Cao Q, Wang Y, Zheng G, Tan TK, et al. Characterization of murine macrophages from bone marrow, spleen and peritoneum. *BMC Immunol* (2013) 14:6. doi:10.1186/1471-2172-14-6
59. Khan T, Muise ES, Iyengar P, Wang ZV, Chandalia M, Abate N, et al. Metabolic dysregulation and adipose tissue fibrosis: role of collagen VI. *Mol Cell Biol* (2009) 29(6):1575–91. doi:10.1128/MCB.01300-08
60. Amano SU, Cohen JL, Vangala P, Tencerova M, Nicoloro SM, Yawe JC, et al. Local proliferation of macrophages contributes to obesity-associated adipose tissue inflammation. *Cell Metab* (2014) 19(1):162–71. doi:10.1016/j.cmet.2013.11.017
61. Hill AA, Anderson-Baucum EK, Kennedy AJ, Webb CD, Yull FE, Hasty AH. Activation of NF-kappaB drives the enhanced survival of adipose tissue macrophages in an obesogenic environment. *Mol Metab* (2015) 4(10):665–77. doi:10.1016/j.molmet.2015.07.005
62. Xu H, Barnes GT, Yang Q, Tan G, Yang D, Chou CJ, et al. Chronic inflammation in fat plays a crucial role in the development of obesity-related insulin resistance. *J Clin Nutr* (2003) 112(12):1821–30. doi:10.1172/jci200319451
63. Wentworth JM, Naselli G, Brown WA, Doyle L, Phipson B, Smyth GK, et al. Pro-inflammatory CD11c+CD206+ adipose tissue macrophages are associated with insulin resistance in human obesity. *Diabetes* (2010) 59(7):1648–56. doi:10.2337/db09-0287
64. Schutze S, Wiegmann K, Machleidt T, Kronke M. TNF-induced activation of NF-kappa B. *Immunobiology* (1995) 193(2–4):193–203. doi:10.1016/S0171-2985(11)80543-7
65. Suganami T, Tanimoto-Koyama K, Nishida J, Itoh M, Yuan X, Mizuarai S, et al. Role of the toll-like receptor 4/NF-kappaB pathway in saturated fatty acid-induced inflammatory changes in the interaction between adipocytes and macrophages. *Arterioscler Thromb Vasc Biol* (2007) 27(1):84–91. doi:10.1161/01.ATV.0000251608.09329.9a
66. Kopp A, Gross P, Falk W, Bala M, Weigert J, Buechler C, et al. Fatty acids as metabolic mediators in innate immunity. *Eur J Clin Invest* (2009) 39(10):924–33. doi:10.1111/j.1365-2362.2009.02185.x
67. Schaeffler A, Gross P, Buettner R, Bollheimer C, Buechler C, Neumeier M, et al. Fatty acid-induced induction of toll-like receptor-4/nuclear factor-κB pathway in adipocytes links nutritional signalling with innate immunity. *Immunology* (2009) 126(2):233–45. doi:10.1111/j.1365-2567.2008.02892.x
68. Engelman JA, Berg AH, Lewis RY, Lisanti MP, Scherer PE. Tumor necrosis factor alpha-mediated insulin resistance, but not dedifferentiation, is abrogated by MEK1/2 inhibitors in 3T3-L1 adipocytes. *Mol Endocrinol* (2000) 14(10):1557–69. doi:10.1210/mend.14.10.0542
69. Hauner H, Petruschke T, Russ M, Rohrig K, Eckel J. Effects of tumour necrosis factor alpha (TNF alpha) on glucose transport and lipid metabolism of newly-differentiated human fat cells in cell culture. *Diabetologia* (1995) 38(7):764–71. doi:10.1007/s001250050350
70. Ryden M, Dicker A, van Harmelen V, Hauner H, Brunnberg M, Perbeck L, et al. Mapping of early signaling events in tumor necrosis factor-alpha-mediated lipolysis in human fat cells. *J Biol Chem* (2002) 277(2):1085–91. doi:10.1074/jbc.M109498200
71. Lafontan M, Langin D. Lipolysis and lipid mobilization in human adipose tissue. *Prog Lipid Res* (2009) 48(5):275–97. doi:10.1016/j.plipres.2009.05.001
72. Bunn RC, Cockrell GE, Ou Y, Thrailkill KM, Lumpkin CK Jr, Fowlkes JL. Palmitate and insulin synergistically induce IL-6 expression in human monocytes. *Cardiovasc Diabetol* (2010) 9:73. doi:10.1186/1475-2840-9-73
73. Chen L, Chen R, Wang H, Liang F. Mechanisms linking inflammation to insulin resistance. *Int J Endocrinol* (2015) 2015:9. doi:10.1155/2015/508409
74. Trayhurn P. Hypoxia and adipose tissue function and dysfunction in obesity. *Physiol Rev* (2013) 93(1):1–21. doi:10.1152/physrev.00017.2012
75. Muir LA, Neeley CK, Meyer KA, Baker NA, Brosius AM, Washabaugh AR, et al. Adipose tissue fibrosis, hypertrophy, and hyperplasia: correlations with diabetes in human obesity. *Obesity (Silver Spring)* (2016) 24(3):597–605. doi:10.1002/oby.21377
76. Fujisaka S, Usui I, Ikutani M, Aminuddin A, Takikawa A, Tsuneyama K, et al. Adipose tissue hypoxia induces inflammatory M1 polarity of macrophages in an HIF-1alpha-dependent and HIF-1alpha-independent manner in obese mice. *Diabetologia* (2013) 56(6):1403–12. doi:10.1007/s00125-013-2885-1
77. Snodgrass RG, Boss M, Zezina E, Weigert A, Dehne N, Fleming I, et al. Hypoxia potentiates palmitate-induced pro-inflammatory activation of primary human macrophages. *J Biol Chem* (2016) 291(1):413–24. doi:10.1074/jbc.M115.686709
78. Yin R, Fang L, Li Y, Xue P, Li Y, Guan Y, et al. Pro-inflammatory macrophages suppress PPARgamma activity in adipocytes via S-nitrosylation. *Free Radic Biol Med* (2015) 89:895–905. doi:10.1016/j.freeradbiomed.2015.10.406
79. Morris DL, Singer K, Lumeng CN. Adipose tissue macrophages: phenotypic plasticity and diversity in lean and obese states. *Curr Opin Clin Nutr Metab Care* (2011) 14(4):341–6. doi:10.1097/MCO.0b013e328347970b

80. Stout RD, Suttles J. Functional plasticity of macrophages: reversible adaptation to changing microenvironments. *J Leukoc Biol* (2004) 76(3):509–13. doi:10.1189/jlb.0504272
81. Stout RD, Suttles J. Immunosenescence and macrophage functional plasticity: dysregulation of macrophage function by age-associated microenvironmental changes. *Immunol Rev* (2005) 205:60–71. doi:10.1111/j.0105-2896.2005.00260.x
82. Kawasaki N, Asada R, Saito A, Kanemoto S, Imaizumi K. Obesity-induced endoplasmic reticulum stress causes chronic inflammation in adipose tissue. *Sci Rep* (2012) 2:799. doi:10.1038/srep00799
83. Xue X, Piao JH, Nakajima A, Sakon-Komazawa S, Kojima Y, Mori K, et al. Tumor necrosis factor alpha (TNFalpha) induces the unfolded protein response (UPR) in a reactive oxygen species (ROS)-dependent fashion, and the UPR counteracts ROS accumulation by TNFalpha. *J Biol Chem* (2005) 280(40):33917–25. doi:10.1074/jbc.M505818200
84. Shan B, Wang X, Wu Y, Xu C, Xia Z, Dai J, et al. The metabolic ER stress sensor IRE1alpha suppresses alternative activation of macrophages and impairs energy expenditure in obesity. *Nat Immunol* (2017) 18(5):519–29. doi:10.1038/ni.3709
85. Suzuki T, Gao J, Ishigaki Y, Kondo K, Sawada S, Izumi T, et al. ER stress protein CHOP mediates insulin resistance by modulating adipose tissue macrophage polarity. *Cell Rep* (2017) 18(8):2045–57. doi:10.1016/j.celrep.2017.01.076
86. Duffaut C, Galitzky J, Lafontan M, Bouloumie A. Unexpected trafficking of immune cells within the adipose tissue during the onset of obesity. *Biochem Biophys Res Commun* (2009) 384(4):482–5. doi:10.1016/j.bbrc.2009.05.002
87. Pirzgalska RM, Seixas E, Seidman JS, Link VM, Sánchez NM, Mahú I, et al. Sympathetic neuron-associated macrophages contribute to obesity by importing and metabolizing norepinephrine. *Nat Med* (2017) 23(11):1309–18. doi:10.1038/nm.4422
88. Czech MP. Macrophages dispose of catecholamines in adipose tissue. *Nat Med* (2017) 23(11):1255–7. doi:10.1038/nm.4440
89. Talukdar S, Oh DY, Bandyopadhyay G, Li D, Xu J, McNelis J, et al. Neutrophils mediate insulin resistance in mice fed a high-fat diet through secreted elastase. *Nat Med* (2012) 18(9):1407–12. doi:10.1038/nm.2885
90. Elgazar-Carmon V, Rudich A, Hadad N, Levy R. Neutrophils transiently infiltrate intra-abdominal fat early in the course of high-fat feeding. *J Lipid Res* (2008) 49(9):1894–903. doi:10.1194/jlr.M800132-JLR200
91. Ferrante AW Jr. The immune cells in adipose tissue. *Diabetes Obes Metab* (2013) 15(Suppl 3):34–8. doi:10.1111/dom.12154
92. Houghton AM, Rzymkiewicz DM, Ji H, Gregory AD, Egea EE, Metz HE, et al. Neutrophil elastase-mediated degradation of IRS-1 accelerates lung tumor growth. *Nat Med* (2010) 16(2):219–23. doi:10.1038/nm.2084
93. Shah TJ, Leik CE, Walsh SW. Neutrophil infiltration and systemic vascular inflammation in obese women. *Reprod Sci* (2010) 17(2):116–24. doi:10.1177/1933719109348252
94. Rouault C, Pellegrinelli V, Schilch R, Cotillard A, Poitou C, Tordjman J, et al. Roles of chemokine ligand-2 (CXCL2) and neutrophils in influencing endothelial cell function and inflammation of human adipose tissue. *Endocrinology* (2013) 154(3):1069–79. doi:10.1210/en.2012-1415
95. Theurich S, Tsaousidou E, Hanssen R, Lempradl AM, Mauer J, Timper K, et al. IL-6/Stat3-dependent induction of a distinct, obesity-associated NK cell subpopulation deteriorates energy and glucose homeostasis. *Cell Metab* (2017) 26(1):171–84. doi:10.1016/j.cmet.2017.05.018
96. Tian Z, Sun R, Wei H, Gao B. Impaired natural killer (NK) cell activity in leptin receptor deficient mice: leptin as a critical regulator in NK cell development and activation. *Biochem Biophys Res Commun* (2002) 298(3):297–302. doi:10.1016/S0006-291X(02)02462-2
97. Wensveen FM, Jelencic V, Valentic S, Sestan M, Wensveen TT, Theurich S, et al. NK cells link obesity-induced adipose stress to inflammation and insulin resistance. *Nat Immunol* (2015) 16(4):376–85. doi:10.1038/ni.3120
98. Lee BC, Kim MS, Pae M, Yamamoto Y, Eberle D, Shimada T, et al. Adipose natural killer cells regulate adipose tissue macrophages to promote insulin resistance in obesity. *Cell Metab* (2016) 23(4):685–98. doi:10.1016/j.cmet.2016.03.002
99. Henegar C, Tordjman J, Achard V, Lacasa D, Cremer I, Guerre-Millo M, et al. Adipose tissue transcriptomic signature highlights the pathological relevance of extracellular matrix in human obesity. *Genome Biol* (2008) 9(1):R14. doi:10.1186/gb-2008-9-1-r14
100. O'Rourke RW, Metcalf MD, White AE, Madala A, Winters BR, Maizlin II, et al. Depot-specific differences in inflammatory mediators and a role for NK cells and IFN-gamma in inflammation in human adipose tissue. *Int J Obes (Lond)* (2009) 33(9):978–90. doi:10.1038/ijo.2009.133
101. O'Rourke RW, Gaston GD, Meyer KA, White AE, Marks DL. Adipose tissue NK cells manifest an activated phenotype in human obesity. *Metabolism* (2013) 62(11):1557–61. doi:10.1016/j.metabol.2013.07.011
102. Bonamichi BDSF, Lee J. Unusual suspects in the development of obesity-induced inflammation and insulin resistance: NK cells, iNKT cells, and ILCs. *Diabetes Metab J* (2017) 41(4):229–50. doi:10.4093/dmj.2017.41.4.229
103. Ying W, Wollam J, Ofrecio JM, Bandyopadhyay G, El Ouarrat D, Lee YS, et al. Adipose tissue B2 cells promote insulin resistance through leukotriene LTB4/LTB4R1 signaling. *J Clin Invest* (2017) 127(3):1019–30. doi:10.1172/JCI90350
104. Winer DA, Winer S, Shen L, Wadia PP, Yantha J, Paltser G, et al. B cells promote insulin resistance through modulation of T cells and production of pathogenic IgG antibodies. *Nat Med* (2011) 17(5):610–7. doi:10.1038/nm.2353
105. Shirakawa K, Yan X, Shinmura K, Endo J, Kataoka M, Katsumata Y, et al. Obesity accelerates T cell senescence in murine visceral adipose tissue. *J Clin Invest* (2016) 126(12):4626–39. doi:10.1172/jci88606
106. Stromnes IM, Goverman JM. Osteopontin-induced survival of T cells. *Nat Immunol* (2007) 8(1):19–20. doi:10.1038/ni0107-19
107. McDonnell ME, Ganley-Leal LM, Mehta A, Bigornia S, Mott M, Rehman Q, et al. B lymphocytes in human subcutaneous adipose crown-like structures. *Obesity (Silver Spring)* (2012) 20(7):1372–8. doi:10.1038/oby.2012.54
108. Sears DD, Hsiao G, Hsiao A, Yu JG, Courtney CH, Ofrecio JM, et al. Mechanisms of human insulin resistance and thiazolidinedione-mediated insulin sensitization. *Proc Nat Acad Sci U S A* (2009) 106(44):18745–50. doi:10.1073/pnas.0903032106
109. Duffaut C, Zakaroff-Girard A, Bourlier V, Decaunes P, Maumus M, Chiotasso P, et al. Interplay between human adipocytes and T lymphocytes in obesity: CCL20 as an adipochemokine and T lymphocytes as lipogenic modulators. *Arterioscler Thromb Vasc Biol* (2009) 29(10):1608–14. doi:10.1161/ATVBAHA.109.192583
110. Feuerer M, Herrero L, Cipolletta D, Naaz A, Wong J, Nayer A, et al. Lean, but not obese, fat is enriched for a unique population of regulatory T cells that affect metabolic parameters. *Nat Med* (2009) 15(8):930–9. doi:10.1038/nm.2002
111. Wu H, Ghosh S, Perrard XD, Feng L, Garcia GE, Perrard JL, et al. T-cell accumulation and regulated on activation, normal T cell expressed and secreted upregulation in adipose tissue in obesity. *Circulation* (2007) 115(8):1029–38. doi:10.1161/CIRCULATIONAHA.106.638379
112. Kintscher U, Hartge M, Hess K, Foryst-Ludwig A, Clemenz M, Wabitsch M, et al. T-lymphocyte infiltration in visceral adipose tissue: a primary event in adipose tissue inflammation and the development of obesity-mediated insulin resistance. *Arterioscler Thromb Vasc Biol* (2008) 28(7):1304–10. doi:10.1161/ATVBAHA.108.165100
113. Nishimura S, Manabe I, Nagasaki M, Eto K, Yamashita H, Ohsugi M, et al. CD8+ effector T cells contribute to macrophage recruitment and adipose tissue inflammation in obesity. *Nat Med* (2009) 15(8):914–20. doi:10.1038/nm.1964
114. Winer S, Chan Y, Paltser G, Truong D, Tsui H, Bahrami J, et al. Normalization of obesity-associated insulin resistance through immunotherapy. *Nat Med* (2009) 15(8):921–9. doi:10.1038/nm.2001
115. Kim JJ, Nottingham LK, Sin JI, Tsai A, Morrison L, Oh J, et al. CD8 positive T cells influence antigen-specific immune responses through the expression of chemokines. *J Clin Invest* (1998) 102(6):1112–24. doi:10.1172/JCI3986
116. Koenen TB, Stienstra R, van Tits LJ, Joosten LA, van Velzen JF, Hijmans A, et al. The inflammasome and caspase-1 activation: a new mechanism underlying increased inflammatory activity in human visceral adipose tissue. *Endocrinology* (2011) 152(10):3769–78. doi:10.1210/en.2010-1480
117. Nomura S, Shouzu A, Omoto S, Nishikawa M, Fukuhara S. Significance of chemokines and activated platelets in patients with diabetes. *Clin Exp Immunol* (2000) 121(3):437–43. doi:10.1046/j.1365-2249.2000.01324.x
118. Mauro C, Smith J, Cucchi D, Coe D, Fu H, Bonacina F, et al. Obesity-induced metabolic stress leads to biased effector memory CD4+ T cell differentiation via PI3K p110delta-Akt-mediated signals. *Cell Metab* (2017) 25(3):593–609. doi:10.1016/j.cmet.2017.01.008

119. Macintyre AN, Finlay D, Preston G, Sinclair LV, Waugh CM, Tamas P, et al. Protein kinase B controls transcriptional programs that direct cytotoxic T cell fate but is dispensable for T cell metabolism. *Immunity* (2011) 34(2):224–36. doi:10.1016/j.immuni.2011.01.012
120. Finlay DK, Rosenzweig E, Sinclair LV, Feijoo-Carnero C, Hukelmann JL, Rolf J, et al. PDK1 regulation of mTOR and hypoxia-inducible factor 1 integrate metabolism and migration of CD8+ T cells. *J Exp Med* (2012) 209(13):2441–53. doi:10.1084/jem.20112607
121. Rocha VZ, Folco EJ, Sukhova G, Shimizu K, Gotsman I, Vernon AH, et al. Interferon-gamma, a Th1 cytokine, regulates fat inflammation: a role for adaptive immunity in obesity. *Circ Res* (2008) 103(5):467–76. doi:10.1161/CIRCRESAHA.108.177105
122. Rocha PM, Barata JT, Teixeira PJ, Ross R, Sardinha LB. Independent and opposite associations of hip and waist circumference with metabolic syndrome components and with inflammatory and atherothrombotic risk factors in overweight and obese women. *Metabolism* (2008) 57(10):1315–22. doi:10.1016/j.metabol.2008.01.003
123. Cheshire JL, Baldwin AS. Synergistic activation of NF-kappaB by tumor necrosis factor alpha and gamma interferon via enhanced I kappaB alpha degradation and de novo I kappaBbeta degradation. *Mol Cell Biol* (1997) 17(11):6746–54. doi:10.1128/mcb.17.11.6746
124. Bourlier V, Bouloumie A. Role of macrophage tissue infiltration in obesity and insulin resistance. *Diabetes Metab* (2009) 35(4):251–60. doi:10.1016/j.diabet.2009.05.001
125. Deng T, Liu J, Deng Y, Minze L, Xiao X, Wright V, et al. Adipocyte adaptive immunity mediates diet-induced adipose inflammation and insulin resistance by decreasing adipose Treg cells. *Nat Commun* (2017) 8(15725):1–11. doi:10.1038/ncomms15725
126. Acosta JR, Douagi I, Andersson DP, Backdahl J, Ryden M, Arner P, et al. Increased fat cell size: a major phenotype of subcutaneous white adipose tissue in non-obese individuals with type 2 diabetes. *Diabetologia* (2016) 59(3):560–70. doi:10.1007/s00125-015-3810-6
127. van Eijkeren RJ, Krabbe O, Boes M, Schipper HS, Kalkhoven E. Endogenous lipid antigens for invariant natural killer T cells hold the reins in adipose tissue homeostasis. *Immunology* (2017) 153(2):179–89. doi:10.1111/imm.12839
128. Huh JY, Park J, Kim JI, Park YJ, Lee YK, Kim JB. Deletion of CD1d in adipocytes aggravates adipose tissue inflammation and insulin resistance in obesity. *Diabetes* (2017) 66(4):835–47. doi:10.2337/db16-1122
129. Lynch L, Michelet X, Zhang S, Brennan PJ, Moseman A, Lester C, et al. Regulatory iNKT cells lack PLZF expression and control T(reg) cell and macrophage homeostasis in adipose tissue. *Nat Immunol* (2015) 16(1):85–95. doi:10.1038/ni.3047
130. Lynch L, Hogan AE, Duquette D, Lester C, Banks A, LeClair K, et al. iNKT cells induce FGF21 for thermogenesis and are required for maximal weight loss in GLP1 therapy. *Cell Metab* (2016) 24(3):510–9. doi:10.1016/j.cmet.2016.08.003
131. Lynch L, O'Shea D, Winter DC, Geoghegan J, Doherty DG, O'Farrelly C. Invariant NKT cells and CD1d(+) cells amass in human omentum and are depleted in patients with cancer and obesity. *Eur J Immunol* (2009) 39(7):1893–901. doi:10.1002/eji.200939349
132. Lynch L, Nowak M, Varghese B, Clark J, Hogan AE, Toxavidis V, et al. Adipose tissue invariant NKT cells protect against diet-induced obesity and metabolic disorder through regulatory cytokine production. *Immunity* (2012) 37(3):574–87. doi:10.1016/j.immuni.2012.06.016
133. Stefanovic-Racic M, Yang X, Turner MS, Mantell BS, Stolz DB, Sumpter TL, et al. Dendritic cells promote macrophage infiltration and comprise a substantial proportion of obesity-associated increases in CD11c+ cells in adipose tissue and liver. *Diabetes* (2012) 61(9):2330–9. doi:10.2337/db11-1523
134. Chen Y, Tian J, Tian X, Tang X, Rui K, Tong J, et al. Adipose tissue dendritic cells enhances inflammation by prompting the generation of Th17 cells. *PLoS One* (2014) 9(3):e92450. doi:10.1371/journal.pone.0092450
135. Pearce EL, Shen H. Generation of CD8 T cell memory is regulated by IL-12. *J Immunol* (2007) 179(4):2074–81. doi:10.4049/jimmunol.179.4.2074
136. Martinez FO, Gordon S. The M1 and M2 paradigm of macrophage activation: time for reassessment. *F1000Prime Rep* (2014) 6:13. doi:10.12703/P6-13
137. Wang N, Liang H, Zen K. Molecular mechanisms that influence the macrophage M1–M2 polarization balance. *Front Immunol* (2014) 5:614. doi:10.3389/fimmu.2014.00614
138. Bertola A, Ciucci T, Rousseau D, Bourlier V, Duffaut C, Bonnafous S, et al. Identification of adipose tissue dendritic cells correlated with obesity-associated insulin-resistance and inducing Th17 responses in mice and patients. *Diabetes* (2012) 61(9):2238–47. doi:10.2337/db11-1274
139. Hannibal TD, Schmidt-Christensen A, Nilsson J, Fransén-Pettersson N, Hansen L, Holmberg D. Deficiency in plasmacytoid dendritic cells and type I interferon signalling prevents diet-induced obesity and insulin resistance in mice. *Diabetologia* (2017) 60(10):2033–41. doi:10.1007/s00125-017-4341-0
140. Ernst MC, Issa M, Goralski KB, Sinal CJ. Chemerin exacerbates glucose intolerance in mouse models of obesity and diabetes. *Endocrinology* (2010) 151(5):1998–2007. doi:10.1210/en.2009-1098
141. Goossens P, Gijbels MJ, Zernecke A, Eijgelaar W, Vergouwe MN, van der Made I, et al. Myeloid type I interferon signaling promotes atherosclerosis by stimulating macrophage recruitment to lesions. *Cell Metab* (2010) 12(2):142–53. doi:10.1016/j.cmet.2010.06.008
142. Pattison MJ, MacKenzie KF, Elcombe SE, Arthur JS. IFNbeta autocrine feedback is required to sustain TLR induced production of MCP-1 in macrophages. *FEBS Lett* (2013) 587(10):1496–503. doi:10.1016/j.febslet.2013.03.025
143. Ghosh AR, Bhattacharya R, Bhattacharya S, Nargis T, Rahaman O, Duttagupta P, et al. Adipose recruitment and activation of plasmacytoid dendritic cells fuel metaflammation. *Diabetes* (2016) 65(11):3440–52. doi:10.2337/db16-0331
144. Morelli AE, Thomson AW. Dendritic cells: regulators of alloimmunity and opportunities for tolerance induction. *Immunol Rev* (2003) 196:125–46. doi:10.1046/j.1600-065X.2003.00079.x
145. Pond CM. Adipose tissue and the immune system. *Prostaglandins Leukot Essent Fatty Acids* (2005) 73(1):17–30. doi:10.1016/j.plefa.2005.04.005
146. Chawla A, Nguyen KD, Goh YPS. Macrophage-mediated inflammation in metabolic disease. *Nat Rev Immunol* (2011) 11(11):738–49. doi:10.1038/nri3071
147. Wu D, Molofsky AB, Liang H, Ricardo-Gonzalez R, Jouihan H, Bando J, et al. Eosinophils sustain adipose alternatively activated macrophages associated with glucose homeostasis. *Science* (2011) 332(6026):243–7. doi:10.1126/science.1201475
148. Schipper HS, Prakken B, Kalkhoven E, Boes M. Adipose tissue-resident immune cells: key players in immunometabolism. *Trends Endocrinol Metab* (2012) 23(8):407–15. doi:10.1016/j.tem.2012.05.011
149. Mohrs K, Wakil AE, Killeen N, Locksley RM, Mohrs M. A two-step process for cytokine production revealed by IL-4 dual-reporter mice. *Immunity* (2005) 23(4):419–29. doi:10.1016/j.immuni.2005.09.006
150. Qiu Y, Nguyen KD, Odegaard JI, Cui X, Tian X, Locksley RM, et al. Eosinophils and type 2 cytokine signaling in macrophages orchestrate development of functional beige fat. *Cell* (2014) 157(6):1292–308. doi:10.1016/j.cell.2014.03.066
151. Liu J, Divoux A, Sun J, Zhang J, Clement K, Glickman JN, et al. Genetic deficiency and pharmacological stabilization of mast cells reduce diet-induced obesity and diabetes in mice. *Nat Med* (2009) 15(8):940–5. doi:10.1038/nm.1994
152. Zhou Y, Yu X, Chen H, Sjöberg S, Roux J, Zhang L, et al. Leptin deficiency shifts mast cells toward anti-inflammatory actions and protects mice from obesity and diabetes by polarizing M2 macrophages. *Cell Metab* (2015) 22(6):1045–58. doi:10.1016/j.cmet.2015.09.013
153. El-Haggar SM, Farrag WF, Kotkata FA. Effect of ketotifen in obese patients with type 2 diabetes mellitus. *J Diabetes Complications* (2015) 29(3):427–32. doi:10.1016/j.jdiacomp.2015.01.013
154. Tzanetakou IP, Katsilambros NL, Benetos A, Mikhailidis DP, Perrea DN. "Is obesity linked to aging?": adipose tissue and the role of telomeres. *Ageing Res Rev* (2012) 11(2):220–9. doi:10.1016/j.arr.2011.12.003
155. Palmer AK, Kirkland JL. Aging and adipose tissue: potential interventions for diabetes and regenerative medicine. *Exp Gerontol* (2016) 86:97–105. doi:10.1016/j.exger.2016.02.013
156. Aw D, Silva AB, Palmer DB. Immunosenescence: emerging challenges for an ageing population. *Immunology* (2007) 120(4):435–46. doi:10.1111/j.1365-2567.2007.02555.x
157. Pawelec G. Hallmarks of human "immunosenescence": adaptation or dysregulation? *Immun Ageing* (2012) 9(1):15. doi:10.1186/1742-4933-9-15
158. Shaw AC, Goldstein DR, Montgomery RR. Age-dependent dysregulation of innate immunity. *Nat Rev Immunol* (2013) 13(12):875–87. doi:10.1038/nri3547

159. Puzianowska-Kuźnicka M, Owczarz M, Wieczorowska-Tobis K, Nadrowski P, Chudek J, Slusarczyk P, et al. Interleukin-6 and C-reactive protein, successful aging, and mortality: the PolSenior study. *Immun Ageing* (2016) 13:21. doi:10.1186/s12979-016-0076-x
160. Nikolich-Žugich J. Aging of the T cell compartment in mice and humans: from no naïve expectations to foggy memories. *J Immunol* (2014) 193(6):2622–9. doi:10.4049/jimmunol.1401174
161. Effros RB. Replicative senescence of CD8 T cells: effect on human ageing. *Exp Gerontol* (2004) 39(4):517–24. doi:10.1016/j.exger.2003.09.024
162. Akbar AN, Fletcher JM. Memory T cell homeostasis and senescence during aging. *Curr Opin Immunol* (2005) 17(5):480–5. doi:10.1016/j.coi.2005.07.019
163. Lang P-O, Mendes A, Socquet J, Assir N, Govind S, Aspinall R. Effectiveness of influenza vaccine in aging and older adults: comprehensive analysis of the evidence. *Clin Interv Aging* (2012) 7:55–64. doi:10.2147/CIA.S25215
164. Sheridan PA, Paich HA, Handy J, Karlsson EA, Hudgens MG, Sammon AB, et al. Obesity is associated with impaired immune response to influenza vaccination in humans. *Int J Obes (Lond)* (2012) 36(8):1072–7. doi:10.1038/ijo.2011.208
165. Huttunen R, Syrjanen J. Obesity and the risk and outcome of infection. *Int J Obes (Lond)* (2013) 37(3):333–40. doi:10.1038/ijo.2012.62
166. Neidich SD, Green WD, Rebeles J, Karlsson EA, Schultz-Cherry S, Noah TL, et al. Increased risk of influenza among vaccinated adults who are obese. *Int J Obes* (2017) 41(9):1324–30. doi:10.1038/ijo.2017.131
167. Mau T, Yung R. Adipose tissue inflammation in aging. *Exp Gerontol* (2017) S0531-5565(17):30714–30713. doi:10.1016/j.exger.2017.10.014
168. Baker DJ, Wijshake T, Tchkonia T, LeBrasseur NK, Childs BG, van de Sluis B, et al. Clearance of p16Ink4a-positive senescent cells delays ageing-associated disorders. *Nature* (2011) 479(7372):232–6. doi:10.1038/nature10600
169. Tchkonia T, Zhu Y, van Deursen J, Campisi J, Kirkland JL. Cellular senescence and the senescent secretory phenotype: therapeutic opportunities. *J Clin Invest* (2013) 123(3):966–72. doi:10.1172/jci64098
170. Lumeng CN, Liu J, Geletka L, Delaney C, Delproposto J, Desai A, et al. Aging is associated with an increase in T cells and inflammatory macrophages in visceral adipose tissue. *J Immunol* (2011) 187(12):6208–16. doi:10.4049/jimmunol.1102188
171. Starr ME, Evers BM, Saito H. Age-associated increase in cytokine production during systemic inflammation: adipose tissue as a major source of IL-6. *J Gerontol A Biol Sci Med Sci* (2009) 64(7):723–30. doi:10.1093/gerona/glp046
172. Bapat SP, Myoung Suh J, Fang S, Liu S, Zhang Y, Cheng A, et al. Depletion of fat-resident Treg cells prevents age-associated insulin resistance. *Nature* (2015) 528(7580):137–41. doi:10.1038/nature16151
173. Flurkey K, Currer JM, Harrison DE. Mouse models in aging research. In: Fox JG, Quimby FW, Barthold SW, Newcomer CE, Smith AL, editors. *The Mouse in Biomedical Research*, 2nd ed. Burlington: Academic Press (2007). p. 637–72.
174. Ortega Martinez de Victoria E, Xu X, Koska J, Francisco AM, Scalise M, Ferrante AW Jr, et al. Macrophage content in subcutaneous adipose tissue: associations with adiposity, age, inflammatory markers, and whole-body insulin action in healthy Pima Indians. *Diabetes* (2009) 58(2):385–93. doi:10.2337/db08-0536
175. Camell CD, Sander J, Spadaro O, Lee A, Nguyen KY, Wing A, et al. Inflammasome-driven catecholamine catabolism in macrophages blunts lipolysis during ageing. *Nature* (2017) 550(7674):119–23. doi:10.1038/nature24022
176. Ghosh AK, Mau T, O'Brien M, Garg S, Yung R. Impaired autophagy activity is linked to elevated ER-stress and inflammation in aging adipose tissue. *Aging (Albany NY)* (2016) 8(10):2525–36. doi:10.18632/aging.101083
177. Ghosh AK, Garg SK, Mau T, O'Brien M, Liu J, Yung R. Elevated endoplasmic reticulum stress response contributes to adipose tissue inflammation in aging. *J Gerontol A Biol Sci Med Sci* (2015) 70(11):1320–9. doi:10.1093/gerona/glu186
178. Ye J, Gao Z, Yin J, He Q. Hypoxia is a potential risk factor for chronic inflammation and adiponectin reduction in adipose tissue of ob/ob and dietary obese mice. *Am J Physiol Endocrinol Metab* (2007) 293(4):E1118–28. doi:10.1152/ajpendo.00435.2007
179. Lahteenvuo J, Rosenzweig A. Effects of aging on angiogenesis. *Circ Res* (2012) 110(9):1252–64. doi:10.1161/circresaha.111.246116
180. Valli A, Harris AL, Kessler BM. Hypoxia metabolism in ageing. *Aging (Albany NY)* (2015) 7(7):465–6. doi:10.18632/aging.100782
181. Soro-Arnaiz I, Li QOY, Torres-Capelli M, Melendez-Rodriguez F, Veiga S, Veys K, et al. Role of mitochondrial complex IV in age-dependent obesity. *Cell Rep* (2016) 16(11):2991–3002. doi:10.1016/j.celrep.2016.08.041
182. Dalmas E, Clement K, Guerre-Millo M. Defining macrophage phenotype and function in adipose tissue. *Trends Immunol* (2011) 32(7):307–14. doi:10.1016/j.it.2011.04.008
183. Fessler J, Ficjan A, Duftner C, Dejaco C. The impact of aging on regulatory T-cells. *Front Immunol* (2013) 4:231. doi:10.3389/fimmu.2013.00231
184. Frasca D, Blomberg BB. Adipose tissue inflammation induces B cell inflammation and decreases B cell function in aging. *Front Immunol* (2017) 8:1003. doi:10.3389/fimmu.2017.01003
185. Frasca D, Diaz A, Romero M, Landin AM, Blomberg BB. High TNF-α levels in resting B cells negatively correlate with their response. *Exp Gerontol* (2014) 0:116–22. doi:10.1016/j.exger.2014.01.004
186. Frasca D, Ferracci F, Diaz A, Romero M, Lechner S, Blomberg BB. Obesity decreases B cell responses in young and elderly individuals. *Obesity (Silver Spring)* (2016) 24(3):615–25. doi:10.1002/oby.21383
187. Tahir S, Fukushima Y, Sakamoto K, Sato K, Fujita H, Inoue J, et al. A CD153+CD4+ T follicular cell population with cell-senescence features plays a crucial role in lupus pathogenesis via osteopontin production. *J Immunol* (2015) 194(12):5725–35. doi:10.4049/jimmunol.1500319
188. Crawford A, Angelosanto JM, Nadwodny KL, Blackburn SD, Wherry EJ. A role for the chemokine RANTES in regulating CD8 T cell responses during chronic viral infection. *PLoS Pathog* (2011) 7(7):e1002098. doi:10.1371/journal.ppat.1002098
189. Strindhall J, Skog M, Ernerudh J, Bengner M, Löfgren S, Matussek A, et al. The inverted CD4/CD8 ratio and associated parameters in 66-year-old individuals: the Swedish HEXA immune study. *Age* (2013) 35(3):985–91. doi:10.1007/s11357-012-9400-3
190. He LK, Liu LH, Hahn E, Gamelli RL. The expression of cyclooxygenase and the production of prostaglandin E2 in neutrophils after burn injury and infection. *J Burn Care Rehabil* (2001) 22(1):58–64. doi:10.1097/00004630-200101000-00012
191. Grainger JR, Wohlfert EA, Fuss IJ, Bouladoux N, Askenase MH, Legrand F, et al. Inflammatory monocytes regulate pathologic responses to commensals during acute gastrointestinal infection. *Nat Med* (2013) 19(6):713–21. doi:10.1038/nm.3189
192. Ahren B, Mansson S, Gingerich RL, Havel PJ. Regulation of plasma leptin in mice: influence of age, high-fat diet, and fasting. *Am J Physiol* (1997) 273(1 Pt 2):R113–20.
193. Li H, Matheny M, Nicolson M, Tumer N, Scarpace PJ. Leptin gene expression increases with age independent of increasing adiposity in rats. *Diabetes* (1997) 46(12):2035–9. doi:10.2337/diab.46.12.2035
194. Sánchez-Rodríguez M, García-Sánchez A, Retana-Ugalde R, Mendoza-Núñez VCM. Serum leptin levels and blood pressure in the overweight elderly. *Arch Med Res* (2000) 31(4):425–8. doi:10.1016/S0188-4409(99)00079-X
195. Wang ZW, Pan WT, Lee Y, Kakuma T, Zhou YT, Unger RH. The role of leptin resistance in the lipid abnormalities of aging. *FASEB J* (2001) 15(1):108–14. doi:10.1096/fj.00-0310com
196. Sapey E, Greenwood H, Walton G, Mann E, Love A, Aaronson N, et al. Phosphoinositide 3-kinase inhibition restores neutrophil accuracy in the elderly: toward targeted treatments for immunosenescence. *Blood* (2014) 123(2):239–48. doi:10.1182/blood-2013-08-519520
197. Devaney JM, Greene CM, Taggart CC, Carroll TP, O'Neill SJ, McElvaney NG. Neutrophil elastase up-regulates interleukin-8 via toll-like receptor 4. *FEBS Lett* (2003) 544(1–3):129–32. doi:10.1016/S0014-5793(03)00482-4
198. Pham CT. Neutrophil serine proteases: specific regulators of inflammation. *Nat Rev Immunol* (2006) 6(7):541–50. doi:10.1038/nri1841
199. Hazeldine J, Lord JM, Hampson P. Immunesenescence and inflammaging: a contributory factor in the poor outcome of the geriatric trauma patient. *Ageing Res Rev* (2015) 24(Pt B):349–57. doi:10.1016/j.arr.2015.10.003
200. Nguyen M, Pace AJ, Koller BH. Age-induced reprogramming of mast cell degranulation. *J Immunol* (2005) 175(9):5701–7. doi:10.4049/jimmunol.175.9.5701
201. Agrawal A, Tay J, Ton S, Agrawal S, Gupta S. Increased reactivity of dendritic cells from aged subjects to self-antigen, the human DNA. *J Immunol* (2009) 182(2):1138–45. doi:10.4049/jimmunol.182.2.1138

202. Myer RG, El Mezayen R, High KP. Prostaglandin E2-dependent IL-23 production in aged murine dendritic cells. *Exp Gerontol* (2010) 45(11):834–41. doi:10.1016/j.exger.2010.06.007
203. Panda A, Qian F, Mohanty S, van Duin D, Newman FK, Zhang L, et al. Age-associated decrease in TLR function in primary human dendritic cells predicts influenza vaccine response. *J Immunol* (2010) 184(5):2518–27. doi:10.4049/jimmunol.0901022
204. Lee SC, Srivastava RM, Lopez-Albaitero A, Ferrone S, Ferris RL. Natural killer (NK): dendritic cell (DC) cross talk induced by therapeutic monoclonal antibody triggers tumor antigen-specific T cell immunity. *Immunol Res* (2011) 50(2–3):248–54. doi:10.1007/s12026-011-8231-0
205. Shi Q, Yin Z, Zhao B, Sun F, Yu H, Yin X, et al. PGE2 elevates IL-23 production in human dendritic cells via a cAMP dependent pathway. *Mediators Inflamm* (2015) 2015:7. doi:10.1155/2015/984690
206. Agrawal A, Agrawal S, Cao JN, Su H, Osann K, Gupta S. Altered innate immune functioning of dendritic cells in elderly humans: a role of phosphoinositide 3-kinase-signaling pathway. *J Immunol* (2007) 178(11):6912–22. doi:10.4049/jimmunol.178.11.6912
207. Pilaro AM, Taub DD, McCormick KL, Williams HM, Sayers TJ, Fogler WE, et al. TNF-alpha is a principal cytokine involved in the recruitment of NK cells to liver parenchyma. *J Immunol* (1994) 153(1):333–42.
208. Krishnaraj R. Senescence and cytokines modulate the NK cell expression. *Mech Ageing Dev* (1997) 96(1–3):89–101. doi:10.1016/S0047-6374(97)00045-6
209. Borrego F, Alonso MC, Galiani MD, Carracedo J, Ramirez R, Ostos B, et al. NK phenotypic markers and IL2 response in NK cells from elderly people. *Exp Gerontol* (1999) 34(2):253–65. doi:10.1016/S0531-5565(98)00076-X
210. Chidrawar SM, Khan N, Chan YLT, Nayak L, Moss PAH. Ageing is associated with a decline in peripheral blood CD56(bright)NK cells. *Immun Ageing* (2006) 3:10. doi:10.1186/1742-4933-3-10
211. Hayhoe RP, Henson SM, Akbar AN, Palmer DB. Variation of human natural killer cell phenotypes with age: identification of a unique KLRG1-negative subset. *Hum Immunol* (2010) 71(7):676–81. doi:10.1016/j.humimm.2010.03.014
212. Almeida-Oliveira A, Smith-Carvalho M, Porto LC, Cardoso-Oliveira J, Ribeiro Ados S, Falcao RR, et al. Age-related changes in natural killer cell receptors from childhood through old age. *Hum Immunol* (2011) 72(4):319–29. doi:10.1016/j.humimm.2011.01.009
213. Bai L, Sagiv Y, Liu Y, Freigang S, Yu KOA, Teyton L, et al. Lysosomal recycling terminates CD1d-mediated presentation of short and polyunsaturated variants of the NKT cell lipid antigen αGalCer. *Proc Natl Acad Sci U S A* (2009) 106(25):10254–9. doi:10.1073/pnas.0901228106
214. Birkholz AM, Girardi E, Wingender G, Khurana A, Wang J, Zhao M, et al. A novel glycolipid antigen for NKT cells that preferentially induces IFN-gamma production. *J Immunol* (2015) 195(3):924–33. doi:10.4049/jimmunol.1500070
215. Chmelař J, Chatzigeorgiou A, Chung K-J, Prucnal M, Voehringer D, Roers A, et al. No role for mast cells in obesity-related metabolic dysregulation. *Front Immunol* (2016) 7:524. doi:10.3389/fimmu.2016.00524
216. Soo MK, Lun M, Wang M, Senyo SE, Guillermier C, Patwari P, et al. Loss of white adipose hyperplastic potential is associated with enhanced susceptibility to insulin resistance. *Cell Metab* (2014) 20(6):1049–58. doi:10.1016/j.cmet.2014.10.010
217. Kusminski CM, Scherer PE. Mitochondrial dysfunction in white adipose tissue. *Trends Endocrinol Metab* (2012) 23(9):435–43. doi:10.1016/j.tem.2012.06.004
218. Mohamed-Ali V, Goodrick S, Rawesh A, Katz DR, Miles JM, Yudkin JS, et al. Subcutaneous adipose tissue releases interleukin-6, but not tumor necrosis factor-alpha, in vivo. *J Clin Endocrinol Metab* (1997) 82(12):4196–200. doi:10.1210/jcem.82.12.4450
219. Lumeng CN, Bodzin JL, Saltiel AR. Obesity induces a phenotypic switch in adipose tissue macrophage polarization. *J Clin Invest* (2007) 117(1):175–84. doi:10.1172/jci29881
220. Atzmon G, Pollin TI, Crandall J, Tanner K, Schechter CB, Scherer PE, et al. Adiponectin levels and genotype: a potential regulator of life span in humans. *J Gerontol A Biol Sci Med Sci* (2008) 63(5):447–53. doi:10.1093/gerona/63.5.447
221. Kawano J, Arora R. The role of adiponectin in obesity, diabetes, and cardiovascular disease. *J Cardiometab Syndr* (2009) 4(1):44–9. doi:10.1111/j.1559-4572.2008.00030.x
222. Zhang Y, Proenca R, Maffei M, Barone M, Leopold L, Friedman JM. Positional cloning of the mouse obese gene and its human homologue. *Nature* (1994) 372(6505):425–32. doi:10.1038/372425a0
223. Weisberg SP, Hunter D, Huber R, Lemieux J, Slaymaker S, Vaddi K, et al. CCR2 modulates inflammatory and metabolic effects of high-fat feeding. *J Clin Invest* (2006) 116(1):115–24. doi:10.1172/jci24335
224. Zeyda M, Gollinger K, Kriehuber E, Kiefer FW, Neuhofer A, Stulnig TM. Newly identified adipose tissue macrophage populations in obesity with distinct chemokine and chemokine receptor expression. *Int J Obes (Lond)* (2010) 34(12):1684–94. doi:10.1038/ijo.2010.103
225. Shah R, Hinkle CC, Ferguson JF, Mehta NN, Li M, Qu L, et al. Fractalkine is a novel human adipochemokine associated with type 2 diabetes. *Diabetes* (2011) 60(5):1512–8. doi:10.2337/db10-0956
226. Polyak A, Ferenczi S, Denes A, Winkler Z, Kriszt R, Pinter-Kubler B, et al. The fractalkine/Cx3CR1 system is implicated in the development of metabolic visceral adipose tissue inflammation in obesity. *Brain Behav Immun* (2014) 38:25–35. doi:10.1016/j.bbi.2014.01.010
227. Morris DL, Oatmen KE, Wang T, DelProposto JL, Lumeng CN. CX3CR1 deficiency does not influence trafficking of adipose tissue macrophages in mice with diet-induced obesity. *Obesity (Silver Spring)* (2012) 20(6):1189–99. doi:10.1038/oby.2012.7
228. Shah R, O'Neill SM, Hinkle C, Caughey J, Stephan S, Lynch E, et al. Metabolic effects of CX3CR1 deficiency in diet-induced obese mice. *PLoS One* (2015) 10(9):e0138317. doi:10.1371/journal.pone.0138317
229. Deiuliis JA, Oghumu S, Duggineni D, Zhong J, Rutsky J, Banerjee A, et al. CXCR3 modulates obesity-induced visceral adipose inflammation and systemic insulin resistance. *Obesity (Silver Spring)* (2014) 22(5):1264–74. doi:10.1002/oby.20642
230. Garcia-Alonso V, Titos E, Alcaraz-Quiles J, Rius B, Lopategi A, Lopez-Vicario C, et al. Prostaglandin E2 exerts multiple regulatory actions on human obese adipose tissue remodeling, inflammation, adaptive thermogenesis and lipolysis. *PLoS One* (2016) 11(4):e0153751. doi:10.1371/journal.pone.0153751
231. Vidal-Puig AJ, Considine RV, Jimenez-Linan M, Werman A, Pories WJ, Caro JF, et al. Peroxisome proliferator-activated receptor gene expression in human tissues. Effects of obesity, weight loss, and regulation by insulin and glucocorticoids. *J Clin Invest* (1997) 99(10):2416–22. doi:10.1172/jci119424
232. Kurki E, Shi J, Martonen E, Finckenberg P, Mervaala E. Distinct effects of calorie restriction on adipose tissue cytokine and angiogenesis profiles in obese and lean mice. *Nutr Metab* (2012) 9(1):64. doi:10.1186/1743-7075-9-64
233. Fabbiano S, Suarez-Zamorano N, Rigo D, Veyrat-Durebex C, Stevanovic Dokic A, Colin DJ, et al. Caloric restriction leads to browning of white adipose tissue through type 2 immune signaling. *Cell Metab* (2016) 24(3):434–46. doi:10.1016/j.cmet.2016.07.023
234. Miller KN, Burhans MS, Clark JP, Howell PR, Polewski MA, DeMuth TM, et al. Aging and caloric restriction impact adipose tissue, adiponectin, and circulating lipids. *Aging Cell* (2017) 16(3):497–507. doi:10.1111/acel.12575
235. Clement K, Viguerie N, Poitou C, Carette C, Pelloux V, Curat CA, et al. Weight loss regulates inflammation-related genes in white adipose tissue of obese subjects. *FASEB J* (2004) 18(14):1657–69. doi:10.1096/fj.04-2204com
236. Kovacikova M, Sengenes C, Kovacova Z, Siklova-Vitkova M, Klimcakova E, Polak J, et al. Dietary intervention-induced weight loss decreases macrophage content in adipose tissue of obese women. *Int J Obes (Lond)* (2011) 35(1):91–8. doi:10.1038/ijo.2010.112
237. Baturcam E, Abubaker J, Tiss A, Abu-Farha M, Khadir A, Al-Ghimlas F, et al. Physical exercise reduces the expression of RANTES and its CCR5 receptor in the adipose tissue of obese humans. *Mediators Inflamm* (2014) 2014:13. doi:10.1155/2014/627150
238. Chen Y-C, Travers RL, Walhin J-P, Gonzalez JT, Koumanov F, Betts JA, et al. Feeding influences adipose tissue responses to exercise in overweight men. *Am J Physiol Endocrinol Metab* (2017) 313(1):E84–93. doi:10.1152/ajpendo.00006.2017
239. Yudkin JS. Inflammation, obesity, and the metabolic syndrome. *Horm Metab Res* (2007) 39(10):707–9. doi:10.1055/s-2007-985898
240. Kawanishi N, Yano H, Yokogawa Y, Suzuki K. Exercise training inhibits inflammation in adipose tissue via both suppression of macrophage infiltration and acceleration of phenotypic switching from M1 to M2 macrophages in high-fat-diet-induced obese mice. *Exerc Immunol Rev* (2010) 16:105–18.

241. Kawanishi N, Niihara H, Mizokami T, Yada K, Suzuki K. Exercise training attenuates neutrophil infiltration and elastase expression in adipose tissue of high-fat-diet-induced obese mice. *Physiol Rep* (2015) 3(9):e12534. doi:10.14814/phy2.12534
242. Gleeson M, Bishop NC, Stensel DJ, Lindley MR, Mastana SS, Nimmo MA. The anti-inflammatory effects of exercise: mechanisms and implications for the prevention and treatment of disease. *Nat Rev Immunol* (2011) 11(9):607–15. doi:10.1038/nri3041
243. Radak Z, Chung HY, Goto S. Systemic adaptation to oxidative challenge induced by regular exercise. *Free Radic Biol Med* (2008) 44(2):153–9. doi:10.1016/j.freeradbiomed.2007.01.029
244. Turner JE. Is immunosenescence influenced by our lifetime "dose" of exercise? *Biogerontology* (2016) 17(3):581–602. doi:10.1007/s10522-016-9642-z
245. Stienstra R, Duval C, Keshtkar S, van der Laak J, Kersten S, Muller M. Peroxisome proliferator-activated receptor gamma activation promotes infiltration of alternatively activated macrophages into adipose tissue. *J Biol Chem* (2008) 283(33):22620–7. doi:10.1074/jbc.M710314200
246. Kratz M, Coats BR, Hisert KB, Hagman D, Mutskov V, Peris E, et al. Metabolic dysfunction drives a mechanistically distinct proinflammatory phenotype in adipose tissue macrophages. *Cell Metab* (2014) 20(4):614–25. doi:10.1016/j.cmet.2014.08.010
247. Shaul ME, Bennett G, Strissel KJ, Greenberg AS, Obin MS. Dynamic, M2-like remodeling phenotypes of CD11c+ adipose tissue macrophages during high-fat diet-induced obesity in mice. *Diabetes* (2010) 59(5):1171–81. doi:10.2337/db09-1402
248. Xu X, Grijalva A, Skowronski A, van Eijk M, Serlie MJ, Ferrante AW Jr. Obesity activates a program of lysosomal-dependent lipid metabolism in adipose tissue macrophages independently of classic activation. *Cell Metab* (2013) 18(6):816–30. doi:10.1016/j.cmet.2013.11.001
249. Zeyda M, Farmer D, Todoric J, Aszmann O, Speiser M, Gyori G, et al. Human adipose tissue macrophages are of an anti-inflammatory phenotype but capable of excessive pro-inflammatory mediator production. *Int J Obes (Lond)* (2007) 31(9):1420–8. doi:10.1038/sj.ijo.0803632

16

Parameters of the Immune System and Vitamin D Levels in Old Individuals

*Amanda Soares Alves[1], Mayari Eika Ishimura[1], Yeda Aparecida de Oliveira Duarte[2] and Valquiria Bueno[1]**

[1] Division of Immunology, DMIP Microbiology, Immunology, and Parasitology, Federal University of São Paulo, São Paulo, Brazil, [2] Division of Epidemiology, Faculdade de Saúde Pública, Universidade de São Paulo, São Paulo, Brazil

***Correspondence:**
Valquiria Bueno
vbueno@unifesp.br

Aim: The increased number of individuals older than 80 years, centenarians, and super-centenarians is not a synonym for healthy aging, since severe infections, hospitalization, and disability are frequently observed. In this context, a possible strategy is to preserve the main characteristics/functions of the immune system with the aim to cause less damage to the organism during the aging process. Vitamin D acts on bone marrow, brain, breast, malignant cells, and immune system and has been recommended as a supplement. We aimed to evaluate whether immune parameters and vitamin D serum levels are correlated.

Methods: We evaluated some features of the immune system using the peripheral blood of individuals older than 80 years ($n = 12$) compared to young subjects ($n = 10$). In addition, we correlated these findings with vitamin D serum levels.

Results: Old individuals presented metabolic parameters of healthy aging and maintained preserved some features of immunity such as CD4/CD8 ratio, and low production of pro-inflammatory cytokines after stimulus. On the other hand, we observed increase in the frequency of myeloid-derived suppressor cells, reduction in circulating leukocytes, in the percentage of total CD8+, and in CD8+ Naïve T cells, in addition to increase in the percentage of CD8+ effector memory re-expressing CD45RA (EMRA) T cells. We found seropositivity for CMV in 97.7%, which was correlated with the decrease of CD8+ Naïve T cells and increase in CD8+ EMRA T cells. Vitamin D levels were insufficient in 50% of old individuals and correlated positively with total CD8+ T cells and negatively with CD8+ EMRA T cells.

Conclusion: In the studied population, longevity was correlated to maintenance of some immune parameters. Considering the limitations of the study as size of the sample and lack of functional assays, it was found that vitamin D in old individuals was correlated to some features of the immune system, mainly in the CD8 compartment.

Keywords: longevity, immunity, vitamin D, myeloid-derived suppressor cells, T cells

INTRODUCTION

In several developed and developing countries, human longevity has been achieved (1–3) but insufficient function of the immune system in the old population leads to severe infections, frequent hospitalizations, and immunization reduced after vaccination (4–6).

Therefore, to reach the longevity with good quality of life, a possible strategy is to preserve the main characteristics/functions of the immune system with the aim to cause less damage to the organism during the aging process. Aging has been associated with lower generation of progenitors from pluripotent hematopoietic stem cells (HSC) located in the bone marrow. In addition, there occurs a myeloid-biased differentiation of HSC due to selection pressures from cell-intrinsic and extrinsic mechanisms (7–10). These factors lead to a decrease in the number of circulating leukocytes and increased frequency in the myeloid lineage. The increase in the frequency of myeloid cells may be the reason for the recently described increase in myeloid-derived suppressor cells (MDSC) in aging individuals. MDSC membrane markers are $CD11b^+$ $CD33^+HLA^-DR^{-/low}$, which can be subtyped in monocytic MDSC ($CD14^+$) or granulocytic ($CD15^+$) MDSC.

The suppressive actions of MDSC are mainly based on the production of arginase-1, reactive oxygen species, nitric oxide (NO), IL-10, and TGF-β1. These cells exert several effects on lymphocytes such as impairment in the antigen presentation and recognition by T cells, deficient B and T cells activation, and accumulation of regulatory T cells (11, 12).

Changes in hematopoiesis have also been related to the decreased percentage of $CD4^+$ and $CD8^+$ T cells in the circulating blood. In addition, the inverted CD4/CD8 ratio was reported by Swedish OCTO and NONA immune longitudinal studies as a blood marker predictive for a high rate of mortality in 2, 4, and 6 years (immune risk profile) (13).

Another aspect of aging is the thymic involution which has been linked to less diversity in the T-cell receptor and decreased frequency of Naive T cells (14, 15), while the peripheral homeostatic proliferation compensates for the T-cell loss (16, 17).

The phenotype of T cells has been used to characterize the immune system status and Hamann et al. (18, 19) proposed that in humans, the $CD8^+$ T cell compartment presents four different phenotypes based on membrane markers and cellular function. The phenotype $CD45RA^+CD27^+$ represents undifferentiated Naive cells and $CD45RA^-CD27^+$ lymphocytes are antigen-experienced T cells (central memory) with increased frequency of lymphotoxicity precursors (CTLp). $CD45RA^+CD27^-$ cells present features of antigen-stimulated cells with cytolytic potential, production of IFN-γ and tumor necrosis factor-alpha (TNF-α), high amounts of perforin and granzyme B, Fas ligand mRNA expressed in abundancy, and cells exerting potent cytotoxic activity without previous *in vitro* stimulation [effector memory re-expressing CD45RA (EMRA)]. $CD45RA^-CD27^-$ T cells are observed in low frequency and express perforin and granzyme B (effector memory). The correlation between aging and increased frequency of $CD8^+CD45RA^+CD27^-$ has been reported. The same phenotypes were identified in different stages of $CD4^+$ T cells mainly during stimulation by viral infections (CMV, EBV, HSV, and VZV) (20, 21).

In order to preserve the functional characteristics of the immune system that could in turn prevent and/or delay age-related diseases, health professionals have proposed physical activity, control of diet, supplements, and probiotics (22–24).

The main actions of vitamin D in bone tissue and the latest reports of its effects on bone marrow, brain, colon, breast, malignant cells, and immune system (25) raised the interest of researchers to investigate the role played by vitamin D in the immunity of old individuals.

Considering that low levels of vitamin D are common in older individuals, some health professionals have recommended vitamin D supplementation to the aging population in general and especially for aged-care residents and critically ill patients (26–28). However, the benefits arising on the immunity with vitamin D supplementation are not consistent in the literature. Upper respiratory infections (URI) in non-hospitalized middle-aged and older individuals with vitamin D supplementation have been associated with a lower incidence of infection (29), discrete decrease of infections events (30), or no alteration in severity and duration of infection (31, 32). In addition, residents of sheltered accommodation supplemented with vitamin D showed increase in URI and duration of symptoms and no changes to the risk or duration of lower respiratory infections (33). However, in patients with antibody deficiency or increased susceptibility to respiratory tract infections (RTI), supplementation with vitamin D was beneficial and associated with fewer episodes of RTI and increased time for first infection compared to placebo group (34).

As the extension of life expectancy is a reality, it is a challenge to understand how the aging population deals with the remodeling of the immune system and if interventions as vitamin D could provide extra years of life with good health. In this study, our goal was to investigate changes that occur in some parameters of the immune system in individuals reaching longevity (80–100 years) and the possible correlation with vitamin D levels.

MATERIALS AND METHODS

The present study is part of a larger epidemiologic survey called the health, well-being, and aging study (SABE), which was coordinated by the Pan-American Health Organization, Washington, and in Brazil by the School of Public Health of the University of São Paulo. From 2000 to 2001, SABE evaluated a sample of 2,143 non-institutionalized individuals, representing 836,204 aging people (60 years and older) living in the municipality of São Paulo, who were selected through multi-stage sampling. In 2006, the School of Public Health continued the survey in São Paulo and transformed it into a multi-cohort study with 1,115 individuals from the previous study who agreed to participate in the follow-up. Since then, the survey has been repeated every 5 years. In this study, the inclusion/exclusion criteria were applied as cited above, except that we used blood only from individuals older than 80 years (male, female) and they were enrolled as their biological samples were received. Young individuals (20–30 years, male and female) were master and Ph.D. students from UNIFESP.

The blood samples were collected with 12 h of fasting (6:00 a.m.–9:00 a.m.) during the summer months (December, January, and February) in Brazil.

The Ethics Committee of the Federal University of São Paulo—UNIFESP approved all procedures (Protocol number 10904).

Peripheral blood mononuclear cells (PBMCs) were isolated using Ficoll–Hypaque density gradient (Amersham Biosciences, Uppsala, Sweden) and centrifugation. Viable cells were counted, adjusted for $2 \times 10^6/100$ µL in 80% fetal bovine serum and 20% dimethylsulfoxide (Sigma, St. Louis, MO, USA), and frozen stored (−80°C) until the phenotyping and cell culture.

Cell Culture

Cells were diluted in RPMI 10, counted, and adjusted for 1×10^6/100 mL. The assessment of cell proliferation was based on a substance (CFSE) that once in the cell cytoplasm halves its content to each cell division. Cells were incubated with 5(6)-carboxyfluorescein acetate (CFSE, CFDA Vybrant IF Cell Tracer Kit Invitrogen) for 10 min. The cells were washed, counted, and adjusted for plating (2×10^5/100 μL of RPMI10 per well). Culture conditions were phytohemagglutinin (PHA$^+$, 5 μg/mL, Sigma) or absence of stimulus (PHA) for 72 h in 5% CO_2, humidity controlled and 37°C. After 3 days of culture, the cell suspension was collected, centrifuged, and the proliferation (CFSE) was measured in flow cytometer (35). The cell culture supernatant was frozen (−80°C) for the measurement of cytokines (ELISA).

Cell Phenotype

The cells were stained with monoclonal antibodies to T-cell phenotype CD3 APC, CD4 PerCP Cy 5.5, CD8 APC Cy7, CD27 FITC, CD45RA PE (eBioscience, CA, USA). The cells were also stained with monoclonal antibodies to MDSC phenotype CD3 APC, CD19 APC, CD56 APC, HLA-DR APC e-fluor 780, CD33 PerCP Cy5.5, CD11b PE, CD14 PE Cy7, CD15 FITC (eBioscience, CA, USA). After 30 min of incubation with monoclonal antibodies, in the dark and at 4°C, the cells were washed with PBS and centrifuged. Living cells (based on forward and side scatter) were acquired in the FACS Canto II using the DIVA software (Becton Dickinson, USA). Further analyses of FACS data were performed using the 9.3 FLOWJO software (Tree Star, USA).

T lymphocytes were characterized as described previously (36).

Naïve: CD3$^+$CD4$^+$CD45RA$^+$CD27$^+$ or CD3$^+$CD8$^+$CD45RA$^+$ CD27$^+$ (Naïve).
Central memory: CD3$^+$CD4$^+$CD45RA$^-$CD27$^+$ or CD3$^+$CD8$^+$ CD45RA$^-$CD27$^+$ (CM).
Effector memory: CD3$^+$CD4$^+$CD45RA$^-$CD27$^-$ or CD3$^+$CD8$^+$ CD45RA$^-$CD27$^-$ (EM).
Effectormemoryre-expressingCD45RA:CD3$^+$CD4$^+$CD45RA$^+$ CD27$^-$ or CD3$^+$CD8$^+$CD45RA$^+$CD27$^-$ (EMRA).

Myeloid-derived suppressor cells were characterized as:

CD3$^-$CD19$^-$CD56$^-$HLA$^-$DR$^{-/low}$CD33$^+$CD11b$^+$CD15$^+$ granulocytic or
CD3$^-$CD19$^-$CD56$^-$HLA$^-$DR$^{-/low}$CD33$^+$CD11b$^+$CD14$^+$ monocytic.

ELISA

The frozen culture supernatants were thawed and cytokines [IL-1, IL-2 α, interleukin-6 (IL-6), IFN-γ, and TNF-α] were evaluated by ELISA assay according to the manufacturer's instructions (DuoSet ELISA Development Systems R&D). ELISA reading PerkinElmer—EnSpire, quantified the samples.

Metabolic Data

Obtained from the databank of SABE study.

Cytomegalovirus IgM and IgG

Serum was previously isolated by centrifugation and frozen stored (−80°C). IgG and IgM levels were measured in serum by electrochemiluminescence immunoassay according to the manufacturer's instructions (cobas® http://e-labdoc.roche.com REF 04784618 190).

Measurement of Vitamin D

Serum of studied individuals was previously isolated by centrifugation and frozen stored (−80°C) until the measurement of vitamin D. 25-Hydroxyvitamin D value was obtained in accordance with the manufacturer's instructions (cobas® http://e-labdoc.roche.com 05894913 190 V7).

Statistics

After testing the variables for normality (Shapiro–Wilk) it was used the unpaired Student's t-test (Vitamin D) or Mann–Whitney

TABLE 1 | Metabolic parameters in old individuals (80–100 years) and reference values of 80-year-old individuals (37).

Metabolic parameters								
Age	**Gender**	**Cholesterol total mg/dL**	**HDL mg/dL**	**Triglycerides mg/dL**	**Glucose mg/dL**	**Urea mg/dL**	**Creatinine mg/dL**	**Albumin mg/dL**
100	F	179	38	183	162	35	0.91	3.1
90	F	224	53	178	80	33	1.09	3.4
90	F	188	73	125	86	42	0.67	3.9
93	M	181	43	47	80	57	0.98	3.9
93	F	186	51	121	93	28	0.93	3.6
88	M	275	68	114	104	36	1.01	4
94	M	177	39	86	71	47	1.26	3.4
90	M	163	43	72	82	30	1.1	3.7
90	M	181	38	135	95	43	1.22	3.9
94	M	132	33	80	90	61	1.97	3.9
91	F	207	63	106	81	41	0.73	4.3
90	F	236	58	109	90	29	0.94	4
Mean ± SD		194.1±37.1	50 ± 13.1	113 ± 40.2	92.8 ± 2	40.2 ± 10.7	1.1 ± 0.3	3.8 ± 0.3
Range		132–275	33–73	47–183	71–162	28–61	0.67–1.97	3.1–4.3
Reference values (37)		108.3–313.2	27.1–104.4	43.8–287.8	126	19.8–89.5	0.52–1.94	3.2–4.7

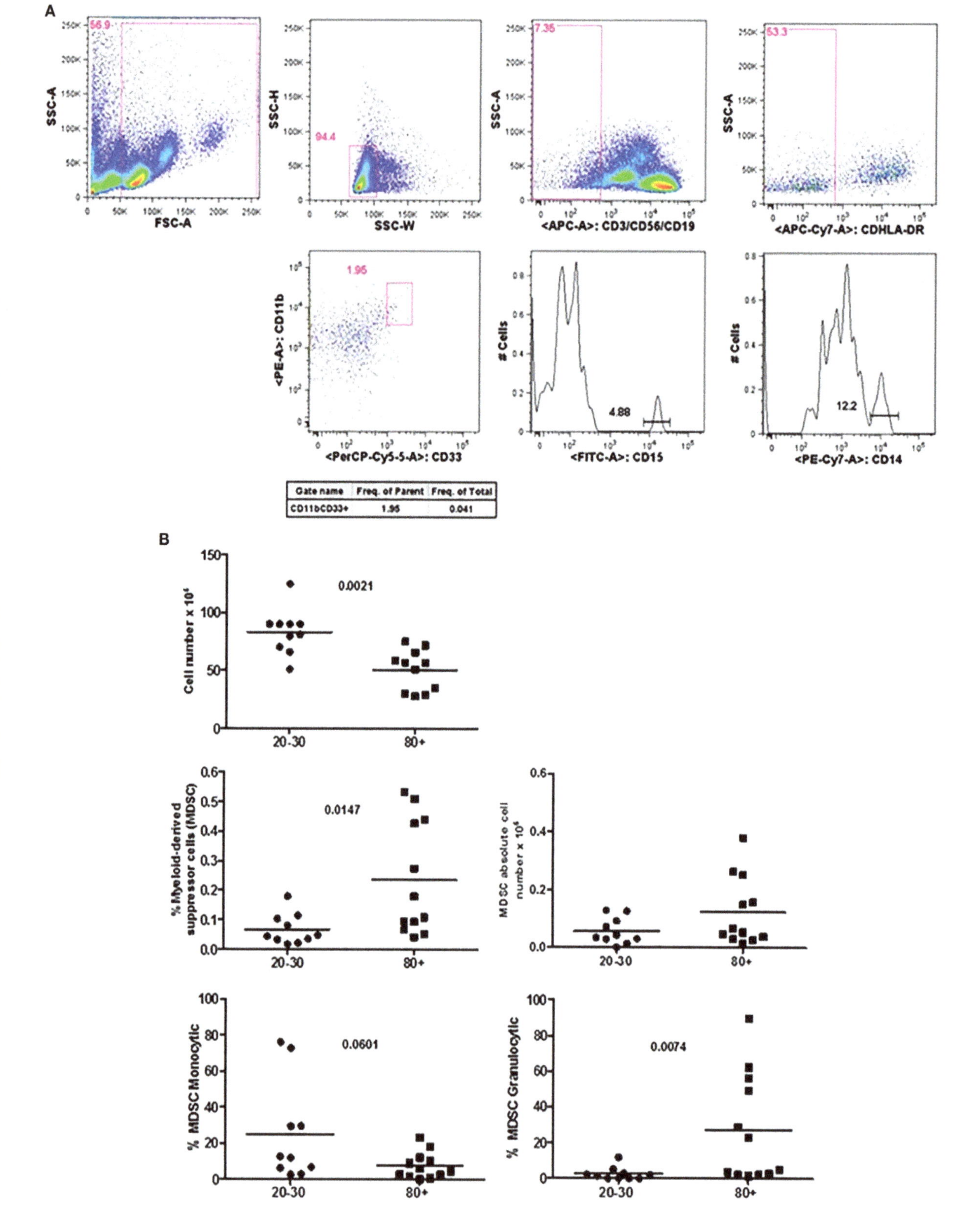

FIGURE 1 | Representative flow cytometry plots showing gate strategy for myeloid-derived suppressor cells (MDSC) frequency. Gate in live cells (FSC-A × SSC-A), doublets exclusion (SSC-H × SSC-W), gate in lineage negative cells ($CD3^{-}CD56^{-}CD19^{-}$), gate in HLA-$DR^{low/neg}$ cells, gate in $CD33^{+}CD11b^{+}$ cells. Gate in granulocytic ($CD15^{+}$) and monocytic ($CD14^{+}$) cells **(A)**. Number of circulating leukocytes, MDSC (% MDSC) frequency, absolute number of MDSC, and frequency of monocytic and granulocytic MDSC in individuals of 20–30 years and 80+ years old individuals **(B)**.

(parameters of the immune system) for comparisons between young and old groups. The correlation between parameters of the immune system and serum levels of IgG (CMV) or vitamin D was performed by Spearman test. Values of $p < 0.05$ were considered statistically significant. All statistical analyses were performed with the aid of the Graph Pad PRISM software (Graph pad, La Jolla, CA, USA).

RESULTS

Young ($n = 10$, 5 male and 5 female, 20–30 years old) and old ($n = 12$, 6 male and 6 female, 80–100 years old) individuals were evaluated. **Table 1** shows some metabolic parameters that highlight the health status of the old population evaluated. In agreement with Helmersson-Karlqvist et al. (37), our old population may be considered healthy for most of the parameters evaluated in spite of great variability observed. Only one female (100 years) presented glucose (162 mg/dL) higher than the reference values established by Helmersson-Karlqvist et al. (37).

Figure 1 shows that old individuals (80–100 years) presented a significantly high percentage of MDSC (%MDSC). However, as this group had a significantly lower number of leukocytes, the absolute cell number of MDSC (leukocytes cell number × percentage of MDSC) was not different compared to young individuals (20–30 years). There was significant predominance of granulocytic MDSC in individuals older than 80 years, while the subtype monocytic was statistically higher in young individuals. The percentage of T CD4$^+$ lymphocytes was similar in both groups while there was a trend toward lower percentage of CD8$^+$ T cells in old individuals ($p = 0.0572$). The CD4/CD8 ratio was significantly higher in old individuals except in a woman (96 years) with the CD4/CD8 ratio inverted (0.542) (**Figure 2**).

The evaluation of T cells phenotypes showed a significantly lower percentage of CD4$^+$ central memory in elderly individuals (**Figure 3**). In the CD8 compartment, Naive cells were statistically less expressed in old individuals and CD8$^+$ EMRA T cells presented significantly higher expression in old individuals

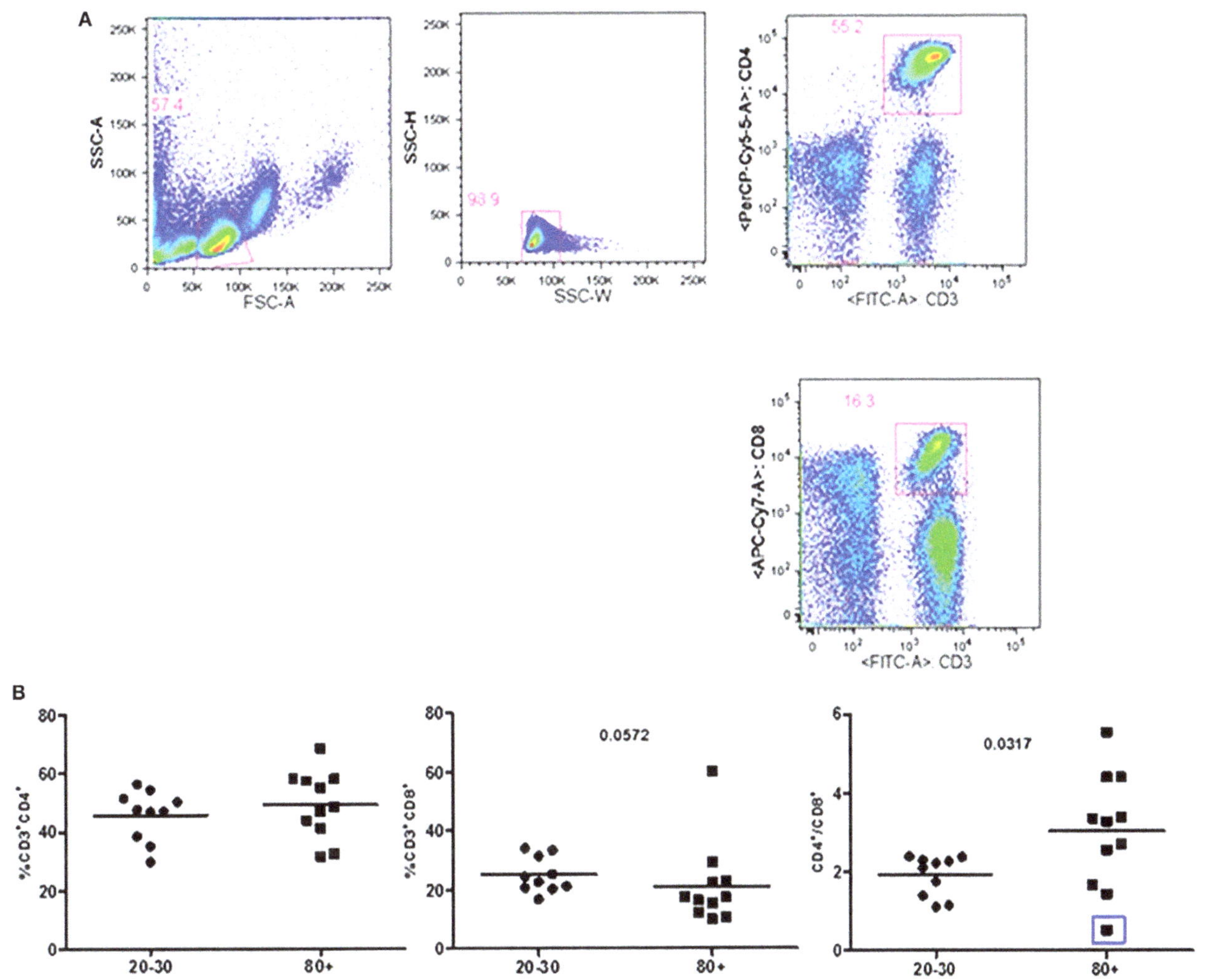

FIGURE 2 | Representative flow cytometry plots showing gate strategy for the frequency of CD4$^+$ and CD8$^+$ T cells. Gate in live lymphocytes (FSC-A × SSC-A), doublets exclusion (SSC-H × SSC-W), gate in CD3$^+$CD4$^+$ T cells, gate in CD3$^+$CD8$^+$ T cells **(A)**. Frequency of T lymphocytes CD3$^+$CD4$^+$, CD3$^+$CD8$^+$, and CD4/CD8 ratio in 20–30 and 80$^+$ years old individuals. The CD4/CD8 ratio lower than 1 (0.542; blue square) **(B)**.

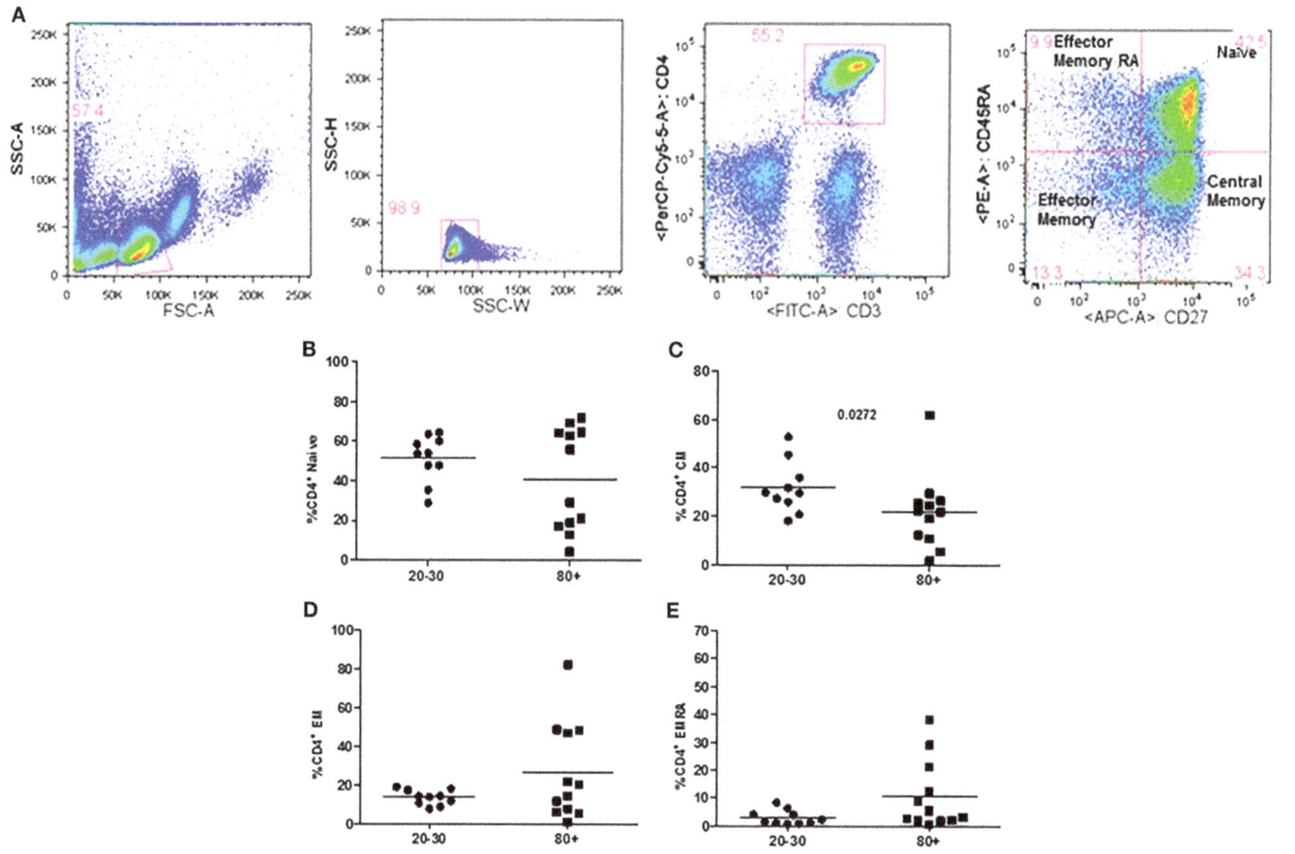

FIGURE 3 | Representative flow cytometry plots showing gate strategy for the frequency of $CD4^+$ T cells phenotype. Gate in live lymphocytes (FSC-A × SSC-A), doublets exclusion (SSC-H × SSC-W), gate in $CD3^+CD4^+$ T cells, gate in $CD45RA^+CD27^+$ (Naïve) T cells, gate in $CD45RA^-CD27^+$ (central memory) T cells, gate in $CD45RA^-CD27^-$ (effector memory), gate in $CD45RA^+CD27^-$ (effector memory re-expressing CD45RA) T cells **(A)**. Percentage (%) of $CD4^+$ T cells phenotypes: Naïve **(B)**, central memory **(C)**, effector memory **(D)**, effector memory RA re-expressing CD45RA **(E)** in 20–30 and 80+ years old individuals.

(**Figure 4**). Considering the functions of T cells after stimulation in culture with PHA, the percentage of proliferation was lower in old individuals both in the compartment $CD4^+$ and $CD8^+$ (**Figure 5**). The production of cytokines was reduced in old individuals with statistical difference for IL-6 and TNF-α (**Figure 6**). As cytomegalovirus infection/latency has been related to immunosenescence, we evaluated IgM and IgG against CMV in serum of old (80–100 years) individuals (**Table 2**) and the possible correlation with immune parameters (**Table 3**).

Table 2 shows that in 12-old individuals evaluated, only one male (88 years old) can be considered negative for cytomegalovirus as the IgM level was <0.7 (0.158) and IgG level was <0.5 (<0.25). In addition, only one male (90 years old) could be considered as recently infected by CMV as the IgM level was >1.0 (1.240) and the IgG level was relatively low (55.85) in comparison to other old individuals studied. Levels of IgG >500 U/mL were observed in four individuals (3 females and 1 male).

The levels of IgG against CMV were negatively correlated ($p = 0.027$) with the percentage of Naïve $CD8^+$T cells. There was a trend of negative correlation ($p = 0.06$) between the percentage of $CD4^+$ central memory T cells and IgG levels (CMV). A trend of positive correlation ($p = 0.055$) between the percentage of $CD8^+$ EMRA T cells and IgG levels (CMV) was observed (**Table 3**).

The next question was whether total vitamin D levels were different in the studied groups (**Figure 7**). Vitamin D levels were lower in old individuals ($p = 0.050$). In 50% ($n = 6$) of aged individuals vitamin D levels were <20 ng/mL (deficiency) and in 90% ($n = 9$) of young individuals vitamin D levels were greater than 20 ng/mL. Insufficiency (21–29 ng/mL) was present in 25% ($n = 3$) of old individuals and 50% ($n = 5$) of young individuals. Sufficient levels (30 ng/mL or more) were observed in 25% ($n = 3$) of aged and 40% ($n = 4$) of young individuals.

It was analyzed whether total vitamin D was correlated with the immunological parameters evaluated previously. We observed correlation of vitamin D levels only for the CD8 compartment (**Table 4**). The percentage of total CD8 T cells was positively correlated ($p = 0.006$) with vitamin D levels in old individuals, whereas there was a trend toward positive correlation ($p = 0.074$) in young individuals. $CD8^+$ effector memory T cells were positively correlated with vitamin D levels in young individuals and $CD8^+$ EMRA T cells were negatively correlated ($p = 0.05$) with vitamin D levels in old individuals.

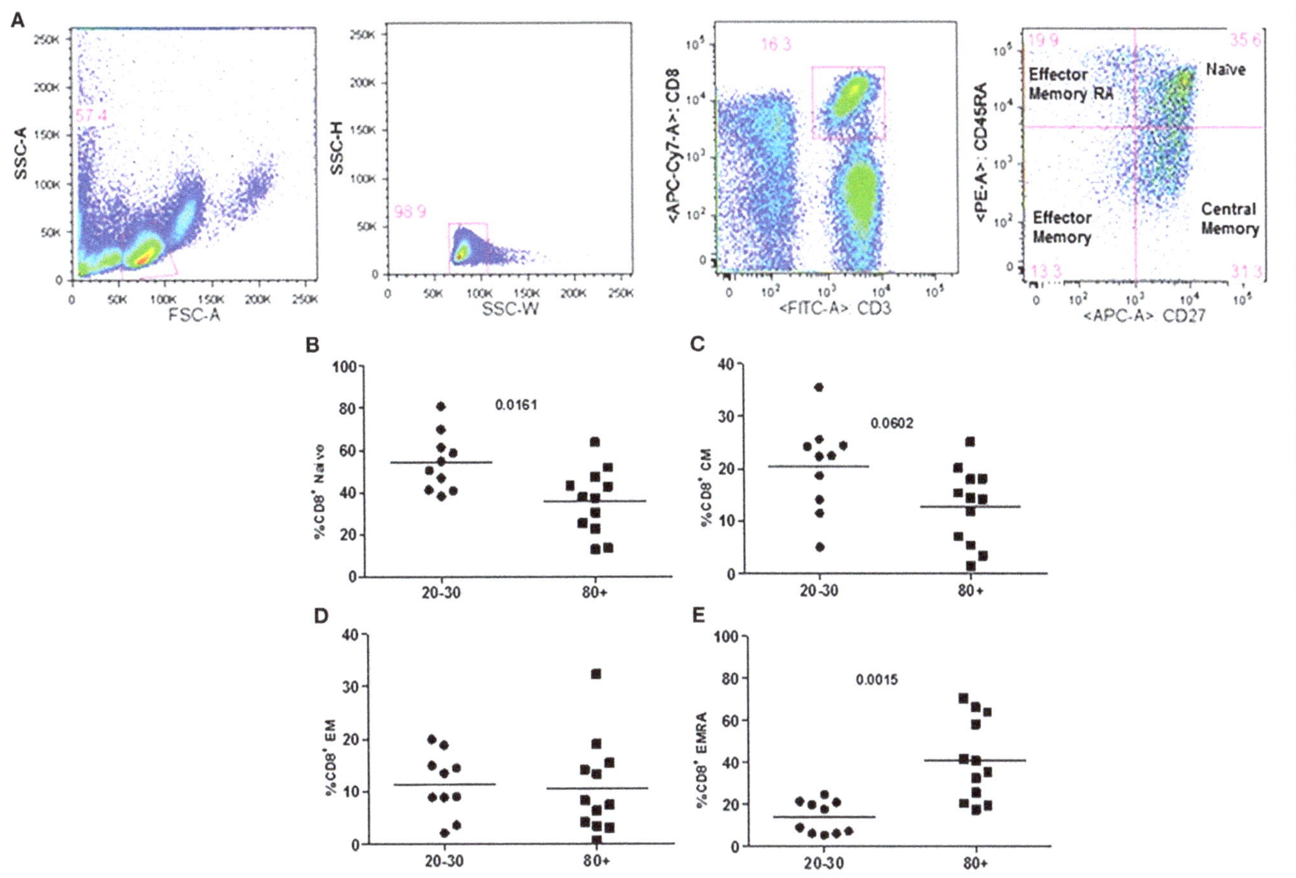

FIGURE 4 | Representative flow cytometry plots showing gate strategy for the frequency of CD8+ T cells phenotype. Gate in live lymphocytes (FSC-A x SSC-A), doublets exclusion (SSC-H x SSC-W), gate in CD3+CD8+ T cells, gate in CD45RA+CD27+ (Naïve) T cells, gate in CD45RA-CD27+ (central memory) T cells, gate in CD45RA-CD27- (effector memory), gate in CD45RA+CD27- (effector memory re-expressing CD45RA) T cells **(A)**. Percentage (%) of CD8+ T cells phenotypes: Naïve **(B)**, central memory **(C)**, effector memory **(D)**, effector memory RA re-expressing CD45RA **(E)** in 20–30 and 80+ years old individuals.

DISCUSSION

Morbidities associated with aging contribute to organ failure that leads to a pathway of poor quality of life and/or death. In addition, the impairment in the protective functions of the immune system promoting infections and tumors, and the increase of inflammatory factors causing tissue damage and contributing for age-related diseases have also been reported in old individuals.

In our study, it was observed that old individuals presented metabolic parameters consistent with healthy aging except for a female (100 years) with blood glucose higher than 126 mg/dL. Our data are in agreement with the report of Helmersson-Karlqvist et al. (37) who have developed reference intervals of metabolic parameters adjusted for very old (80 years) individuals.

Despite our studied population could be considered healthy, we observed characteristics reported as immune senescence.

Myeloid-derived suppressor cells were only recently described as potential markers of the aging process, since these cells were initially associated with tumor development (12). We observed in old individuals that MDSC were present in high percentage with predominance of the granulocytic subtype. It has been reported that the accumulation of MDSC with aging may contribute to some of the immune disorders and pathologies observed in older adults (12). In aging individuals, Verschoor et al. observed a significant increase in the frequency of MDSC compared to young adults in addition to the higher number of MDSC in older individuals with frailty and previous history of cancer (11). In addition to the increased percentage of MDSC, our old population presented decreased number of circulating leukocytes, reduced percentage of total CD8+ and CD8+ Naïve T cells, and increase in the percentage of terminally differentiated CD8+ EMRA T cells. Significant changes in the phenotype and function occurred mainly in CD8+ T cells in these individuals and are in agreement with the literature (38–43). In addition, it has been shown that the homeostatic proliferation is less effective for CD8 than for CD4 Naïve T cells (44).

In old individuals, it has been shown that many aspects of immunosenescence are related to the seropositivity for cytomegalovirus (CMV). However, it seems that the effects of CMV in the immune system of healthy old individuals are dependent on the increased latency of the virus (45, 46). In our study, 11 out of 12 old individuals were seropositive for CMV and four individuals presented

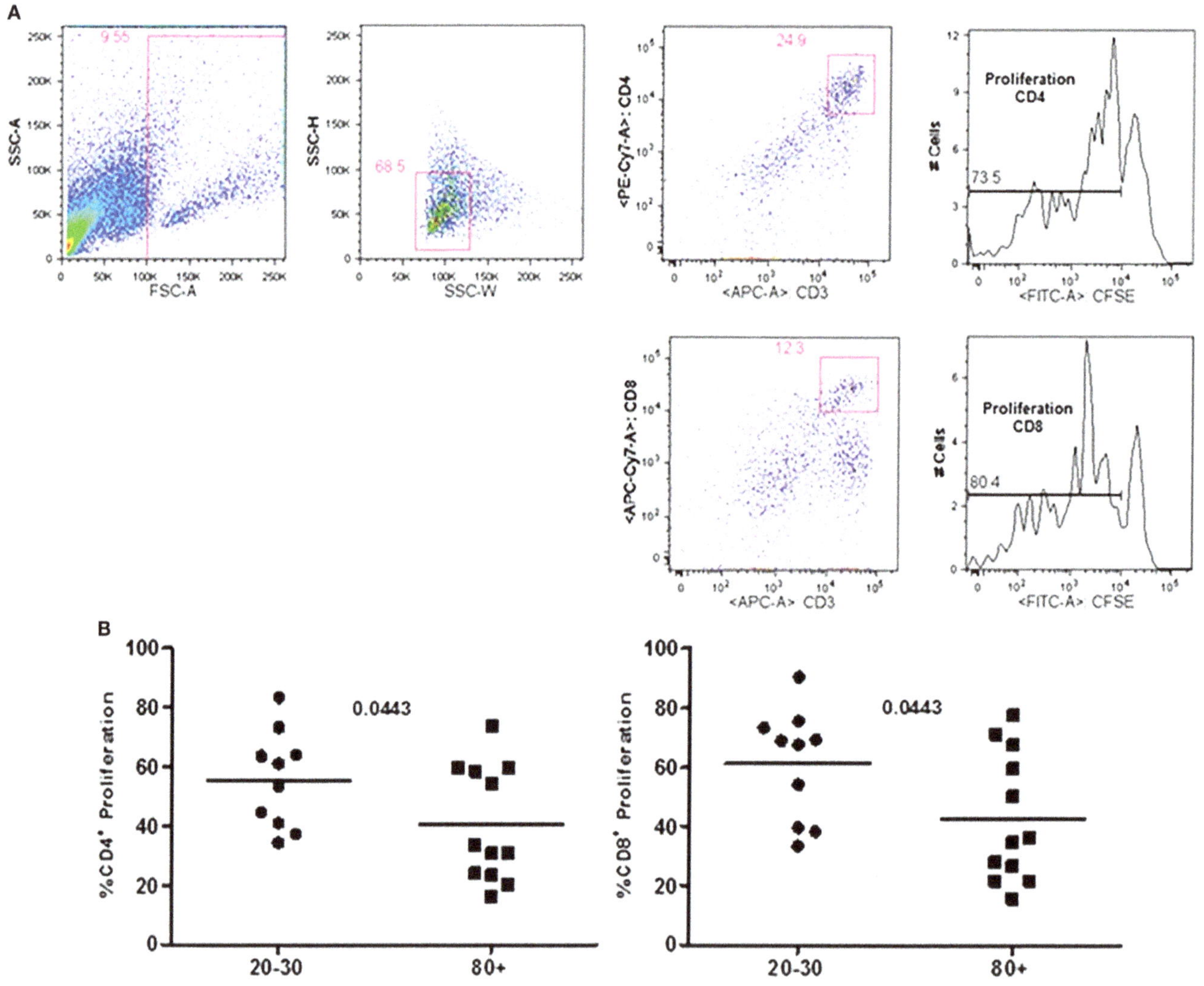

FIGURE 5 | Representative flow cytometry plots showing gate strategy for the frequency of proliferation in CD4⁺ and CD8⁺ T cells after stimulus with phytohemagglutinin (PHA) in culture. Gate in live cells (FSC-A x SSC-A), doublets exclusion (SSC-H x SSC-W), gate in CD3⁺CD4⁺ T cells, gate in the decrease of CFSE, gate in CD3⁺CD8⁺ T cells, gate in the decrease of CFSE **(A)**. Percentage of CD3⁺CD4⁺ and CD3⁺CD8⁺ T cells proliferation after stimulus with PHA according to age: 20–30 and 80+ years old **(B)**.

IgG levels >500 U/mL. The seropositivity to CMV was correlated with the decrease of Naïve CD8⁺ T cells and with a trend toward decrease in CD4⁺ central memory T cells and increase in CD8⁺ EMRA T cells. The impact of CMV infection/latency in immunity can exacerbate the features of immunosenescence. However, some of the features reported in literature were not in agreement with our studied old individuals such as the decrease in Naïve CD4⁺ T cells and CD4/CD8 ratio in addition to the increase in CD4⁺ and CD8⁺ central memory, CD8⁺ effector memory T cells, and pro-inflammatory cytokines (39, 47, 48). These differences may be due to the small number of individuals and great variability observed in the frequency of cell subtypes and cytokine production in our study population. Nonetheless, it cannot be ruled out by the possibility that the features preserved in immune system and observed in the old individuals studied are the key to achieve the longevity (13, 49, 50). Arai et al. (49) found in two different Japanese cohorts ($n = 1{,}554$) evaluating very old individuals (85–99 years), centenarians, and individuals ≥105 years that the lowest levels of inflammation correlated with the main indicators markers of successful aging, such as survival, capability, and cognition.

In old individuals, we observed lower rates of proliferation in CD4 and CD8 compartments in addition to the reduced levels of cytokines after stimulation with PHA. In association, we found lower percentage of CD4⁺ central memory T cells, which have been described as highly proliferative, and producers of IL-2 (13, 49–53). Corroborating with our data, Whisler et al. (51) showed that in *in vitro* there were diminished proliferative capacity and decreased production of IL-2 after stimulation with

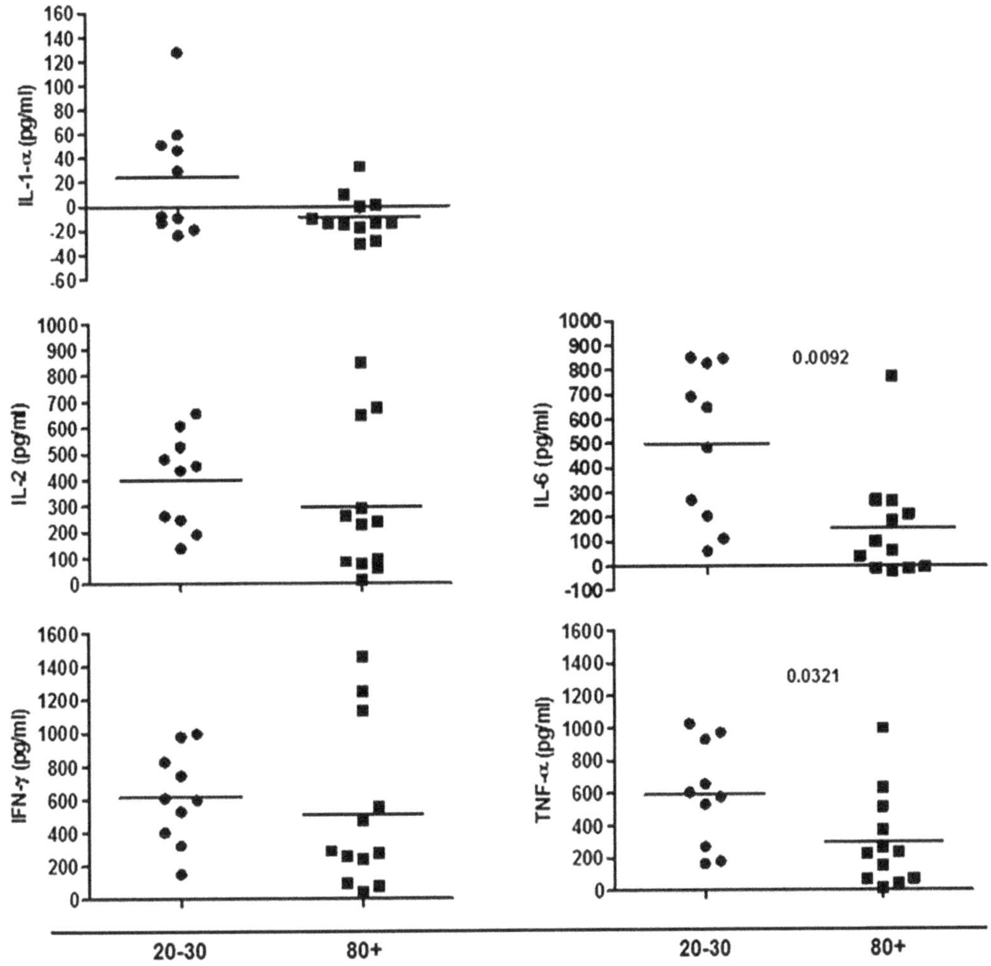

FIGURE 6 | Cytokines produced by cells in culture under phytohemagglutinin stimulus according to age: 20–30 and 80+ years old.

TABLE 2 | Serum levels of IgM and IgG to cytomegalovirus in old (80–100 years) individuals.

Age	Gender	IgM	IgG
100	F	0.159	>500
90	F	0.296	240.60
90	F	0.164	>500
93	M	0.237	316.30
93	F	0.160	31.36
88	M	0.158	<0.25
94	M	0.436	153.90
90	M	1.240	55.85
90	M	0.189	>500
94	M	0.157	180.60
91	F	0.488	>500
90	F	0.428	87.39

IgM cutoff index negative: <0.7; indeterminate: 0.7–0.99; positive: ≥1.0.
IgG negative <0.5 U/mL; indeterminate: 0.5–0.99 U/mL; positive: ≥1.0 U/mL.

PHA in 7 out of 12 old individuals evaluated (mean age 78 years) in association with deficient activation of transcriptional factor AP-1 and nuclear factor of activated T cells.

Others have reported that age interferes negatively with the expansion of T cells due to telomere erosion (52, 53). On the other hand, after vaccination with live attenuated virus varicella zoster Qi et al. (54) observed that the majority of activated T cells were $CD4^+$ and age (50–70 years) did not interfere with the expansion of antigen-specific T cells. However, the long-lived memory T cells (production of IFN-γ *in vitro*) decreased from day 14 to 28 post-vaccination.

The study of Shahid et al. (55) showed reduced expression of IFN-γ and granzyme B in $CD8^+$ T cells of older adults vaccinated against influenza.

Our findings show that despite the common features of immune senescence presented by old individuals, they managed to achieve longevity.

Health professionals have proposed alternatives to circumvent age-associated diseases, such as physical activity, diet control, supplements, and probiotics (22–24). Vitamin D has been recommended due to its action on the immunity, but data from literature are inconclusive regarding the benefits of supplementation with vitamin D.

TABLE 3 | IgG levels against cytomegalovirus and correlation with parameters of the immune system in old (80–100 years) individuals.

Parameters	*r* Spearman	*p*
Cell number × 10^5	−0.164	0.6054
% Myeloid-derived suppressor cells (MDSC) ($CD33^+CD11b^+$)	0.071	0.8267
MDSC absolute cell number × 10^5	0.046	0.883
% CD15 MDSC	−0.267	0.397
% CD14 MDSC	−0.377	0.225
% $CD3^+CD4^+$	−0.209	0.532
% $CD3^+CD8^+$	0.107	0.753
CD4/CD8	−0.191	0.566
% Proliferation $CD4^+$	0.259	0.410
% Proliferation $CD8^+$	0.085	0.792
% $CD4^+$ Naïve	−0.135	0.673
% $CD4^+$ central memory	−0.559	0.06
% $CD4^+$ effector memory	0.295	0.347
% $CD4^+$ effector memory RA	0.499	0.100
% $CD8^+$ Naïve	−0.648	0.027
% $CD8^+$ central memory	−0.420	0.174
% $CD4^+$ effector memory	0.085	0.792
% $CD8^+$ effector memory RA	0.573	0.055
IL-1α	−0.346	0.276
IL-2	0.025	0.941
Interleukin-6	0.143	0.652
IFN-γ	0.110	0.731
Tumor necrosis factor-alpha	0.075	0.818
Vitamin D	0.302	0.336

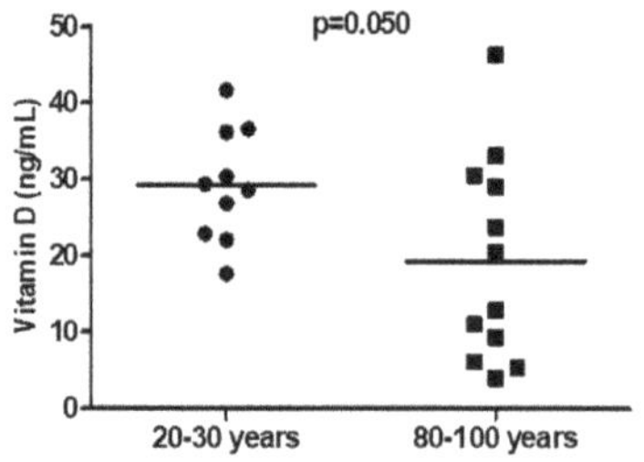

Parameter	Median (variation)	p
Vitamin D (20-30 years old)	29.0 (17.7 - 41.7) ng/mL	
Vitamin D (80-100 years old)	16.7 (4.01 - 46.4) ng/mL	0.050

FIGURE 7 | Vitamin D [25(OH)D3] levels in young (*n* = 10; 20–30 years) and old (*n* = 12; 80–100 years) individuals.

The US Endocrine Society defined vitamin D levels of 20 ng/mL or less as deficiency, 21–29 ng/mL as insufficiency, and 30 ng/mL or more as sufficiency (56). However, suboptimal levels of vitamin D have been reported worldwide and depending on the lifestyle and environmental conditions, hypovitaminosis D could be observed in all age groups (57). In old adults, the diminished sun exposure, skin atrophy with decreased amounts of the precursor 7-dehydrocholesterol, and the reduced content of vitamin D in the diet leads to lower serum levels of vitamin D (58, 59). In accordance, blood samples were collected in summer and yet we observed that 50% of individuals older than 80 years showed vitamin D deficiency, while the insufficiency was observed in 50% of young individuals.

In innate immunity, macrophages and dendritic cells can convert vitamin D3 on biological active 1,25OH (60). In addition, immune cells also express the vitamin D receptor (VDR) and thus 1,25OH can act on immune microenvironment in paracrine and autocrine pathways (61).

Human monocytes activated through TLR upregulate the expression of genes associated with the conversion of 25OH to 1,25OH (Cyp27B1) and VDR. The addition of vitamin D to monocytes in culture leads to upregulation of VDR downstream genes, such as the antimicrobial cathelicidin (62–64). In opposition, it was observed that in adaptive immunity, vitamin D added in culture abolished the production of IFN-γ and IL-17 by $CD4^+$ memory T cells co-cultured with activated dendritic cells (pneumococci products) (65). Accordingly, Rode et al. (66) found that human $CD4^+$ T cells stimulated with CD3/CD28 beads in the presence of 25OH or 1,25OH present reduced production of IFN-γ.

In this study, there was a trend toward negative correlation between the absolute number of MDSC and vitamin D levels ($r = -0563$ $p = 0.089$) in young individuals. This is an important finding, since there was a higher percentage of MDSC in old individuals with predominance of the granulocytic phenotype ($CD33^+CD11b^+CD15^+$) that has been associated with some types of cancer in humans. In addition, these cells have recently been associated with frailty and Alzheimer's disease (11, 67).

Interventions to circumvent the MDSC increase have been proposed such as the use of vitamin D to induce the differentiation of non-mature suppressive myeloid cells into mature effector non-suppressive cells (68). In patients (49–71 years old) with head and neck cancer, vitamin D3 (20, 40, 60 μg/day) decreased the number of progenitor cells with suppressive phenotype, promoted the proliferation of T cells after *in vitro* stimulation, and increased the levels of effector cytokines (IL-12 and IFN-γ) (69).

Regarding to the $CD4^+$ T cell compartment there was no correlation with the levels of vitamin D which is in agreement with literature data showing that for young adults, vitamin D levels (70), or supplement (71, 72) previously to vaccination did not cause enhanced humoral immunity that is dependent of $CD4^+$ T cells help. However, Khoo et al. (73) showed that during winter the level of vitamin D decreases and is associated with lower percentage of Naive $CD4^+$ T cells suggesting a role played by vitamin D in this cell compartment.

Our data points for correlation of vitamin D levels with some parameters of $CD8^+$ T cells. In old individuals, vitamin D had a positive correlation with total $CD8^+$ T cells. Considering that we observed a trend toward lower percentage of $CD8^+$ T cells in old individuals (**Figure 2**), vitamin D could be beneficial in preventing the decrease of this cell subtype. In young individuals, vitamin D levels correlated positively with the frequency of $CD8^+$ effector memory T cells.

Another important result was the negative correlation between vitamin D and CD8 EMRA T cells in old individuals suggesting that higher levels of vitamin D would be linked to less

TABLE 4 | Vitamin D [25(OH)D3] levels and correlation with parameters of the immune system in young (20–30 years) and old (80–100 years) individuals.

Parameters	*r* Spearman 20–30 years	*p*	*r* Spearman 80–100 years	*p*
Cell number × 10^5	0.012	0.973	−0.182	0.571
% Myeloid-derived suppressor cells (MDSC) ($CD33^+CD11b^+$)	−0.527	0.117	0.370	0.235
MDSC absolute cell number × 10^5	−0.563	0.089	0.181	0.571
% CD15 MDSC	0.281	0.431	0.167	0.602
% CD14 MDSC	−0.176	0.626	0.168	0.602
% $CD3^+CD4^+$	0.442	0.200	0.190	0.574
% $CD3^+CD8^+$	0.588	0.074	0.764	0.006
CD4/CD8	−0.090	0.803	−0.547	0.082
% Proliferation $CD4^+$	0.345	0.328	−0.238	0.457
% Proliferation $CD8^+$	0.236	0.511	−0.126	0.697
% $CD4^+$ Naïve $CD3^+CD4^+CD45RA^+CD27^+$	−0.109	0.764	−0.027	0.931
% $CD4^+$ central memory $CD3^+CD4^+CD45RA^-CD27^+$	−0.079	0.829	0.287	0.366
% $CD4^+$ effector memory $CD3^+CD4^+CD45RA^-CD27^-$	−0.042	0.907	0.028	0.931
% $CD4^+$ effector memory RA $CD3^+CD4^+CD45RA^+CD27^-$	0.150	0.701	−0.192	0.548
% $CD8^+$ Naïve $CD3^+CD8^+CD45RA^+CD27^+$	−0.297	0.405	0.378	0.269
% $CD8^+$ central memory $CD3^+CD8^+CD45RA^-CD27^+$	0.236	0.511	0.462	0.131
% $CD8^+$ effector memory $CD3^+CD8^+CD45RA^-CD27^-$	0.697	0.025	0.260	0.467
% $CD8^+$ effector memory RA $CD3^+CD8^+CD45RA^+CD27^-$	0.188	0.603	−0.552	0.050
IL-1α (pg/mL)	−0.472	0.169	0.505	0.094
IL-2 (pg/mL)	0.030	0.934	−0.266	0.404
Interleukin-6 (pg/mL)	−0.151	0.676	−0.246	0.442
IFN-γ (pg/mL)	−0.491	0.150	−0.014	0.966
Tumor necrosis factor-alpha (pg/mL)	0.212	0.556	−0.133	0.681

accumulation of cells that have been described as a marker of senescence (74, 75).

There was no correlation of vitamin D levels and proliferation of T cells ($CD4^+$ and $CD8^+$) or production of cytokines after stimulation with PHA. In agreement, the addition of vitamin D to culture of T cells stimulated with CD3 and CHO-CD80 cell line did not increase the proliferative capacity (individuals from 32 to 57 years old) (76). In addition, PBMCs stimulated *in vitro* in the presence of vitamin D showed diminished IFN-γ and increased IL-4 production in culture supernatant (77).

Aging has been related to chronic low-grade inflammation (inflammaging) with increased levels of circulating C-reactive protein (CPR), IL-6, and TNF-α. The InCHIANTI study found that individuals ($n = 867$, mean age 75.1 years) with vitamin D levels lower than 31.4 nmol/L presented high circulating IL-6, but not TNF-α, IL-1α, and IL-18 (78).

The English Longitudinal Study of Aging assessed community-dwelling individuals ($n = 5,870$, 50–80 years) and reported that low levels of 25OH (≤30 nmol/L) were negatively associated with CPR (79). A follow-up of old individuals ($n = 23$, 55–86 years) for 12 months showed that vitamin D levels were significantly lower in the winter with an increase in the number of individuals presenting deficiency. In the same season, there was a significant increase of circulating IL-6, IL-8, IL-β-1, MCP-1, and TNF-α (80). The low-grade chronic inflammation has been associated with aging-related diseases, and suboptimal levels of vitamin D have been related to chronic diseases/overall mortality (81–84), suggesting that adequate levels of vitamin D could benefit the aging population.

Despite the size of the sample be a limitation of the study and not allow more detailed statistical analyses, after testing the variables for normality and applying the adequate statistics, we obtained some important results. We found that the old population evaluated could be considered healthy based on the metabolic parameters. In this sample, 11 out of 12 were CMV^+ and still maintained preserved some features of immunity such as CD4/CD8 ratio, and low production of inflammatory cytokines after stimulus. On the other hand, we observed increased frequency of MDSC, reduced number of circulating leukocytes, reduced percentage of total $CD8^+$ and Naïve $CD8^+$ T cells, and increased percentage of terminally differentiated $CD8^+$EMRA T cells. CMV^+ was correlated with the decrease of $CD8^+$ Naïve T cells and increase in $CD8^+$ EMRA T cells. Vitamin D levels were insufficient in 50% of old individuals and correlated positively with total $CD8^+$ T cells and negatively with CD8 EMRA T cells. Our next step is to develop an *ex vivo* model to study the action of vitamin D in $CD4^+$ and $CD8^+$ T cells, associated phenotypes, proliferation, and cytokines production.

CONCLUSION

In the studied population, longevity was correlated to maintenance of some immune parameters. Considering the limitations of the study as size of the sample and lack of functional assays showing the direct effect of vitamin D in immunity, it was found that vitamin D in old individuals was correlated to some features of the immune system, mainly in the CD8 compartment.

ETHICS STATEMENT

This study was carried out in accordance with the recommendations of "UNIFESP CEP Committee of Ethics in Research" with written informed consent from all subjects. All subjects gave written informed consent in accordance with the Declaration of

Helsinki. The protocol was approved by the "CEP Committee of Ethics in Research."

AUTHOR CONTRIBUTIONS

All authors contributed significantly to this study and have read and approved the submitted manuscript. AA—laboratorial experiments, data analysis, figures. MI—laboratorial experiments. YD—SABE coordinators of study teams responsible for recruitment and sample collection. VB—laboratorial experiments and data analysis, figures, manuscript writing, and primary responsibility for final content.

ACKNOWLEDGMENTS

To Gianni Saints by statistical analysis, Rosani TS Silva (Central Laboratory—UNIFESP) for the measurement of IgM and IgG levels against CMV, FAPESP (Fundação de Amparo à Pesquisa do Estado de São Paulo) financial support (Project 2014/50261-8).

REFERENCES

1. World Population Ageing 2013. *Economic and Social Affairs*. New York: United Nations (2013). 111 p. Available from: http://www.un.org/en/development/desa/population/publications/pdf/ageing/WorldPopulationAgeing2013.pdf (Accessed: July 21, 2016).
2. OECD. *Health at a Glance 2015: OECD Indicators*. Paris: OECD Publishing (2015). 220 p. doi:10.1787/health_glance-2015-en
3. Passarino G, De Rango F, Montesanto A. Human longevity: genetics or lifestyle? It takes two to tango. *Immun Ageing* (2016) 13:12. doi:10.1186/s12979-016-0066-z
4. Sahyoun NR, Lentzner H, Hoyert D, Robinson NK. Trends in causes of death among the elderly. *Aging Trends* (2001):1–10.
5. Kaplan V, Angus DC, Griffin MF, Clermont G, Scott Watson R, Linde-Zwrible WT. Hospitalized community-acquired pneumonia in the elderly: age- and sex related patterns of care and outcome in the United States. *Am J Respir Crit Care Med* (2002) 165(6):766–72. doi:10.1164/ajrccm.165.6.2103038
6. Thompson WW, Shay DK, Weintraub E, Brammer L, Cox N, Anderson LJ, et al. Mortality associated with influenza and respiratory syncytial virus in the United States. *JAMA* (2003) 289:179–86. doi:10.1001/jama.289.2.179
7. Rossi DJ, Bryder D, Seita J, Nussenzweig A, Hoeijmakers J, Weissman IL. Deficiencies in DNA damage repair limit the function of haematopoietic stem cells with age. *Nature* (2007) 447(7145):725–9. doi:10.1038/nature05862
8. Ju Z, Jiang H, Jaworski M, Rathinam C, Gompf A, Klein C, et al. Telomere dysfunction induces environmental alterations limiting hematopoietic stem cell function and engraftment. *Nat Med* (2007) 13(6):742–7. doi:10.1038/nm1578
9. Wagner W, Horn P, Bork S, Ho AD. Aging of hematopoietic stem cell is regulated by the stem cell niche. *Exp Gerontol* (2008) 43(11):974–80. doi:10.1016/j.exger.2008.04.007
10. Elias HK, Bryder D, Park CY. Molecular mechanisms underlying lineage bias in aging hematopoiesis. *Semin Hematol* (2017) 54(1):4–11. doi:10.1053/j.seminhematol.2016.11.002
11. Verschoor CP, Johnstone J, Millar J, Dorrington MG, Habibagahi M, Lelic A, et al. Blood CD33(+)HLA-DR(−) myeloid-derived suppressor cells are increased with age and history of cancer. *J Leukoc Biol* (2013) 93:633–7. doi:10.1189/jlb.0912461
12. Bueno V, Sant'Anna OA, Lord JM. Ageing and myeloid-derived suppressor cells: possible involvement in immunosenescence and age-related disease. *Age (Dordr)* (2014) 36(6):9729. doi:10.1007/s11357-014-9729-x
13. Strindhall J, Nilsson BO, Löfgren S, Ernerudh J, Pawelec G, Johansson B, et al. No immune risk profile among individuals who reach 100 years of age: findings from Swedish NONA immune longitudinal study. *Exp Gerontol* (2007) 42(8):753–61. doi:10.1016/j.exger.2007.05.001
14. Palmer DB. The effect of age on thymic function. *Front Immunol* (2013) 4:316. doi:10.3389/fimmu.2013.00316
15. Dixit VD. Impact of immune-metabolic interaction on age-related thymic demise and T cell senescence. *Semin Immunol* (2012) 24:321–30. doi:10.1016/j.smim.2012.04.002
16. Surh CD, Sprent J. Homeostasis of naïve and memory T cells. *Immunity* (2008) 29:848–62. doi:10.1016/j.immuni.2008.11.002
17. Fry TJ, Mackall CL. The many faces of IL-7:from lymphopoiesis to peripheral T cell maintenance. *J Immunol* (2005) 174:6571–6. doi:10.4049/jimmunol.174.11.6571
18. Hamman D, Baars PA, Rep MH, Hooibrink B, Kerkhof-Garde SR, Klein MR, et al. Phenotypic and functional separation of memory and effector human CD8+ T cells. *J Exp Med* (1997) 186(9):1407–18. doi:10.1084/jem.186.9.1407
19. Hamman D, Konstense S, Wolthers KC, Otto SA, Baars PA, Miedema F, et al. Evidence that human CD8+ CD45RA+CD27- are induced by antigen and evolve through extensive rounds of division. *Int Immunol* (1999) 11(7):1027–33. doi:10.1093/intimm/11.7.1027
20. Libri V, Azevedo RI, Jackson SE, Di Mitri D, Lachmann R, Fuhrmann S, et al. Cytomegalovirus infection induces the accumulation of short-lived, multifunctional CD4+CD45RA+CD27- T cells: the potential involvement of interleukin-7 in this process. *Immunology* (2011) 132(3):326–39. doi:10.1111/j.1365-2567.2010.03386.x
21. Di Mitri D, Azevedo RI, Henson SM, Libri V, Riddell NE, Macaulay R, et al. Reversible senescence in human CD4+CD45RA+CD27− memory T cells. *J Immunol* (2011) 187(5):2093–100. doi:10.4049/jimmunol.1100978
22. Dato S, Crocco P, D'Aquila P, de Rango F, Bellizzi D, Rose G, et al. Exploring the role of genetic variability and lifestyle in oxidative stress for healthy aging and longevity. *Int J Mol Sci* (2013) 14(8):16443–72. doi:10.3390/ijms140816443
23. Logan SL, Spriet LL. Omega-3 fatty acid supplementation for 12 weeks increases resting and exercise metabolic rate in healthy community-dwelling older females. *PLoS One* (2015) 10(12):e0144828. doi:10.1371/journal.pone.0144828
24. Maijó M, Clements SJ, Ivory K, Nicoletti C, Carding SR. Nutrition, diet and immunosenescence. *Mech Ageing Dev* (2014) 13(6–137):116–28. doi:10.1016/j.mad.2013.12.003
25. Bikle D. Nonclassic actions of vitamin D. *J Clin Endocrinol Metab* (2009) 94(1):26–34. doi:10.1210/jc.2008-1454
26. MacDonell SO, Miller JC, Harper MJ, Waters DL, Houghton LA. Vitamin D status and its predictors in New Zealand aged-care residents eligible for a government-funded universal vitamin D supplementation programme. *Public Health Nutr* (2016) 19(18):3349–60. doi:10.1017/S1368980016001683
27. Moyersoen I. Intake of fat-soluble vitamins in the Belgian population: adequacy and contribution of foods, fortified foods and supplements. *Nutrients* (2017) 9(8):1–22. doi:10.3390/nu9080860
28. Walker P. Prevalence of vitamin D supplement use in Australian residential aged care facilities in November 2014. *BMC Res Notes* (2017) 10(1):385. doi:10.1186/s13104-017-2721-7
29. Ginde AA, Blatchford P, Breese K, Zarrabi L, Linnebur SA, Wallace JI, et al. High-dose monthly vitamin D for prevention of acute respiratory infection in older long-term care residents: a randomized clinical trial. *J Am Geriatr Soc* (2017) 65(3):496–503. doi:10.1111/jgs.14679
30. Avenell A, Cook JA, Maclennan GS, Macpherson GC. Vitamin D supplementation to prevent infections: a sub-study of a randomised placebo-controlled trial in older people. *Age Ageing* (2007) 36(5):574–7. doi:10.1093/ageing/afm091
31. Li-Ng M, Aloia JF, Pollack S, Cunha BA, Mikhail M, Yeh J, et al. A randomized controlled trial of vitamin D3 supplementation for the prevention of symptomatic upper respiratory tract infections. *Epidemiol Infect* (2009) 137(10):1396–404. doi:10.1017/S0950268809002404
32. Murdoch DR, Slow S, Chambers ST, Jennings LC, Stewart AW, Priest PC, et al. Effect of vitamin D3 supplementation on upper respiratory tract infections in healthy adults: the VIDARIS randomized controlled trial. *JAMA* (2012) 308(13):1333–9. doi:10.1001/jama.2012.12505

33. Martineau AR, Hanifa Y, Witt KD, Barnnes NC, Hooper RL, Patel M, et al. Double-blind randomised controlled trial of vitamin D3 supplementation for the prevention of acute respiratory infection in older adults and their carers (ViDiFlu). *Thorax* (2015) 70(10):953–60. doi:10.1136/thoraxjnl-2015-206996
34. Bergman P, Norlin AC, Hansen S, Björkhem-Bergman L. Vitamin D supplementation to patients with frequent respiratory tract infections: a post hoc analysis of a randomized and placebo-controlled trial. *BMC Res Notes* (2015) 8:391. doi:10.1186/s13104-015-1504-2
35. Lyons AB, Parish CR. Determination of lymphocyte division by flow cytometry. *J Immunol Methods* (1994) 171(1):131–7. doi:10.1016/0022-1759(94)90236-4
36. Geginat J, Sallusto F, Lanzavecchia A. Cytokine-driven proliferation and differentiation of human naïve, central memory, and effector memory CD4(+) T cells. *J Exp Med* (2001) 194(12):1711–9. doi:10.1084/jem.194.12.1711
37. Helmersson-Karlqvist J, Ridefelt P, Lind L, Larsson A. Reference values for 34 frequently used laboratory tests in 80-year-old men and women. *Maturitas* (2016) 92:97–101. doi:10.1016/j.maturitas.2016.07.015
38. Weinberger B, Lazuardi L, Weiskirchner I, Keller M, Neuner C, Fischer KH, et al. Healthy aging and latent infection with CMV lead to distinct changes in CD8+ and CD4+ T-cell subsets in the elderly. *Hum Immunol* (2007) 68(2):86–90. doi:10.1016/j.humimm.2006.10.019
39. Van Epps P, Banks R, Aung H, Betts MR, Canaday DH. Age-related differences in polyfunctional T cell responses. *Immun Ageing* (2014) 11:14. doi:10.1186/1742-4933-11-14
40. Geginat J, Lanzavecchia A, Sallusto F. Proliferation and differentiation potential of human CD8+ memory T-cells subsets in response to antigen or homeostatic cytokines. *Blood* (2003) 101(11):4260–6. doi:10.1182/blood-2002-11-3577
41. van der Geest KS, Abdulahad WH, Teteloshvili N, Tete SM, Peters JH, Horst G, et al. Low-affinity TCR engagement drives IL-2-dependent post-thymic maintenance of naïve CD4+ T cells in ageing humans. *Aging Cell* (2015) 14(5):744–53. doi:10.1111/acel.12353
42. Kock S, Larbi A, Derhovanessian E, Ozcelik D, Naumova E, Pawelec G. Multiparameter flow cytometric analysis of CD4 and CD8 T cell subsets in young and old people. *Immun Ageing* (2008) 5:6. doi:10.1186/1742-4933-5-6
43. Teixeira D, Ishimura ME, Longo-Maugéri IM, Lebrão ML, Duarte YAO, Bueno V. Biological markers changes at the very early stage of ageing (60–65 years). Is there a gender-related effect? *Aging Sci* (2015) 3:132. doi:10.4172/2329-8847.1000132
44. Goronzy JJ, Fang F, Cavanagh MM, Qi Q, Weyand CM. Naïve T cells maintenance and function in human aging. *J Immunol* (2015) 194:4073–80. doi:10.4049/jimmunol.1500046
45. Wertheimer AM, Bennett MS, Park B, Uhrlaub JL, Martinez C, Pulko V, et al. Aging and cytomegalovirus (CMV) infection differentially and jointly affect distinct circulating T cell subsets in humans. *J Immunol* (2014) 192(5):2143–55. doi:10.4049/jimmunol.1301721
46. Jackson SE, Sedikides GX, Okecha G, Poole EL, Sinclair JH, Wills MR. Latent cytomegalovirus (CMV) does not detrimentally alter T cell responses in healthy old, but increased latent CMV carriage is related to expanded CMV-specific T cells. *Front Immunol* (2017) 8:733. doi:10.3389/fimmu.2017.00733
47. Wikby A, Maxson P, Olsson J, Johansson B, Ferguson FG. Changes in CD8 and CD4 lymphocyte subsets, T cell proliferation responses and non-survival in the very old: the Swedish longitudinal OCTO-immune study. *Mech Ageing Dev* (1998) 102(2–3):187–98. doi:10.1016/S0047-6374(97)00151-6
48. Strindhall J, Skog M, Ernerudh J, Bengner M, Löfgren S, Matussek A, et al. The inverted CD4/CD8 ratio and associated parameters in 66-years old individuals: the Swedish HEXA immune study. *Age (Dordr)* (2013) 35(3):985–91. doi:10.1007/s11357-012-9400-3
49. Arai Y, Martin-Ruiz CM, Takayama M, Abe Y, Takebayashi T, Koyasy S, et al. Inflammation, but not telomere length, predicts successful ageing at extreme old age: a longitudinal study of semi-supercentenarians. *EBioMedicine* (2015) 2(10):1549–58. doi:10.1016/j.ebiom.2015.07.029
50. Bucci L, Ostan R, Giampieri E, Cevenini E, Pini E, Scurti M, et al. Immune parameters identify Italian centenarians with a longer five-year survival independent of their health and functional status. *Exp Gerontol* (2014) 54:14–20. doi:10.1016/j.exger.2014.01.023
51. Whisler RL, Beiging L, Chen M. Age-related decreases in IL-2 production by human T cells are associated with impaired activation of nuclear transcriptional factors AP-1 and NF-AT. *Cell Immunol* (1996) 169(2):185–95. doi:10.1006/cimm.1996.0109
52. Kaszubowska L. Telomere shortening and ageing of the immune system. *J Physiol Pharmacol* (2008) 59 Suppl 9:169–86.
53. Sharpless NE, DePinho RA. Telomeres, stem cells, senescence and cancer. *J Clin Invest* (2004) 113(2):160–8. doi:10.1172/JCI20761
54. Qi Q, Cavanagh MM, Le Saux S, Wagar LE, Mackey S, Hu J, et al. Defective T memory cell differentiation after varicella zoster vaccination in older in review individuals. *PLoS Pathog* (2016) 12(10):e1005892. doi:10.1371/journal.ppat.1005892
55. Shahid Z, Kleppinger A, Gentleman B, Falsey AR, McElhaney JE. Clinical and immunologic predictors of influenza illness among vaccinated older adults. *Vaccine* (2010) 28:6145–51. doi:10.1016/j.vaccine.2010.07.036
56. Bischoff-Ferrari HA, Giovannucci E, Willett WC, Dietrich T, Dawson-Hughes B. Estimation of optimal serum concentrations of 25-hydroxyvitamin D for multiple health outcomes. *Am J Clin Nutr* (2006) 84(1):18–28. doi:10.1093/ajcn/84.1.18
57. Mithal A, Wahl DA, Bonjour JP, Burckhardt P, Dawson-Hughes B, Eisman JA, et al. Global vitamin D status and determinants of hypovitaminosis D. *Osteoporos Int* (2009) 20(11):1807–20. doi:10.1007/s00198-009-0954-6
58. Godar DE, Pope SJ, Grant WB, Hokick MF. Solar UV doses of young Americans and vitamin D3 production. *Environ Health Perspect* (2012) 120(1):139–43. doi:10.1289/ehp.1003195
59. MacLaughlin J, Holick MF. Aging decreases the capacity of human skin to produce vitamin D3. *J Clin Invest* (1985) 76(4):1536–8. doi:10.1172/JCI112134
60. Gottfried E, Rehli M, Hahn H, Holler E, Andreesen R, Kreutz M. Monocyte derived cells express CYP27A1 and convert vitamin D3 into its active metabolite. *Biochem Biophys Res Commun* (2006) 349(1):209–13. doi:10.1016/j.bbrc.2006.08.034
61. Wu S, Ren S, Nguyen L, Adams JS, Hewison M. Splice variants of the CYP27b1 gene and the regulation of 1,25-dihydroxyvitamin D3 production. *Endocrinology* (2007) 148(7):3410–8. doi:10.1210/en.2006-1388
62. Liu PT, Stenger S, Li H, Wenzel L, Tan BH, Krutzik SR, et al. Toll-like receptor triggering of a vitamin D-mediated human antimicrobial response. *Science* (2006) 311(5768):1770–3. doi:10.1126/science.1123933
63. Wong HJ, Ye XJ, Ng TB. Cathelicidins: peptides with antimicrobial, immunomodulatory, anti-inflammatory, angiogenic, anticancer and procancer activities. *Curr Protein Pept Sci* (2013) 14(6):504–14. doi:10.2174/13892037113149990067
64. Lowry MB, Guo C, Borregaard N, Gombart AF. Regulation of the human cathelicidin antimicrobial peptide gene by 1α,25-dihydroxyvitamin D3 in primary immune cells. *J Steroid Biochem Mol Biol* (2014) 143:183–91. doi:10.1016/j.jsbmb.2014.02.004
65. Olliver M, Spelming L, Hiew J, Meyer-Hoffert U, Henriques-Normark B, Bergman P. Immunomodulatory effects of vitamin D on innate and adaptive immune responses to Streptococcus pneumonia. *J Infect Dis* (2013) 208(9):1474–81. doi:10.1093/infdis/jit355
66. Rode AKO, Kongsbak M, Hansen MM, Lopez DV, Levring TB, Woetmann A, et al. Vitamin D counteracts *Mycobacterium tuberculosis*-induced cathelicidin downregulation in dendritic cells and allows Th1 differentiation and IFNγ secretion. *Front Immunol* (2017) 8:656. doi:10.3389/fimmu.2017.00656
67. Le Page A, Garneau H, Dupuis G, Frost EH, Larbi A, Witkowski JM. Differential phenotypes of myeloid-derived suppressor and T regulatory cells and cytokine levels in amnestic mild cognitive impairment subjects compared to mild Alzheimer diseased patients. *Front Immunol* (2017) 8:783. doi:10.3389/fimmu.2017.00783
68. Najjar YG, Finke JH. Clinical perspectives on targeting of myeloid derived suppressor cells in the treatment of cancer. *Front Oncol* (2013) 3:49. doi:10.3389/fonc.2013.00049
69. Lathers DM, Clark JI, Achille NJ, Young MR. Phase 1B study to improve immune responses in head and neck cancer patients using escalating doses of 25-hydroxyvitamin D3. *Cancer Immunol Immunother* (2015) 53:422–30. doi:10.1007/s00262-003-0459-7
70. Peelen E, Rijkers G, Meerveld-Eggink A, Meijvis S, Vogt M, Cohen Tervaert JW, et al. Relatively high serum vitamin D levels do not impair the antibody response to encapsulated bacteria. *Eur J Clin Microbiol Infect Dis* (2013) 32(1):61–9. doi:10.1007/s10096-012-1714-7
71. Kriesel JD, Spruance J. Calcitriol (1,25-cihydroxy-vitamin D3) coadministered with influenza vaccine does not enhance humoral immunity in human volunteers. *Vaccine* (1999) 17(15–16):1883–8. doi:10.1016/S0264-410X(98)00476-9

72. Heine G, Drozdenki G, Lahl A, Unterwalder N, Mei H, Volk HD, et al. Efficient tetanus toxoid immunization on vitamin D supplementation. *Eur J Clin Nutr* (2011) 65(3):329–34. doi:10.1038/ejcn.2010.276
73. Khoo AL, Koenen HJPM, Chai LYA, Sweep FCJ, Netea MG, van der Vem AJAM, et al. Seasonal variation in vitamin D3 levels is paralleled by in review changes in the peripheral blood human T cell compartment. *PLoS One* (2012) 7(1):e29250. doi:10.1371/journal.pone.0029250
74. Saule P, Trauet J, Dutriez V, Lekeux V, Dessaint JP, Labalette M. Accumulation of memory T cells from childhood to old age: central and effector memory cells in CD4(+) versus effector memory and terminally differentiated memory cells in CD8(+) compartment. *Mech Ageing Dev* (2006) 127(3):274–81. doi:10.1016/j.mad.2005.11.001
75. Apoil PA, Puissant-Lubrano B, Congy-Jolivet N, Peres M, Tkzczuk J, Roubinet F, et al. Influence of age, sex and HCMV-serostatus on blood lymphocyte subpopulations in healthy adults. *Cell Immunol* (2017) 314:42–53. doi:10.1016/j.cellimm.2017.02.001
76. Liaskou E, Jeffrey L, Chanouas D, Soskic B, Seldin MF, Harper L, et al. Genetic variation at the CD28 locus and its impact on expansion of proinflammatory CD28 negative cells in healthy individuals. *Sci Rep* (2017) 7(1):7652. doi:10.1038/s41598-017-07967-2
77. Cantorna MT, Snyder L, Lin YD, Yang L. Vitamin D and 1,25(OH)2D regulation of T cells. *Nutrients* (2015) 7(4):3011–21. doi:10.3390/nu7043011
78. De Vita F, Lauretani F, Bauer J, Bautmans I, Shardell M, Cherubini A, et al. Relationship between vitamin D and inflammatory markers in older individuals. *Age* (2014) 36:9694. doi:10.1007/s11357-014-9694-4
79. Oliveira C, Biddulph JP, Hirani V, Schneider IJC. Vitamin D and inflammatory markers: cross-sectional analysis using data from the English Longitudinal Study of Ageing (ELSA). *J Nutr Sci* (2017) 6:e1. doi:10.1017/jns.2016.37
80. Elizondo-Montemayor L, Castillo EC, Rodriguez-López C, VillarrealCalderón JR, Gómez-Carmona M, Tenorio-Martínez S, et al. Seasonal variation in vitamin D is association with age, inflammatory cytokines, anthropometric parameters, and life style factors in older adults. *Mediators Inflamm* (2017) 2017:5719461. doi: 10.1155/2017/5719461
81. Ferrucci L, Corsi A, Lauretani F, Bandinelli S, Bartali B, Taub DD, et al. The origins of age-related proinflammatory state. *Blood* (2005) 105(6):2294–9. doi:10.1182/blood-2004-07-2599
82. Franceschi C, Bonafè M, Valensin S, Olivieri F, De Luca M, Ottaviani E, et al. Inflamm-aging. An evolutionary perspective on in review immunosenescence. *Ann N Y Acad Sci* (2000) 908:244–54. doi:10.1111/j.1749-6632.2000.tb06651.x
83. Pradhan AD, Manson JE, Rifai N, Buring JE, Ridker PM. C-reactive protein, interleukin 6, and risk of developing type 2 diabetes mellitus. *JAMA* (2001) 286:327–34. doi:10.1001/jama.286.3.327
84. Il'yasova D, Colbert LH, Harris AB, Bauer DC, Satterfield S, Kritchevsky SB. Circulating levels of inflammatory markers and cancer risk in the health aging and body composition cohort. *Cancer Epidemiol Biomarkers Prev* (2005) 14:2413–8. doi:10.1158/1055-9965.EPI-05-0316

17

Excess of Mortality in Adults and Elderly and Circulation of Subtypes of Influenza Virus in Southern Brazil

*André Ricardo Ribas Freitas[1] and Maria Rita Donalisio[2]**

[1] Department of Social Medicine, School of Medicine San Leopoldo Mandic, Campinas, Brazil, [2] Department of Public Health, School of Medical Sciences, University of Campinas, Campinas, Brazil

Correspondence:
Maria Rita Donalisio
rita.donalisio@gmail.com

Purpose: In the elderly population, the influenza infection and its clinical complications are important causes of hospitalization and death, particularly, in longer-lived age. The objective of this study is to analyze the impact of influenza virus circulation on mortality in the elderly and adults, in years with different predominant virus strains.

Methods: We performed a time trend study to evaluated excess of mortality for pneumonia and influenza, respiratory disease, and all-causes in southern region of Brazil, from 2002 to 2015. After considering other models, we opted for Serfling regression. Excess of death rates per 100,000 inhabitants were analyzed in specific age groups (24–59, 60–69, 70–79, ≥80 years) and by year of occurrence. Mortality information were taken from Brazilian Mortality Information System and etiological data were accessed in Sentinel Virological Surveillance database, getting the weekly positivity of the immunofluorescence tests for influenza A (H1N1, H3N2), and B.

Results: In southern Brazil, there is an evident seasonal pattern of all death outcomes among different age groups in the dry and cold season (April–September). The highest excess mortality rates occurs among older, particularly in years of circulation of influenza AH3N2, especially among people ≥80 years, in 2003 and 2007—years of great severity of influenza activity. After 2009, with the introduction of the pandemic influenza AH1N1, we observed a lower impact on the mortality of the elderly compared to <60 years.

Discussion: A cross reactivity antibody response from past exposure probably provided protection against disease in the elderly. Despite not controlling for comorbidities, climate, and vaccination, for the >70 years, ratio of respiratory diseases excess mortality rates between AH1N1 (2009) and severe year of H3N2 (2007) shows protection in the pandemic year and great vulnerability during AH3N2 virus predominance.

Conclusion: The reduced immune response to infection, and to vaccination, and presence of comorbidities recommend a special attention to this age group in Brazil. Besides medical assistance, the timeliness of vaccine campaigns, its composition, and etiological surveillance of respiratory diseases are some of the preventive and public health measures.

Keywords: influenza, excess of mortality, influenza AH3N2, influenza AH1N1, pandemic, elderly, Serfling regression model

INTRODUCTION

Human influenza viruses can cause diseases through many direct and indirect pathological effects. Consequences are destruction of infected cells, release of cytokines leading to fever, malaise, damage to respiratory epithelium and pulmonary parenchyma, and pneumonia. It includes secondary bacterial infections because of tissue damage and exacerbation of preexisting comorbidities such as cardiovascular and renal diseases, diabetes, or chronic lung disease (1–3).

The rates of hospitalization and mortality associated with influenza are higher among patients with chronic diseases, children under 1 year and after 65 years of age (4, 5). With the aging population in recent decades, the raw number of hospitalizations and deaths related to pneumonia and influenza tends to increase (4), this phenomenon has been observed also in Brazil (6, 7). However, the impact and severity of influenza virus circulation depend in part, on the strain that predominates in the season each year.

Due to the lack of laboratory confirmation, influenza-associated morbidity and mortality are often classified as pneumonia, other respiratory diseases, or other causes. Given the difficulty of directly measuring influenza morbidity and mortality, time series models are used to elucidate disease patterns in various age groups. Trends are usually determined by means of statistical inference, based on seasonal coincidence of the occurrence of certain diseases or death and laboratory confirmation of the viral circulation (4, 8).

Different approaches, with and without the quantification of the proportion of viral isolates, can produce average estimates of excess deaths associated with the circulation of certain viral variants (9–11). Viral surveillance data, hospitalization, or death indicators are particularly useful for the study of influenza in the tropics, as seasonality may be less evident (11–13). Serfling regression has been used to analyze excess of mortality related with respiratory virus circulation (7, 14–16). Despite some limitations (17), the inclusion of sinusoidal terms in weekly regression may reduce spurious correlation between influenza occurrence and death (18, 19). It is particularly useful when no other covariables are available, and with small samples of viral sentinel surveillance data (18). Poisson regression and the generalized linear model (GLM) can produce more specific estimates and support adjustments for variables (temperature, humidity, comorbidities, other circulations of viruses), although they require a more robust and consistent virological surveillance and cannot be used for pandemics (4).

In Brazil, surveillance for influenza syndromes was implemented in 2000, monitoring the occurrence of respiratory viruses (influenza A and B, parainfluenza 1, 2, and 3, respiratory syncytial virus, adenovirus). The Brazilian Ministry of Health provides vaccination coverage annually since 1999 for seniors and some risk groups, with vaccine coverage of the elderly population at around 80% in southern Brazil, the region with the highest coverage of the country. Despite the adequate coverage, protective titers after vaccination (HI ≥ 0) are consistently lower with poorer cell mediate and antibody responses in the elderly comparing to adults (20).

Considering the vulnerability of the elderly to influenza virus infection, and the lack of studies on its repercussion in Brazil, the objective of this study was to analyze the impact of different strains of Influenza A virus circulation. We analyzed particularly the most predominant variants (AH1N1 and AH3N2) on excess of mortality in the adults and elderly of different age groups in a region with marked seasonality of respiratory diseases in Brazil.

MATERIALS AND METHODS

Local of Study

This is a time trend study to evaluated excess of mortality from 2002 to 2015 in southern region of Brazil (states of Paraná, Santa Catarina e Rio Grande do Sul), total area is 576,774,31 km^2, population is 27,386,891 inhabitants with subtropical climate (Köppen-Geiger classification Cfa). We choose these states for analysis because of the consistent seasonal pattern of influenza, as well as the availability and quality of etiological data from the virological surveillance system in that region.

Mortality Data and Population

For the mortality rates of specific age groups (24–59, 60–69, 70–79, and ≥80 years) and death causes, we took data from Brazilian Mortality Information System. Causes are classified according to International Causes of Death ICD-10 revision, pneumonia, and influenza (ICD J 10 to J18.9), respiratory diseases (ICD J00 to J99), and all-cause (excluding external causes of mortality).

We obtained population of each year and age group from Instituto Brasileiro de Geografia e Estatística-IBGE from the Census-2010, and population estimates for the following years.

National Viral Surveillance Data

Etiologic information of flu-like syndrome was accessed in database of the National Sentinel Virological Surveillance System. It has data from 128 sentinel units distributed in all regions of the country—North (21 units), Northeast (26 units), Southeast (34 units), South (38 units), and Central West (9 units). Surveillance is performed through the systematic collection of weekly samples of nasopharyngeal secretions from patients who present flu-like syndrome. Reference laboratories process samples by using indirect immunofluorescence (IIF), with tests for influenza A and B, parainfluenza 1, 2, and 3, respiratory syncytial virus, and adenovirus. A portion of the samples is submitted to polymerase chain reaction tests to identify the virus genotype.

We calculated the laboratory positivity indicator using weekly positive results of IIF divided by the total of weekly valid tests, i.e., excluding the results within inadequate samples (not enough biological material, improper storage, incorrect material in the sample) or inconclusive results (no valid results).

Influenza vaccination coverage (%) of southern region from 2002 to 2015 was obtained from Brazilian National Program of Immunization data base (DATASUS).

Definition of Influenza Epidemic Periods

The criteria used to define the period of increase of influenza activity was when the positivity of the samples tested exceeded twice the annual mean of the weekly positivity of samples processed by surveillance, during two consecutive weeks.

In the year 2009, we consider the period officially recognized by the Brazilian Ministry of Health as epidemic by the influenza AH1N1pmd2009 strain, due to irregularity of the sample collection by the sentinel surveillance system at the end of epidemic.

Statistical Analysis

We calculated the weekly mortality rates by age group using the number of deaths per group of causes divided by the estimated population in the middle of the year multiplied by 100,000.

We constructed a Serfling cyclical regression model (14) for weekly data applied to each age group and causes of death (pneumonia and influenza, respiratory diseases, and all causes), as seen in others studies (7, 15), to estimate baseline of predicted deaths in the absence of influenza epidemics.

To fit regression, we used period of 13 years (from 2002 to 2015), excluding the weeks of epidemics periods. A cyclical linear regression was adjusted with the equation:

$$\begin{aligned} Y = {} & \beta 0 + \beta 1 * t + \beta 2 * t2 + \beta 3 * t3 + \beta 4 * \sin(2 * \pi * t / 52.17) \\ & + \beta 5 * \cos(2 * \pi * t / 52.17) + \beta 6 * \sin(4 * \pi * t / 52.17) \\ & + \beta 7 * \cos(4 * \pi * t / 52.17) + e1, \end{aligned}$$

where Y is the mortality rate, β is the coefficients of regression, t is time in weeks, and t^2 and t^3 are variables for adjusting the secular trend of the disease. We used of sine and cosine for adjust of annual and semiannual periodic components.

After adjusting a linear regression and define the expected mortality rate, we delimited 95% upper confidence limit of the baseline as the reference threshold in the absence of influenza epidemics. We calculated the excess of deaths as the observed mortality minus the expected mortality in the periods when mortality was above 95% of the confidence interval during epidemics periods.

We also present ratios of excess mortality rates among years of predominant circulation of influenza strains AH3N2 (mean and years of severity), AH1N1 pre-pandemic, and AH1N1 post-pandemic for each age group.

For data compilation, we used Microsoft Office Excel 2007, and for statistical analysis, SPSS for Windows, version 24.0.

RESULTS

Table 1 shows the proportion of positivity of the IIF nasopharyngeal samples and the annual prevalence of strains of influenza in the period. Before 2009, the year of entry of the pandemic strain AH1N1pmd 2009, there was a predominance of influenza AH3N2 in the years 2003 to 2007. After 2009, there is alternation of strains in the southern Brazil. Annual elderly vaccination coverage in southern region is high and homogeneous, around 80%, and even higher in the recent years.

There is an evident seasonal pattern of deaths from pneumonia and influenza, respiratory diseases, and all-causes among the elderly in different age groups in the dry, cold months (April–September) in southern region (**Figure 1**).

We note a progressive increase in the rates of excess deaths (of all outcomes) with increasing age, especially among those older than 70 years. In the pre-pandemic years with dominance of the AH1N1 strain, the excess of mortality rates associated with influenza were relatively low, compared to years of prevalence of AH3N2 strain (**Table 2**). Among those over 80 years, the ratio of excess mortality rates between 2009 and the years with dominium of H3 strains was less than one. This ratio suggests that this age group was spared in the 2009 pandemic. However, in years of predominance of strain H3, excess of mortality rate of all causes in this group were 449.6 per 100,000 (corresponding to 1,598 obits), 5, and 8.2 times greater than the same rate in years of circulation of H1N1 in pre- and post-pandemic period, respectively.

Among adults (24–59 years), we observe a large excess of deaths rates during the 2009 pandemic (953 obits), which correspond to 7.1 excess deaths from all causes, and 99 excess mortality from respiratory diseases associated with viral infection in every 100,000 individuals of the age group. The ratio between excess mortality rates due to pneumonia/influenza in the pandemic year (2009) and the mean rate of the period was 12 times higher among the youngest (**Table 2**).

TABLE 1 | Specimens collected, positive proportion, and predominant subtypes of influenza between 2002 and 2016 in the sentinel units of southern Brazil.

Years	Samples	Positive samples	% indirect immunofluorescence positive	AH1N1	AH3N2	Not subtyped	B	Virus Predom.	% Vac. Coverage
2002	186	23	12			8	15	H1/B	75.3
2003	355	41	12			37	4	H3	73.0
2004	474	52	11			47	5	H3	75.6
2005	383	15	4			14	1	H3	72.7
2006	676	94	14			72	22	H3	84.0
2007	800	127	16			122	5	H3	71.1
2008	1,018	129	13			60	69	H1/B	71.4
2009	540	112	21			91	21	H1/B	76.9
2010	949	142	15			62	80	H1/B	77.1
2011	1,104	175	16			129	46	H3	82.9
2012	1,514	138	9			106	32	H1/B	96.5
2013	3,728	926	25	320	229	0	377	H1/B	91.8
2014	5,249	815	16	73	660	10	72	H3	91.4
2015	5,752	854	15	109	390	19	336	H3	93.7

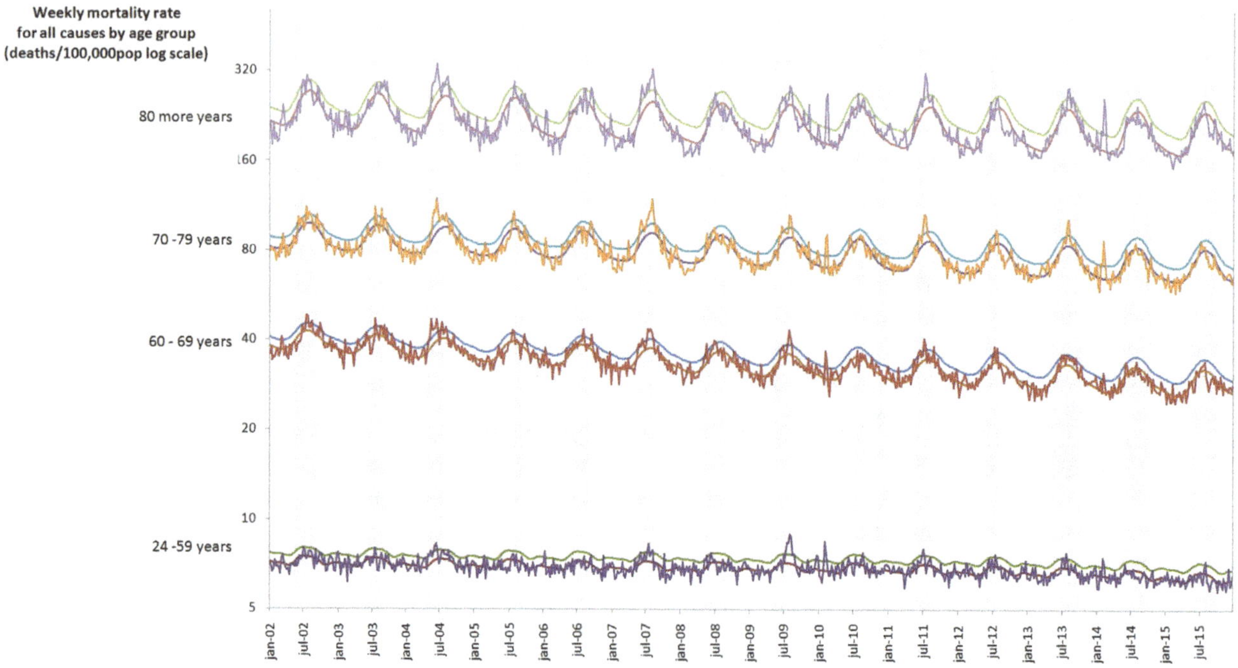

FIGURE 1 | Weekly mortality rate by age group (deaths/100,000) log scale in southern regions of Brazil, 2002–2015. Colored lines are age groups and gray columns are the seasons of influenza.

Rates of excess mortality by pneumonia and influenza and respiratory diseases are lower than all causes in all age groups, but particularly high in older than 80 years (**Table 2**).

DISCUSSION

The results highlight the great vulnerability of elderly to influenza AH3N2, especially among older than 70 years in severe years of influenza activity, like 2003 and 2007. The study also shows the lower impact of influenza AH1N1pdm 2009 in this age group compared to younger. Risk of dying among the elderly in years of circulating AH3N2 influenza has been reported in several parts of the world (9, 10, 21, 22); however, in Brazil, there are no recent estimates available. Few studies analyze the circulation and impact of influenza in tropical and subtropical regions (6, 7, 9–11). Influenza B virus is also associated with severe disease (23); however, this variant did not circulate with intensity during the study years in Brazil.

Although the elderly are the most vulnerable group to viral respiratory infections, we found relative small excess of deaths in years of circulating AH1N1 pre pandemic (2002 and 2008). Study comparing excess deaths from respiratory diseases in the elderly in Latin America shows stable rates (mean of 89.4 per 100,000 inhabitants) in southern Brazil between 1998 and 2008 (pre-pandemic Flu A-H1N1), although higher in Brazil than in other countries (24). In the USA and in European countries, influenza seasons dominated by subtype AH3N2 are typically associated with mortality two to three times higher than in seasons with predominance of AH1N1 (prior to pandemic strain 2009) and of influenza B viruses (9, 10, 19, 25).

When all causes of death are studied, the overall mortality associated with influenza among elderly exceeds that observed in younger age group. It should be considered that all causes mortality is a non-specific measure and a distant outcome of influenza infection. However, it is difficult to determine which group of causes of death could better characterize the influenza burden in mortality. By choosing only the respiratory causes, we may underestimate clinical complications of pulmonary viral infection (e.g., cardiovascular). Therefore, in this study, we analyzed all causes, respiratory, and pneumonia and influenza deaths.

The unfavorable evolution of infection in the elderly is possibly due to the prevalence of comorbidities, deficiencies in defense mechanisms, and poor antibody response to vaccination, as cell-mediated and humoral responses limit severity of disease (26). Patients with chronic diseases are more susceptible to infection due to decline of the immune function through inflammatory mechanisms, hindering the mucosal barrier, and the adaptive and innate immunological defense mechanisms (27).

The immune response to infection in the elderly tend to be delayed and weak, with prolonged inflammatory responses, which involves different types of host reaction, mainly to clearance virus. The exacerbations of these mechanisms may induce immune-mediated pathology causing tissue damage (28). Cytokine high serum levels of IL-6, TNF-a, IFN-g and sIL-2R, chemokines IP-10, MCP-1, and monokine induced by IFN-g (MIG), are associated with severe clinical cases and lung damage (29).

Immunological abnormalities in people with diabetes, chronic respiratory diseases, cardiopathy, or other chronic diseases have increased risk of severe infection and bad prognosis (19). For example, there is the consistent association of influenza infection

TABLE 2 | Excess mortality rate (per 100,000 population) and excess deaths (absolute number) according to influenza virus subtypes prevalent in southern Brazil, 2002–2015.

		24–59		60–69		70–79		≥80	
		Excess mort rate	**Exc. deaths**	**Exc. mort rate**	**Exc. deaths**	**Exc. mort rate**	**Exc. deaths**	**Exc. mort rate**	**Exc. deaths**
Mean of annual excess mortality during all period	Pnm and Flu	0.2	27	0.8	17	2.9	29	20.2	85
	Resp	0.4	57	3.8	64	12.3	113	37.2	143
	All causes	1.3	176	13.0	214	37.0	331	116.5	422
Mean of annual excess mortality in H1/B pre-pandemic years (2002 and 2008)	Pnm and Flu	0.0	0	0.4	7	2.1	19	2.2	9
	Resp	0.0	0	3.5	54	7.4	59	15.4	42
	All causes	0.9	118	13.1	201	35.7	287	88.3	255
Excess mortality during 2009	Pnm and Flu	2.5	331	3.2	57	12.0	113	20.5	82
	Resp	5.2	698	7.4	129	17.6	167	7.3	29
	All causes	7.1	953	21.0	368	58.6	555	125.1	501
Mean of annual excess mortality in H1/B pos-pandemic years (2010, 2012, and 2013)	Pnm and Flu	0.4	60	1.5	31	4.2	44	17.3	83
	Resp	0.7	99	3.0	62	14.3	150	21.5	102
	All causes	0.9	129	5.6	116	16.6	178	54.6	262
Mean of excess mortality during H3 years (2003, 2004, 2005, 2006, 2007, 2011, 2014, 2015)	Pnm and Flu	0.0	4	0.6	12	2.1	22	27.4	112
	Resp	0.1	13	4.1	66	12.6	111	50.6	191
	All causes	1.2	148	15.1	240	42.3	371	145.6	514
Excess mortality during severe H3 epidemics (2007)	Pnm and Flu	0.0	0	0.6	10	2.1	19	49.5	176
	Resp	0.2	24	8.5	138	32.5	288	134.2	477
	All causes	2.9	375	35.6	576	136.1	1,209	449.6	1,598
Relative risk 2009/mean of period	Pnm and Flu	12.6		3.8		4.1		1.0	
	Resp	12.4		1.9		1.4		0.2	
	All causes	5.3		1.6		1.6		1.1	
Relative risk 2009/mean of H3 years	Pnm and Flu	83.9		5.6		5.6		0.7	
	Resp	49.2		1.8		1.4		0.1	
	All causes	6.2		1.4		1.4		0.9	
Relative risk 2009/severe H3 epidemics	Pnm and Flu	#		5.5		5.6		0.4	
	Resp	28.3		0.9		0.5		0.1	
	All causes	2.5		0.6		0.4		0.3	

Exc., excess; Pnm and FLU, pneumonia and influenza; Resp, Respiratory causes International Causes of Deaths ICD chapter J (J10–J18.9).
 # - Relative risk has no valid value as denominator is zero.

with cardiovascular mortality, particularly acute myocardial infarction (30). In part, it is attributed to altering endothelial function due to an acute inflammatory and procoagulant stimulus during viral infection (31, 32). Clinical complications of diabetes triggered by influenza infection cause impairment of leukocyte function and increase post-infection colonization rates resulting in poor prognosis in the elderly (33, 34).

In young people and adults, in 2009, the emerging influenza AH1N1 strain had a notable impact on the mortality of people up to 59 years in various parts of the world, including Brazil (7, 25, 35, 36). Excess mortality of individuals aged 24–59 years in the state of São Paulo, Brazil was identified during the pandemic AH1N1 virus (7). Pregnant women adults with metabolic conditions, including obesity, chronic respiratory disease, and other chronic diseases were significantly associated with severe acute respiratory syndrome and the lethality in Brazil (37). Our study showed a 41.5-fold higher rate of mortality from pneumonia and influenza in adults (24–59 years) in the pandemic year AH1N1 than the average of years with predominance of AH3N2 circulation in southern region.

In addition to the clinical severity and the large portion of the affected population, pandemics affect age groups in different ways (38). While only 10% of deaths from seasonal influenza occur among those under 65 years of age, in the pandemics of 1918, 1957–1958, and 1968, this proportion was 95, 40, and 50%, respectively (39). Therefore, pandemics tend to affect a larger proportion of young people than seasonal influenza. In this study, higher rates of death due to pneumonia, influenza, respiratory, and all causes were observed among those aged 24–59 years in 2009.

One explanation for the higher mortality observed among the youngest is that they would be more prone to the situation known as "cytokine storm," i.e., a dysfunctional overproduction of cytokines that would lead to diffuse damage to the respiratory tract with severe and potentially lethal systemic repercussions (40). Viral replication and production of inflammatory mediators seem to be involved in the pathogenesis of infection with influenza A H1N1pmd2009, hindering the clearance of virus in lung tissue and leading to pathologic lesions (41).

Another explanation for the lower mortality in the elderly is that they were exposed previously to antigens of the pandemic virus. Hancock et al. (42) suggested a cross-reactive antibody response to 2009 pandemic AH1N1. Similarities between AH1N1 antigen from 2009 and 1918 were detected. This last virus strain has not circulated since 1958 (39), when the AH1N1 strain was displaced by AH2N2 (Asian flu). At that time, AH1N1viral circulation occurred mainly in children, the current elderly of 2009.

The emergence of the AH3N2 strain in the pandemic year 1968 (Hong Kong flu) affected several age groups. This new strain resulted from a large genetic mutation (shift) recombining virus material of the circulating AH2N2 with the avian H3, of Asian origin, resulting in the new variant AH3N2 (38).

In 2002–2003, under selective pressure an antigenic small mutation (drift), resulted in A/Fujian/411/02(H3N2) a strains emerged after a "jump" in genes evolution of Hemagglutinin and Neuraminidase proteins of virus surface (43, 44). The circulation of the Fujian strain had a great impact on the mortality from pneumonia in several parts of the world in 2003–2004 and 2004–2005 (22) and in Brazil (45). In 2007, a new drift resulted in influenza AH3N2 detected in south Brazil (46) also affecting hospitalizations and deaths in various parts of the world (47). We observed high rates of excess mortality in the elderly, in the years of 2003 and 2007.

Limitations of this study refer mainly to the ecological analysis of pooled data. We did not analyze individual information regarding comorbidities and history of vaccination that could be important confounders influencing mortality (17). We just had the overall annual vaccination coverage which were in general, around 80% in the period. Estimates of the number of deaths (all causes, respiratory, and pneumonia-influenza) supposedly related to influenza may be inaccurate in inferring the impact of respiratory viruses. Correlations in time series studies may produce spurious associations, especially between all causes of death and influenza infection, due to the distance between cause and outcome, and to multiple components of the obits. Serfling addresses part of this limitation by introducing sinusoidal terms in equation, since non-influenza mortality is not expected to coincide exactly with sinusoidal pattern (14, 19). Moreover, excess mortality of pneumonia, respiratory diseases, and all causes can be considered as an alert to surveillance of viral respiratory diseases, such as a sentinel indicator to be investigated (4, 48). Although all causes mortality is a non-specific indicator, it does not underestimate the complications of chronic diseases associated with influenza (4). Despite the influenza component in all causes mortality is small, the indicator can be considered an indirect measure, a warning, useful in epidemiological monitoring.

Another limitation is the lack of robust etiologic data from virological surveillance in the years 2002–2012, which could lead to imprecision in the analyses; however, the data on the predominance strains in the southern region are reliable, and influenced the composition of the vaccine of each season.

Considering the option for the analysis model, Serfling linear regression may produce different estimates when compared with other models (Poisson, ARIMA, and GLM) (9, 10); Poisson and ARIMA models produce higher mortality estimates than Serfling, and Serfling higher than GLM, especially among the elderly (16, 17, 21). We chose Serfling model because we do not have robust virological surveillance data, before 2013, and the study period includes a pandemic year (4).

Besides, in this study, we did not analyze climatic variables (minimum temperatures and relative air humidity) that could also interfere with viral transmission and increase the impact of the disease, particularly in the elderly.

In conclusion, probably previous exposures to influenza AH1N1 in the past influenced the mortality of Brazilian elderly in 2009, despite the vulnerability of this age group to clinical complications. For the >70 years, we observe higher excess mortality rates (of all outcomes) in severe year of AH3N2 circulation (2003, 2007). It is also worth noting that vaccination has been associated with the prevention of death particularly at age 65 (49). Therefore, the high elderly vaccination cover in southern Brazil may have attenuated excess of mortality estimated, although the immune response is limited among those.

More attention should be given to the circulation of influenza AH3N2 in subtropical regions in Brazil. The reduced immune response to infection and to vaccination, and associated comorbidities recommend a special attention to this age group. Besides medical assistance, the timeliness of vaccine campaigns, its composition, and etiological surveillance of respiratory diseases in the region are some of the preventive and public health measures.

AUTHOR CONTRIBUTIONS

Both authors made contributions to the conception of the work, acquisition, analysis, interpretation of data, and writing the manuscript.

ACKNOWLEDGMENTS

We thank Ana Claudia Medeiros de Souza (General Coordination of Information and Epidemiological Analyzes - Brazilian Health Ministry) and Walquiria Aparecida Ferreira de Almeida (Influenza Technical Group - Brazilina Health Ministry).

REFERENCES

1. Center for Disease Control and Prevention. Prevention and control of influenza: recommendations of the Advisory Committee on Immunization Practices (ACIP). *MMWR Recomm Rep* (2002) 51:1–31.
2. Reichert TA, Simonsen L, Sharma A, Pardo SA, Fedson DS, Miller MA. Influenza and the winter increase in mortality in the United States, 1959–1999. *Am J Epidemiol* (2004) 160(5):492–502. doi:10.1093/aje/kwh227
3. Glezen WP, Greenberg SB, Atmar RL, Piedra PA, Couch RB. Impact of respiratory virus infections on persons with chronic underlying conditions. *JAMA* (2000) 283(4):499–505. doi:10.1001/jama.283.4.499
4. Thompson WW, Comanor L, Shay DK. Epidemiology of seasonal influenza: use of surveillance data and statistical models to estimate the burden of disease. *J Infect Dis* (2006) 194(S2):S82–91. doi:10.1086/507558
5. Chiu SS, Lau YL, Chan KH, Wong WHS, Peiris JM. Influenza-related hospitalizations among children in Hong Kong. *N Engl J Med* (2002) 347(26):2097–103. doi:10.1056/NEJMoa020546
6. Francisco PMSB, Donalisio MR, Marín-León L. Trends in mortality from respiratory diseases among the elderly and the influenza vaccine intervention, 1980–2009. *Rev Panm Salud Publica* (2013) 34(3):155–61.
7. Freitas ARR, Francisco PMSB, Donalisio MR. Mortality associated with influenza in tropics, state of Sao Paulo, Brazil, from 2002 to 2011: the pre-pandemic, pandemic, and post-pandemic periods. *Influenza Res Treat* (2013) 2013:696274. doi:10.1155/2013/696274
8. Nicoll A, Ciancio BC, Lopez-Chavarrias V, Mølbak K, Pebody R, Pedzinski B, et al. Influenza-related deaths – available methods for estimating numbers and detecting patterns for seasonal and pandemic influenza in Europe. *Euro Surveill* (2012) 17(18):20162. doi:10.2807/ese.17.18.20162-en
9. Nunes B, Viboud C, Machado A, Ringholz C, Rebelo-de-Andrade H, Nogueira P, et al. Excess mortality associated with influenza epidemics in Portugal, 1980 to 2004. *PLoS One* (2011) 6(6):e20661. doi:10.1371/journal.pone.0020661
10. Nunes B, Natário I, Carvalho ML. Time series methods for obtaining excess mortality attributable to influenza epidemics. *Stat Methods Med Res* (2011) 20:331–45. doi:10.1177/0962280209340201

11. Yang L, Ma S, Chen PY, He JF, Chan KP, Chow A, et al. Influenza associated mortality in the subtropics and tropics: results from three Asian cities. *Vaccine* (2011) 29(48):8909–14. doi:10.1016/j.vaccine.2011.09.071
12. Viboud C, Alonso WJ, Simonsen L. Influenza in tropical regions. *PLoS Med* (2006) 3(4):e89. doi:10.1371/journal.pmed.0030089
13. Alonso WJ, Viboud C, Simonsen L, Hirano EW, Daufenbach LZ, Miller MA. Seasonality of influenza in Brazil: a traveling wave from the Amazon to the subtropics. *Am J Epidemiol* (2007) 165(12):1434–42. doi:10.1093/aje/kwm012
14. Serfling RE. Methods for current statistical analysis of excess pneumonia-influenza deaths. *Public Health Rep* (1963) 78(6):494–506. doi:10.2307/4591848
15. Simonsen L, Reichert TA, Viboud C, Blackwelder WC, Taylor RJ, Miller MA. Impact of influenza vaccination on seasonal mortality in the US elderly population. *Arch Intern Med* (2005) 165(3):265–72. doi:10.1001/archinte.165.3.265
16. López-Cuadrado MS, Jiménez-Jorge S, Savulescu AC, Larrauri A. Influenza-related mortality in Spain, 1999–2005. *Gac Sanit* (2012) 26:325–9. doi:10.1016/j.gaceta.2011.09.033
17. Thomas RE. Is influenza-like illness a useful concept and an appropriate test of influenza vaccine effectiveness? *Vaccine* (2014) 32:2143–9. doi:10.1016/j.vaccine.2014.02.059
18. Thompson WW, Weintraub E, Dhankhar P, Cheng PY, Brammer L, Meltzer MI, et al. Estimates of US influenza-associated deaths made using four different methods. *Influenza Other Respi Viruses* (2009) 3:37–49. doi:10.1111/j.1750-2659.2009.00073.x
19. Thompson WW, Shay DK, Weintraub E, Brammer L, Cox N, Anderson LJ, et al. Mortality associated with influenza and respiratory syncytial virus in the United States. *JAMA* (2003) 289(2):179–86. doi:10.1001/jama.289.2.179
20. Murasko DM, Bernstein ED, Gardner EM, Gross P, Munk G, Dran S, et al. Role of humoral and cell-mediated immunity in protection from influenza disease after immunization of healthy elderly. *Exp Gerontol* (2002) 37(2–3):427–39. doi:10.1016/S0531-5565(01)00210-8
21. Lemaitre M, Carrat F, Rey G, Miller M, Simonsen L, Viboud C. Mortality burden of the 2009 A/H1N1 influenza pandemic in France: comparison to seasonal influenza and the A/H3N2 pandemic. *PLoS One* (2012) 7(9):e45051. doi:10.1371/journal.pone.0045051
22. Russell CA, Jones TC, Barr IG, Cox NJ, Garten RJ, Gregory V, et al. The global circulation of seasonal influenza A (H3N2) viruses. *Science* (2008) 320(5874):340–6. doi:10.1126/science.1154137
23. Su S, Chaves SS, Perez A, D'Mello T, Kirley PD, Yousey-Hindes K, et al. Comparing clinical characteristics between hospitalized adults with laboratory-confirmed influenza A and B virus infection. *Clin Infect Dis* (2014) 59(2):252–5. doi:10.1093/cid/ciu269
24. Souza MDFMD, Widdowson MA, Alencar AP, Gawryszewski VP, Aziz-Baumgartner E, Palekar R, et al. Trends in mortality from respiratory disease in Latin America since 1998 and the impact of the 2009 influenza pandemic. *Bull World Health Organ* (2013) 91(7):525–32. doi:10.2471/BLT.12.116871
25. Dawood FS, Iuliano AD, Reed C, Meltzer MI, Shay DK, Cheng PY, et al. Estimated global mortality associated with the first 12 months of 2009 pandemic influenza A H1N1 virus circulation: a modelling study. *Lancet Infect Dis* (2012) 12:687–95. doi:10.1016/S1473-3099(12)70121-4
26. La Gruta NL, Turner SJ. T cell mediated immunity to influenza: mechanisms of viral control. *Trends Immunol* (2014) 35(8):396–402. doi:10.1016/j.it.2014.06.004
27. McElhaney JE, Kuchel GA, Zhou X, Swain SL, Haynes L. T-cell immunity to influenza in older adults: a pathophysiological framework for development of more effective vaccines. *Front Immunol* (2016) 7:41. doi:10.3389/fimmu.2016.00041
28. La Gruta NL, Kedzierska K, Stambas J, Doherty PC. A question of self-preservation: immunopathology in influenza virus infection. *Immunol Cell Biol* (2007) 85:85–92. doi:10.1038/sj.icb.7100026
29. Jong MD, Simmons CP, Thanh TT, Hien VM, Smith GJ, Chau TN, et al. Fatal outcome of human influenza A (H5N1) is associated with high viral load and hypercytokinemia. *Nat Med* (2006) 12:1203–7. doi:10.1038/nm1477
30. Warren-Gash C, Smeeth L, Hayward AC. Influenza as a trigger for acute myocardial infarction or death from cardiovascular disease: a systematic review. *Lancet Infect Dis* (2009) 9(10):601–10. doi:10.1016/S1473-3099(09)70233-6
31. Harskamp RE, van Ginkel MW. Acute respiratory tract infections: a potential trigger for the acute coronary syndrome. *Ann Med* (2008) 40:121–8. doi:10.1080/07853890701753672
32. Madjid M, Awan I, Ali M, Frazier L, Casscells W. Influenza and atherosclerosis: vaccination for cardiovascular disease prevention. *Expert Opin Biol Ther* (2005) 5:91–6. doi:10.1517/14712598.5.1.91
33. Drell DW, Notkins AL. Multiple immunological abnormalities in patients with type 1 (insulin dependent) diabetes mellitus. *Diabetologia* (1987) 30:132–43. doi:10.1007/BF00274217
34. Smith SA, Poland GA. Use of influenza and pneumococcal vaccines in people with diabetes. *Diabetes Care* (2000) 23(1):95–108. doi:10.2337/diacare.23.1.95
35. Green HK, Andrews N, Fleming D, Zambon M, Pebody R. Mortality attributable to influenza in England and Wales prior to, during and after the 2009 pandemic. *PLoS One* (2013) 8(12):e79360. doi:10.1371/journal.pone.0079360
36. Van Kerkhove MD, Vandemaele KAH, Shinde V, Jaramillo-Gutierrez G, Koukounari A, Donnelly CA, et al. Risk factors for severe outcomes following 2009 influenza A (H1N1) infection: a global pooled analysis. *PLoS Med* (2011) 8:e1001053. doi:10.1371/journal.pmed.1001053
37. Oliveira WK, Carmo EH, Penna GO, Kuchenbecker RS, Santos HB, Araujo WN, et al. Pandemic H1N1 influenza in Brazil: analysis of the first 34,506 notified cases of influenza-like illness with severe acute respiratory infection (SARI). *Euro Surveill* (2009) 14(42):19362. doi:10.2807/ese.14.42.19362-en
38. Simonsen L, Clarke MJ, Schonberger LB, Arden NH, Cox NJ, Fukuda K. Pandemic versus epidemic influenza mortality: a pattern of changing age distribution. *J Infect Dis* (1998) 178(1):53–60. doi:10.1086/515616
39. Simonsen L, Viboud C, Taylor RJ, Miller MA. Epidemiology of influenza and its control. In: Rappuoli R, Del Giudice G, editors. *Influenza Vaccines for the Future*. 2nd ed. Basel: Springer (2011). p. 27–55.
40. Kobasa D, Jones SM, Shinya K, Kash JC, Copps J, Ebihara H, et al. Aberrant innate immune response in lethal infection of macaques with the 1918 influenza virus. *Nature* (2007) 445(7125):319. doi:10.1038/nature05495
41. Gao R, Bhatnagar J, Blau DM, Greer P, Rollin DC, Denison AM, et al. Cytokine and chemokine profiles in lung tissues from fatal cases of 2009 pandemic influenza A (H1N1): role of the host immune response in pathogenesis. *Am J Pathol* (2013) 83(4):1258–68. doi:10.1016/j.ajpath.2013.06.023
42. Hancock K, Veguilla V, Lu X, Zhong W, Butler EN, Sun H, et al. Cross-reactive antibody responses to the 2009 pandemic H1N1 influenza virus. *N Engl J Med* (2009) 361(20):1945–52. doi:10.1056/NEJMoa0906453
43. Bragstad K, Nielsen LP, Fomsgaard A. The evolution of human influenza A viruses from 1999 to 2006: a complete genome study. *Virol J* (2008) 5(1):40. doi:10.1186/1743-422X-5-40
44. Chi SX, Bolar TV, Zhao P, Tam JS, Rappaport R, Cheng S. Molecular evolution of human influenza A/H3N2 virus in Asia and Europe from 2001 to 2003. *J Clin Microbiol* (2005) 43:6130–2. doi:10.1128/JCM.43.12.6130-6132.2005
45. Oliveira TFDMS, Yokosawa J, Motta FC, Siqueira MM, da Silveira HL, Queiróz DAO. Molecular characterization of influenza viruses collected from young children in Uberlandia, Brazil—from 2001 to 2010. *BMC Infect Dis* (2015) 15(1):71. doi:10.1186/s12879-015-0817-z
46. Straliotto SM, Gregianini TS, Baccin TG, Motta FC, Siqueira M. Virus influenza detectados no estado do Rio Grande do Sul durante, 2006 e 2007. *Bol Saúde* (2009) 23(1):57–62.
47. Center for Disease Control and Prevention. Influenza activity – United States and worldwide, 2007–08 season. *MMWR Recomm Rep* (2008) 2757(25):692–7.
48. Simonsen L, Clarke J, Williamson GD, Stroup DF, Arden NH, Schonberger LB. The impact of influenza epidemics on mortality: introducing a severity index. *Am J Public Health* (1997) 87(2):1944–50. doi:10.2105/AJPH.87.12.1944
49. Foppa IM, Cheng PY, Reynolds SB, Shay DK, Carias C, Bresee JS, et al. Deaths averted by influenza vaccination in the US during the seasons 2005/06 through 2013/14. *Vaccine* (2015) 33(26):3003–9. doi:10.1016/j.vaccine.2015.02.042

Permissions

All chapters in this book were first published by Frontiers; hereby published with permission under the Creative Commons Attribution License or equivalent. Every chapter published in this book has been scrutinized by our experts. Their significance has been extensively debated. The topics covered herein carry significant findings which will fuel the growth of the discipline. They may even be implemented as practical applications or may be referred to as a beginning point for another development.

The contributors of this book come from diverse backgrounds, making this book a truly international effort. This book will bring forth new frontiers with its revolutionizing research information and detailed analysis of the nascent developments around the world.

We would like to thank all the contributing authors for lending their expertise to make the book truly unique. They have played a crucial role in the development of this book. Without their invaluable contributions this book wouldn't have been possible. They have made vital efforts to compile up to date information on the varied aspects of this subject to make this book a valuable addition to the collection of many professionals and students.

This book was conceptualized with the vision of imparting up-to-date information and advanced data in this field. To ensure the same, a matchless editorial board was set up. Every individual on the board went through rigorous rounds of assessment to prove their worth. After which they invested a large part of their time researching and compiling the most relevant data for our readers.

The editorial board has been involved in producing this book since its inception. They have spent rigorous hours researching and exploring the diverse topics which have resulted in the successful publishing of this book. They have passed on their knowledge of decades through this book. To expedite this challenging task, the publisher supported the team at every step. A small team of assistant editors was also appointed to further simplify the editing procedure and attain best results for the readers.

Apart from the editorial board, the designing team has also invested a significant amount of their time in understanding the subject and creating the most relevant covers. They scrutinized every image to scout for the most suitable representation of the subject and create an appropriate cover for the book.

The publishing team has been an ardent support to the editorial, designing and production team. Their endless efforts to recruit the best for this project, has resulted in the accomplishment of this book. They are a veteran in the field of academics and their pool of knowledge is as vast as their experience in printing. Their expertise and guidance has proved useful at every step. Their uncompromising quality standards have made this book an exceptional effort. Their encouragement from time to time has been an inspiration for everyone.

The publisher and the editorial board hope that this book will prove to be a valuable piece of knowledge for researchers, students, practitioners and scholars across the globe.

List of Contributors

Miriam G. Jasiulionis
Laboratory of Ontogeny and Epigenetics, Pharmacology Department, Universidade Federal de São Paulo, São Paulo, Brazil

Guy A. M. Berbers, Susana Fuentes and Anne-Marie Buisman
Centre for Infectious Disease Control (Cib), National Institute for Public Health and the Environment (RIVM), Bilthoven, Netherlands

Marieke van der Heiden
Centre for Infectious Disease Control (Cib), National Institute for Public Health and the Environment (RIVM), Bilthoven, Netherlands
Department of Rheumatology and Clinical Immunology, University of Groningen, University Medical Centre Groningen, Groningen, Netherlands

Annemieke M. H. Boots
Department of Rheumatology and Clinical Immunology, University of Groningen, University Medical Center Groningen, Groningen, Netherlands

Menno C. van Zelm
Department of Immunology, Erasmus MC, Rotterdam, Netherlands
Department of Immunology and Pathology, Monash University and Alfred Hospital, Melbourne, VIC, Australia

Paulo Rodrigues-Santos
Faculty of Medicine, Institute of Immunology, University of Coimbra, Coimbra, Portugal
Laboratory of Immunology and Oncology, Center for Neuroscience and Cell Biology, University of Coimbra, Coimbra, Portugal
Faculty of Medicine, Center of Investigation in Environment, Genetics and Oncobiology - CIMAGO, University of Coimbra, Coimbra, Portugal

Jani Sofia Almeida and Patricia Couceiro
Laboratory of Immunology and Oncology, Center for Neuroscience and Cell Biology, University of Coimbra, Coimbra, Portugal
Faculty of Medicine, Center of Investigation in Environment, Genetics and Oncobiology - CIMAGO, University of Coimbra, Coimbra, Portugal

Vera Alves and Manuel Santos-Rosa
Faculty of Medicine, Institute of Immunology, University of Coimbra, Coimbra, Portugal
Faculty of Medicine, Center of Investigation in Environment, Genetics and Oncobiology - CIMAGO, University of Coimbra, Coimbra, Portugal

Raquel Tarazona
Immunology Unit, University of Extremadura, Cáceres, Spain

Nelson López-Sejas, Carmen Campos, Corona Alonso and Rafael Solana
Department of Immunology, Instituto Maimónides de Investigación Biomédica de Córdoba - Reina Sofia University Hospital - University of Córdoba, Córdoba, Spain

Lenka Ruzičková and Paulo Freitas-Tavares
Hematology Service, Coimbra Hospital and Universitary Centre, Coimbra, Portugal

Kornelis S. M. van der Geest, Gerda Horst and Elisabeth Brouwer
Department of Rheumatology and Clinical Immunology, University of Groningen, University Medical Center Groningen, Groningen, Netherlands

Bart-Jan Kroesen
Department of Laboratory Medicine, University of Groningen, University Medical Center Groningen, Groningen, Netherlands

Wayel H. Abdulahad
Department of Pathology and Medical Biology, University of Groningen, University Medical Center Groningen, Groningen, Netherlands

Carmen Vida, Irene Martinez de Toda, Antonio Garrido and Mónica De la Fuente
Facultad de Biología, Universidad Complutense de Madrid, Madrid, Spain
Instituto de Investigación Hospital Universitario 12 de Octubre (i+12), Madrid, Spain

Eva Carro and José Antonio Molina
Instituto de Investigación Hospital Universitario 12 de Octubre (i+12), Madrid, Spain
Centro de Investigación Biomédica en Red sobre Enfermedades Neurodegenerativas (CIBERNED), Madrid, Spain

Ling Huang, Michiel G. H. Betjes, Mariska Klepper, Carla C. Baan and Nicolle H. R. Litjens
Department of Internal Medicine, Erasmus MC, University Medical Center Rotterdam, Nephrology and Transplantation, Rotterdam, Netherlands

Anton W. Langera
Department of Immunology, Erasmus MC, University Medical Center Rotterdam, Rotterdam, Netherlands

Stella Lukas Yani, Michael Keller, Franz Leonard Melzer, Birgit Weinberger, Luca Pangrazzi and Beatrix Grubeck-Loebenstein
Department of Immunology, Institute for Biomedical Aging Research, University of Innsbruck, Innsbruck, Austria

Sieghart Sopper
Clinic for Haematology and Oncology, Tyrolean Cancer Research Institute, Medical University of Innsbruck, Innsbruck, Austria

Klemens Trieb
Department of Orthopedic Surgery, Hospital Wels-Grieskirchen, Wels, Austria

Monia Lobina, Valeria Orrù, Edoardo Fiorillo and Francesco Cucca
Istituto di Ricerca Genetica e Biomedica (IRGB), Consiglio Nazionale delle Ricerche (CNR), Monserrato, Italy

Irene Maeve Rea
School of Medicine, Dentistry and Biomedical Science, Queens University Belfast, Belfast, United Kingdom
Northern Ireland Centre for Stratified Medicine, Biomedical Sciences Research Institute, University of Ulster, C-TRIC Building, Altnagelvin Area Hospital, Londonderry, United Kingdom
Care of Elderly Medicine, Belfast Health and Social Care Trust, Belfast, United Kingdom

Susan E. McNerlan
Regional Genetics Service, Belfast Health and Social Care Trust, Belfast, United Kingdom

David S. Gibson, Victoria McGilligan and H. Denis Alexander
Northern Ireland Centre for Stratified Medicine, Biomedical Sciences Research Institute, University of Ulster, C-TRIC Building, Altnagelvin Area Hospital, Londonderry, United Kingdom

Owen A. Ross
Department of Neuroscience, Mayo Clinic, Jacksonville, FL, United States
Department of Clinical Genomics, Mayo Clinic, Jacksonville, FL, United States
School of Medicine and Medical Science, University College Dublin, Dublin, Ireland

Tamas Fulop and Aurélie Le Page
Research Center on Aging, Graduate Program in Immunology, Faculty of Medicine and Health Sciences, University of Sherbrooke, Sherbrooke, QC, Canada

Anis Larbi
Singapore Immunology Network (SIgN), Biopolis, Agency for Science Technology and Research (A*STAR), Singapore, Singapore

Eric H. Frost
Department of Infectious Diseases and Microbiology, Faculty of Medicine and Health Sciences, University of Sherbrooke, Sherbrooke, QC, Canada

Gilles Dupuis
Department of Biochemistry, Graduate Program in Immunology, Faculty of Medicine and Health Sciences, University of Sherbrooke, Sherbrooke, QC, Canada

Alan A. Cohen
Department of Family Medicine, Faculty of Medicine and Health Sciences, University of Sherbrooke, Sherbrooke, QC, Canada

Jacek M. Witkowski
Department of Pathophysiology, Medical University of Gdańsk, Gdańsk, Poland

Claudio Franceschi
Italian National Research Center on Aging, Department of Experimental Pathology, University of Bologna, Bologna, Italy

Daniela Frasca and Bonnie B. Blomberg
Department of Microbiology and Immunology, University of Miami Miller School of Medicine, Miami, FL, United States

Roberto Paganelli
Dipartimento di Medicina e Scienze dell'Invecchiamento, Università degli Studi 'G. d'Annunzio' Chieti-Pescara, Chieti, Italy

Marion Hendriks, Ronald H. J. Jacobi and Josine van Beek
Centre for Infectious Disease Control, National Institute for Public Health and the Environment, Bilthoven, Netherlands

Sara P. H. van den Berg and Debbie van Baarle
Centre for Infectious Disease Control, National Institute for Public Health and the Environment, Bilthoven, Netherlands
Laboratory of Translational Immunology, Department of Immunology, University Medical Center Utrecht, Utrecht University, Utrecht, Netherlands

Albert Wong
Department of Statistics, Informatics and Mathematical Modelling, National Institute for Public Health and the Environment, Bilthoven, Netherlands

Nato Teteloshvili, Gerjan Dekkema, Peter Heeringa, Pytrick Jellema, Debora de Jong, Anke van den Berg and Joost Kluiver
Department of Pathology and Medical Biology, University of Groningen, University Medical Center Groningen, Groningen, Netherlands

Martijn Terpstra and Klaas Kok
Genetics, University of Groningen, University Medical Center Groningen, Groningen, Netherlands

John P. Campbell and James E. Turner
Department for Health, University of Bath, Bath, United Kingdom

Fabiano Pinheiro da Silva and Marcel Cerqueira César Machado
Laboratório de Emergências Clínicas, Faculdade de Medicina FMUSP, Universidade de São Paulo, São Paulo, Brazil

William Trim, James E. Turner and Dylan Thompson
Department for Health, University of Bath, Bath, United Kingdom

Amanda Soares Alves, Mayari Eika Ishimura, and Valquiria Bueno
Division of Immunology, DMIP Microbiology, Immunology, and Parasitology, Federal University of São Paulo, São Paulo, Brazil

Yeda Aparecida de Oliveira Duarte
Division of Epidemiology, Faculdade de Saúde Pública, Universidade de São Paulo, São Paulo, Brazil

André Ricardo Ribas Freitas
Department of Social Medicine, School of Medicine San Leopoldo Mandic, Campinas, Brazil

Maria Rita Donalisio
Department of Public Health, School of Medical Sciences, University of Campinas, Campinas, Brazil

Index

www.ingramcontent.com/pod-product-compliance
Lightning Source LLC
LaVergne TN
LVHW082148200926
848484LV00008B/2126